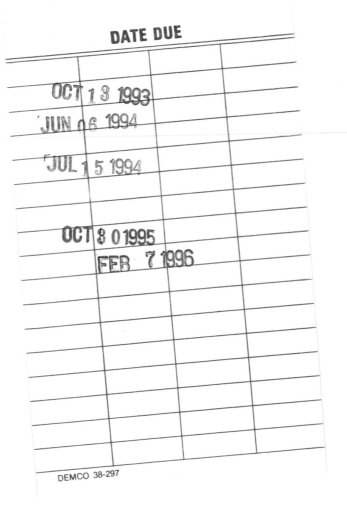

DATE DUE

OCT 1 3 1993		
JUN 06 1994		
JUL 1 5 1994		
OCT 3 0 1995		
FEB 7 1996		

DEMCO 38-297

ATLAS OF

Female Infertility Surgery

Robert B. Hunt, MD
Clinical Instructor;
Department of Obstetrics and Gynecology;
Harvard Medical School,
Boston, Massachusetts

Second edition

With 688 illustrations, 64 in 4-color

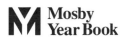
Mosby
Year Book

St. Louis Baltimore Boston Chicago London Philadelphia Sydney Toronto

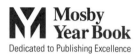
Mosby
Year Book
Dedicated to Publishing Excellence

Senior Editor: Stephanie Manning
Editorial Assistant: Colleen Boyd
Project Manager: Carol Sullivan Wiseman
Production Editor: Lisa D. Cohen
Designer: Julie Taugner
Illustrator: Jean Kanski Bittl

Second edition
Copyright © 1992 by Mosby–Year Book, Inc.
A Mosby imprint of Mosby–Year Book, Inc.

Previous editions copyrighted 1986

Printed in the United States of America

Mosby–Year Book, Inc.
11830 Westline Industrial Drive,
St. Louis, Missouri 63146

NOTICE
Every effort has been made to ensure that the surgical procedures herein are accurate and in accord with the standards accepted at the time of publication. As new research and experience broaden our knowledge, however, changes in treatment and procedures occur. The authors assume no liability in either the misapplication or misuse of these procedures.

Library of Congress Cataloging in Publication Data

Atlas of female infertility surgery / [edited by] Robert B. Hunt. —
  2nd ed.
     p. cm.
   Includes bibliographical references and index.
   ISBN 0-8151-4739-2
   1. Infertility, Female—Surgery. 2. Microsurgery. I. Hunt,
Robert B.
   [DNLM: 1. Infertility, Female—surgery. 2. Microsurgery. WP 570
A881]
RG201.A85 1992
618.1′78059—dc20
DNLM/DLC
for Library of Congress   91-37520
                                      CIP

92 93 94 95 96 GW/MV 9 8 7 6 5 4 3 2 1

Contributors

Hugo A. Acuna, MD
General Surgeon
Department of General Surgery
Mayo Regional Hospital, Dover—Foxcroft, Maine

Ronald E. Batt, MD
Clinical Associate Professor of Gynecology
Department of Gynecology—Obstetrics
State University of New York at Buffalo

Michael Alan Bermant, MD
Plastic and Reconstructive Surgeon
St. Elizabeth's Hospital
Utica, New York

Diane N. Clapp, BSN, RN
Medical Information Counselor
National Resolve, Inc.
Arlington, Massachusetts

Brian M. Cohen, MB ChB, MD
Clinical Professor
Department of Obstetrics and Gynecology
The University of Texas Southwestern Medical Center

Stephen M. Cohen, MD
Associate Professor of Obstetrics and Gynecology
Director of Reproductive Endocrinology
Department of Obstetrics and Gynecology
University of Massachusetts Medical School
Worcester, Massachusetts

Marian D. Damewood, MD
Associate Professor and Director
In-Vitro Fertilization Program
Department of Gynecology and Obstetrics
Division of Reproductive Endocrinology
Johns Hopkins University School of Medicine
Baltimore, Maryland

David G. Diaz, MD
Director, In-Vitro Fertilization
Martin Luther Hospital
Anaheim, California
Former Fellow, Reproductive Endocrinology
Harvard Medical School
Boston, Massachusetts

Carlton A. Eddy, PhD
Associate Professor
Department of Obstetrics and Gynecology
The University of Texas Health Science Center at San Antonio

James F. Green, MEd
Director Media Production
Department of Media Production
New England Baptist Hospital
Boston, Massachusetts

Martha E. Griffin, RN MSN, CS
Psychiatric Clinical Specialist
Founder, Resolve of The Bay State
Staff, Brigham and Women Hospital
Boston, Massachusetts

Jerome J. Hoffman, MD, FACS, FACOG
Director, Research in Reproductive Physiology
The Mount Sinai Medical Center of Greater Miami
Fort Lauderdale, Florida

Gary Holtz, MD
Clinical Associate Professor
Department of Obstetrics and Gynecology
Medical University of South Carolina
Charleston, South Carolina

Robert B. Hunt, MD
Clinical Instructor
Department of Obstetrics and Gynecology
Harvard Medical School
Boston, Massachusetts

Jeremy V. Kredentser, MD
Head, Section of Reproductive Endocrinology and
Infertility
Obstetrics and Gynaecology
University of Manitoba
Winnipeg, Manitoba, Canada

Fung Lam, MD, FACOG
Assistant Clinical Professor
Department of Obstetrics, Gynecology, and
Reproductive Sciences
University of California—San Francisco

W. Dwayne Lawrence, MD
Associate Professor and Chief of Anatomic Pathology
Department of Pathology
Detroit Medical Center and Wayne State University
School of Medicine
Detroit, Michigan

Carl J. Levinson, MD
Clinical Professor
Department of Obstetrics, Gynecology and
Reproductive Sciences
University of California—San Francisco

Dan C. Martin, MD
Clinical Associate Professor
Department of Obstetrics and Gynecology
University of Tennessee, Memphis

Howard A. Pattinson, MB, MRCOG
Assistant Professor
Department of Obstetrics and Gynaecology
University of Calgary
Calgary, Alberta, Canada

Harry Reich, MD, FACOG
Clinical Associate Professor
Department of Obstetrics and Gynecology
Baystate Medical Center (Western Campus of Tufts
University School of Medicine)
Springfield, Massachusetts

Jacques E. Rioux, MD, MPH
Professor
Department of Obstetrics and Gynaecology
University of Laval
Cite Universitaire, Ste-Foy, Quebec
Canada

John A. Rock, MD
Professor Gynecology—Obstetrics and Pediatrics
Department of Gynecology and Obstetrics
The Johns Hopkins University School of Medicine
Baltimore, Maryland

Hans W. Schlosser, MD
Department of Obstetrics and Gynecology
The Microsurgical Center
University of Dusseldorf
Dusseldorf, West Germany

Robert E. Scully, MD
Professor
Department of Pathology
Massachusetts General Hospital
Harvard Medical School
Boston, Massachusetts

Raymond E. Shively, MD
Associate Clinical Professor of Surgery (Plastic
Surgery)
Department of Surgery
St. Louis University
St. Louis, Missouri

Alvin M. Siegler, MD
Clinical Professor
Department of Obstetrics and Gynecology
State University of New York
Health Science Center at Brooklyn

Patrick J. Taylor, MD
Chairman
Department of Obstetrics and Gynaecology
St. Paul's Hospital
Vancouver, B.C. Canada

Amy S. Thurmond, MD
Director of Women's Imaging Services
Director of Ultrasound
Oregon Health Sciences University
Portland, Oregon

Salvador M. Udagawa, MD
Chief of Surgery
St. Francis Hospital
Buffalo, New York

Hugo C. Verhoeven, MD
Department of Obstetrics and Gynecology
The Microsurgical Center
University of Dusseldorf
Dusseldorf, West Germany

James M. Wheeler, MD, MPH
Assistant Professor
Department of Obstetrics and Gynecology
Baylor College of Medicine
Houston, Texas

I dedicate this atlas to my late father,
James,
for inspiring me to work hard
and to my mother,
Marie,
for teaching me to be gracious to others.

Preface

....

As an instructor in microsurgical and surgical laparoscopy courses for the past decade, I have come to realize the need for the attendees to have a resource book to review details of particular procedures. The purpose of this book is to achieve that goal.

In addition to a very detailed description of microsurgical procedures, I have dedicated a chapter to operative laparoscopy. In keeping with the first edition, I have retained chapters on pelvic physiology and pathology, as well as complications, the use of adjunctive agents, and photography. Furthermore, I have expanded and updated the list of vendors and have included updated informed consent sheets.

Although this book may have many foibles, and perhaps I have left out items that should have been included and incorporated others that should have been omitted, I have done my best to provide a reference for my colleagues that will result in the finest reconstructive surgery possible.

ACKNOWLEDGMENTS

My wife and son, Kate and Jamie, relinquished 1 year of weekends to allow me to put together the second edition of this atlas. To them I am most grateful.

A debt of appreciation goes to my contributors for their writings. Without their efforts, this book would have missed the mark as a comprehensive surgical atlas. Of greatest assistance has been my editor, Sarah Jeffries, who took care of literally thousands of items in preparation of this second edition. My artist, Jean Kanski-Bittl, updated old and created new drawings to keep the atlas current. Jim Green did most of the photography. My staff, Judy Nelson and Marlene Rivkin, did all mailings, assisted in the research, and helped in countless other ways

Carol Grill at New England Baptist Hospital and Paula Skalinski at Faulkner Hospital were of immense help in looking up catalog numbers and providing instruments to be photographed or drawn. Likewise, the staff at Mosby–Year Book, headed by Stephanie Manning, were most patient and supportive.

Also, I thank Doctors Jordan Phillips, Wolf H. Utian, Brian Cohen, and Ganson Purcell for inviting me to instruct in their microsurgical and surgical laparoscopy workshops. Finally, I wish to acknowledge my colleagues for inspiring me to continue to refine techniques and my patients for challenging me with difficult surgical problems.

Robert B. Hunt

ATLAS OF

Female Infertility Surgery

Contents

··

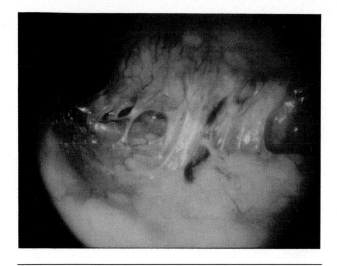

Plate 1
Hysteroscopic view of intrauterine adhesions before division.
Courtesy Jacques Hamou, Paris.

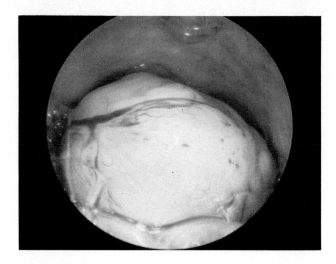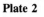

Plate 2
Hysteroscopic view of a large submucous myoma before resection. Courtesy Jacques Hamou, Paris.

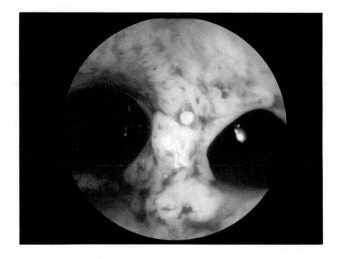

Plate 3
Hysteroscopic view of a uterine septum before surgical correction. Courtesy Jacques Hamou, Paris.

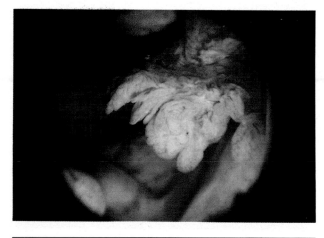

Plate 4
Underwater laparoscopic view of the fimbriae, demonstrating hydroflotation with Ringer's lactate solution. Courtesy Robert B. Hunt, Boston.

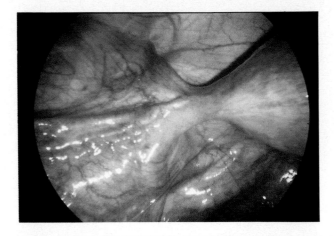

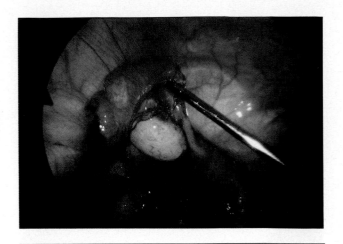

Plate 5
Extensive adhesions of the left adnexa. Courtesy Robert B. Hunt, Boston.

Plate 6
A left salpingoovariolysis has been completed laparoscopically. This woman achieved a successful pregnancy shortly after the procedure (same patient as in Plate 5). Courtesy Robert B. Hunt, Boston.

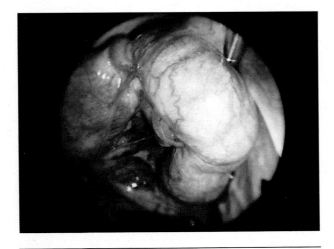

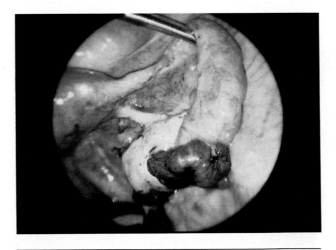

Plate 7
A right hydrosalpinx. Courtesy Robert B. Hunt, Boston.

Plate 8
Adhesions were resected and a salpingostomy performed laparoscopically (same patient as in Plate 7). Courtesy Robert B. Hunt, Boston.

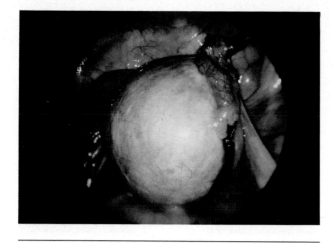

Plate 9
A persistent cyst of the right ovary. Courtesy Robert B. Hunt, Boston.

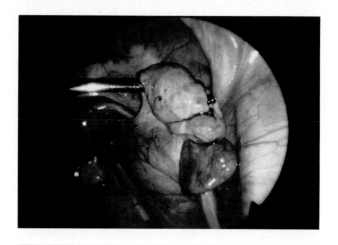

Plate 10
The follicular cyst was resected laparoscopically (same patient as in Plate 9). Courtesy Robert B. Hunt, Boston.

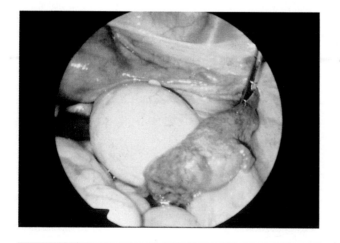

Plate 11.
A right ovary containing a dermoid. Courtesy Robert B. Hunt, Boston.

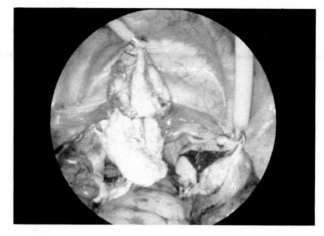

Plate 12
Laparoscopic removal of the dermoid (same patient as in Plate 11). Courtesy Robert B. Hunt, Boston.

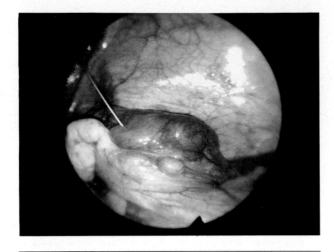

Plate 13
Dilute vasopressin is injected into the mesosalpinx of the right fallopian tube adjacent to the right ampullary pregnancy. Courtesy Robert B. Hunt, Boston.

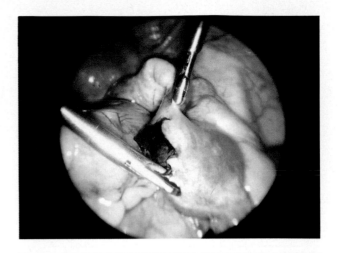

Plate 14
An incision is made over the pregnancy with scissors (same patient as in Plate 13). Courtesy Robert B. Hunt, Boston.

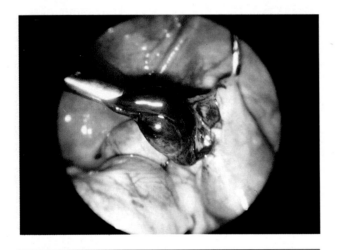

Plate 15
Removal of the ectopic gestation (same patient as in Plate 13). Courtesy Robert B. Hunt, Boston.

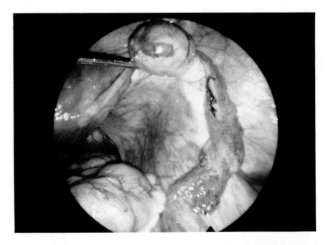

Plate 16
The tubal procedure is complete. Note the corpus luteum of pregnancy (same patient as in Plate 13). Courtesy Robert B. Hunt, Boston.

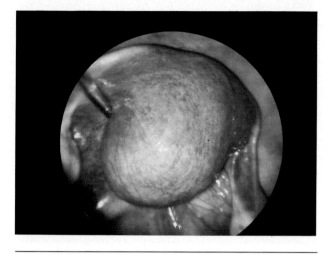

Plate 17
An intramural myoma. Courtesy Robert B. Hunt, Boston.

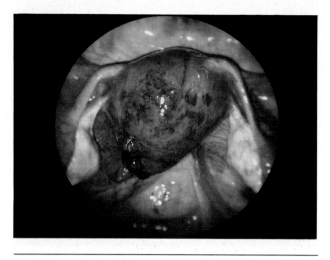

Plate 18
A laparoscopic myomectomy was performed and the defect closed with 4-0 polydioxanone (same patient as in Plate 17). Courtesy Robert B. Hunt, Boston.

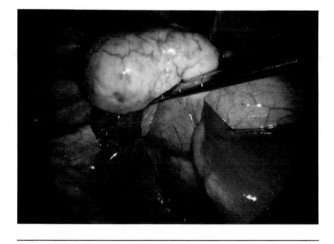

Plate 19
Laparoscopic view of a polycystic ovary. Courtesy Robert B. Hunt, Boston.

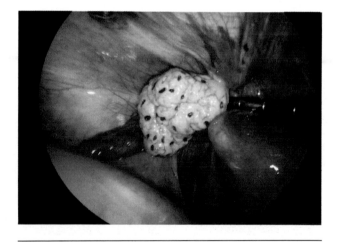

Plate 20
Multiple follicles have been drained laparoscopically by the CO_2 laser (same patient as in Plate 19). Courtesy Robert B. Hunt, Boston.

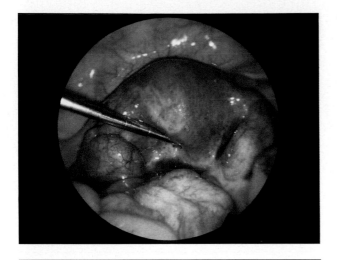

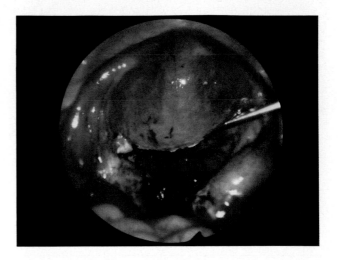

Plate 21
An acute pelvic abscess. Courtesy Robert B. Hunt, Boston.

Plate 22
The pelvic abscess has been drained, the abscess wall debrided, and pelvic structures separated by aquadissection (same patient as in Plate 21). Courtesy Robert B. Hunt, Boston.

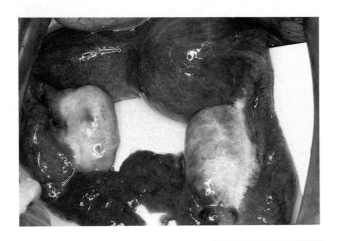

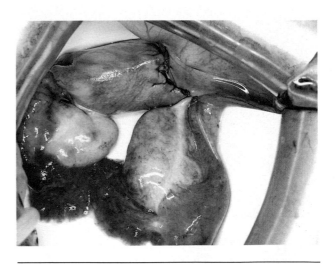

Plate 23
A left unicornuate uterus with an expanded and noncommunicating right uterine horn. Courtesy Robert B. Hunt, Boston.

Plate 24
The right uterine horn has been excised (same patient as in Plate 23). Courtesy Robert B. Hunt, Boston.

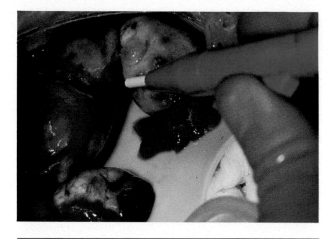

Plate 25
This patient has a septate uterus and a history of two spontaneous abortions. A Tompkins metroplasty is shown. After the myometrium is infiltrated with 5 U dilute vasopressin, the uterus is incised in the midline electrosurgically. Courtesy Robert B. Hunt, Boston.

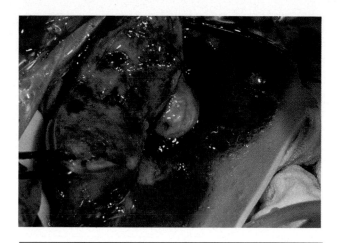

Plate 26
A previously placed intrauterine catheter marks the inferior margin of the septum (same patient as in Plate 25). Courtesy Robert B. Hunt, Boston.

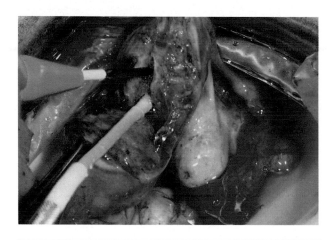

Plate 27
A dissecting rod is placed inside the right uterine horn and the septum incised to its fundal limit (same patient as in Plate 25). Courtesy Robert B. Hunt, Boston.

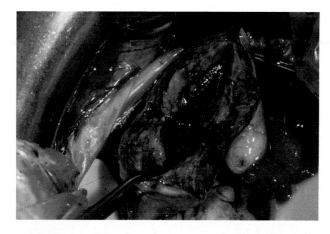

Plate 28
The process is repeated on the left uterine horn. The two uterine horns have been converted into a single cavity. Note the septum ends very near the intramural portion of the fallopian tube (same patient as in Plate 25). Courtesy Robert B. Hunt, Boston.

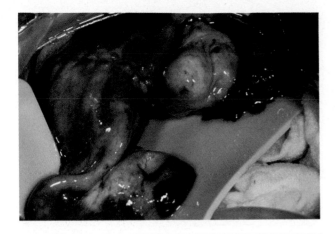

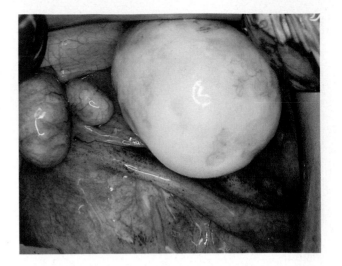

Plate 29

The myometrium is closed in three layers. Interrupted 2-0 or 3-0 absorbable material is selected for the two deeper layers. Polydioxanone is an excellent choice since it glides through tissue easily. It is best to begin the sutures inferiorly and place the anterior and posterior sutures alternately to achieve symmetric closure. Great care is taken to avoid compromising the intramural portion of the fallopian tube. The first layer is placed to include the inner one-half of the myometrium but excludes the serosa. The second layer includes the outer one-half of the myometrium but excludes the endometrium. The third layer is closed with a running suture of 4-0 material and incorporates the serosa and superficial myometrium. Oxidized cellulose (Interceed) may be placed over the suture line. The patient is instructed to avoid pregnancy for 3 months and deliver by elective cesarean section. This patient subsequently delivered a healthy infant by cesarean section (same patient as in Plate 25). Courtesy Robert B. Hunt, Boston.

Plate 30

A uterus markedly distorted by myomata. Courtesy Robert B. Hunt, Boston.

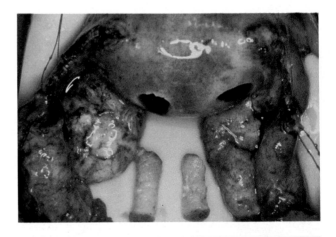

Plate 32

Bilateral pathologic cornual occlusion developed after pelvic infection. The intramural tubal segments were severely sclerosed. A bilateral tubal implantation after the method of Levinson was performed. Note the tubal segments are bivalved, with flaps held with 3-0 synthetic absorbable material. A 1-cm Cohen reamer was used to develop implantation sites. An intrauterine catheter was used to expand the uterine cavity to facilitate use of the reamer. Courtesy Robert B. Hunt, Boston.

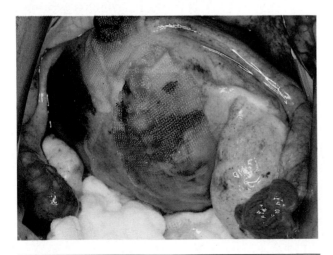

Plate 31

A multiple myomectomy has been performed and oxidized cellulose (Interceed) applied to the incision sites to diminish postoperative adhesion formation (same patient as in Plate 30). Courtesy Robert B. Hunt, Boston.

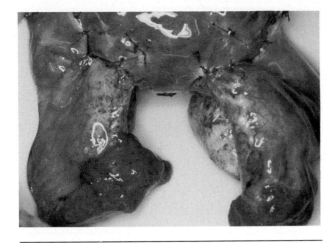

Plate 33
The fallopian tubes have been implanted and the sutures holding the respective tubal flaps are tied. Additional 3-0 absorbable sutures have been placed to approximate the tubal serosa to the uterine serosa at the implantation sites to relieve all tension. The cornual areas have also been closed over with serosa. If the uterus is retroverted, a suspension procedure should be considered (same patient as in Plate 11). Courtesy Robert B. Hunt, Boston.

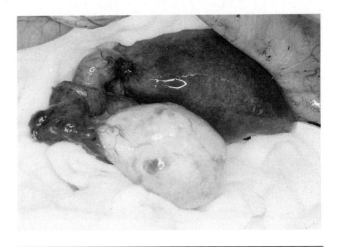

Plate 34
This woman had left cornual occlusion from endometriosis. She had previously undergone a right salpingoophorectomy. Courtesy Robert B. Hunt, Boston.

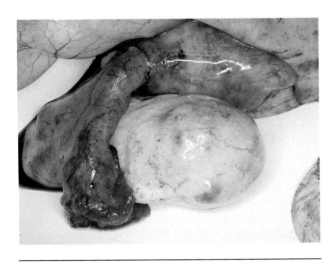

Plate 35
A left cornual anastomosis has been accomplished. The patient achieved an intrauterine pregnancy shortly after the procedure (same patient as in Plate 34). Courtesy Robert B. Hunt, Boston.

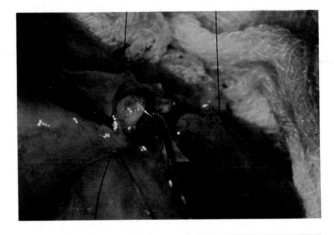

Plate 36
This patient, who had undergone tubal ligation performed by coagulation, wanted to conceive again. Fibrosed segments of the tube have been resected, 6-0 stay sutures positioned, and a 9-0 suture placed extramucosally in the proximal segment in the 6 o'clock position. Courtesy Robert B. Hunt, Boston.

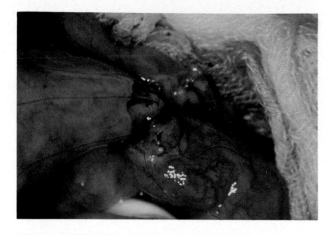

Plate 37
The stay sutures and 6 o'clock suture have been tied and three additional 9-0 sutures placed extramucosally (same patient as in Plate 36). Courtesy Robert B. Hunt, Boston.

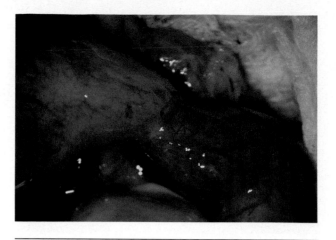

Plate 38
The inner sutures have been tied and the serosa has now been closed with interrupted 8-0 nylon sutures (same patient as in Plate 36). Courtesy Robert B. Hunt, Boston.

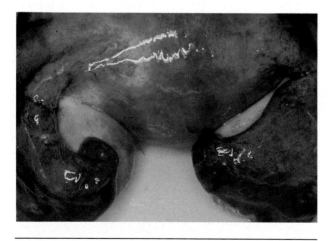

Plate 39
The anastomosis is complete. Note that additional 6-0 sutures were tied to alleviate any tension and to close the mesosalpinx (same patient as in Plate 36). This patient subsequently delivered a healthy infant. Courtesy Robert B. Hunt, Boston.

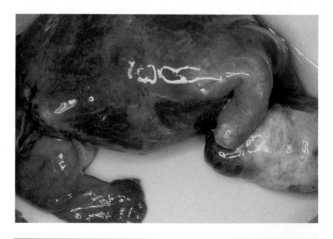

Plate 40
This 31-year-old woman underwent tubal coagulation by unipolar technique 6 years previously and desired a reversal. Note the complete absence of the right ampulla and severe fibrosis of the left cornu. This emphasizes the importance of a preoperative laparoscopy for patients having had tubal ligation by this method. Courtesy Robert B. Hunt, Boston.

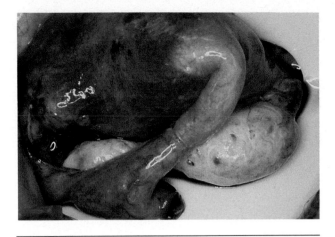

Plate 41
The two-layer anastomosis is completed using the right isth-mus and the left ampulla. Tension is alleviated by suturing the utero-ovarian ligaments to the posterior surface of the uterus with 3-0 synthetic permanent sutures (same patient as in Plate 40). The patient subsequently delivered a healthy in-fant. The fertility surgeon must be innovative. Courtesy Robert B. Hunt, Boston.

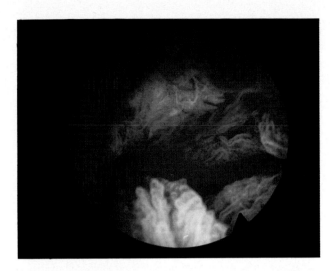

Plate 42
Ampullary tubal mucosa seen at tuboscopy after salpingos-tomy. Note the ampullary folds, indicating a favorable prog-nosis for pregnancy. Courtesy Robert B. Hunt, Boston.

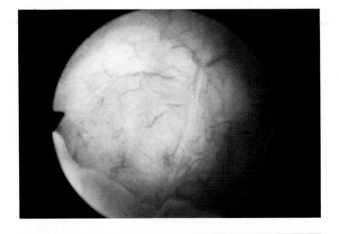

Plate 43
Absent ampullary tubal mucosa seen at tuboscopy after sal-pingostomy, indicating a poor prognosis for pregnancy. Courtesy Robert B. Hunt, Boston.

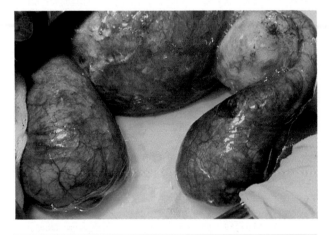

Plate 44
Typical appearance of a bilateral hydrosalpinx (sactosalpinx). Courtesy Hugo C. Verhoeven, Dusseldorf.

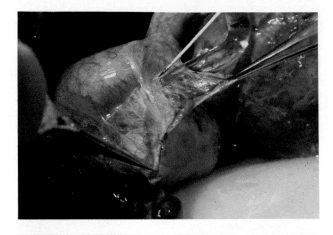

Plate 45
Adhesions are resected from the fallopian tubes and ovaries with a microelectrode over the dissecting rod (same patient as in Plate 44). Courtesy Hugo C. Verhoeven, Dusseldorf.

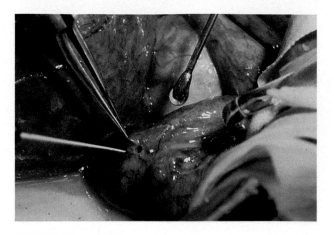

Plate 46
The surgeon opens the distal end of the right fallopian tube electrosurgically (same patient as in Plate 44). Courtesy Hugo C. Verhoeven, Dusseldorf.

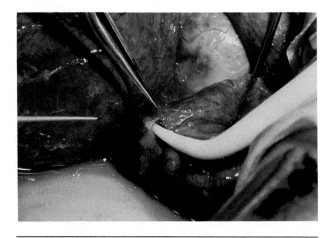

Plate 47
The opening is enlarged with the microelectrode (same patient as in Plate 44). Courtesy Hugo C. Verhoeven, Dusseldorf.

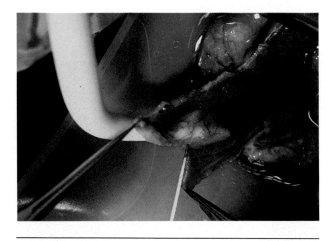

Plate 48
The fallopian tube is everted and radial incisions are made between the mucosal folds. Hemostasis is achieved by bipolar coagulation (same patient as in Plate 44). Courtesy Hugo C. Verhoeven, Dusseldorf.

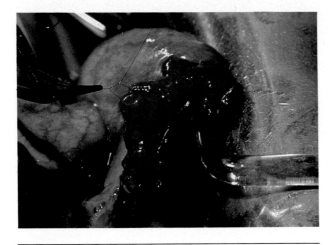

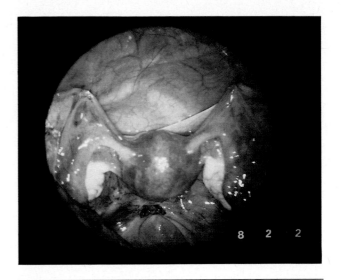

Plate 49
The sutures of the serosa of the newly created mucosal flaps
are sutured to the serosa of the fallopian tube, completing
the salpingostomy (same patient as in Plate 44). The procedure is repeated on the contralateral side. Eversion after the
method of Kosasa could have been performed alternatively.
Courtesy Hugo C. Verhoeven, Dusseldorf.

Plate 50
This patient underwent laparoscopic uterosacral nerve ablation and round ligament suspension. Note there is no kinking
of the tubes. Courtesy Robert B. Hunt, Boston.

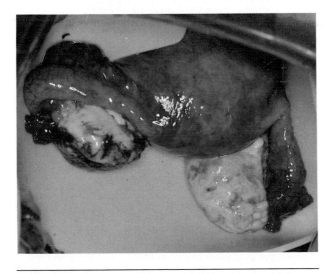

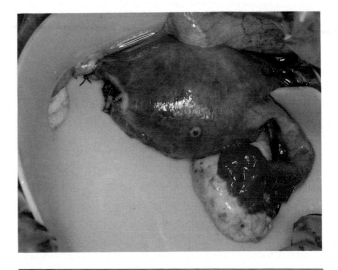

Plate 51
The left tube and ovary are afflicted with severe endometriosis. Courtesy Robert B. Hunt, Boston.

Plate 52
The left tube and ovary have been excised and triplication of
the round ligaments accomplished. Bipolar coagulation was
used instead of sutures on the mesovarium and mesosalpinx
(same patient as in Plate 51). Courtesy Robert B. Hunt,
Boston.

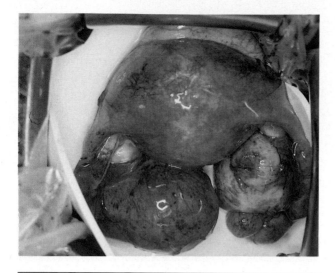

Plate 53
This woman had an inoperable left tube and bipolar obstruction of the right tube. Courtesy Robert B. Hunt, Boston.

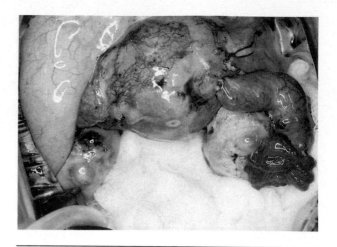

Plate 54
A left salpingectomy and a right distal salpingostomy with cornual anastomosis have been performed. The patient subsequently delivered a healthy infant (same patient as in Plate 53). Courtesy Robert B. Hunt, Boston.

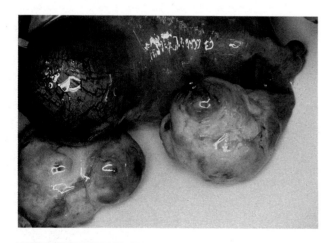

Plate 55
This left cornual pregnancy developed after in vitro fertilization. Courtesy Robert B. Hunt, Boston.

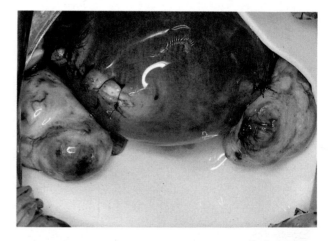

Plate 56
The ectopic pregnancy has been excised and a partial right salpingectomy accomplished (same patient as in Plate 55). Courtesy Robert B. Hunt, Boston.

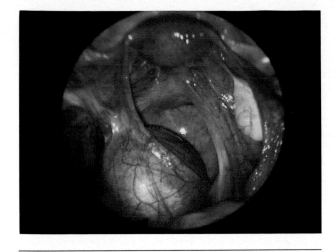

Plate 57
A large paratubal cyst of the left mesosalpinx. Courtesy Robert B. Hunt, Boston.

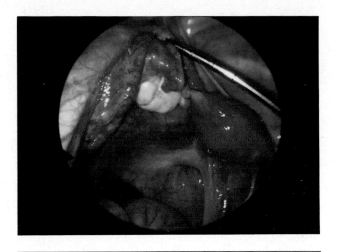

Plate 58
The cyst has been resected laparoscopically (same patient as in Plate 57). Courtesy Robert B. Hunt, Boston.

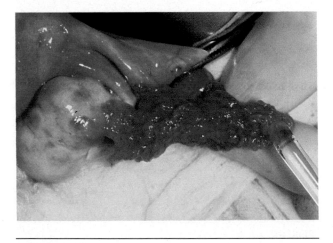

Plate 59
Accessory fimbrial folds occupy the space between the true fimbriae and the ovary. Courtesy Brian M. Cohen, Dallas.

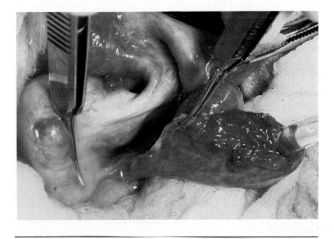

Plate 60
The accessory fimbrial folds have been excised under magnification using the microelectrode and bipolar coagulation. The fimbria ovarica is repaired to establish normal anatomic relationships between the fallopian tube and ovary (same patient as in Plate 59). Courtesy Brian M. Cohen, Dallas.

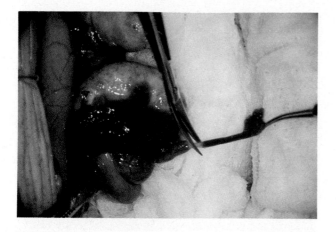

Plate 61
A rudimentary accessory oviduct is excised at the site of bipolar coagulation. Courtesy of Brian M. Cohen, Dallas.

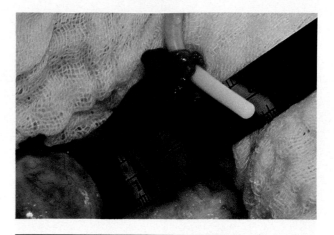

Plate 62
Distal tubal accessory ostium. The fimbria ovarica is 4 cm in length. Courtesy Brian M. Cohen, Dallas.

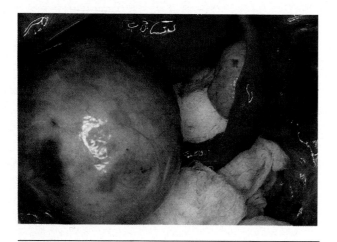

Plate 63
A left ovarian endometrioma. Courtesy Robert B. Hunt, Boston.

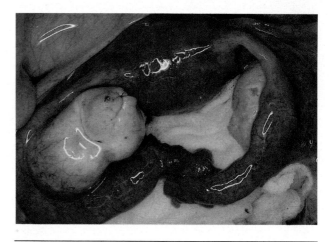

Plate 64
The endometrioma has been resected (same patient as in Plate 63). Courtesy Robert B. Hunt, Boston.

BASIC SCIENCE

1

Anatomy and Physiology of the Fallopian Tube

JEROME J. HOFFMAN

Until recently the fallopian tube was conceptualized as a fundamentally simple conduit through which spermatozoa ascended by means of their own propulsive efforts to encounter ova that descended by a peristaltic mechanism resembling that of the intestinal tract. The resulting zygote was then thought to have moved toward implantation by the same simple means. With so undeveloped a concept, it is not surprising that reparative surgery had been considered unsuccessful until the mid 1970s when substantive advances in technique and understanding began to change expectations. Concomitantly, the clinical observations, which were inevitably harvested from a marked increase in tubal surgery, carried with them the implications of a vastly more complex fallopian physiology that had been suspected. To that point, efforts to replace the oviduct were not only futile but reflected the naivete of the earlier era. Several things were tried, including polyethylene cylinders,[1,2] the vermiform appendix,[3] and even arterial grafts.[4,5] Attempts were made to eliminate the fallopian tube altogether by implanting the ovary into the uterine cavity.[6,7] Despite a recently published design for an "artificial fallopian tube,"[8] the use of an artificially fertilized zygote and a microinfusion pump to infuse the incubated zygote into the uterus only serves to underscore the complexity of the myriad functions of the oviduct.

When Rubin published the success he had achieved with the reestablishment of patency after the first tubal insufflation in 1920,[9,10] patency not only became a primary object but the entire object until the inception of the present era. It is important to note that despite the incremental increase in our knowledge of ovum and sperm transport, we are still unable to assay tubal function. Today (just as in Rubin's day), we are able to evaluate only tubal patency.[11] Despite an attempt to evaluate the feasibility of transport with radionuclide hysterosalpingography,[12] this statement must be as fundamentally true today as it was in 1979. Nevertheless, it is indisputable that the surgeon's knowledge of current facts regarding the anatomy and physiology of the oviduct and a conscientious attempt to respect and preserve these facts have helped considerably in achieving the desired clinical results.

ANATOMY

Not until there was considerable literature on the reanastomosis of tubal segments to reverse prior sterilization was the true significance of tubal length appreciated. The average length of the human tube (excluding the intramural portion) has been variously cited as between 7 and 11 cm. The intramural (also known as the interstitial) portion is tortuous and capable of changing shape; its length is 1 to 2 cm. Although we have no convincing evidence of a "long tube" syndrome in infertility, it has been suspected. There is, however, ample evidence that a foreshortened oviduct has an impact on fertility. It seems to have been confirmed that a fallopian tube shortened to less than 3 cm overall is incompatible with conception.[13] It also appears that the total length of the oviduct must be more than 8 cm to be compatible with success after the attempted reversal of a fimbriectomy. An inverse ratio of successful outcome to tubal length was reported,[14] and the same sort of inverse ratio was related to length of time required to achieve a viable intrauterine pregnancy.[15] Other factors being equal, overall tubal length has been shown to provide a more proficient prognostic variable than ampullary length, as long as fimbriae are present and the ampulla measures at least 1 cm.[16] Rabbit studies demonstrated 50% infertility when the entire isthmus was excised and absolute infertility when more than 60% of the ampulla was removed.[17]

Despite this finding, however, small numbers of successful pregnancies have been reported when little more than the infundibulum, including the fimbriae, and the isthmus remained.

Tubal segments
Intramural tube

Traversing the distance between the uterine cornu and the termination of the isthmus is the intramural or interstitial tube. It is the narrowest portion of the oviduct, measuring between 0.4 and 0.5 mm, and is surrounded by three muscle layers that are essentially myometrial. These consist of an inner circular, a middle oblique, and an outer longitudinal layer, each of which responds differently to the same prostaglandin fractions[18] (Figures 1-1 and 1-2). The mucosa is unique in that it contains a large number of secretory elements and is more abundantly ciliated than the isthmus. On sectioning, its lumen is tortuous and thrown into crypts, which may only reflect the contractility of the surrounding muscularis after extirpation. As near as can be determined, the normal length of the intramural tube is between 1.5 and 2.0 cm in both the extirpated and the in vivo uterus.

A striking feature of the muscularis surrounding the intramural tube is its marked vascularity[19] (Figure 1-3). The vascular network, deriving branches from both the ovarian and uterine circulation, has been a source of speculation by some authors who believe it capable of intermittent compression of the intramural tube.

Isthmus

In a strict sense the tubocornual junction should be the joint at which the intramural tube meets the uterine cornu. For surgical purposes, the term *tubocornual junction* refers to the juncture of the intraabdominal portion of the tube with the intramural tube. The isthmus extends from this point to the most proximal portion of the ampulla, a distance of approximately one third the total tube.

The stout muscularis of the isthmus consists of an outer longitudinal layer from which some of the fibers extend into the broad ligament at its distal extremity, a thick inner circular layer that is somewhat oblique, and a thinner longitudinal layer that attenuates as it approaches the ampulla and is evidenced by a few fibrils in the lamina propria. On transection, the lumen of the isthmus, which measures between 2 mm and 230 μm in diameter, is characterized by a distinctive division into four crypts, giving it a cruciate appearance (Figure 1-4).

As in other portions of the oviduct, the mucosa consists of four types of cells: peg, indifferent, secretory, and ciliated. Only the last two appear to play a role in ovum transport.[20] It has been shown in the *Macaca mulatta* (crab-eating Macaca) that in the preovulatory period there is profuse secretion of glycoprotein into the isthmus, the physical characteristics of which might be supposed to

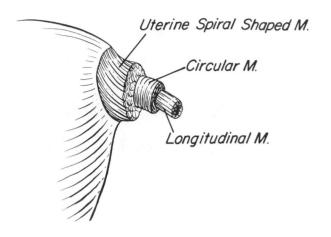
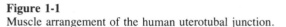

Figure 1-1
Muscle arrangement of the human uterotubal junction.

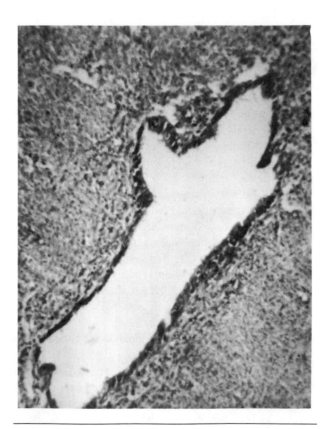

Figure 1-2
High-power view of the intramural tube. Note the thick longitudinal muscularis.

exert an influence on ovum transport.[21] The oviductal fluids have also been described as a transudate containing other components such as bicarbonate, which may be essential to respiration in the transported cell and has been credited with creating a pH of 7.5 to 8.0[22]; urea, which may be used as a protein precursor; inositol, which

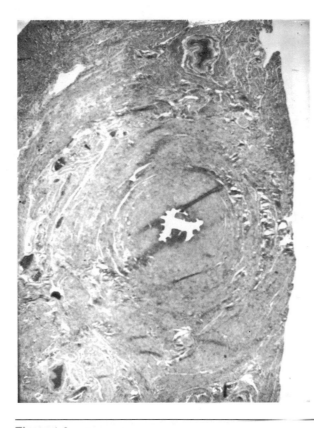

Figure 1-3
Intramural tube. Note vascularity in the surrounding muscularis.

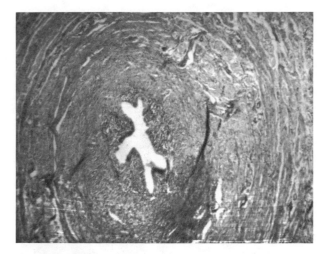

Figure 1-4
Cross section of the isthmus of the fallopian tube. Note the cruciate appearance of the lumen and the thickness of the circular muscularis.

appears in some species to prevent birth defects; and various ions. It has been found that oviductal fluid displays a potassium concentration significantly greater than plasma and a calcium ion concentration significantly below that of plasma.[23] The ciliated cells are relatively sparse, constituting about 54% of the cellular make-up of the isthmus.[24]

The ampulla

The distal two thirds of the oviduct is the markedly widened and exuberantly lined ampullary segment (Figure 1-5). It extends from the ampullary-isthmal junction (AIJ) to the vestibule to which the fimbriae lead. Its diameter measures approximately 1 cm. In this segment the secretory elements are outnumbered by the ciliated cells, which constitute about 79% of the fimbriae and 74% of the ampulla. The ciliated cells tend to be located at the apices and sides of the mucosal folds (Figure 1-6). They are columnar and have approximately 250 kinocilia in rows at the apex of the cell. Absence of cilia as the result of prior inflammatory disease or diminution of their preponderance to below 50% of observable cell types may be expected to result in infertility (Figure 1-7) and is frequently associated with flattened mucosal folds, as well as a diminution of secretory elements.[25] Currently,

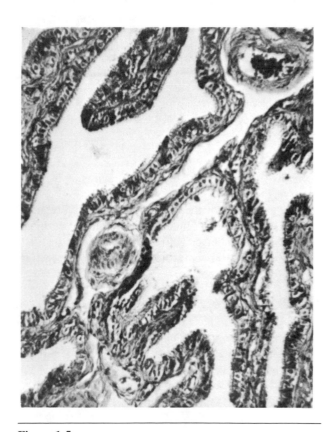

Figure 1-5
High-power view of the tubal ampulla.

there is no agreement on the potential for cilial regeneration, although some appears to take place.[26] Equally, the proximity of the tube to the ovary by attachment to the fimbria ovarica or to the tubo-ovarian ligament is

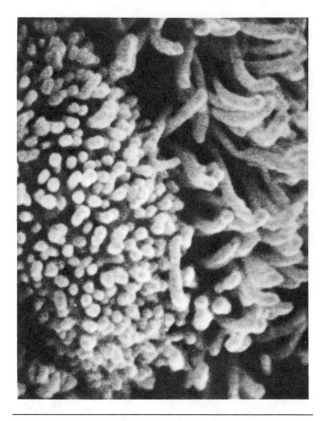

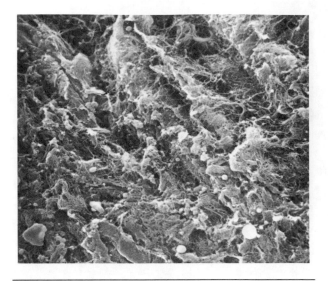

Figure 1-7
Scanning electron microscopic view of deciliation and fibrosis of rabbit ampulla after 7 days of indwelling polyethylene stent.

Figure 1-6
Scanning electron microscopy of cilia in the ampulla of the tube. There is profuse ciliation at the crest of the folds, with secretory predominance in the depressions.

accredited with varying degrees of importance by some observers.

The muscularis of the ampulla is considerably attenuated. The two longitudinal layers are almost vestigial, while the circular layer between is so thinned that it is a challenge to the surgeon who does not wish to penetrate the mucosa with a needle.

Circulation

The fallopian tube has an arcuate circulation. In examining many specimens, Diamond[19] found considerable consistency in the circulatory pattern. As it enters the mesosalpinx, the tubal branch of the uterine artery decussates into two branches, one coursing the entire length of the tube and the other extending over the uterine fundus and cornu (Figure 1-8). Just under the isthmus the tubal artery divides into two branches, one superior and the other inferior, that rejoin as they anastomose with a major branch of the ovarian artery. As the tubal artery runs along inferiorly to the tube, it sends forth small branches that supply the tube and its serosa. Distally, these distinct vessels become a complex network of arterioles that extends to the fimbriae and joins the ovarian artery. The ovarian artery courses toward the ovary and sends off anastomotic branches not only to the ovary but to the tubal artery as well. The veins follow a similar pattern. Ovarian veins deprived of their drainage to the parauterine complex by ligation may be observed to dilate and pool to a greater degree than the uterine complex.

Nerve supply

The sympathetic and parasympathetic nerves of the fallopian tube do not appear to be as crucial to tubal function as was once supposed.[27] Despite the contention of several theoreticians that the time course of ovum transport is under neural control, the denervated tube does not appear to suffer any deprivation of function. Nevertheless, the tubal musculature is richly supplied by the parasympathetic nerves of the pelvic plexus and the vagus, as well as the inferior mesenteric plexus and the cervicovaginal plexus. The tubal muscularis appears to respond to a number of stimuli in a much more complex fashion than the innervation would appear to suggest.

Pain sensation in the tube is derived from T11 and T12 and the upper lumbar nerves, a fact worth remembering while performing tubal ligations under low spinal or local anesthesia.

PHYSIOLOGY OF THE HUMAN OVIDUCT

Although there are still large gaps in our knowledge of the processes that take place within the human oviduct, our understanding is constantly developing. This is the result of the continuing pursuit of animal experimentation and by indirect observation of the various approaches and their results in tubal surgery and, to some degree,

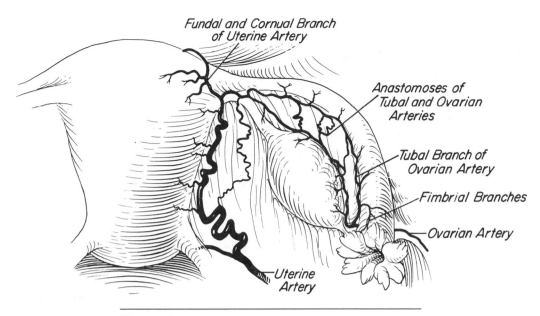

Figure 1-8
Arterial blood supply of the fallopian tube.

in vitro fertilization (IVF) and gamete intrafallopian transfer (GIFT).

Sperm transport and capacitation

In primates, seminal plasma has not been found to pass the cervix after coitus.[28] Spermatozoa can reach the ampulla in as little as 1½ hours. However, how they cover this distance so rapidly is unknown. It is also unknown why high-volume and low-count specimens are consistently subfertile. Nonmotile sperm are capable of ascent (albeit more slowly than motile sperm, which can reach the isthmus in as little as 5 minutes) and usually reach the ampulla in about 6 hours. In humans, unlike some other species, ciliary action does not seem to supply a cogent explanation. In fact, the thick preovulatory mucus in the isthmus provides a milieu in which the cilia are caught up and largely immobilized.[29] Whether sperm transport is aided by fluid currents in an environment made turbulent by muscle contractions is yet to be determined.[20] Although the nuances of sperm capacitation within the oviduct, which has been shown to be species specific,[22] is better understood in species other than humans, it is hoped that increased experience in IVF and GIFT will enhance the understanding of this process.

Fertilization

The oviductal environment appears to provide for the metabolic needs of spermatozoa. Although we have extensive knowledge of the electrolytes and nonelectrolytes and their variability in the fallopian tube, it is evident that other factors, which have not yet been appreciated and have become a part of the process in the in vitro phenomenon,[30] enhance fertilization in the in vivo en-

vironment. Although spermatozoa have been recovered still motile from the oviduct after 72 hours, no reliable data exist on the fertilization life of the spermatozoa.

Ovum pick-up

In 1852, Meigs[31] described ovum pick-up by the fimbriae, or the *morsus diaboli* ("devil's bit") in which he conceptualized that the ovum was seized by a joint effort of suction, vermicular movement, and ciliary action that conveyed it to the uterus. After that date the concept appeared frequently in the literature. Some aspects of that contention, although simplistic, are possibly not far from the truth.

It has been demonstrated in laparoscopy that the human egg, extruded in cumulus from the graafian follicle, is surrounded by fimbriae that frame the infundibulum. The muscle fibers in the tubo-ovarian ligament, as well as those in the mesosalpinx, visibly contract.[32] Although it is difficult to prove that there is suction into the tube, experiments with catheters in the human oviduct have shown negative pressure of 1 mm Hg during antiperistaltic activity.[32] The prevalence of ciliated mucosal cells at the tubal ostium has been variously cited at 50% to 79%. These cells are in constant abovarian motion and appear to be responsible for the rapid transmittal of the ovum to the ampullary-isthmal junction.

It is to be noted that pregnancies certainly occur when there is only one ovary and a contralateral tube, so that some ovum pick-up may be expected to occur from the cul-de-sac. Given this anatomic situation in the presence of infertility, a number of pregnancies have been achieved by microsurgical transposition of the tube to a position of approximation to the ovary.[33]

Transport of the ovum and zygote

The time course of ovum transport in the human has been definitely established as 80 hours, 72 of which are spent in the ampulla.[34] By performing salpingectomies for sterilization on a number of women in planned relation to their time of ovulation, as determined by endocrinologic criteria, these authors located the ovum in its aduterine progress along the oviduct. This was done by tying the oviduct in four equidistant locations and then searching out the ovum in one of three areas thus demarcated. Similar research performed in the rhesus monkey and the baboon revealed virtually identical results.[16] When radioactive surrogate ova, however, are transmitted through the oviducts of these primates, the results are erratic, possibly attributable to the fact that the primate egg, unlike the more commonly used rabbit model (which is surrounded by a mucoid substance only), travels in cumulus.[35]

Just as there are marked structural differences between the ampulla and the isthmus, the means by which they propel the ovum along its course differ. After its pickup at the infundibulum, the egg travels rapidly in 1 or 2 hours to the ampullary-isthmal junction where, for unknown reasons, it remains for the requisite 72 hours awaiting fertilization.[37] The presence of an adequate complement of cilia seems to be vital to this progression.[36] No patients with less than 54% fimbrial cilia were able to conceive.[34] Significant deciliation was demonstrated after tubal sterilization, ectopic pregnancy, as well as pelvic inflammatory disease.[38] This latter contention has been borne out by a number of observers[25,39] and probably explains the high prevalence of infertility and tubal pregnancy in these instances. It is especially interesting to note that the simple presence of adequately numerous cilia in the mucosa appears to be at least as important as their motility. Women with Kartagener's syndrome, a clinical triad of bronchitis, sinusitis, and rhinitis, which is due to the absence of dynein "arms" rendering the cilia immotile, are able to conceive.[40] This appears to support the theory that other biases can propel the ovum effectively, providing that it has an adequate surface over which to ride. The theory that the presence of tubal surfactant is essential has been advanced.[41]

There is no doubt, however, that when motile, the cilia are integral to transport in the ampulla. At 7.3 beats/sec with an aduterine motion, the rhythm of each cell is metachromal, or individually derived.[24] There is no question of the direction of beat. In animal experiments in which a vascularized segment of ampulla was excised and then reanastomosed after having been turned 180 degrees, it was evident that surrogate eggs, influenced by the contradirectionality of the two segments, lined up on the anastomosis line and were incapable of further progress.[42] In succeeding experiments in another laboratory, several of the animals were able to conceive after

a longer interval, the presumption being that after a more extended period the cilia are capable of reprogramming.[43] This contention remains unsubstantiated.

In any event, considering the functioning muscularis, the secretory activity within the mucosal folds, as well as the active cilia on the ridges, it is safe to assume that ovum transport in the ampulla is the result of forces that come into play when a particle moves through a turbulent mucociliary system. This is a rheologic phenomenon longer appreciated and better known to those who have studied it in relation to the trachea and bronchi than it is to gynecologists.

The AIJ has been the subject of much study and speculation, but its exact mechanisms are still unknown. At first it was believed that the ovum was delayed in its entrance to the isthmus because of sphincteric action induced by neural control. This theory was abandoned not only because the AIJ presented none of the characteristics of a true sphincter, but because denervation of the area, such as could be seen in the transposition of an animal tube, did not negate the phenomenon. Furthermore, extirpation of the anatomic AIJ in animals resulted in a perfectly functional new physiologic AIJ once the anastomosis had been completed.[44] The same result was observed in humans after reanastomosis in which the previous Pomeroy sterilization bilaterally excised the anatomic AIJ (Figure 1-9). Recently there has been an increased appreciation of the thick glycoprotein secretions that occur in the isthmus in the periovulatory period,[21] which have been postulated to exert an influence on the retention of the egg in the appreciably less viscous environment of the ampulla, allowing it to pass after dissipation of that physical block.

Thus once it enters the isthmus, the egg is in a fluid milieu that has become markedly less viscid. It is then subjected to a number of influences that constitute an aduterine bias, the exact nature of which is elusive. Certainly the simplistic notion that the egg or zygote is moved along by peristaltic action, much like a bolus of food, is not tenable. Electrical bursts inducing muscle activity in the circular muscle are local, whereas in the longitudinal muscle, numerous bursts of similar amplitude seem to occur longitudinally at the same time.[45] Thus it appears that intrinsic pacemakers work in a random fashion. These were demonstrated in in vitro specimens and do not appear to vary with age.[46] It appears that they exert an influence on the egg only in its immediate vicinity. Inasmuch as these pacemakers transmit in short directions, a back-and-forth action is induced in which the ovum or zygote is pushed in one direction or another. Since, however, about 40% of the isthmus nearest the uterus displays relative electrical inactivity after ovulation (at least in the rabbit), there is a collecting zone in which muscle activity is not sufficient to drive the ovum in the opposite direction. By itself, this is not

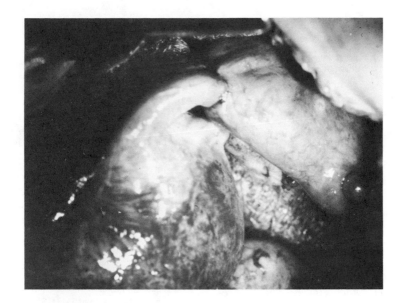

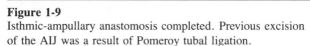

Figure 1-9
Isthmic-ampullary anastomosis completed. Previous excision
of the AIJ was a result of Pomeroy tubal ligation.

enough to explain isthmal transport. When prostaglandin $F_{2\alpha}$ was given to women before sterilization, it did not appreciably affect ovum transport,[47] although it could significantly add to the amplitude of muscle contractions and was noted to increase the diameter of the tube.[48] Although a number of pharmacologic agents, such as norepinephrine, isoproterenol, oxytocin, indomethacin, and the progesterone-inhibitory substance RU-486,[49] have been shown to strongly influence the amplitude of tubal contractions, no definitive observations on their influence on transport has yet appeared.

It is noteworthy, however, that the endocrine influences on transport have been well established. In rabbits, the speed, tone, and amplitude of muscle contractions are affected by the administration of prostaglandins only after prior conditioning with progesterone. In addition, "tubal locking" with estrogen, a phenomenon that delays the progress of the ovum in the ampulla, is capable of being reversed with progesterone. The antiestrogenic effect of clomiphene alters ovum transport, resulting in premature arrival of eggs into the rat uterus.[50] All of this would seem to indicate that whatever the nature of the complex factors in transport along the oviduct, there is a necessary overlay of hormonal influence on the collected phenomena.[45]

It should be remembered that foreshortening of the isthmus exerts no discernible influence over conception as long as the overall length of the tube is within the previously mentioned acceptable bounds.[14] Unlike the ampulla, when a 1-cm vascularized segment of isthmus in the rabbit is excised and turned 180 degrees, fertility is not significantly impaired.[51]

There remains a strong implication that the uterotubal junction and the intramural tube may play a role in transport and in implantation not yet fully identified and probably underresearched. The intramural tube does possess a uniqueness not only in the previously mentioned differential responses of the surrounding muscle layers but also in the fact that it is both heavily ciliated and generously endowed with secretory lining. A valuable clue may well be contained in the fact that the results of both uterotubal anastomosis[15] and posterior implantations of the Peterson-Behrman type[44] were far improved over the older implantation methods that excised the intramural tube.

Most of the large series of implantations in which the intramural tube was extirpated with a cork borer or knife excision achieved success rates, as reckoned in intrauterine pregnancies, of little more than 10% to 25%.[52] The exception was Shirodkar,[53,54,55] who claimed results in excess of 36%, a feat that almost no one else could approach. In a series of posterior implantations that retained the intramural tube, the success rate rose to 50%[56] and even ascended to as high as 75% in sterilization reversals.[57] Historically, it was Ehrler[58] who pointed out that the intramural tube generally resisted the effects of inflammatory disease or salpingitis nodosa. He attempted tubo-uterine anastomosis, which failed when performed by relatively crude macroscopic means. The resilience of the form and function of that portion of the oviduct is well demonstrated by the contemporary successes of balloon dilatation of the tubo-ovarian junction. There was a report of spontaneous recanalization of a cornual tubal obstruction after an IVF pregnancy,[59] again pointing toward the fact that, in that area, one is dealing with a forgiving structure with some unique properties.

What possible influence could the retention of the intramural tube have on increasing the pregnancy rates of the procedures in question? The profusion of cilia, beating in an aduterine direction, might logically be expected to convey the yield of the amply supplied secretory elements. Could this be offering a contribution to the uterine milieu for implantation? Is there a significant role to be played by the differentially contractile surrounding musculature? These questions still do not have definitive answers.

SUMMARY

Clinicians now have a ready solution to many of the difficult questions presented in reproductive failure. Certainly, IVF and GIFT provide a solution that was not available in the previous era when concern with the rehabilitation of the imperfect fallopian tube was at its highest. Nevertheless, further understanding of the functioning of the oviduct in its vital role in transport could lead to simpler, less invasive therapeutic approaches that are more successful than current "test-tube" modalities. Except in the instance of critical foreshortening and complete nonpatency, there appear to be few absolutes when dealing with the fallopian tube. The undeniable differences between species (e.g., humans are the only animals that sustain tubal pregnancies) and the obvious impossibility of in-depth human experimentation, have militated against simple answers in many clinical situations. Even at this point, we cannot emphasize too strongly that we have not yet devised a test for tubal function as opposed to mere patency. In the meticulous recording of the procedures, findings, and results of tubal surgery, a few answers are to be extrapolated. At least we have a clear idea of many of the questions to be answered. Many of the explanations to be supplied by animal experimentation could also provide information involving the complex processes of fertilization and support in the oviduct, which might further benefit the results not only of tubal repair but also of the technology involved in IVF and GIFT, as well as in future modalities.

REFERENCES

1. Wood C, Leeton J, and Taylor R: A preliminary design and trial of an artificial human tube, *Fertil Steril* 22:446-450, 1971.
2. Cross RG and Erskine CA: A new operation for the construction of a fallopian tube, *Lancet* 1:777-778, 1956.
3. O'Neill JJ: The use of the vermiform appendix as a fallopian tube, *Am J Obstet Gynecol* 95:219-222, 1966.
4. Davids AM and Bellwin A: A reconstruction of fallopian tubes by vein and artery transplants, *Fertil Steril* 5:525-533, 1954.
5. Schein CJ and Ferreria R: Use of autogenous arterial grafts for the experimental reconstruction of fallopian tubes, *Am J Obstet Gynecol* 71:206-211, 1956.
6. Estes WL Jr: Ovarian implantation, *Surg Gynecol Obstet* 38:394-398, 1924.
7. Estes WL Jr: Implantation of an ovary, *Ann Surg* 82:475-482, 1925.
8. Hunter SK et al: Developing an artificial fallopian tube: successful in vitro trial in mice, *Fertil Steril* 53:1083-1086, 1970.
9. Rubin IC: Nonoperative determination of patency of fallopian tubes in sterility, *JAMA* 74:1017, 1920.
10. Rubin IC: *Uterotubal insufflation*, St. Louis, 1947, The CV Mosby Co.
11. Hoffman JJ: The tubal factor in infertility. In Givens JR (ed): *The infertile female*, Chicago, 1979, Year Book Medical Publishers.
12. Brundin J et al: Radionuclide hysterosalpingography for measurement of human oviductal function, *Int J Gynecol Obstet* 28:53-59, 1989.
13. Cantor B and Rigall FC: The choice of sterilizing procedure according to its potential reversibility with microsurgery, *Fertil Steril* 31:9-12, 1979.
14. Silber SJ and Cohen R: Microsurgical reversal of female sterilization: the role of tubal length, *Fertil Steril* 33:598-601, 1980.
15. Gomel V: Microsurgical reversal of female sterilization: a reappraisal, *Fertil Steril* 33:587-597, 1980.
16. Pauerstein CJ and Eddy CA: Applied tubal physiology. In Muldoon TA, Mabesh B, and Perez-Ballister B (eds): *Recent advances in fertility research*, New York, 1981, Alan R. Liss.
17. Land JA: Tubal microsurgery. II. Experimental use, *Gynecol Obstet Invest* 23:145-150, 1987.
18. Wilhelmsson L and Lindblom B: Adrenergic responses of the various smooth muscle layers at the human uterotubal junction, *Fertil Steril* 33:280-282, 1980.
19. Diamond E: A microsurgical study of the blood supply of the uterine tube and ovary. In Phillips JM (ed): *Microsurgery in gynecology*, Downey, Calif, 1977, American Association of Gynecologic Laparoscopists.
20. Hoffman JJ: The fallopian tube: an upsurge of interest, *Curr Probl Obstet Gynecol* 136:292-308, 1980.
21. Jansen RPS and Bajpai VK: Periovulatory glycoprotein secretion in the macaque fallopian tube, *Am J Obstet Gynecol* 147:598-608, 1983.
22. Leese HJ: The formation and function of oviduct fluid, *J Reprod Fertil* 82:843-856, 1988.
23. Borland RM et al: Elemental composition of fluid in the human fallopian tube, *J Reprod Fertil* 58:479-482, 1980.
24. Critoph FN and Dennis KJ: Ciliary activity in the human oviduct, *Obstet Gynecol Surv* 32:602-603, 1977.
25. Patton DL et al: A comparison of the fallopian tube's response to overt and silent salpingitis, *Obstet Gynecol* 73:622-630, 1989.
26. Brenner RM: Renewal of oviductal cilia during the menstrual cycle of the rhesus monkey. In Hafez ESE and Blanda RJ (eds): *Comparative biology and methodology*, Chicago, 1969, University of Chicago Press.
27. Black DL: *Ovum transport and fertility regulations*, Copenhagen, 1976, Scriptions.
28. Asch RH, Balmaceda J, and Pauerstein CJ: Failure of seminal plasma to enter the uterus and oviducts of the rabbit following artificial insemination, *Fertil Steril* 28:671-673, 1977.
29. Jansen RPS: Cyclic changes in the human fallopian tube isthmus and their functional importance, *Am J Obstet Gynecol* 136:292-308, 1980.
30. Suzuki S et al: Gamete-oviduct interactions. Presented to the Fallopius International Society, Acapulco, 1989.
31. Meigs CD: *Obstetrics, the science and the art*, Philadelphia, 1852, Blanchard & Lea.
32. Maia HS and Coutinho EM: Peristalsis and antiperistalsis of the human fallopian tube during the menstrual cycle, *Biol Reprod* 2:305-314, 1970.
33. DeCherney A and Naftolin F: Homotransplantation of the human fallopian tube: report of a successful case and description of a technique, *Fertil Steril* 34:14-16, 1980.

34. Croxatto HB et al: Studies on the duration of egg transport by the human oviduct: ovum location at various intervals following luteinizing hormone peak, *Am J Ostet Gynecol* 132:629-634, 1978.

35. Eddy CA and Hodgson BJ: Tubal research: today's findings and a look at the future, *Contemp Obstet Gynecol* 8:5, 1976.

36. Land JA et al: Ovum transport after microsurgical anastomosis of the rabbit oviduct, *J Reprod Med* 32:104-106, 1987.

37. Brosens IA and Vasquez G: Fimbrial microbiopsy, *J Reprod Med* 16:171-178, 1976.

38. Vasquez G et al: Tubal lesions subsequent to sterilization and their relation to fertility after attempts at reversal, *Am J Obstet Gynecol* 138:86-92, 1980.

39. Russell JB: The etiology of tubal pregnancy, *Clin Obstet Gynecol* 30:181-189, 1987.

40. Jean Y et al: Fertility of a woman with nonfunctional ciliated cells in the fallopian tubes, *Fertil Steril* 31:349-350, 1949.

41. Egberts J: Letter. *Fertil Steril* 47:361-362, 1987.

42. Eddy CA et al: The role of cilia in fertility: an evaluation by selective modification of the rabbit oviduct, *Am J Obstet Gynecol* 132:814-821, 1978.

43. McComb P and Gomel V: The effect of segmental ampullary reversal on the subsequent fertility of the rabbit, *Fertil Steril* 31:83-85, 1979.

44. Winston RML, Frantzen C, and Oberti C: Oviduct function following resection of the ampullary-isthmic junction (abstr), *Fertil Steril* 28:284, 1977.

45. Talo A and Hodgson BJ: Spike bursts in rabbit oviduct I: effect of ovulation, *Am J Physiol* 234:E430-438, 1980.

46. Nadasy GI et al: Spontaneous periodic contraction of the ampullar segment of the human fallopian tube in vitro, *Acta Physiol Hung* 72:13-21, 1988.

47. Croxatto HB et al: Effect of 15(S)-15-methyl prostaglandin F_2-alpha on human oviductal motility and ovum transport, *Fertil Steril* 30:408-414, 1978.

48. Laszlo A et al: Effect of pharmacological agents on the activity of the circular and longitudinal smooth muscle layers of human fallopian tube ampullary segments, *Acta Physiol Hung* 72(1):123-133, 1988.

49. Nozaki M and Nakamura G: Effects of RU-486 on the mechanical properties of rabbit fallopian tubes, *Asia Oceania J Obstet Gynaecol* 14:120-135, 1988.

50. Gupta JS and Roy SK: The effect of clomiphene on nuclear estrogen receptors of the fallopian tube during ovum transport in rabbits, *Endocrinol Res* 15:339-353, 1989.

51. Eddy CA, Hoffman JJ, and Pauerstein CJ: Pregnancy following segmental isthmic reversal of the rabbit oviduct, *Experientia* 32:1194-1196, 1976.

52. Kistner RW and Patton GW Jr: *Atlas of infertility surgery*, Boston, 1975, Little, Brown & Co.

53. Shirodkar VN: Factors influencing the results of salpingostomy, *Int J Fertil* 2:361-365, 1961.

54. Shirodkar VN: *Contributions to obstetrics and gynaecology*, Edinburgh, 1960, E & S Livingstone.

55. Shirodkar VN: Further experiences in tuboplasty, *Aust N Z J Obstet Gynaecol Surv* 15:680, 1960.

56. Peterson EP, Musich JR, and Behrman SJ: Uterotubal implantation and obstetric outcome after previous sterilization, *Am J Obstet Gynecol* 128:662-667, 1977.

57. Levinson CJ: Implantation procedures for intramural obstruction, *J Reprod Med* 26(7):347-351, 1981.

58. Ehrler P: The intramural tube anastomosis (a contribution to the treatment of sterility), *Zentralbl Gynaekol* 85:393-400, 1963.

59. Confino E, Friberg J, and Gleicher N: Spontaneous recanalization of cornual tubal occlusion following a pregnancy achieved by in vitro fertilization, *Fertil Steril* 49:723-725, 1988.

2

Pathology of the Fallopian Tube

W. DWAYNE LAWRENCE

ROBERT E. SCULLY

Although the fallopian tube is affected by many diseases, this chapter is restricted to those that cause infertility or may be encountered during surgery to investigate or treat infertility. These diseases include acute, chronic, and granulomatous inflammatory processes and their sequelae; endometriosis and endosalpingiosis; benign tumors; and congenital anomalies. Malignant neoplasms involving the tube are not discussed.

INFLAMMATORY DISEASES
Acute salpingitis

Inflammatory diseases of the fallopian tube are an important cause of infertility. Historically, acute salpingitis has been attributed to the gonococcus *Neisseria gonorrhoeae* in most cases; studies of pelvic inflammatory disease (PID), however, have implicated other organisms,[1-4] including streptococci, staphylococci, coliform bacilli, anaerobic bacteria, *Chlamydia* and *Mycoplasma* organisms, and Herpes simplex virus alone or in combination. Chlamydial infection of the fallopian tubes has been increasingly recognized as an important pathogen in the development of acute salpingitis. In fact, *Chlamydia trachomatis* currently is regarded as the most frequent cause of PID in the United States.

Studies have demonstrated a high prevalence of silent chlamydial colonization of the tubal mucosa in infertile women.[5] Indeed, 6 of 34 asymptomatic, infertile women without distal tubal occlusion had isolates of *C trachomatis* in at least one tube in the absence of clinical signs of pelvic infection. To examine the role of chronic active chlamydial infection on fertility, tubal and endometrial biopsies and cultures were performed on 52 women undergoing a tubal procedure for infertility.[6] Positive cultures were obtained from either or both sites in 15% of the patients; 80% of the women with positive fallopian tube cultures also had positive endometrial cultures. Of

interest, culture-positive patients had been treated with standard antichlamydial antibiotics. Neither the endometrial nor the tubal biopsy specimens had a specific histopathologic lesion. The authors concluded that chronic active chlamydial infection frequently is associated with fallopian tube–related infertility, that the infection may persist in the face of standard therapy for these organisms, and that endometrial biopsy and culture may be an effective means of detecting the pathogen.

Experimental studies in mice infected with a human genital tract isolate of *C. trachomatis* showed that it could induce infertility by producing salpingitis.[7] Ova were not transported to the tubes, and ciliary activity was markedly impaired or absent. Ultrastructural studies suggested that *Chlamydia*-induced tubal damage was secondary to severe mucosal congestion and edema and loss of ciliated tubal epithelial cells, both of which could result in a diminished ability to transport the ovum to and through the tube. In addition, recovery of ciliary function, restoration of relatively normal fine structural architecture, and luminal patency were still associated with defective ovum transport.

Furthermore, the prevalence of immunoglobulin G (IgG) and IgM antibodies against *C. trachomatis* was significantly higher in infertile patients with fallopian tube abnormalities than in control pregnant patients.[8] Despite the fact that all the tubal cultures were negative, these workers believe that a close association existed between infertility of tubal etiology and an immune response to *C. trachomatis*. These results were substantiated in women in the so-called infertility belt of central Africa, in whom tubal occlusion, most likely related to infection, was present in approximately 83% of infertile patients.[9] Such patients had a significantly higher prevalence of serum chlamydial antibodies at a titer of 164 or higher than a control group of women with normal tubes.

Gonococci are thought to enter the tubes by upward

spread along mucosal surfaces. The disease begins with an acute endocervicitis, followed by a transient endometritis and finally salpingitis. In contrast, streptococci, staphylococci, and coliform bacilli enter the tubes by way of the lymphatics or blood vessels, especially after an abortion or pregnancy, and result in an initial perisalpingitis with subsequent spread throughout the wall of the tube. Since the mucosa is less severely inflamed and bilateral involvement is much less frequent, infections caused by these organisms result in infertility much less often than infection of gonococcal origin.

Gross pathology

The acutely inflamed tube exhibits the following abnormalities to varying degrees depending on the severity of the process: enlargement with edema of the wall and surrounding tissue, fiery red discoloration of the serosal surface, and an adherent purulent or fibrinopurulent exudate. In severe disease, which is usually of gonococcal origin, purulent exudate may distend the lumen of the tube and ooze from its fimbriated end. If the fimbriated end has been occluded as a result of previous acute inflammatory episodes, the tube acquires a sausagelike appearance. Adherence to adjacent organs and tissues often occurs. If the infection spreads to the ovary a tubo-ovarian abscess may form, appearing typically as a large mass in which the distinction between the tube and ovary may be difficult; sectioning may reveal numerous locules containing foul-smelling purulent exudate.

Acute salpingitis caused by nongonococcal organisms typically results in an enlarged edematous tube without a significant accumulation of purulent exudate within the lumen; the diffuse edema may impart a brawny consistency to the wall and surrounding tissue.

Microscopic pathology

Acute gonococcal salpingitis is characterized by vascular engorgement and edema of the mucosal folds. An infiltrate of polymorphonuclear leukocytes is confined to the plicae in the early stages; subsequently, these cells migrate into the lumen to form a purulent exudate, which often includes fibrin; transmural spread of inflammation occurs in severe cases (Figures 2-1 and 2-2). Focal sloughing of mucosal tissue into the lumen and interadherence of inflamed plicae may be observed. In pyosalpinx the wall is usually markedly thinned and the lumen filled with polymorphonuclear leukocytes and cellular debris; the plicae may be shortened and contain acute, as well as chronic, inflammatory cells, including lymphocytes and plasma cells.

Nongonococcal acute salpingitis caused by streptococci, staphylococci, and coliform bacilli is characterized by acute inflammation of the perisalpingeal tissue with extension into the muscularis in some cases, but with relative sparing of the mucosa. The infiltrate often has a prominent perivascular distribution.

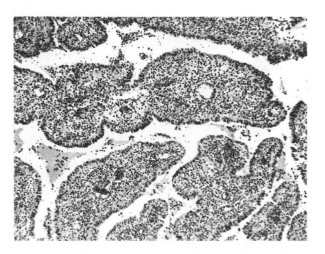

Figure 2-1
Acute salpingitis. The plicae contain numerous acute inflammatory cells, some of which have migrated into the lumen.

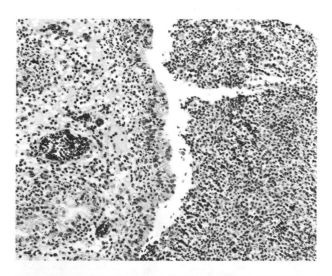

Figure 2-2
Acute salpingitis. Polymorphonuclear leukocytes are abundant in the plicae and form a purulent exudate within the tubal lumen. Plical blood vessels are engorged.

Chronic salpingitis

The changes observed in chronic salpingitis are generally the result of repeated episodes of acute salpingitis, which alter normal anatomic relationships.

One study of chronic salpingitis compared the degree of tubal damage in two groups of infertile women, one with a history of clinically recognized salpingitis (overt PID) and the other with apparently silent salpingitis.[10] The degree of morphologic damage was similar in both groups and included flattening of the plicae, extensive deciliation, and degeneration of secretory epithelial cells.

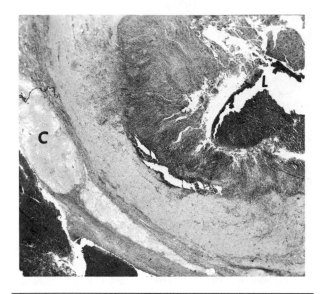

Figure 2-3
Tubo-ovarian abscess. The tubal lumen *(L)* exhibits loss of its lining epithelium and replacement by a densely cellular acute and chronic inflammatory infiltrate. The outer rim of ovary containing two corpora albicanta *(C)* is densely adherent to the fibrotic wall of the tube.

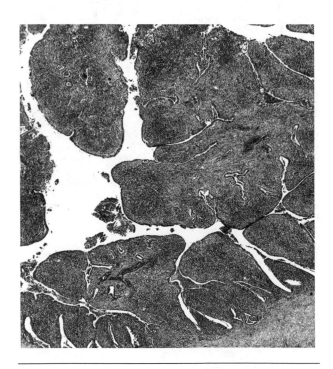

Figure 2-4
Chronic salpingitis. The tubal plicae are shortened, blunted, and swollen by a dense infiltrate of chronic inflammatory cells. Pinching off of interplical spaces to form pseudoglandular structures is seen in the lower left corner.

Ciliary beat frequency of the epithelial cells as measured by laser light–scattering spectroscopy was decreased significantly in both overt and silent PID.

So-called silent inflammation apparently may exist in grossly normal-appearing fallopian tubes.[11] Although a normal laparoscopic examination in an infertile patient is considered by some investigators to be sufficient evidence for normal tubal function, some of these women have had an ectopic pregnancy in spite of a previously "normal" laparoscopy. Thorough examination of total salpingectomy specimens from 8 of these patients showed low-grade salpingitis in areas away from the ectopic pregnancy. This finding suggests that grossly normal-appearing tubes at laparoscopy does not rule out the presence of significant microscopic disease, which may result in an ectopic pregnancy or "idiopathic" infertility.

Gross pathology

The only gross evidence of mild chronic salpingitis may be the presence of focal fibrous adhesions between the tube and ovary. In severe disease the tube may be enlarged and markedly distorted, with extensive adhesions to ovary and adjacent tissues. The ampulla may be converted into a blind sac if the fimbriae have coalesced with obliteration of the ostium; the purulent exudate may resolve, with transformation of a pyosalpinx into a hydrosalpinx. The latter is characterized by a thin, translucent wall, especially in the ampullary portion, a smooth, glistening external surface, which has a network of delicate vessels, and a content of clear fluid. Torsion followed by infarction occasionally occurs. Some authors[12] subclassify hydrosalpinx into simplex and follicularis types, depending on whether the tubal lumen is unilocular or multilocular. A tubo-ovarian abscess (Figure 2-3) may similarly resolve to form a tubo-ovarian cyst.

Microscopic pathology

In the resolving phase of acute salpingitis, the polymorphonuclear leukocytes in the plicae are replaced progressively by lymphocytes and plasma cells, which eventually predominate. Typically, the delicate complex arrangement of the mucosal folds is lost and they are replaced by shortened, blunted plicae, the stromal cores of which are fibrotic and contain chronic inflammatory cells (Figure 2-4). The epithelium lining the thickened plicae may be cuboidal or low columnar and inactive in appearance. Fibrous organization of the exudate that led to interadherence of plicae during one or more previous acute episodes has typically resulted in pinching off of rounded pseudoglandular spaces, or "follicles," which no longer communicate with the lumen (Figure 2-5). Occasionally the epithelium assumes a proliferative pseudopapillary pattern, pseudoglandular structures may penetrate the muscle layer, and mesothelial cells may become incorporated within the fibrotic tissue that has replaced

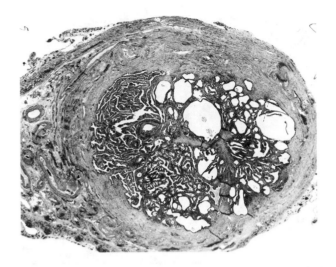

Figure 2-5
Chronic follicular salpingitis. The tubal lumen contains variably sized follicle-like spaces.

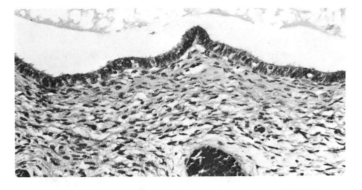

Figure 2-6
Hydrosalpinx, simple type. The lining epithelium consists of low columnar cells, some of which are ciliated. The wall is fibrous and the lumen contains a granular precipitate.

the serosa. These changes may lead to an erroneous diagnosis of adenocarcinoma, but the presence of severe, chronic inflammation and fibrosis and the absence of significant nuclear atypicality enable one to identify the cellular proliferation as reactive.

In the simple type of hydrosalpinx, the epithelium is usually low cuboidal to flattened, the wall is fibrous, and the plicae are generally few and small; some plicae, however, may be well preserved and lined by normal-appearing epithelium (Figure 2-6). In cases of hydrosalpinx follicularis, the architecture is that of follicular salpingitis, with the pseudoglandular structures distended with fluid (Figure 2-7).

GRANULOMATOUS SALPINGITIS
Tuberculosis

Granulomatous salpingitis may be secondary to a number of infectious and noninfectious agents. By far the most common cause is the tubercle bacillus, either *Mycobacterium tuberculosis* or *M. bovis*. Although tuberculous salpingitis is not a common cause of infertility in the United States, it accounts for a number of cases in less well-developed countries. In a study of patients with genital tuberculosis, the fallopian tubes were involved in 90% to 100% of the women.[13] The true frequency of tuberculous salpingitis in the United States is difficult to determine; earlier investigations based on histologic examination of excised adnexa indicated that it had been decreasing, probably as a result of antituberculous chemotherapy.[12] More recent workers have suggested, however, that tuberculous salpingitis may be diagnosed with increasing frequency in the future because of the influx of immigrants from developing countries.[14]

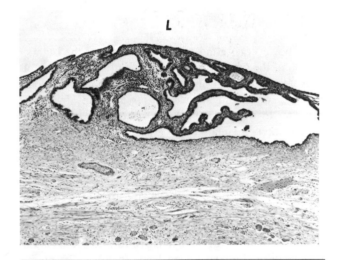

Figure 2-7
Hydrosalpinx, follicular type. The tubal lumen *(L)* is lined by a flattened mucosa composed of follicle-like spaces of variable size that form pseudoglandular structures.

Sexual transmission of the tubercle bacillus is rare and probably never results in tubal involvement. The most common route of tubal infection is blood stream dissemination from a primary focus, usually pulmonary. Hematogenous or lymphatic dissemination from a primary infection of the intestine or urinary bladder is relatively rare. Bilateral tubal involvement occurs in 90% of patients, resulting in a high probability of sterility.

Gross pathology

The gross appearance of tuberculous salpingitis depends on its severity. Early or mild infections may be manifested by irregular thickening or nodularity of the wall, sometimes simulating salpingitis isthmica nodosa. The

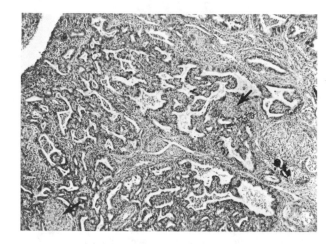

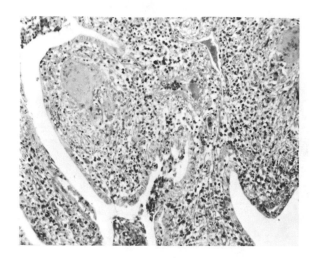

Figure 2-8
Tuberculous salpingitis. The plicae contain tubercles *(arrows)* with associated hyperplasia of the tubal epithelium simulating adenocarcinoma.

Figure 2-9
Tuberculous salpingitis. Tubercles are composed of multinucleated giant cells, lymphocytes, and histiocytes.

latter, however, is almost always confined to the isthmic portion of the tube, which is infrequently the sole site of tuberculous infection. Indeed, the severity of tuberculous involvement is said to increase progressively from the proximal to the distal portion of the tube.[15] Although some workers maintain that a grossly diseased tube with preservation of the fimbriae and an open ostium is highly suggestive of tuberculous salpingitis,[14] others reported that the ostia are obliterated in 50% to 85% of patients.[15,16] In the so-called adhesive form of tuberculous salpingitis, dense fibrous adhesions develop between the tube and ovary with destruction of the fimbriae and closure of the ostium. In the exudative form, accumulation of exudate within the lumen leads to tubal distention, simulating pyosalpinx.[12] Enlargement and saclike distention may impart a "tobacco-pouch" appearance. The recognition of caseous material within the lumen or studding of the serosal surface by tubercles may alert the surgeon or pathologist to the correct diagnosis, but the nature of the infection is frequently unsuspected by either on gross examination.

Microscopic pathology

The initial lesions are mucosal tubercles, which are aggregates of epithelioid histiocytes and multinucleated giant cells of the Langhans type (Figures 2-8 and 2-9). The former cells may predominate, with relatively few of the latter present. Careful investigation reveals caseation necrosis of some tubercles in most cases. Schaumann bodies, similar to those occurring in the granulomas of sarcoidosis, are often encountered in tuberculous granulomas as well. The inflammatory process spreads from the mucosa into the muscularis and serosa. Coalescence of tubercles and progressive caseation necrosis result in

mucosal destruction and rupture of caseous material into the lumen. The tubal epithelial cells may undergo marked hyperplasia, which in some cases mimics adenocarcinoma. The diagnosis of tuberculous salpingitis should be confirmed by the demonstration of acid-fast bacilli by appropriate stains or culture.

Actinomycosis

Actinomycosis of the fallopian tube is rare.[17] The causative organism is *Actinomyces israelii*, an anaerobic bacterium indigenous to the oral cavity and gastrointestinal tract. Infection may occur as a complication of gastrointestinal actinomycosis or after instrumentation of the uterus, including insertion of an intrauterine contraceptive device and therapeutic abortion.[18]

Gross pathology

According to one investigation,[19] actinomycosis of the genital tract is most frequent in the adnexa; approximately 4% of the infections are bilateral, 38% right-sided, and 18% left-sided. The tube may be simply enlarged, without obvious signs of inflammatory disease, or may exhibit the usual manifestations of PID, including the formation of numerous tubo-ovarian adhesions and a tubo-ovarian abscess. Sectioning of the inflammatory mass reveals replacement of the tube or the tube and ovary by a cavity with a shaggy lining and a content of purulent material. Examination of the pus may reveal characteristic small yellow flecks, sulfur granules, which are colonies of actinomyces. Fistulas invading the bowel, bladder, or skin may form.

Microscopic pathology

Microscopic examination reveals characteristic colonies that correspond to the sulfur granules within the abscesses

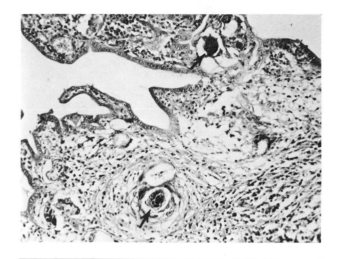

Figure 2-10
Schistosomiasis. The tubal plicae contain several ova *(arrows)* of *S. hematobium*. The ova have induced a reactive fibrosis, and a chronic inflammatory infiltrate is present within the connective tissue cores of the plicae.

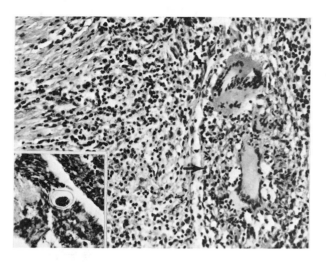

Figure 2-11
Enterobius vermicularis infection. A pseudotubercle *(arrow)* contains multinucleated giant cells, histiocytes, and chronic inflammatory cells. *(Inset)* An ovum is surrounded by necrotic debris.

or in their walls. The granules may be composed of one mycelial colony or several that have coalesced. The central portion is a dense amorphous tangle of fibrils; at the periphery, the filaments are less dense and radiate outward. Some of the filaments have club-shaped ends. The organisms are typically gram positive and nonacid fast.[20] Numerous lymphocytes, plasma cells, and histiocytes, some of which may form epithelioid aggregates, are present within the wall of the abscess cavity. Caseation necrosis is not seen. Long-standing inflammation may be associated with granulation tissue formation and fibrosis of the wall.

Schistosomiasis

Tubal schistosomiasis (bilharziasis) is common in some parts of the world but rare in the United States. In Africa and the Near East, the disease is endemic, with *Schistosoma haematobium* being the usual infective organism. In an autopsy study, approximately one of five African women had tubal schistosomiasis,[21] and genital involvement was demonstrated in every case of schistosomiasis because of *S. haematobium* in African women.[22] In contrast to *S. japonicum* and *S. mansoni,* the other schistosomes that infect humans, *S. haematobium* typically migrates to the venous plexuses of the pelvis and urinary bladder and therefore is the agent most commonly responsible for genital and tubal disease. *S. mansoni* and *S. japonicum* rarely involve the female genital tract.

Pathology

The gross findings in tubal schistosomiasis may be unimpressive, or the wall may be scarred or nodular since the deposition of ova results in fibrosis. A granulomatous

reaction is induced by the ova, which are deposited in the lumina of veins. The venous walls are destroyed by enzymatic digestion, with extravasation of the ova. The granulomas may simulate those of tuberculosis, containing multinucleated giant cells, epithelioid histiocytes, and chronic inflammatory cells (Figure 2-10). It has been stated that an ovum, or at least a portion of one, is almost always identifiable within a schistosomal granuloma if serial sections are made.[23] The ova of each of the three species of schistosomes differ in size and structure, permitting their specific identification.

Oxyuriasis

Oxyuris *(Enterobius vermicularis)* infection of the fallopian tube is probably secondary to migration of the pinworm from the lower genital tract.

Pathology

The tube may be focally nodular because the worm has become embedded in the wall and both it and its ova have elicited fibrosis[24]; seeding of the pelvic peritoneum by ova may result in lesions that simulate tubercles. Occasionally, a severe inflammatory reaction results in a tubo-ovarian abscess. Microscopic examination of the nodular areas reveals fragments of the worm or its ova in varying degrees of preservation surrounded by necrotic debris (Figure 2-11). The ova measure approximately 55×25 μm and are flattened along one side. The cellular infiltrate may include large numbers of eosinophils, and occasionally Charcot-Leyden crystals are found. Foreign body giant cells may be present, but Langhans' giant cells are characteristically absent. The necrotic tissue is surrounded by granulation tissue and fibrous tissue. The

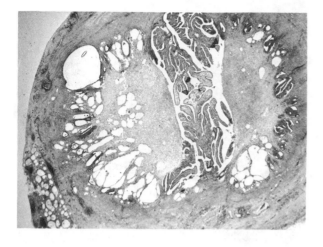

Figure 2-12
Salpingitis resulting from foreign material. The lumen shows marked narrowing by a granulomatous reaction to an oily contrast medium (*clear spaces*). Serosal involvement is seen in the lower left corner.

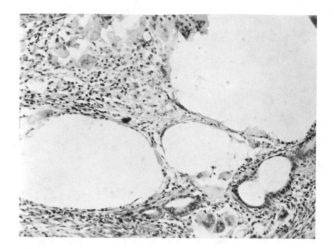

Figure 2-13
Higher magnification of Figure 2-12 shows foreign body giant cells surrounding the droplets of contrast medium. The spaces are clear due to loss of lipid during histologic processing.

granulomas have been designated pseudotubercles because of their resemblance to true tubercles.

Salpingitis resulting from foreign material

Salpingitis may be secondary to a variety of irritative agents introduced into the genital tract, including lubricant jellies used for vaginal examinations, mineral oil applied on cervical dilators, and powder containing talc or starch[12,25,26]; contrast media used in the radiographic investigation of infertility, especially media with a viscous oil base, have also been implicated. Although salpingitis secondary to contrast media has been said to impair fertility, some investigators have questioned the validity of this conclusion, since the tubal epithelium in some cases appears unaltered on microscopic examination, and some patients who have had these studies subsequently conceived.[27]

Gross pathology

Gross examination of a tube inflamed as a result of introduction of foreign material may reveal yellow discoloration or a chocolate-brown appearance of the mucosa, suggesting endometriosis. The peritoneal surface of the tube may have a similar appearance, giving rise to the erroneous diagnosis of endometriosis.

Microscopic pathology

Numerous foamy histiocytes may accumulate in the tubal mucosa in response to the introduction of oil-based contrast media or their vehicles; the contrast media may elicit a foreign body giant cell reaction, which involves not only the tubal lumen but also the serosa (Figures 2-12 and 2-13). One group designated this lesion lipoid sal-

pingitis but regarded it as nonspecific, having encountered it in patients who had no history of hysterosalpingography; in these cases the lesion was suspected of being postinfectious.[27] Rubin[28] also reported the occasional presence of "lipoidal granulomas" in women with gonococcal and tuberculous salpingitis. In one of these patients, a single intracellular acid-fast bacillus was found on serial sections, and she returned 2 years later with cavitary pulmonary tuberculosis. Consequently, thorough investigation of lesions with the histologic picture of lipoid salpingitis should be undertaken to rule out tuberculosis and other infectious causes.

OTHER FORMS OF GRANULOMATOUS SALPINGITIS

Sarcoidosis and Crohn's disease[25] have been reported rarely as causes of granulomatous salpingitis. Tubal involvement in the former occurs as part of a systemic disease and in the latter more commonly as a result of proximity of the tube to an involved segment of intestine.

Salpingitis isthmica nodosa

The term *salpingitis isthmica nodosa* (SIN) refers to unilateral or bilateral nodular thickening of the isthmic portion of the tube, in which diverticula lined by tubal epithelium penetrate into the muscle layer. Although SIN has been reported rarely in postmenopausal women, it is almost always encountered in women of reproductive age. In a large combined retrospective and prospective study of this disorder in patients with and without tubal pregnancy, the mean age at the time of diagnosis was 26 years.[29] In a more recent study of approximately 600

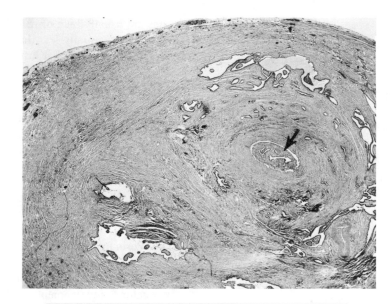

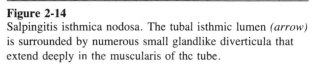

Figure 2-14
Salpingitis isthmica nodosa. The tubal isthmic lumen *(arrow)*
is surrounded by numerous small glandlike diverticula that
extend deeply in the muscularis of the tube.

ectopic pregnancies, 6% were associated with some degree of tubal diverticula,[30] the most florid examples of which were associated with isthmic nodularity and periglandular myohypertrophy, the features associated with typical salpingitis isthmica nodosa. These workers suggested that tubal diverticula may form a spectrum of histopathologic appearances, varying greatly in their number, distribution, depth of mural extension, and association with periglandular myohypertrophy. The number of diverticula varied from less than 10 in 40% of patients to more than 100 in 10%; in most of the latter group, myohypertrophy and isthmic nodularity (so-called SIN) was present. Since all the cases were associated with an ectopic pregnancy, however, even a few diverticula may be a risk factor for ectopic pregnancy or infertility. One third of ectopic pregnancies associated with diverticula were complicated by tubal rupture. It is probable that the fertilized ovum was carried through a diverticulum to an intramural location where implantation occurred.

In a study of obstructive SIN, the tubal lumen was narrowed in all women and was unidentifiable by endoscopy in one third of them.[31] The finding of at least mild chronic inflammation in all patients led these workers to conclude that SIN may result from an acute inflammatory irritant leading to tubal spasm and muscular hypertrophy. Almost one half of these patients had high titers of serum antibodies to *Chlamydia*. Ultrastructural studies by these authors showed that the intramural glandlike structures were lined by cells similar to those of fallopian tube epithelium.

To our knowledge, SIN has not been described in infants and young children, but bilateral involvement was reported in a 12-year-old postmenarchal girl, who also had clear-cell carcinoma of the endocervix, benign glandular inclusions in pelvic lymph nodes, and endosalpingiosis; her clinical history was suspicious for intrauterine drug exposure.[32] The authors speculated that the various proliferative lesions were secondary to a developmental defect induced by a teratogenic agent. Other investigators[33] postulated a developmental background for SIN in older patients, since ipsilateral uterine adenomyosis frequently accompanies unilateral disease. The finding of uterine adenomyosis in association with SIN has led some authors to argue that the latter is a tubal analog of the former. Additional evidence for this viewpoint is the occasional presence of stroma of endometrial type around the epithelial elements of SIN.

Gross pathology

As the name implies, the isthmus is occupied by one to several nodules varying in size from barely perceptible to 2 cm in diameter. The adjacent uterine cornu may be involved as well. The sectioned surfaces of the nodules are firm and rubbery, suggesting hypertrophied muscle; recognition of glandular elements within the nodules depends on their quantity and the extent of dilatation.

Microscopic pathology

Microscopic examination reveals a nodule or nodules of smooth muscle containing glandlike structures that are irregularly dispersed in the tubal wall (Figure 2-14). Se-

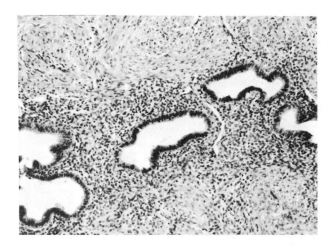

Figure 2-15
Serosal endometriosis. Endometrial-type glands are surrounded by condensed endometrial stroma.

rial sectioning has disclosed communication of the lumina of the "glands" with the lumen of the tube. Most of the nodularity is due to hyperplasia of smooth muscle, which is most prominent in the immediate vicinity of the glands. The "glandular" epithelium simulates that of the tube, being low columnar to cuboidal and containing occasional ciliated cells. Despite the inflammatory causation implied by the term *SIN,* significant numbers of acute or chronic inflammatory cells are absent, and granulation tissue and fibrosis, frequent concomitants of other types of salpingitis, are seen only rarely. Although unilateral SIN may be accompanied by acute and chronic salpingitis of infectious origin and its sequelae, the infection often spares the tube involved by SIN, reinforcing the conclusion that the two disorders are unrelated.

ENDOMETRIOSIS
Endometriosis

Infertility is reported to be present in at least one third of patients with endometriosis, as a result of a variety of mechanisms, one of which is tubal involvement by the disease.[34] Some have suggested that endometriotic foci within the tube or ovary may initiate an inflammatory response that impedes tubal function.[35] Others, however, have claimed that no relationship exists between tubal inflammation and endometriosis.[36] Endometriosis of the tube is divided into two categories: disease with predominant serosal involvement and disease that affects primarily the mucosa.

Serosal endometriosis
Gross pathology

The gross appearance of serosal endometriosis varies depending on its degree of activity and chronicity. Active lesions are usually blue or red and may appear as small spots or cysts, usually less than 0.5 cm in diameter, on the serosal surface; similar lesions may be present on the surface of the ovary. Chronic endometriosis is characterized by fibrosis and often dense adhesions to the ovary and surrounding tissues. The tube may be greatly distorted and kinked, with impairment of its motility. Older endometriotic cysts may contain thick, dark brown blood similar to that found within chocolate cysts of the ovary.

Microscopic pathology

In the typical example of an active lesion, endometrial-type glands are surrounded by endometrial stroma containing small, thin-walled blood vessels (Figure 2-15). Hemosiderin from past episodes of bleeding may be present within and around the lesion. The process is found most commonly in the serosa, and, according to one investigator,[37] involvement of the muscle layer is unusual. Older lesions are characterized by scarring and the deposition of blood pigment in histiocytes; residual glands of the endometrial type may be present within the scar tissue.

Endometrial polyps and ectopic endometrium of the tubal mucosa

Some authors classify endometrial polyps and ectopic endometrium in the tubal mucosa (mucosal endometriosis) as distinct from tubal endometriosis of the serosal type, and the former lesions have been the subject of separate investigations. The frequency of tubal endometrial polyps (TEP) is difficult to determine, since many of the series of cases in the literature are based on radiographic studies of women investigated for infertility, and some of these reports are not documented or are only incompletely documented pathologically. In two large hysterosalpingographic studies of TEP,[38,39] the frequency ranged from 1.2% to 2.5%; in a histopathologic study of 300 hysterectomy specimens, these lesions were found in the interstitial portion of the tube in 11%.

The association of polyps with infertility is controversial. Although they are usually discovered in the course of an infertility study, some patients have conceived despite their presence.[39,40] In one report, the mean duration of infertility appeared to become longer with increasing size of the polyps, although excision in patients with larger polyps did not result in subsequent pregnancy.[41] Some polyps have obstructed the tubal lumen partially or completely, but this complication is rare.[38,42]

Some investigators[43] believe that endometrial polyps of the tube arise from isolated foci of endometrium that are occasionally present in the interstitial portion of the tube. In one study,[38] endometrial mucosa was found in the interstitial segment either completely or partially lining the lumen in about 25% of 300 hysterectomy specimens. Endometrial mucosa may be seen occasionally in the extrauterine portion of the tube as well.[44] The involvement is usually unilateral. Although some investigators believe that ectopic endometrial mucosa in the tube does not affect fertility, it was suggested that it may obstruct the lumen of the interstitial portion of the tube.[45] This conclusion was supported by disappearance of the obstruction as demonstrated by hysterosalpingographic examination with subsequent conception in two of five patients after treatment with danazol.

Serosal endometriosis may accompany both ectopic tubal endometrium and TEP. In two studies,[40,41] pelvic endometriosis was found in approximately 40% of women with TEP, although other studies indicated no increase in the frequency of extrauterine endometriosis in these patients.[38,43]

Gross pathology

Because of their small size, TEPs are rarely recognized on gross examination, although they may be associated with slight distention of the lumen of the interstitial segment on section. In both hysterosalpingographic and pathologic studies, these lesions have ranged from 0.1 to 1.3 cm in length and 0.3 to 0.4 cm in width. They generally have a smooth outline with a free, rounded surface pointed toward the fimbriated end. Attachment to the tubal wall is commonly by a broad sessile base. The polyps are typically pale and resemble the surrounding mucosa, except that their tips are sometimes red. They are primarily single and unilateral, but in one study, two polyps were found in one tube, and in one woman both tubes contained two polyps.[40] Some investigators reported bilateral polyps in infertile women.[46,41]

Microscopic pathology

Tubal endometrial polyps are composed of mucosa of the endometrial type (Figure 2-16). In most cases, the endometrial tissue is nonfunctioning, but occasionally secretory and decidual changes are seen; in postmenopausal women senile atrophy may be observed.

BENIGN NEOPLASMS

Benign neoplasms of the fallopian tube are rare. As in other sites in the female genital tract, the tumors may be of epithelial, mesothelial, mesenchymal, mixed, or rarely, other origins.

Epithelial tumors

Only a few examples of adenomas or papillomas have been reported[47,48]; one of them, the metaplastic papillary lesion, has been encountered almost exclusively during the last trimester of pregnancy.[49] Papillomas, which are incidental microscopic findings in most cases, consist of thin, delicately branching papillae with fibrovascular stromal cores and a nonciliated, columnar epithelial lin-

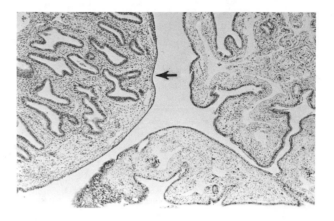

Figure 2-16
Tubal endometrial polyp (mucosal endometriosis) *(arrow)* protruding into the lumen. Endometrial-type glands are present within the polyp. Tubal plicae are present at right and below.

ing.[25,47,48] The metaplastic papillary lesion resembles an ovarian serous papillary tumor of borderline malignancy, except that most of its cells have abundant eosinophilic cytoplasm; some of them may contain mucin. It is debatable whether or not this lesion is neoplastic, but peritoneal implants have not been reported and follow-up information to date has disclosed no evidence of recurrence after removal.

Adenomatoid tumor

Adenomatoid tumors are the most common benign neoplasms of the fallopian tube, which, after the uterus, is the most frequent site of their occurrence. At least one reported example was associated with an ectopic pregnancy,[50] in which case the neoplasm was near the uterus, proximal to the implantation site, a location similar to that of other benign tumors associated with ectopic pregnancy.

Adenomatoid tumors, which are usually incidental findings at surgery, rarely exceed 1 to 2 cm in diameter. They are nodular and well circumscribed, and their sectioned surfaces are gray to yellow and firm. Transmural involvement of the tube is common and the tumor may bulge into the lumen, narrowing it (Figure 2-17).

Microscopic examination reveals a tumor in the muscle layer and serosa characterized by small clusters of vacuolated cells as well as small, cleftlike or oval spaces lined by low cuboidal to flattened cells; the spaces contain slightly basophilic fluid; smooth muscle may be a prominent component, and aggregates of lymphocytes may also be present (Figure 2-18). The cellularity of the lesion may lead to an erroneous diagnosis of low-grade carcinoma, but the bland nuclei and rarity of mitotic figures are diagnostic of its benign nature. The tumor may grow

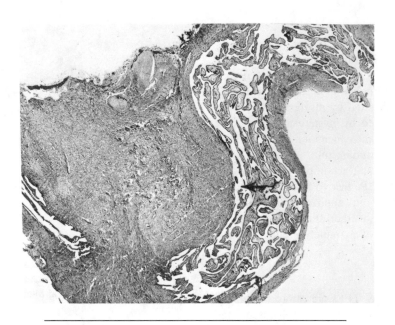

Figure 2-17
Adenomatoid tumor bulges into and distorts the tubal lumen
(arrow).

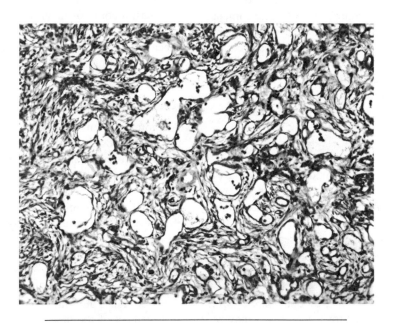

Figure 2-18
Adenomatoid tumor. Small oval to cleftlike spaces are lined
by flattened cells.

into the stromal cores of the plicae, but spares the overlying epithelium. In some cases, continuity between the
cells lining the spaces and the overlying mesothelium has
been observed.[51] Special stains for glycogen usually show
no appreciable amounts, but mucin and hyaluronic acid
have been demonstrated both within the tumor cells and
the gland lumina. These observations favor a mesothelial
origin of the tumor, as does the presence of desmosomes,
tonofilaments, and microvilli on ultrastructural examination.[52]

Soft tissue tumors

Although benign soft tissue tumors of the fallopian tube are rare, they are more common than benign epithelial tumors, and include leiomyomas, fibromas, hemangiomas,[52-54] and very rare lymphangiomas, lipomas, and ganglioneuromas.[55-57]

Leiomyomas are unexpectedly infrequent in the tube in view of the common origin and continuity of the uterine and tubal musculature. Most tubal leiomyomas are asymptomatic. Rare examples have been associated with tubal pregnancy; in one case an ectopic pregnancy was accompanied by a 3-cm tubal leiomyoma that obstructed the lumen more proximally.[58] Tubal leiomyomas are usually single and small, although one weighed 13 kg and was 56 cm in diameter, and another weighed 2 kg.[59,60] As in the uterus, these tumors may be intramural, submucosal, or subserosal, sometimes hanging by a thin pedicle.

Most of them arise in the proximal portion of the tube and only rarely has the distal portion, particularly the infundibulum and fimbriated end, been involved. Early workers emphasized the propensity for a location in the interstitial segment of the tube,[61] but the distinction between a myometrial and a tubal origin is difficult at this site. Microscopic examination reveals findings similar to those of leiomyomas at other locations, with interlacing bundles of eosinophilic, spindle-shaped cells containing cigar-shaped nuclei. Tubal leiomyomas may exhibit hyaline and other degenerative changes similar to those seen in uterine leiomyomas.

Adenofibromas

Several papillary adenofibromas of the tube have been reported. They may occur in any portion of the organ, but in at least three reports they were at the fimbriated end.[32,62,63] In one patient the tumors were bilateral; two successful pregnancies followed their removal.[32] On gross examination, the tube may appear swollen. Sectioning discloses a soft, spongy, cystic mass obliterating the lumen. The tumor usually contains clear fluid, and the cyst lining exhibits numerous small excrescences. Microscopic examination reveals numerous small papillae that are composed of dense fibromatous tissue, which often resembles an ovarian fibroma, and a lining of cuboidal to low columnar epithelium, which typically contains numerous ciliated cells (Figure 2-19).

Other Benign Tumors

Other benign neoplasms include dermoid cysts and mature solid teratomas.[48,64,65] The former are usually small and appear within the lumen of the distal portion attached to the mucosa by a thin pedicle. In an early review of the literature, Aaron[66] reported that approximately 45% of patients with a tubal dermoid cyst were sterile. These lesions have also been reported in association with ec-

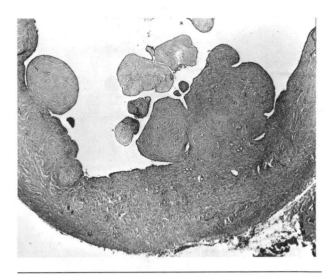

Figure 2-19
Adenofibroma. Blunt papillary, fibromatous excrescences project into the tubal lumen.

topic pregnancy.[67] On pathologic examination, dermoid cysts of the tube are similar to those found elsewhere and contain several mature tissues, which usually represent all three embryonic layers.

ENDOSALPINGIOSIS

The term *endosalpingiosis,* coined by Sampson in 1930, is the currently accepted designation for the presence of tubal-type epithelium in extramucosal locations in the female genital tract and elsewhere in the abdomen. The lesions of endosalpingiosis may occur in the muscular and serosal layers of the tubes, in the ovaries, uterus, and omentum, and on peritoneal surfaces elsewhere in the pelvis. On gross examination, they may appear as cysts that are usually less than 0.5 cm in diameter and contain clear fluid. Microscopic examination discloses small, rounded, glandlike inclusions lined by epithelium resembling that of the fallopian tube (Figures 2-20 and 2-21). All the cell types of the tube may be present, with ciliated cells a prominent feature. Occasionally, the epithelium is thrown into complex papillary projections. The nuclei appear bland, and mitotic figures are almost never seen.

All 16 patients with omental endosalpingiosis in one series had tubal inflammatory disease, leading these authors to postulate tubal epithelial sloughing secondary to inflammation as the most probable cause.[68] In support of this premise, seven of the patients had a diagnosis of primary or secondary infertility and had undergone tubal lavage, another factor that may have resulted in omental implantation of tubal tissue. Two other associations of endosalpingiosis, however, suggest in situ metaplasia of

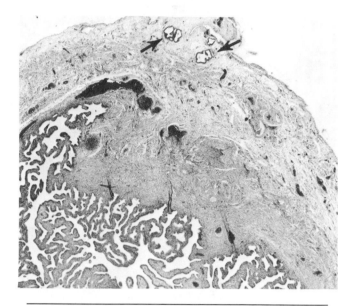

Figure 2-20
Endosalpingiosis. Small, rounded, glandlike structures *(arrows)* are present in the tubal serosa.

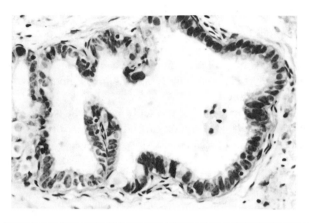

Figure 2-21
Endosalpingiosis. Low columnar, tubal-type epithelium lines the glandlike structures.

mesothelium as a mechanism of development of this lesion: the occasional transitions that are observed between endosalpingiosis and endometriosis, which would be difficult to explain on the basis of implantation; and the common association of endosalpingiosis with serous borderline tumors of the ovary, which some observers believe reflects a field change in the pelvic mesothelium. An alternative explanation of some examples of the latter association is maturation of implants of the ovarian neoplasm.

In the original report of Sampson,[69] the term *postsalpingectomy endosalpingiosis* was used to designate an outgrowth of tubal epithelium into the operative site after salpingectomy or tubal sterilization. Examination of 147 tubal stumps or residual portions of tube from 100 patients revealed this process in 112. Occasionally, the tubal sprouts extended into the surrounding tissues, including the ovary, intestinal tract, and abdominal wall. The cornua from 100 hysterectomy specimens that had not been subjected to prior tubal operations were examined as controls, and only 16 of them showed a similar phenomenon. Two of the patients in Sampson's series had an ectopic pregnancy in the tubal stump.

Observation of the relationship of endosalpingiosis to ectopic pregnancy after laparoscopic tubal coagulation revealed that electrocoagulation of the proximal portion of the tube activated the epithelium, resulting in endosalpingiosis of the muscle layer of the tube or the uterine cornu.[70] In some cases, the tubal epithelium penetrated through the serosa with the formation of tuboperitoneal or uteroperitoneal fistulas. It is possible that such fistulas allow the egress of sperm into the peritoneal cavity, where a recently discharged ovum could be fertilized and implant on the omentum or within the ampulla. The activated endosalpinx assumed several forms, including a tubal type that resembled SIN except for an absence of muscle proliferation, an endometrial type similar to adenomyosis, or a combination of the two. Dye injection studies showed that the glands connected with the tubal lumen. Coagulation of more distal segments of the tube usually resulted in fibrosis without activation of the epithelium.

CONGENITAL ANOMALIES

Much of our knowledge concerning congenital anomalies of the fallopian tube has been engendered by the advent of gynecologic microsurgery and its emphasis during the 1970s.[71] Consequently, more attention has been devoted to them in the gynecology, rather than the pathology, literature. In one study concerning the microsurgical reconstruction of the tube affected by such anomalies,[71] the cases included (1) elongation of the fimbria ovarica, (2) accessory tubal ostia, and (3) enlarged paratubal cysts (see p. 2-17). Of these, approximately two thirds were represented by elongation of the fimbria ovarica. This condition was defined as unilateral or bilateral elongation of the ovarian-fimbrial attachment, with the tubal ostium being situated more than 4 cm from its fimbriated attachment to the ovary. Accessory tubal ostia were less common (28%); those occurring within 1 cm of the primary ostium were designated as terminal types and those in the middle or distal ampulla, more than 1 cm from the primary ostium, were designated as ampullary types. All have been found exclusively on the antimesenteric border of the tube and some have been bilateral.

Other congenital malformations of the tube, including unilateral absence, atresia of the lumen, absence of various segments,[72] duplication, and multiple lumina, may be discovered in the investigation of women with infertility. These anomalies may be associated with other malformations of the urogenital tract. Probably the most frequent congenital anomaly of significance is the absence of derivatives of one müllerian duct, that is, one tube and the ipsilateral uterine horn; this condition is often associated with absence of the ipsilateral kidney.

Atresia of the tubal lumen occurs most often in the isthmus.[37] Although the myosalpinx appears normal, the tubal epithelium is absent. The midportion of one tube in a 26-year-old woman was represented by concentrically arranged fibromuscular tissue without a lumen.[73] Small disorganized portions of a lumen were present in the segment immediately proximal to the defect. More proximal and distal portions of the tube appeared normal, but there was no contralateral tube, ovary, or broad ligament. In another case report, a bicornuate uterus with one rudimentary noncanalized horn was associated with an ipsilateral, partially atretic tube.[74]

Tubal duplications have been described. An operation for an ectopic pregnancy in a 22-year-old woman disclosed duplication of the left tube associated with a single uterus and single right tube.[75] The left tubes were separated at the fimbriated ends by a peritoneal fold but joined before entering the cornu; both of them were patent. Accessory tubes may be more common than generally appreciated; in one report, they were removed over a 2-year period from 14 patients undergoing various elective gynecologic procedures for reasons unrelated to the accessory tubes.[76] All of them were attached to the ampullary portion of the normal tube and ranged in length from 1.5 to 3 cm. They were cylindric and were composed of fibromuscular tissue without a lumen; their distal portions terminated in fimbriated ends containing ciliated cells. Other investigators, however, noted that some accessory tubes have lumina (Scully RE and Lawrence WD, personal observations, 1990). The accessory fimbriae could contribute to infertility by capturing ova and preventing their entry into the main tube and the uterine cavity, resulting in an ectopic pregnancy. Multiple lumina of the tube have also been described.[12] Since multiple infoldings of the tubal lumen occur during embryogenesis, persistence of more than one of them could explain these anomalies.

Another rare anomaly that has been described in infertile women is the convoluted fallopian tube. Fourteen cases were encountered in a series of 83 tuboplasty procedures.[77] Histologic study revealed muscular hypoplasia, leading the author to hypothesize poor peristalsis as a factor contributing to infertility. Ten patients with convoluted fallopian tubes had been included in the category of idiopathic infertility, with patent tubes by hysterosalpingography.[78] In surgery, the fimbriae and ovarian ligaments were measured and retrograde insufflation was carried out. Eight patients had elongated accessory ligaments of the ovaries and tubes, six had increased convolutions of the tube beneath a laterally shortened and scarred broad ligament, and two had accessory fimbriae. Retrograde insufflation revealed dilated areas within the tubes that were apparently devoid of muscle.

The potential importance of alterations in normal cilia in ovum transport is emphasized by two studies. In one investigation, an infertile patient with Kartagener's syndrome was shown by ultrastructural studies to have microtubular defects in both respiratory and tubal cilia.[79] In the other, transmission electron microscopy showed an identical appearance of cilia in both the respiratory and reproductive tracts of an infertile woman with Kartagener's syndrome; cilia were immotile in both tracts as well.[80] These workers concluded that the infertility of patients with Kartagener's syndrome is explained by the dyskinetic motion of tubal cilia, and that normal ciliation of the endosalpinx is essential for reproduction.

In contrast, ultrastructural and morphometric studies on endosalpingeal biopsy specimens from both fertile and infertile women revealed no relation between the percentage of ciliated cells and fertility.[81] Although the authors stated that normal ciliation does not appear to be essential for reproductive success, their studies were carried out with a scanning electron microscope rather than with a transmission electron microscope. Accordingly, study of the surface ultrastructure would not have identified internal abnormalities such as the aforementioned microtubular defect. Furthermore, one cannot infer normal ciliary activity from the study of static scanning electron micrographs.

Paratubal cysts

The most common paratubal cyst is the hydatid of Morgagni, which typically appears as one or more cysts hanging by a thin pedicle or pedicles from the fimbriated end of the tube. Although hydatids are usually less than 1 cm in diameter, rare examples grow to a considerable size and may undergo torsion. The cysts are thin walled and contain clear serous fluid (Figure 2-22). They are lined by pseudostratified columnar epithelium. Ciliated cells are present, and, according to one report,[82] the nonciliated cells may show cyclic changes; infoldings resembling those of the normal tube occasionally are observed.

Infertile women who had large, cystically dilated paratubal cysts (of wolffian origin) accounted for the minority of patients with infertility and congenital anomalies.[71] Such cysts grossly distorted the mesosalpinx and displaced the tubal ostium away from the ipsilateral ovary.

Despite the almost invariable presence of mesonephric rests adjacent to the tubes, mesonephric cysts are less

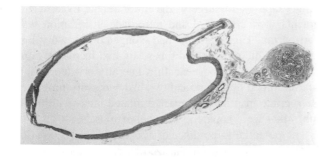

Figure 2-22
Paratubal cyst. The wall is fibrotic and the lumen is distended by fluid. No communication with the tubal lumen is present.

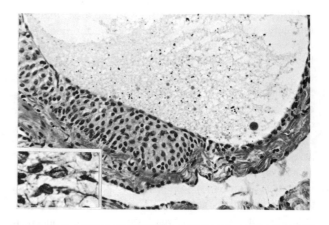

Figure 2-23
A cystic Walthard nest is partially lined by a transitional-type epithelium that flattens to a single layer in one area. *(Inset)* Characteristic coffee-bean appearance of nuclei in a Walthard nest.

common than those of müllerian origin. No mesonephric cysts measured greater than 3 cm in diameter in a study of parovarian tumors.[83] On microscopic examination, the cyst lining is a single layer of low columnar to cuboidal cells with a paucity or absence of ciliated cells; smooth muscle may form a prominent component of the wall.[25]

Walthard nests

On gross inspection of the tubal serosa, Walthard nests appear as cystic or solid yellow-tan nodules, usually 0.1 to 0.2 cm in diameter. They are sometimes misinterpreted as tubercles or other granulomas, particularly when they are numerous.[84] Rarely, these lesions are seen in the ovary or elsewhere on the pelvic peritoneum.

On microscopic examination, the cells forming the nests resemble those of transitional epithelium; their nuclei are ovoid and contain single longitudinal grooves, creating a coffee-bean appearance. The nests may be solid or cystic; the cysts are lined by stratified or single, flattened cells, and their lumina contain granular eosinophilic precipitate (Figure 2-23). The innermost portion of the lining epithelium may be composed of mucinous epithelial cells.[85] Walthard nests apparently arise by metaplasia from the mesothelial covering of the tube. They have no clinical significance.

REFERENCES

1. Chow AW et al: The bacteriology of acute pelvic inflammatory disease, *Am J Obstet Gynecol*, 122(7):876-879, 1975.
2. Thadapalli H, Gorbach SL, and Keith L: Anaerobic infections of the female genital tract: bacteriologic and therapeutic aspects, *Am J Obstet Gynecol* 117:1034-1040, 1973.
3. Thompson SE III et al: The microbiology and therapy of acute pelvic inflammatory disease in hospitalized patients, *Am J Obstet Gynecol* 136:179-186, 1980.
4. Barton IG et al: Isolation and characterization of two strains of herpesvirus hominis type I from fallopian tubes, *J Med Microbiol* 15(1):63-71, 1982.
5. Marana R et al: High prevalence of silent chlamydia colonization of the tubal mucosa in infertile women, *J Fertil Stertil* 88(1):295-305, 1990.
6. Shepard MK and Jones RB: Recovery of *Chlamydia trachomatis* from endometrial and fallopian tube biopsies in women with infertility of tubal origin, *Fertil Steril* 52(2):232-238, 1989.
7. Tuffrey M et al: Correlation of infertility with altered tubal morphology and function in mice with salpingitis induced by a human genital-tract isolate of *Chlamydia trachomatis, J Reprod Fertil* 88(1):295-305, 1990.
8. Anestad G et al: Infertility and chlamydial infection, *Fertil Steril* 46(3):412-416, 1986.
9. Collet M et al: Infertility in central Africa: infection is the cause, *Int J Gynaecol Obstet* 26(3):423-428, 1988.
10. Patton DL et al: A comparison of the fallopian tube's response to overt and silent salpingitis, *Obstet Gynecol* 73(4):622-630, 1989.
11. Cumming DC et al: Microscopic evidence of silent inflammation in grossly normal fallopian tubes with ectopic pregnancy, *Int J Fertil* 33:(5):324-328, 1988.
12. Woodruff JD and Pauerstein CJ: *The fallopian tube: structure, function, pathology, and management,* Baltimore, 1969, Williams & Wilkins.
13. Schaefer G: Tuberculosis of the female genital tract, *Clin Obstet Gynecol* 13:965-998, 1970.
14. Bateman BG et al: Genital tuberculosis in reproductive-age women: a report of two cases, *J Reprod Med* 31(4):287-290, 1986.
15. Hall JE: *Applied gynecologic pathology,* New York, 1963, Appleton-Century-Crofts.
16. Jedberg H: A study on genital tuberculosis in women, *Acta Obstet Gynecol Scand* 31(suppl 1):1-176, 1950.
17. Braby HH, Dougherty CM, and Mickal A: Actinomycosis of the female genital tract, *Obstet Gynecol* 23:580-583, 1964.
18. Dische FE et al: Tubo-ovarian actinomycosis associated with intrauterine contraceptive devices, *J Obstet Gynaecol Br Commonw* 81:724-729, 1974.
19. Paalman RJ, Dockerty MB, and Mussey RD: Actinomycosis of ovaries and fallopian tubes, *Am J Obstet Gynecol* 58:419-431, 1949.
20. Dowell VR Jr and Sonnenwirth AC: Gram-positive, anaerobic, non-spore-forming bacilli. In Jarett L and Sonnenwirth AC (eds): *Gradwohl's clinical laboratory methods and diagnosis,* vol. 2, St. Louis, 1980, The CV Mosby Co.
21. Frost O: Bilharzia of the fallopian tube, *S Afr Med J* 49(30):1201-1203, 1975.

22. Gelfand M et al: Distribution and extent of schistosomiasis in female pelvic organs with special reference to the genital tract, as determined at autopsy, *Am J Trop Med Hyg* 20:846-849, 1971.

23. Arean VM: Manson's schistosomiasis of the female genital tract, *Am J Obstet Gynecol* 72:1038-1053, 1956.

24. Symmers WS: Pathology of oxyuriasis, *Arch Pathol* 50:475-516, 1950.

25. Wheeler JE: Pathology of the fallopian tube. In Kurman RJ (ed): *Blaustein's pathology of the female genital tract,* ed 3, New York, 1987, Springer-Verlag.

26. Campbell JS et al: Mineral oil granulomas of the uterus and parametrium and granulomatous salpingitis with Schaumann bodies and oxalate deposits, *Fertil Steril* 15:278-289, 1964.

27. Elliott GB, Brody H, and Elliott KA: Implications of "lipoid salpingitis," *Fertil Steril* 16:541-548, 1965.

28. Rubin IC: Lipoidal granuloma in fallopian tubes localized by intrauterine diodrast injection, with special reference to the value of follow-up x-ray films, *Radiology* 33:350-353, 1939.

29. Majmudar B, Henderson PH III, and Semple E: Salpingitis isthmica nodosa: a high-risk factor for tubal pregnancy, *Obstet Gynecol* 62(1):73-78, 1983.

30. Lawrence WD, Ramirez N, and Ginsburg KA: Tubal diverticula associated with ectopic pregnancy. A clinicopathologic analysis of 38 cases, *Lab Invest* 60:52A, 1989.

31. Punnonen R and Soderstrom KO: Inflammatory etiology of salpingitis isthmica nodosa: a clinical, histological and ultrastructural study, *Acta Eur Fertil* 17(3):199-203, 1986.

32. Chen KTK: Bilateral papillary adenofibromas of the fallopian tubes, *Am J Clin Pathol* 75:229-231, 1981.

33. Wrork DH and Brokers AC: Adenomyosis of fallopian tube, *Am J Obstet Gynecol* 44:412-432, 1942.

34. Kistner RW: Infertility with endometriosis: plan of therapy, *Fertil Steril* 13:237-245, 1962.

35. Surrey ES and Halme J: Endometriosis as a cause of infertility, *Obstet Gynecol Clin North Am* 16(1):79-91, 1989.

36. Forrest J, Buckley CH, and Fox H: Pelvic endometriosis and tubal inflammatory disease, *Int J Gynecol Pathol* 3:343, 1984.

37. Craig JM: The pathology of infertility, *Pathol Annu* 10:299-328, 1975.

38. Lisa JR, Gioia JD, and Rubin IC: Observations on the interstitial portion of the fallopian tube, *Surg Gynecol Obstet* 99:159-169, 1954.

39. David MP, Ben-Zwi D, and Langer L: Tubal intramural polyps and their relationship to infertility, *Fertil Steril* 35:526-531, 1981.

40. Fernstrom I and Lagerlof B: Polyps in the intramural part of the fallopian tube, *J Obstet Gynaecol Br Commonw* 71:681-691, 1964.

41. Gordts S, et al: Microsurgical resection of intramural tubal polyps, *Fertil Steril* 40(2):258-259, 1983.

42. Philip E and Huber H: Die Entstenhung der Endometriose, gleichzeitig ein Beitrag zur Pathologie des interstitiellen Tubenabschnittes, *Zentralbl Gynaekol* 63:7-40, 1939.

43. David MP and Soferman N: Tubal polyps: report of four cases, *Int Surg* 49:348-353, 1968.

44. Rubin IC, Lisa JR, and Trinidad S: Further observations on ectopic endometrium of the fallopian tube, *Surg Gynecol Obstet* 103:469-474, 1956.

45. Ayers JWT: Hormonal therapy for tubal occlusion: danazol and tubal endometriosis. *Fertil Steril* 38(6):748-750, 1982.

46. Stangel JJ, Chervenak FA, and Mouradian-Davidian M: Microsurgical resection of bilateral fallopian tube polyps, *Fertil Steril* 35:580-582, 1981.

47. Doleris A and Macrez F: Endosalpingeal papillomas, *Gynecology* 3:289-308, 1898.

48. Green TH and Scully RE: Tumors of the fallopian tube, *Clin Obstet Gynecol* 5:886-906, 1962.

49. Saffos RO, Rhatigan RM, and Scully RE: Metaplastic papillary tumor of the fallopian tube—a distinctive lesion of pregnancy, *Am J Clin Pathol* 74(2):232-236, 1980.

50. Honore LH and Korn GW: Coexistence of tubal ectopic pregnancy and adenomatoid tumor, *J Reprod Med* 17(6):342-344, 1976.

51. Pauerstein CJ, Woodruff JD, and Quinton SW: Developmental patterns in "adenomatoid lesions" of the fallopian tube, *Am J Obstet Gynecol* 100:1000-1007, 1968.

52. Ferenczy A, Fenoglio J, and Richart RM: Observations on benign mesothelioma of the genital tract (adenomatoid tumor). A comparative ultrastructural study, *Cancer* 30:244-260, 1972.

53. Seidner HM and Thompson JR: Fibroma of the fallopian tube, *Am J Obstet Gynecol* 79:32-33, 1960.

54. Patel DR, Kawalek R, and Iger J: Cavernous hemangioma of the fallopian tube, *Int Surg* 58:420-421, 1973.

55. Sanes S and Warner R: Primary lymphangioma of the fallopian tube, *Am J Obstet Gynecol* 37:316-321, 1939.

56. Dede JA and Janovski NA: Lipoma of the uterine tube—a gynecologic rarity, *Obstet Gynecol* 22:461-467, 1963.

57. Weber DL and Fazzini E: Ganglioneuroma of the fallopian tube; a heretofore unreported finding, *Acta Neuropathol* 16:173-175, 1970.

58. Moore OA, Waxman M, and Udoffia C: Leiomyoma of the fallopian tube: a cause of tubal pregnancy, *Am J Obstet Gynecol* 134(1):101-102, 1979.

59. Crissman JD and Handwerker D: Leiomyoma of uterine tube: Report of a case, *Am J Obstet Gynecol* 126(8):1046, 1976.

60. Stringer SW: Leiomyofibroma of the fallopian tube, *NY State J Med* 48:1621, 1948.

61. Kopf H and Fukas M: Myofibroma of the tube, *Zentralbl Gynaekol* 62:1552-1554, 1938.

62. Silverman AY, Artinian B, and Sabin M: Serous cystadenofibroma of the fallopian tube: a case report, *Am J Obstet Gynecol* 130(5):593-595, 1978.

63. de la Fuente AA: Benign mixed mullerian tumour—adenofibroma of the fallopian tube, *Histopathology* 6(5):661-666, 1982.

64. Hurd JK Jr: Benign cystic teratoma of the fallopian tube, *Obstet Gynecol* 52(3):362-364, 1978.

65. Mazzarella P, Okagaki T, and Richart RM: Teratoma of the uterine tube. A case report and review of the literature, *Obstet Gynecol* 39:381-388, 1972.

66. Aaron JB: Dermoid cyst in the uterine tube: a case report with a review of the literature, *Am J Obstet Gynecol* 42:1080-1086, 1941.

67. Zelinger BB, Grinvalsky H, and Fields C: Simultaneous dermoid cyst of the tube and ectopic pregnancy, *Obstet Gynecol* 15:340-343, 1960.

68. Zinsser KR and Wheeler JE: Endosalpingiosis in the omentum: a study of autopsy and surgical material, *Am J Surg Pathol* 6:109-117, 1982.

69. Sampson JA: Postsalpingectomy endometriosis (endosalpingiosis), *Am J Obstet Gynecol* 20:443-480, 1930.

70. McCausland A: Endosalpingiosis ("endosalpingoblastosis") following laparoscopic tubal coagulation as an etiologic factor in ectopic pregnancy, *Am J Obstet Gynecol* 143(1):12-24, 1982.

71. Cohen BM: Microsurgical reconstruction of congenital tubal anomalies, *Microsurgery* 8(2):68-77, 1987.

72. Wanerman J, Wulwick R, and Brenner S: Segmental absence of the fallopian tube, *Fertil Steril* 46(3):525-527, 1986.

73. Richardson DA: Segmental absence of the mid-portion of the fallopian tube, *Fertil Steril* 37(4):577-579, 1982.

74. Farber M and Mitchell GW Jr: Bicornuate uterus and partial atresia of the fallopian tube, *Am J Obstet Gynecol* 134(8):881-883, 1979.

75. Daw E: Duplication of the uterine tube, *Obstet Gynecol* 42:137-138, 1973.

76. Beyth Y and Kopolovic J: Accessory tubes: A possible contributing factor in infertility, *Fertil Steril* 38(3):382-383, 1982.

77. Moore-White M: Evolution of tubal plastic operations, *Int J Fertil* 5:237-250, 1960.

78. Cohen BM and Katz M: The significance of the convoluted oviduct in the infertile woman, *J Reprod Med* 21(1):31-35, 1978.

79. Lurie M et al: Ciliary ultrastructure of respiratory and fallopian tube epithelium in a sterile woman with Kartagener's syndrome. A quantitative estimation, *Chest* 95(3):578-581, 1989.

80. McComb P et al: The oviductal cilia and Kartagener's syndrome, *Fertil Steril* 46(3):412-416, 1986.

81. Marchini M et al: Ultrastructure of endosalpingeal biopsies in infertile patients: Correlation with reproductive success, *Int J Gynecol Obstet* 27(2):239-245, 1988.

82. Bransilver BR, Ferenczy A, and Richart RM: Female genital tract remnants: an ultrastructural comparison of hydatid of Morgagni and mesonephric ducts and tubules, *Arch Pathol* 96:255-261, 1973.

83. Genadry R, Parmley T, and Woodruff JD: The origin and clinical behavior of the parovarian tumor, *Am J Obstet Gynecol* 129:873-880, 1977.

84. Case Records of the Massachusetts General Hospital (case no. 37121): *N Engl J Med* 244(12):445-448, 1981.

85. Bransilver BR, Ferenczy A, and Richart RM: Brenner tumors and Walthard cell nests, *Arch Pathol* 98:76-86, 1974.

PREOPERATIVE ASSESSMENT

3

Psychologic Response of the Infertile Couple

MARTHA E. GRIFFIN

DIANE N. CLAPP

Infertility represents a life crisis to the couple experiencing it; suddenly they are forced to face a life goal that is blocked. Often the couple has practiced birth control and consciously made a decision to start a family based on such factors as economic security, purchase of a home, and the like. When this choice does not go according to the plan, the result can be devastating, with increased tension and anxiety and a tendency to become emotionally depleted.

In addition, by the very nature of infertility this crisis can last for years. Couples often reflect that it feels as though their lives are on hold, which is confirmed as they watch with envy their contemporaries producing second and third children.

Infertility involves loss of an image of bearing and raising a biologic child, of experiencing pregnancy, of control over one's life, and loss of privacy in terms of sexual intimacy and of having one's body being probed and tested. Infertility is, in fact, the death of a dream, which involves a typical grief response: surprise, denial, isolation, anger, guilt, sadness, and resolution.

STAGES OF GRIEF

Physicians often first see a couple or individual in the surprise and denial stages after a conclusive finding of an organic cause for infertility. The couple may seek several medical opinions at this point, in an effort to find a magical solution or in the hopes that the initial physician did not make the correct diagnosis.

Both physician and staff can help in this stage by not fostering denial with false hope and by letting individuals and couples determine how quickly they want surgery or supporting them in seeking a second opinion. Couples may need to use the denial stage to let the diagnosis settle in, to assimilate it, and recognize the possible impact it could have on their lives.

Denial often gives way to isolation, and the couple pulls back from friends and family members who were once a source of support. The partners then must deal with their sadness alone, in a world of pregnancy stimuli. There may be isolation also between husband and wife, especially when there is repeated pregnancy loss, as each may grieve separately and silently. Isolation can take another form as the result of the medical work-up. Thus it is essential that infertility be treated as the couple's problem. Both partners should be urged to come to every appointment, and the man should be included in discussion concerning surgical or medical management of his partner's condition. Putting the couple in touch with a local support group, introducing them to Resolve, Inc. as a resource for information, and providing literature to underscore and elucidate medical aspects that were previously discussed are ways to enhance the pair's knowledge and understanding of infertility as it relates to them.

During the isolation stage, couples or individuals begin to experience feelings of anger, guilt, and depression. Anger may be directed at the medical world in general and their doctor in particular. The couple feels they are no longer in control of their bodies. Sexual activity is dictated, painful tests are necessary, drugs can cause side effects, and surgery may be required that necessitates a recuperative period away from career or job. These are of the major reasons for anger and a sense of noncontrol.

If anger is not expressed, depression and helplessness may result directly from feelings of lack of control and frustration. The inability to make decisions about treatment and a sense that nothing is enjoyable any more, that there is a hollowness in their lives, are often clues to a couple's depression and associated repressed anger. Unfortunately, patients at this stage are the most difficult to deal with. It is helpful to provide an opportunity for the couple to ventilate their feeling. This often means sitting and talking with either partner or the two together under as near normal conditions as possible, and discussing the difficult aspects of the experience. A straightforward approach often allows a couple to share their sadness and anger. Some couples do not feel comfortable ventilating to a physician, but the nurse can be an excellent resource. This person can offer additional information and clarification concerning physician's orders, tests to be performed, drug dosage schedules, and so on.

Thus to both partners are made available the pertinent facts of their case. They are then better able to make informed decisions regarding the important aspects of treatment. Such education can significantly defuse the couple's anger and increase patient compliance with therapy. Avoiding long periods of noncontact is also helpful in reducing anger. Having women check in by phone to validate the treatment plan after the onset of a menstrual cycle is extremely helpful and provides a sense of continuity and hope. There are times when it may be beneficial for the couple to take a break from the work-up or treatment as basal body temperatures, regulated intercourse, and frequent medical appointments begin to deplete their energy. The physician may not only agree with such a break but may in fact prescribe it, thus demonstrating the couple's right to take some control over this experience.

Another emotion that frequently occurs with anger is guilt. Partners attempt to find the reasons for their infertility, often reexamining their lives looking for a cause-and-effect explanation. The best intervention by a physician at this stage is to be honest about the cause and effect and to dispel myths. Discussing what both persons perceive to be a cause of their infertility opens up communications. It is important to reassure them that the anxiety and stress they may be feeling are not the cause of their infertility, but rather the result of a frustrating experience. That anxiety and stress are causes rather than effects is a thought that arises in the minds of many, if not all, couples experiencing infertility.

It helps to talk openly with women whose infertility is due to adhesions resulting from pelvic infection or use of an intrauterine device. One must keep in mind that the infection or method of birth control may have been acquired or used with another partner. In these situations, guilt and isolation between partners is difficult to supercede.

Gradually the individual partners and/or couple will begin to address their loss and grief. This is an important step toward resolution and essential before moving on to alternatives, such as adoption or child-free living. It is

at this stage that many express feeling most vulnerable, emotional, and sad. In many cases, however, it is difficult for couples to know when to start grieving. This is especially true when surgery has been successful but no pregnancy results. Grieving is more easily facilitated when the diagnosis is conclusive.

A delicate and difficult question involves when to tell couples that there is no more to be done and it is time to look at alternatives. The physician must hold out hope for success, but it is also necessary to help couples be realistic. The physician should acknowledge the importance of the couple's own choice and avoid the natural collision of values that can occur with professional advice to wait for a future scientific breakthrough. Many infertility specialists find it helpful to ask couples how they feel about their treatment, and affirm at any time they can say enough is enough.

Physicians should also help the couple evaluate the new technologies, emotional resources, and their need to have a biologic child. Giving the partners articles to read both pro and con often is helpful in preventing false hopes or potential futile attempts that only prolong resolving their problem. Often during this stage, there is subtle or overt disagreement between the man and woman to terminate treatment. A typical example is the woman who does not want more surgery and prefers to look at alternatives, but her spouse is eager to do everything possible. Referral to a therapist or a counselor who is familiar with the stresses of this infertility crisis is helpful in such cases.

Resolution, the final stage, involves working through the first six stages and emerging with a sense of self intact. Couples must abandon a dream and what is generally thought of as a God-given right. They must then separate the issue of pregnancy from that of being parents. If it becomes clear that having a child is their main desire and that the means to that end not the primary issue, adoption may be an excellent alternative.

Physicians should remember the decision to adopt is not easy for a couple to make; nor is the procedure simple to implement. In many states it can take five to eight years to adopt an infant, and the financial expense can be high. Also, once again the couple will be tested, scored, and asked to prove their worthiness to be parents.

Offering general information about local adoption agencies is helpful, but mainly, the couple should not feel abandoned by the physician at this stage. Usually an important relationship has developed, and abrupt termination is painful. Urging the couple to stay in touch is essential.

RESOURCES

Successful treatment for infertility need not be seen only in terms of a live biologic child. Despite the fact that, even with all our modern medical and surgical technologic advances, four to five million people will remain infertile physiologically, most infertility can be resolved emotionally. To make this possible, however, it is necessary to use all available resources.

Resolve, Inc. is a national nonprofit organization established exclusively to help individuals and couples experiencing infertility. Support is extended through counseling, medical referrals, and providing educational material. Local chapters also sponsor women's and couples' support groups. They are small—5 to 10 individuals or 3 to 5 couples—and are run by Resolve-recommended clinicians who are prepared usually at a master's degree level. These groups are support-oriented versus therapy-directed and rely on participants to have intact, basically healthy personalities. Their infertility diagnoses are mixed. The groups provide an atmosphere of exchange for individuals and couples who establish close bonds with each other as they face and come to terms with the problem of infertility.

SUGGESTED READING

For Physicians

Menning BE: Counseling infertile couples, *Contemp Obstet Gynecol* 13:101-108, 1979.

Reading AE and Kerin J: Psychologic aspects of providing infertility services, *J Reprod Med* 34:861-871, 1981.

For Patients

Bolles EB: *The Penguin adoption handbook,* New York, 1984, Penguin Books.

Harkness C: *The infertility book: a comprehensive medical and emotional guide,* San Francisco, 1987, Volcano Press.

Menning BE: *Infertility: a guide for the childless couple,* ed 2, New York, 1988, Prentice-Hall.

Perloe M and Christie LG: *Miracle babies and other happy endings,* New York, 1986, Rawson.

Salzer LP: *Infertility: how couples can cope,* Boston, 1986, G.K. Hall.

Patient Resources

Resolve, Inc.
5 Water Street
Arlington, MA 02174

The Endometriosis Association
8585 North 76th Place
Milwaukee, WI 53223

OPERATIVE PREPARATIONS

4

Laboratory Practice of Microsurgery

CARLTON A. EDDY
ROBERT B. HUNT

Gynecologic microsurgery is now firmly established as a valid and useful technique that has widespread application. It is a highly developed skill that demands a significant degree of neuromuscular eye-hand coordination and ideally, an awareness of and appreciation for the need to restore genital anatomy and adnexal spatial relationships if fertility is to be reestablished.

Microsurgery does not require unique talents, but does require proper instruction and adequate practice to achieve and maintain a desirable level of proficiency. Attendance at one or several courses cannot of itself confer the necessary competence, but it does provide a realistic introduction to the technique, its requirements, and the associated problems that are usually encountered. Without these insights and mastery of the mechanical aspects, simply purchasing a set of microsurgical instruments, arranging for a surgical microscope, and prematurely embarking on the first clinical microsurgery case will, in the words of Robert Winston, "result in embarrassment for the surgeon, boredom and irritation of the theater staff, and trauma to the patient."

The proper setting in which to acquire microsurgical skills, therefore, is not the operating theater as apprentice to a practicing microsurgeon, but the laboratory, which offers the opportunity to perfect one's own skills and achieve required competence. Viewing and surgically manipulating living tissue while using the surgical microscope in the laboratory produce an immediate awareness of the delicacy of tissue and the ease with which iatrogenic trauma may be produced. It is noteworthy that the majority of microsurgeons in gynecology who pioneered the development and use of mirosurgery perfected their mechanical skills and acquired their physiologic point of view in the laboratory. Ideally, after mastering the mechanical aspects of microsurgery in the laboratory, the surgeon should focus on its application by observing and assisting a skilled microsurgeon. Only after becoming familiar with the clinical demands of the procedure should the fledgling microsurgeon undertake to perform the technique—initially in uncomplicated, straightforward cases, followed by progressively more challenging ones.

Gynecologic surgery historically has been considered bold, sanguine, and at times, even flamboyant. It has exemplified the trial-and-error approach whereby many different ways of solving a given problem are evolved, each of which relies heavily upon the tissue's ability to heal and an organ's rather extensive functional reserve. Thus there exist numerous surgical resolutions for a host of given gynecologic procedures—all undertaken with suitable reliance on the surgeon's ability (and historical precedent) to manipulate tissue freely and extensively without regard for minimizing iatrogenic trauma. Dissections tend to be defined and limited only by anatomic planes, and ties are made by hand with large-caliber sutures embracing substantial masses of tissue opposed with sufficient tension to make accidental overstress and suture breakage a common event.

In marked contrast, gynecologic microsurgery is precise and delicate, requires visualization of fine detail under magnification, and is conducted within technical and physiologic constraints imposed by the small margin for error consistent with successful outcome. It is these special problems of working under magnification and making consistent, controlled, fine movements that constitute the technical demands of microsurgery.

As with any precise and demanding technique, different people will achieve different levels of competence and at different rates of speed. It would be totally arbitrary to assign any given number of hours as being required to become a skilled microsurgeon. The majority of prospective microsurgeons achieve a creditable level of competence in response to a reasonable investment of time and effort. This chapter is meant to serve as a guide to allow readers to develop the latent skills they already possess, while avoiding many of the pitfalls and frustrations that exist. A systematic approach is used, starting with the most basic aspect of the technique and progressing through increasingly more difficult tasks. It is important not to allow tunnel vision to develop, whereby prospective microsurgeons strive merely to equip themselves with a set of cookbook instructions to be blindly and dogmatically applied, or to program themselves to perform mechanically whenever circumstances dictate that patients be viewed through the surgical microscope. What surgeons should seek to acquire is a new and therapeutically useful skill that will ultimately benefit the patient when it is successfully integrated into surgeons' existing insights, sensibilities, and clinical skills.

WORK AREA

An appropriate laboratory work area for acquiring and maintaining microsurgical skills need not be large or extensively equipped. Required are sufficient space for surgical microscope, a comfortable, nonreclining seat of adjustable height, and an uncrowded workspace, preferably the top of a sturdy table under which the surgeon's legs will conveniently fit (Figure 4-1). The height of the work surface should be such that one need not stretch one's legs to reach the floor or stoop over to reach the surgical microscope and work surface. The surgeon should achieve a comfortable sitting posture with the back erect and the height of the seat adjusted so that it is not necessary to stretch the neck or hunch over to reach the eyepieces. The shoulders should be comfortably squared and the feet spread and placed in front without stretching to reach the floor (Figure 4-2). There should be sufficient space for a cautery unit, for working with live animals, and for miscellaneous items such as syringes for irrigation and cotton rolls or swabs for removing fluids from the surgical field. The work area should be free of extraneous distractions so the surgeon can work undisturbed at a comfortable pace. Access to a laboratory set up to perform animal microsurgery is ideal; barring this, an office corner or an area at home can serve.

EQUIPMENT

There is a wide variety of operating microscopes, microsurgical instruments, electrosurgery units, suture-needle combinations, and ancillary equipment such as suction/irrigating devices, oviduct stabilizing clamps, and intraluminal probes and stents. Under development are hand-held lasers, tissue adhesive dispensers, and tubal stapling devices for one-step end-to-end tubal anastomosis. Acquisition of equipment should be based on need, functional design, durability, and cost rather than on whim or salesmanship.

Surgical microscope

A variety of surgical microscopes differing greatly in price and functional features is now available. Magnification with high resolution and bright coaxial illumination are hallmarks of quality surgical microscopes and are essential for visualizing tissue adequately to determine the extent of pathology, identify anatomic features,

and avoid iatrogenic trauma during surgery. Relatively inexpensive bench-top models exist (Figures 4-3 and 4-4) with reduced capabilities, but with the same excellent optical qualities and illumination systems as the more expensive and complex floor-mounted models. Bench-top microscopes generally are equipped with manual controls for step-wise magnification changes and fine focusing. Most feature a range of interchangeable objective lenses to alter the working distance between lens and subject. These same manually controlled surgical microscopes may be mounted on floor stands for clinical use (Figures 4-5 and 4-6).

The more expensive models have foot-pedal controls for coarse and fine focus adjustment and for magnification changes in step-wise or continuous (zoom) fashion. They may be fitted with a variety of angulated and articulated extension arms for optimum positioning of the microscope over the patient, while the bulky, counterbalanced base, with all of its electronic circuitry, remains conveniently positioned away from the surgeon and the operating table. Optional features can include a foot-pedal-activated device for changing the position of the microscope in the X-Y plane over the patient. Whether complex and expensive or simple and moderately priced, all surgical microscopes function according to the same basic laws of physics. Differences relate basically to electronic and mechanical options, many of which are superfluous in the laboratory, where simpler equipment is certainly appropriate. If one does not have ready access to a surgical microscope, the coupling piece and stand of a colposcope may easily be modified so it may be used in an upright position for microsurgery training.

Microsurgical instruments

The choice of instruments is a personal matter, with the design and configuration of each reflecting the specific needs of each microsurgeon. Clearly, there is no universal set of instruments ideally suited for all surgeons, even those who perform similar types of microsurgery. It is wasted effort to struggle with inappropriately designed instruments or those unsuited to the individual surgeon, when a different configuration would allow greater comfort and the subtle movement necessary to ensure the most precise, efficient procedure. It is advisable for each surgeon to compare the relative merits of different instruments under actual use. Only then can individuals establish the optimal combination of length, weight, handle shape, opening pressure, and functional configuration. The same types of instruments (if not the same instruments) used for training and in the laboratory should be used in the operating room because they have a natural and familiar feel.

The basic complement required in the laboratory includes a needle holder, a pair of microscissors, and a pair of forceps (Figure 4-7). Because the surgeon will be working in the pelvis under circumstances in which

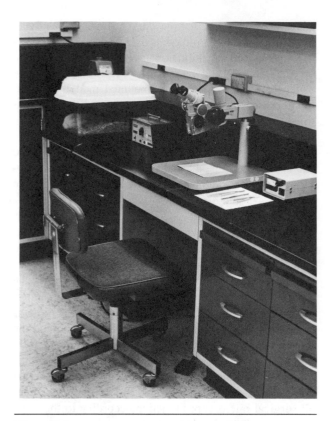

Figure 4-1
Typical laboratory station with bench-top surgical micro-scope, adjustable chair, and cut-out to accommodate legs and feet, and with ample bench-top space for cautery unit, illu-mination system, rheostat, surgical instruments, and miscel-laneous pieces of equipment. The location is in a corner away from traffic, allowing work to proceed undisturbed at an individual pace.

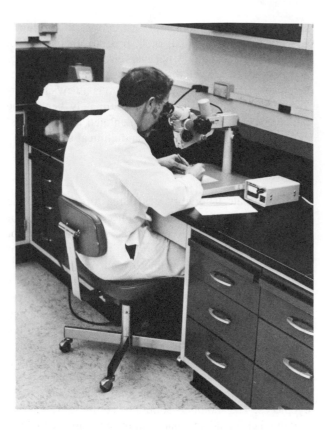

Figure 4-2
Proper seating position with back erect, shoulders squared, eyepieces well accessible, and hands, wrists, and forearms supported.

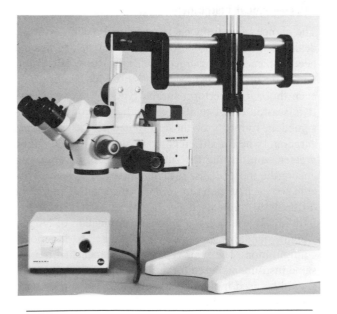

Figure 4-3
Manually adjustable bench-top surgical microscope with integral light source. Courtesy E. Leitz, Inc.

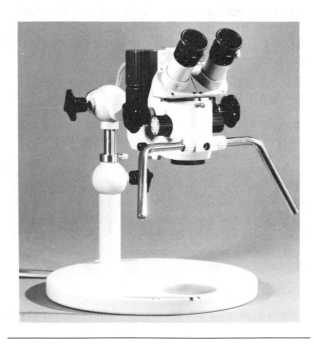

Figure 4-4
Bench-top manually adjustable, surgical microscope, OPMI 1. Courtesy Carl Zeiss, Inc.

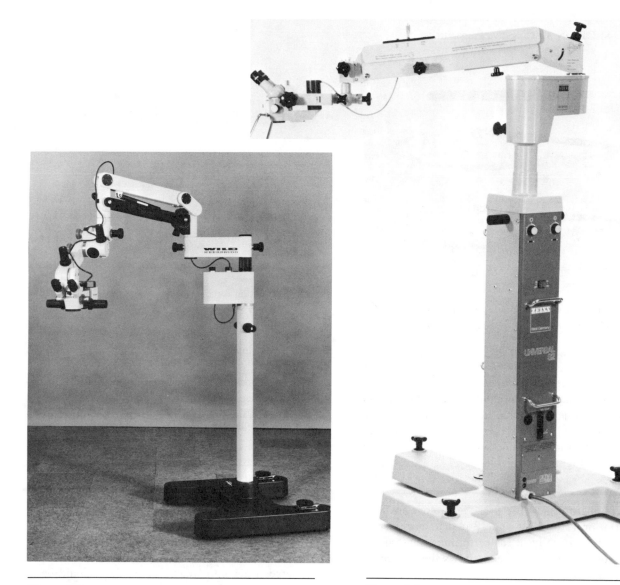

Figure 4-5
Floor-mounted surgical microscope with articulated arm.
Courtesy E. Leitz, Inc.

Figure 4-6
Surgical microscope mounted on floor stand. Courtesy Carl
Zeiss, Inc.

it may not always be possible to mobilize the uterus or
adnexa up to the level of the anterior abdominal wall, it
is advantageous to acquire and train with instruments at
least 15 cm long that allow access to the pelvic viscera
while allowing the fine, finger-tip control necessary for
microsurgery.

Great care should be taken in the use, cleaning, and
storage of instruments. They will quickly, and often permanently, lose their precision and usefulness if abused
in any way. They must never be balanced on their tips
as a means of positioning them in the hand, or brushed
against a drape or each other to clean their tips. They
should be washed individually after use and stored with
their tips protected by a short length of rubber tubing or
similar material placed over their ends. Ideally, they
should be stored in one of the metal instrument cases
available in several sizes from instrument manufacturers.

These cases can be autoclaved together with the set of
instruments placed inside them. Such cases keep the instruments safely separated from each other and, more
important, from the heavy and potentially damaging macrosurgery instruments in a laparotomy pack.

Electrosurgery units

Diathermy is an integral part of gynecologic microsurgery; however, it is quite distinct from the more traditional use of what has come to be referred to generically
as the Bovie unit. The precise, pinpoint, low-power coagulation or cutting done through the operating microscope is a far cry from the method of grasping a bleeding
site with a hemostat and placing the electrode against it.
The units used in microsurgery combine fine-tipped unipolar electrocoagulation needles and bipolar forceps
with solid-state power units capable of delivering low-

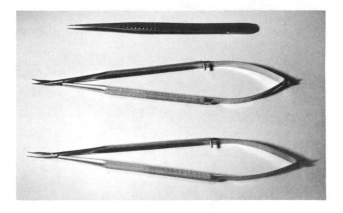

Figure 4-7
Basic instruments used for laboratory training in microsurgery. From top to bottom: forceps, scissors, needle holder.

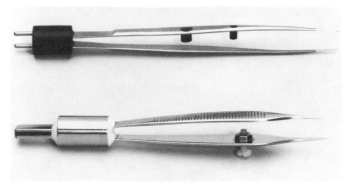

Figure 4-8
Bipolar coagulating forceps.

power currents that limit cutting or coagulation to very small areas of tissue. The microsurgeon should train with bipolar and unipolar electrosurgery units with power settings low enough to accommodate the requirements of microsurgery (Figures 4-8 and 4-9).

Sutures

Sutures for microsurgical use in the laboratory are commonly 10-0 or 11-0 (22-µ and 18-µ diameter, respectively). Either size is ideal for performing anastomosis of rat femoral blood vessels and allows the full development of microsurgical skills. The type of needle most commonly used with such suture is a taper-point, ⅜ circle with a wire diameter ranging from 30 to 150 µ. Passing this type of needle through tissue demands more skill than does the use of cutting or spatulated needles, but produces far less tissue trauma. Cutting needles should be restricted to penetrating tissue tougher than that of the oviduct, such as the uterus or ovarian cortex.

Microsurgical suture is nonreactive and may be absorbable or inert, monofilament, or braided. Each has its own physical properties and handling characteristics. It is therefore advisable to gain experience using all types. All are appropriate for use in infertility surgery, so the choice can be based entirely on personal preference. Multisuture dispensing packets of nonsterile microsuture for laboratory use are commercially available from the major suture manufacturers (see Appendix B).

ADJUSTING THE MICROSCOPE

The first step in adjusting the microscope is to turn on its light source. If it is equipped with an automatic rheostat, the light intensity will automatically increase or decrease as magnification is increased or decreased. If the light must be manually adjusted, care should be taken

that sufficient intensity is maintained as magnification is changed.

Each eyepiece diopter scale should be adjusted to zero and each eyepiece pushed all the way in and firmly seated in its tube. The interpupillary distance should be adjusted so that the two images fuse to form a single image. Unless the microscope is parfocal, the surgeon will have to refocus the microscope each time the magnification is changed. This is frustrating for the surgeon, adds operating time, and ultimately increases the patient's bill. To render the microscope parfocal, the following steps are suggested:

1. Reduce magnification to the lowest setting and adjust the diopter of each eyepiece to zero. If the surgeon plans to wear glasses, they should be in place.
2. The surgeon places an object on which to focus, such as the print on a package of sutures, on a flat surface beneath the microscope objective.
3. The left eye is closed and the microscope adjusted so that the right eye is sharply focused on the print. The diopter setting remains at zero.
4. With the left eye still closed, the magnification of the microscope is increased to its maximum, and the microscope is refocused to bring the print into sharp focus, leaving the diopter setting at zero.
5. With the left eye still closed, the magnification is reduced to its minimum, and the diopter of the right eyepiece is rotated until the print is sharply focused.
6. Steps 3 through 5 are repeated, this time with the right eye closed and the left one open.

At this time the microscope should be parfocal, meaning it should remain in focus at all magnifications. The surgeon should note the diopter settings for the right and left eyepieces, making certain the diopters are set at these numbers in subsequent cases. It should not be necessary to go through these steps each time the same microscope is used by the same surgeon.

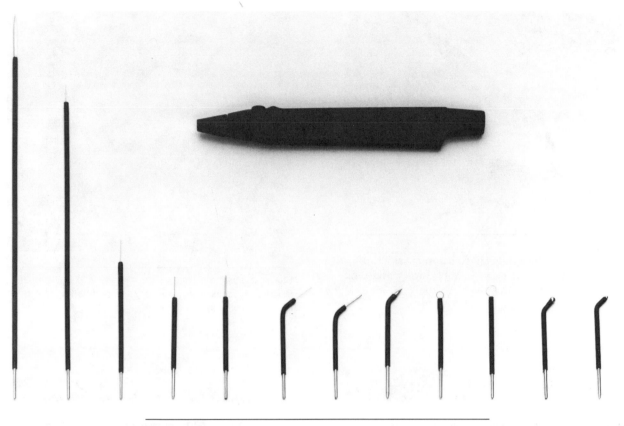

Figure 4-9
Unipolar coagulator handle with various insulated unipolar electrodes.

While operating, the surgeon should always keep the area of interest centered in the optical field—this is the area of brightest illumination and sharpest optical quality. Since the field of view and depth of focus decrease as magnification increases, one must learn to become familiar with and comfortable working at all magnifications. High magnifications are used for critical examination of tissue and accurate placement of sutures. Lower magnifications are used for tying sutures after placement, when a larger field of view and greater depth of focus are needed. As familiarity with the use of the microscope and assessment of spatial relationships improve, it will be possible to bring the tips of the instruments automatically to whatever spot in the field is chosen without taking the eyes away from the eyepiece or "hunting" in broad sweeps of the hand beneath the objective lens.

CONTROL OF UNWANTED MOVEMENT

Microsurgical technique consists of a small number of straightforward, if not simple, steps through which meticulous restoration of anatomy can be achieved. In general, the rules and aims of general surgery pertain to microsurgery; they are just more precise and meticulous and, of course, are performed on a much smaller scale.

The basic mechanical tasks are the ability to place sutures accurately into tissue and tie them so they reapproximate the normal anatomy without distortion.

Most people's reaction to performing hitherto basic surgical tasks, such as tying a suture, through the microscope is one of dismay. The surgical microscope removes all proprioceptive cues and replaces them with solely visual input. Surgeons will initially lose all sense of familiarity with what they are doing and with it, most, if not all, control over movements. The need to accomplish manipulations consistently with a precision of a thousandth of an inch under such circumstances can be quite challenging. In practical terms, microsurgery translates into a battle against unwanted movement.

Hand tremor is present in everyone. The tips of the fingers of an outstretched, unsupported hand exhibit a tremor with an amplitude ranging from less than a millimeter in some individuals to several millimeters and above in others. Such tremors may have a frequency ranging from several to as many as 30 vibrations per second. While this degree of tremor, or more aptly, normal physiologic, uncontrolled movement, is consistent with acceptable macrosurgical performance, uncontrolled movements as slight as 0.5 mm can render accurate placement or tying of microsutures impossible. Factors that promote

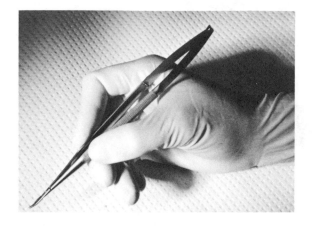

Figure 4-10
Precision grip method of holding microsurgical instruments. This grip allows positive, stable, and sensitive fingertip control of the instruments.

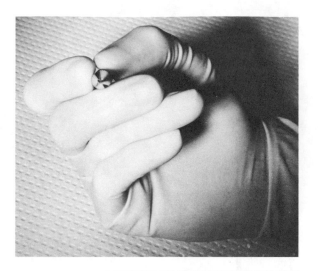

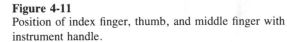

Figure 4-11
Position of index finger, thumb, and middle finger with instrument handle.

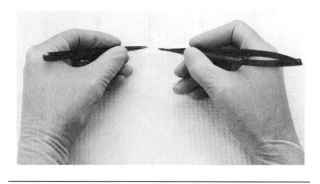

Figure 4-12
Position of hands during microsurgery. Note that both hands are supported along the entire ulnar border and that the tips of both instruments are maintained in close proximity to each other.

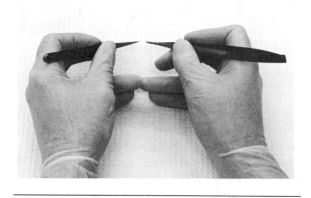

Figure 4-13
Additional stabilization gained by opposing the tips of the ring fingers.

or eliminate tremor are therefore central to the learning process. These may be divided into constitutional, conditional, and intraoperative factors.

Constitutional factors refer to a person's physical and emotional makeup and how well the individual is endowed to meet and carry out the demands of microsurgery. Provided there are no major neuromuscular, orthopedic, or visual deficits and there exists a willingness to invest the necessary time and effort, most people can achieve a creditable level of skill.

Conditional factors refer to the demands placed on the surgeon's skills and the state of physical fitness at the time of surgery. Unlike constitutional factors, which are largely unalterable, one's levels of proficiency and of well-being can be modified by appropriate training and attention to life-style. A great deal of comment has been

made concerning what preparations are required and what activities should be avoided before performing microsurgery. To dictate in general, dogmatic, and arbitrary terms the acceptable behavior necessary to perform skillfully would be meaningless on an individual basis. An appropriate rule of thumb is to moderate behavior that tends to detract from performance, such as excessive use of alcohol and other depressants, engaging in strenuous physical excercise 24 hours before surgery, and placing oneself in high-anxiety situations; while maximizing those factors that promote peak performance, such as having the necessary level of skill demanded by a given case, being adequately rested, and not having to rush to accommodate operating room scheduling or attend to other matters, such as patients in labor.

Intraoperative factors are concerned with how the surgeon actually carries out microsurgery. They relate to such immediate consideration as how adequately the hands and forearms are supported, how comfortably the surgeon is seated, how well the microscope is adjusted, choice of appropriately designed instruments, and adequacy of exposure of the structures on which surgery is being performed.

The most effective way to deal with excessive uncontrolled movement of the hands is to hold the instruments in the so-called external precision grip and to have sufficient support of the forearms and hands. Microsurgical instruments are held like writing instruments (Figure 4-10). The forward portion of the instrument is cradled by the tips of the thumb and index and middle fingers, which in turn are rested on the slightly indented ring and little fingers (Figure 4-11). The butt end of the instrument extends beyond and is cradled in the anatomic snuff box, or pressure-sensitive patch of skin between the base of the thumb and index finger. This arrangement furnishes mechanical support for the instrument and also provides sensory information of the position and pressure exerted by the instrument. The hands should be slightly supinated and the instruments pointed into the surgical field without any tension or torque in the wrists. The hands should be relaxed and supported along the entire ulnar border from the edges of the little finger to the elbow. The hands are positioned in proximity to each other so that the tips of the instruments can be manipulated in unison in a co-ordinated fashion (Figure 4-12). For additional support, the hands may be positioned so that the tips of the ring and/or little fingers touch (Figure 4-13).

SUTURING TECHNIQUES
Positioning the needle in the needle holder

The needle should be held perpendicular to the jaws of the needle holder, several needle thicknesses in from the tips of the holder, to prevent it from being inadvertently ejected and lost in the operative field. The needle should be grasped about two thirds back from the point (Figure 4-14). This is a balanced position that allows maximum control of the needle.

There are two ways of picking up and positioning the needle. One may simply grasp the needle with the forceps and, through a series of hand-offs between the forceps and needle holders, correctly position it. An alternative technique is to grasp the suture with the forceps several needle lengths behind the needle, balance the point of the needle on the work surface, and grasp the needle in the appropriate location with the needle holder.

Placing practice sutures
Glove rubber

Accurate, atraumatic placement of sutures is the sine qua non of microsurgery and is possible through a combination of surgical skill and adequate visualization. The

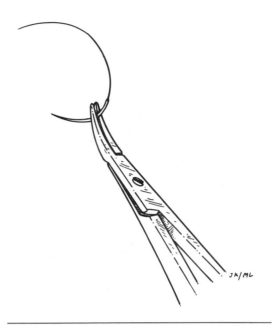

Figure 4-14
Proper position of the needle in the needle holder.

ease with which one passes a needle through tissue is dependent on skill and the judicious use of counterpressure, needle angulation during passage, the size of the needle and its point configuration, and the density and thickness of the tissue. Insight and training are best acquired by undertaking progressively more difficult tasks, starting with suturing incisions in glove rubber, an exercise that also furnishes the opportunity to learn how to tie sutures under the microscope.

A flat sheet of surgical rubber, several inches square and taped around its edges to a piece of cardboard, makes an excellent learning aid. Such practice boards are now available commercially from Xomed, Inc. (see Appendix B). The cardboard should be taped to the surface of the work area to prevent unwanted movement. In the middle of the area illuminated by the microscope light source, an oblique incision should be made through the rubber with a scalpel from the upper left quadrant to the lower right quadrant (opposite orientation for left-handed persons). This orientation is easiest to work with and automatically places the instruments in the position that is most natural and easiest to manipulate.

Placing the sutures. After a packet of microsuture is opened, the needle should be grasped with the needle holder, either under the microscope or using the naked eye. To avoid breaking the suture or pulling it off the needle, one should grasp the needle, not the suture, and carefully pull it out of the foam or rubber block in which it is embedded. The needle is then brought into the operative field and positioned correctly in the needle holder (Figure 4-14). The cut in the rubber sheet is now closed with a series of interrupted sutures.

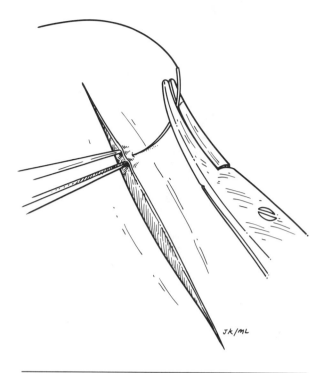

Figure 4-15
Use of forceps for supplying counterpressure against downward passage of the needle.

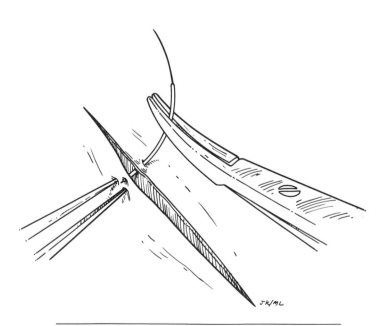

Figure 4-16
Symmetric placement of the needle through edges of glove rubber with counterpressure against upward passage of the needle.

Under high magnification, the point of the needle should be placed on the right side of the cut, three or four needle widths from the edge. After placement of the points of the forceps beneath the rubber on either side of the needle tip, the needle should be driven through the rubber with the needle holder while upward counterpressure is exerted with the tips of the forceps (Figure 4-15). After the rubber has been penetrated by the point of the needle, the tips of the forceps are withdrawn from beneath the right edge. The needle should then be passed further through the rubber sheet and its tip positioned at a corresponding point on the left edge. The tips of the forceps should be positioned on top of the rubber sheeting on either side of the needle point to provide downward counterpressure for the emerging needle (Figure 4-16). Passage of the needle should encompass equal amounts of glove rubber on the right and left sides, and the orientation of the needle should be perpendicular to the axis of the incision. To complete passage, the needle should be regrasped with the needle holder in the normal fashion just behind the point, taking care to avoid damaging its sharp point. It is rotated following its curvature as it is pulled through the rubber sheet. If pulled straight across, the needle's curved configuration will cause the tissue to tear. The forceps should be used to provide counterpressure and to stabilize the tissue while the needle is being pulled through (Figure 4-17). These steps limit trauma to that created by passage of the needle, and avoid the crushing and tearing caused by grasping tissue with forceps or improperly passing the needle. There is an initial and almost universal desire to grasp tissue with the forceps and to squeeze with excessive force in an attempt to gain control of the instruments. This technique should be abandoned as soon as possible. As more control is developed with increased practice, the surgeon will find that the instruments work best and that the finest movements are made when minimal pressure is used.

The needle should be released and the microscope adjusted to low magnification for tying. The suture is grasped a short distance behind the needle and pulled in a straight direction across the incision, with the tip of the forceps used to guide the suture and prevent it from snagging or pulling and enlarging the needle hole. By pulling on the suture itself, the chance of inadvertently separating the needle from the suture if a snag does occur (a common occurrence during the early stages of learning) is avoided, since the suture itself is stronger than its connection with the needle. As the suture is pulled farther and the tips of the needle holder begin to leave the field, there is no need to release the suture and regrasp it to keep the instrument in view. Instead, one should simply continue to pull, taking care to watch the progress of the suture and to avoid inadvertently pulling it entirely out of the rubber material. A short piece should be left for tying. The needle may either be released and allowed to remain outside the field of view or it may be brought

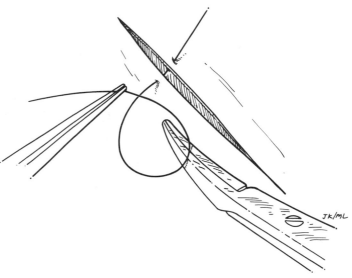

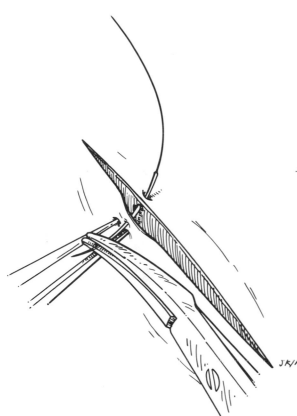

Figure 4-17
Use of the needle holder to grasp the emerging needle tip preparatory to pulling the needle through glove rubber. Forceps supply counterpressure.

Figure 4-18
Technique of forming a loop with the suture. The suture should emerge from the bottom or from the side of the forceps facing the operator. There should be ample length of suture to form a loop that allows easy movement of the needle holder to grasp the short end of the suture.

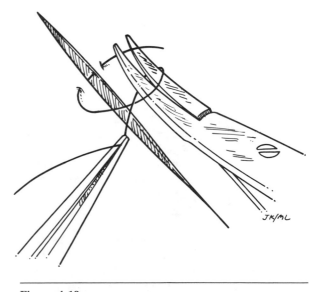

Figure 4-19
Grasping the short end of the suture. Forceps exert upward tension on the suture loop to prevent slippage while maneuvering the needle holder to grasp the suture end.

back into the field and positioned out of the way on the periphery while the suture is tied.

Tying the suture. After correct placement, the short end of the suture will protrude from the rubber to the right of the incision and the long piece from the left. With the forceps in the left hand, the long piece of suture should be grasped far enough back from the rubber sheet so a loop may conveniently be formed. Too short a length will result in a loop too small to work with, while too long a length will be unwieldy and will tend to tangle. The suture should emerge from the bottom of the forceps or from the side facing the surgeon. The tips of the forceps and those of the needle holder (or a second pair of forceps) in the right hand are then brought in proximity to the short suture. This will simplify matters once the actual tying is begun, since it will not be necessary to search for the short end. The forceps should be moved toward the incision, causing a loop to form naturally, or one can form the loop by moving the tips of the forceps in a circular fashion around the tips of the needle holder (Figure 4-18). The short suture end is then grasped with the needle holder and both ends of the suture are pulled,

letting the loop fall off the needle holder tips (Figure 4-19) and taking care to have the resulting half-knot lie flat. The knot should be tight enough just to bring the edges of the incision together.

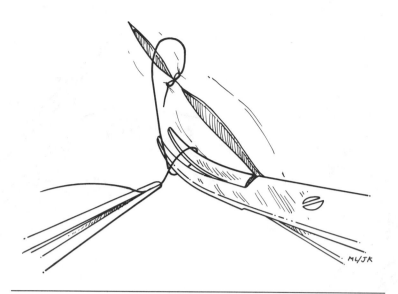

Figure 4-20
Tying of second half-knot. All knots should be placed to lie flat when tied.

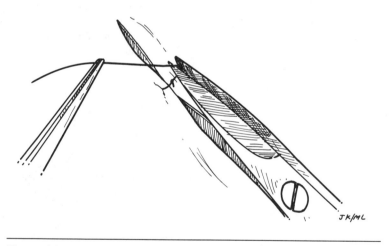

Figure 4-21
Cutting the suture after the third and final half-knot is tied. The suture should be cut under tension, not while it is lying loose or flat on the tissue surface.

If the short end of the suture is too short, the surgeon risks inadvertently pulling it out of the rubber sheet, particularly if the loop is also too small and in the resulting struggle the loop is enlarged at the expense of the short end. The surgeon may also accidentally allow the loop to slip off the tips of the needle holder while attempting to grasp the short end. This can be avoided by being conscious of the need to keep the loop seated around the jaws of the needle holder and be exerting upward tension on the suture with the forceps until the short end is grasped. If difficulty is experienced in grasping the short end, it is usually too short, angled inconveniently, lying flat against the surface of the rubber sheet, or not visible.

It is unwise to increase one's frustration by continually and unsuccessfully trying to grasp the suture with the same futile movements. Rather, the surgeon should stop, bring the short end into the proper position, and only then resume knot tying.

After the first knot is tied, the suture should not be released with the left-handed forceps. There is no need or advantage to releasing and regrasping the suture repeatedly during each step in the knot-tying procedure. Instead, the surgeon should proceed directly to tie the second half-knot as the first: forming a loop, grasping the short end through the loop, and pulling both ends of the suture, letting the loop slip off the needle holder

(Figure 4-20). The second half-knot should also lie flat and be fitted snugly up against the first but without obliterating the small circle of suture visible through the rubber sheeting. This practice will avoid devitalizing tissue.

The third and final half-knot is then placed. It can be tied tightly, since it locks the knot against itself, not against the tissue. If the tie has been made correctly, the suture may be cut at the knot. Each suture strand should be cut separately (Figure 4-21). If short pieces remain, they will be appropriately oriented, perpendicular to the incision.

If the needle has been positioned off the field of view, the suture is simply grasped and dragged across the field until the needle reappears and is repositioned in the needle holder as described previously. If the needle has remained visible off to the edge of the field, it is simply picked up and repositioned. The next suture may now be placed, spacing the sutures about a millimeter apart. As experience is gained, an objective assessment of the surgeon's progress may be made by timing how long it takes to place a given number of sutures.

After achieving reasonable competence in this exercise, the surgeon should change the orientation of the incision so that it crosses the field horizontally. This will necessitate flexing the wrist and rotating needle-holder tips counterclockwise. Next, the incision should be rearranged vertically and finally, obliquely, the orientation being from the upper right to the lower left quadrant. These various orientations will provide the opportunity to expand the necessary range of movements with the instruments so that the surgeon's movements become less mechanical and better coordinated. The successful microsurgeon must be able to place sutures efficiently and to position them consistently and precisely in as relaxed a manner as possible.

Rubber Tubing

Suturing glove rubber is basically a two-dimensional exercise. An added dimension is provided by soft rubber tubing of narrow diameter, which not only allows the above exercise to be performed but also provides the opportunity to rejoin a tubular structure.

Short lengths of tubing (3 to 6 cm long, 1 to 2 mm in diameter) are stapled to a flat piece of cardboard oriented as above. Using a scalpel, a cut is made between the staples perpendicular to the long axis of the tubing, transecting it. The cut edges are then anastomosed by placing a series of interrupted sutures around the entire circumference. Sutures are placed through the full thickness of the wall into the lumen. The so-called six o'clock or inferior suture is placed first, since it is the most difficult technically to place and will quickly become visually inaccessible if other sutures are placed and tied first. The same rules apply as with glove rubber. The suture must

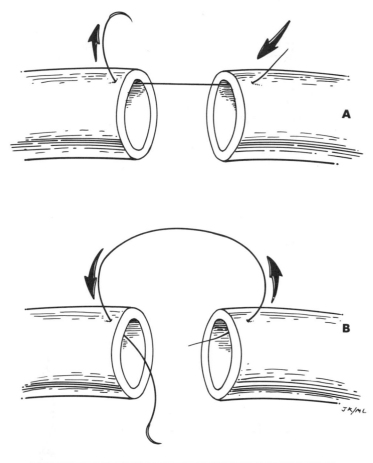

Figure 4-22
Sequence of suture placement and orientation in rubber tubing. **A,** Correct technique. **B,** Such placement would require knots being tied inside the lumen.

be placed so that the knot lies flat and outside the lumen. This is accomplished by passing the needle into the lumen from the outside toward the inside of the cut end of the tubing on the right, followed by passing it from the inside to the outside of the opposite segment of the tubing. If the process were reversed, the knot would have to be tied on the inside (Figure 4-22). Depending on the luminal diameter and the wall thickness of the tubing, four to six sutures equidistantly spaced around the perimeter of the tubing will adequately reapproximate the ends. If the lumen is wide and the walls are thin, additional sutures may be needed. In general, the number of sutures to be placed in any structure should be sufficient to reestablish the normal anatomic relationship of the parts joined. Although it may technically be feasible to place additional sutures, care should be taken to avoid overpowering the tissue. Apart from the added manipulation and possible trauma, excess numbers of sutures may restrict blood flow and devitalize tissue.

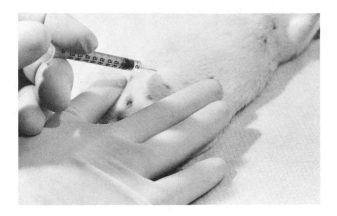

Figure 4-23
Intraperitoneal injection.

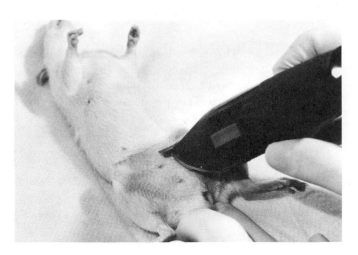

Figure 4-24
The rat abdomen is shaved.

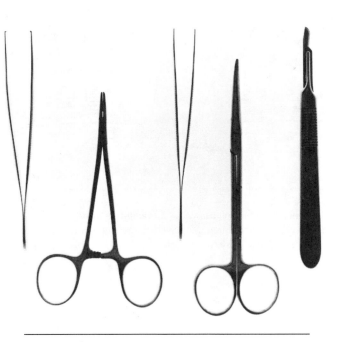

Figure 4-25
Instruments used for conventional dissection: *(left to right)* toothed forceps, plastic needle carrier, smooth forceps, small Metzenbaum scissors, and standard scalpel handle with no. 15 blade.

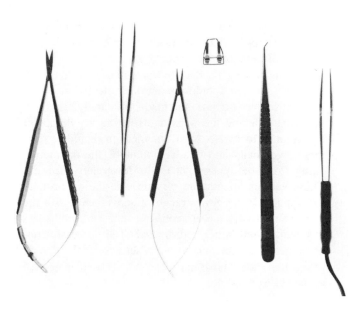

Figure 4-26
Microsurgical instruments: *(left to right)* scissors, straight jeweler's forceps, needle carrier, vascular clamp, angled jeweler's forceps, and fine bipolar forceps.

ANIMAL MODELS

Those fortunate enough to have access to laboratory animals can obtain living tissue on which to work. This will introduce the added dimension of blood flow and the need to achieve hemostasis. Iatrogenically induced trauma causes bleeding and leads eventually to obliteration of the anatomy if the trauma is extensive and excessive. Thus working with living tissue is of great value in realistically imparting the degree of skill necessary to undertake gynecologic microsurgery in humans.

Rat femoral artery and vein models

Performing anastomosis on rat femoral artery and vein models is an excellent exercise. It has numerous advantages: the rat is inexpensive, resistant to infection, and a relatively easy animal on which to work. The procedure demands precise technique, can be performed in approximately 1½ hours, and does not require the presence of an assistant.

At the time the supply house delivers them, each adult female rat weighs approximately 200 gm. Each rat un-

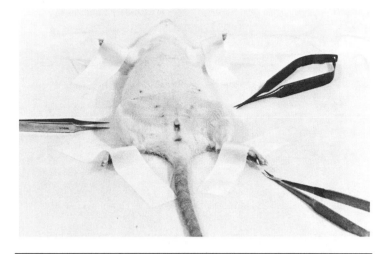

Figure 4-27
Position of anesthetized rat and instruments.

dergoes two procedures—one on each femoral artery—over a period of several weeks. One can note which groin is being operated on by placing a small notch in the ipsilateral ear of the anesthetized animal. After all surgery has been performed, the rats are killed with enflurane or fluothane.

Induction of Anesthesia

After being weighed, the animal is placed in a large glass container that holds a sponge saturated with a nonexplosive anesthetic agent such as fluothane or enflurane. As soon as it has stopped voluntary activity (usually in about 1 minute), it is removed, even if it appears to be awake, because it is not able to survive several seconds of overexposure.

The rat is placed supine and is injected without delay (Figure 4-23). The anesthetic of choice is sodium pentobarbital (Nembutal-Veterinary), which is available in multidose vials containing 60 mg per ml. This may conveniently be diluted 1:10 in saline and administered in a dose of 6 mg per 100 gm body weight. The preferred route of administration is intraperitoneal injection. The tip of a 25-gauge needle (tuberculin syringe) is inserted through the abdominal wall immediately inferior to the umbilicus. After insertion of the needle, the tip should be withdrawn slightly to ensure that it is free in the peritoneal cavity and not in the wall or lumen of the gut. The calculated volume of anesthetic is then administered. The animal should be returned to its cage until anesthesia is achieved, generally within 2 to 10 minutes. If necessary, additional anesthetic can be injected intraperitoneally in 0.1-ml increments. Care must be taken not to give excess sodium pentobarbital. The greatest risk to these animals is not infection but death from overdose.

If it is not possible to determine the animal's weight accurately, a succession of small doses may be given and the effect titrated by noting the progressive decline of response to a pain stimulus delivered with toothed forceps to the interdigital webs of a paw. Surgically anesthetized animals demonstrate refractoriness to pain, rhythmic abdominal breathing, and a strong pulse palpable in the thorax. When the rat is asleep, its abdomen is shaved with a standard electric razor (Figure 4-24).

Instruments used for conventional dissection consist of toothed forceps, plastic needle carrier, smooth forceps, small Metzenbaum scissors, and a standard scalpel handle with a no. 15 blade (Figure 4-25). Microsurgical instruments are scissors, straight and angled jeweler's forceps, needle carrier, vascular clamp, and a fine bipolar forceps (Figure 4-26). The clamp shown is a Louisville clamp.* The anesthetized rat is loosely taped to a breadboard that has been wrapped with an absorbent, heavy drainage pad (Figure 4-27). Silk tape is excellent because it sticks well. Instruments are positioned so that their points are directed toward the proposed site of surgery. A beaker of saline solution and a syringe are at hand to keep the tissues moist. Figures 4-28 and 4-29 show a femoral artery procedure in progress.

The surgeon draws the planned incision with a marking pen, beginning at the anterior junction of the thigh and trunk, and curving around on the abdominal wall to end at the posterior junction of the thigh and trunk (Figure 4-30). This allows space for developing a flap to expose the femoral triangle.

Conventional technique

The surgeon fixes the skin with the thumb and forefinger of the opposite hand and makes an incision through the skin, following the pen line (Figure 4-31). The skin is

---

*Catalog no. 65172, Edward Weck & Company, Inc.

Text cont'd on p. 50.

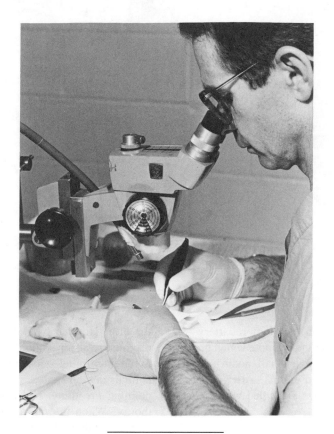

Figure 4-28
Femoral artery surgery.

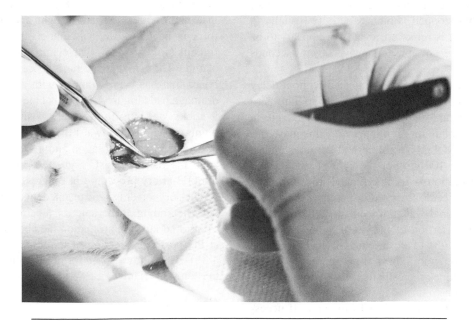

Figure 4-29
Close-up of instruments used in Figure 4-28. A pencil grip is necessary to use these miniature instruments properly.

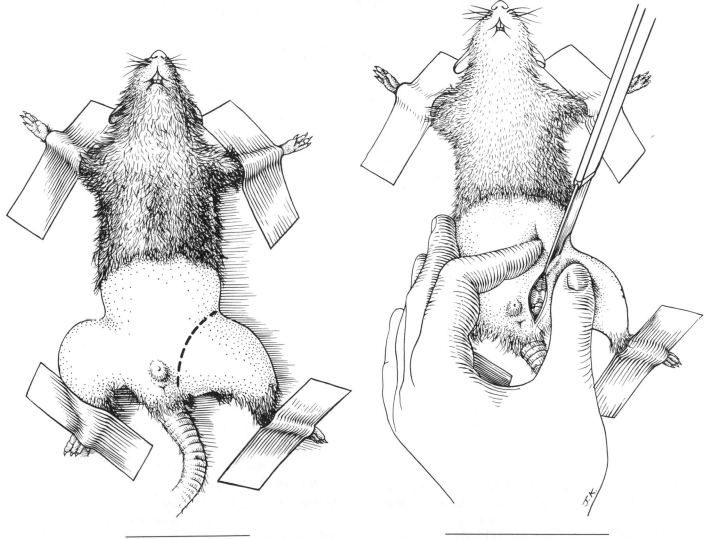

Figure 4-30
Line of planned incision.

Figure 4-31
Incision is made on the pen line.

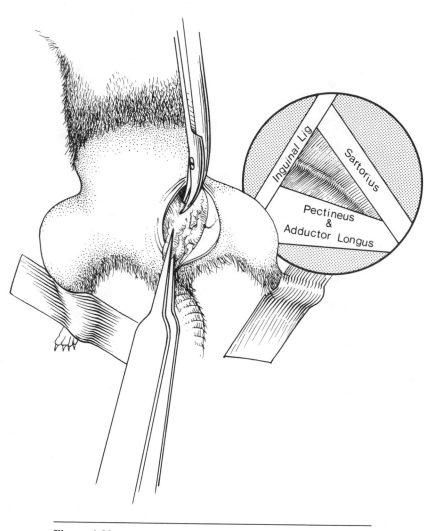

Figure 4-32
Dissection of subcutaneous tissue to expose the femoral triangle.

extremely mobile, and only by following the line can a proper flap be developed. Subcutaneous tissue is dissected away from the abdominal muscles with a toothed forceps and Metzenbaum scissors (Figure 4-32). The flap is developed laterally exposing the femoral triangle. Bleeding is controlled with bipolar forceps.

Using a conventional needle carrier, the surgeon places a suture of 3-0 monofilament material in a figure-of-eight manner through the inguinal ligament, allowing satisfactory traction of the rectus muscles medially to expose the triangle. The surgeon must avoid small arterioles, particularly medially. A damp sponge keeps the flap moist and retracted laterally. The needle carrier is used to retract the inguinal ligament. Either permanent or absorbable sutures may be used (Figure 4-33). There is now ample exposure of the triangle (Figure 4-34) with a viable flap laterally. With this technique, the surgeon will not need an assistant.

Microsurgical technique

At this point, the surgeon converts to a microsurgical technique. Using either straight or curved microscissors and straight jeweler's forceps, the surgeon places a linear incision along the femoral vein, incising the femoral sheath for the full length of the triangle (Figure 4-35). Tissue is brushed away beneath the sheath before incising it to identify small bleeders. Most of these are very small and stop bleeding spontaneously. The surgeon places traction lateral to the femoral nerve trunks and carefully incises between the nerve trunks and femoral artery (Figure 4-36). These trunks must not be damaged. Using an angulated jeweler's forceps, the femoral artery and vein are lifted gently anteriorly, and the deep femoral artery and deep femoral vein are each identified, separated, and coagulated with bipolar forceps and sharply divided (Figure 4-37). This completely frees the vessels from the floor of the femoral triangle. The surgeon lifts the vessel

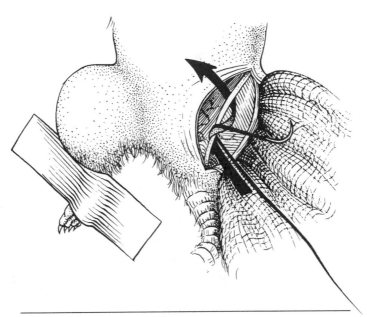

Figure 4-33
Figure-of-eight placement of sutures through the inguinal ligament.

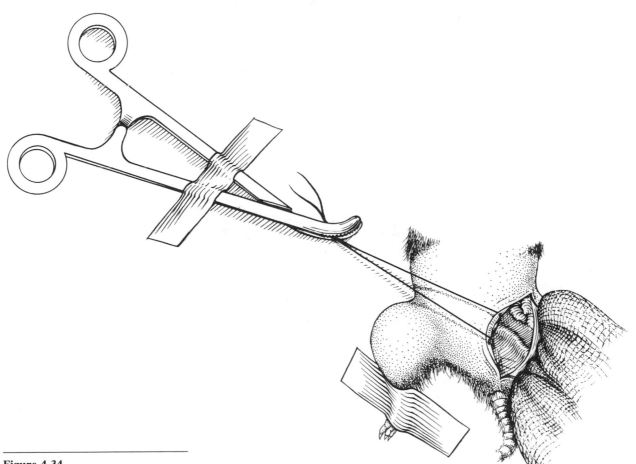

Figure 4-34
Exposure of the inguinal triangle.

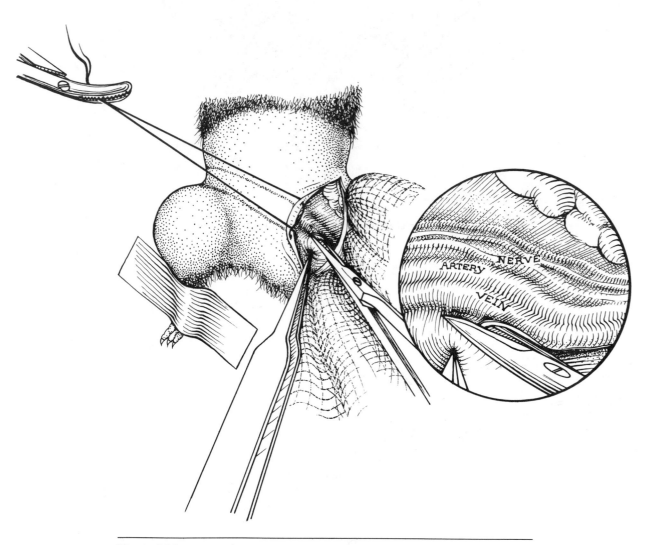

Figure 4-35
Using microsurgical technique, the femoral sheath is incised along the femoral vein.

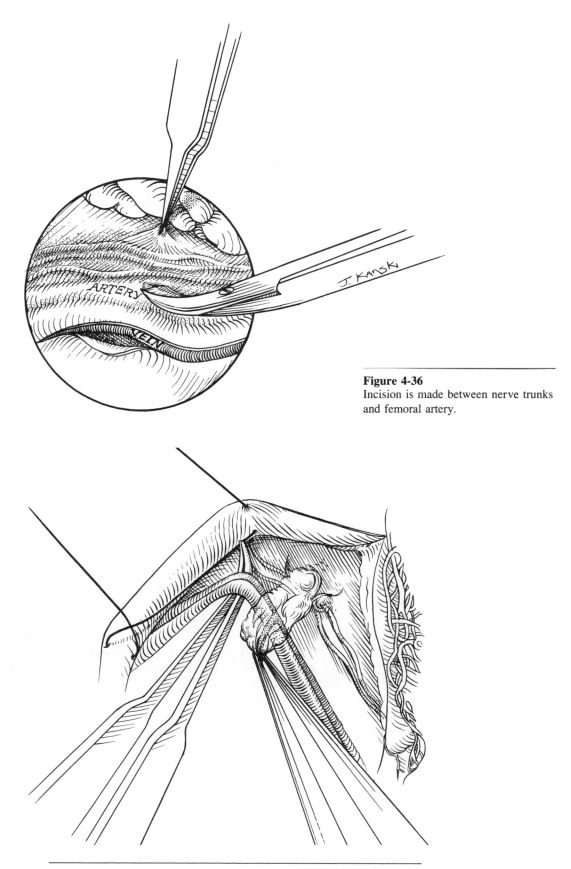

Figure 4-36
Incision is made between nerve trunks and femoral artery.

Figure 4-37
The femoral artery and vein are freed from the floor of the femoral triangle.

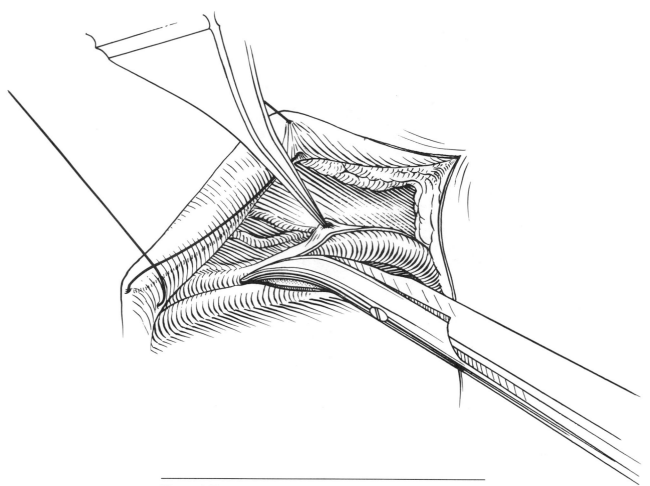

Figure 4-38
The femoral artery is separated carefully from the femoral vein.

anteriorly by its adventitia and by sharp dissection, separates the artery from the vein (Figure 4-38). This must be done with great care, since the femoral vein will rupture easily. Small tears in the femoral vein may be controlled by pressure. If the defect is large and not controlled by pressure, it may be necessary to sacrifice the vein with bipolar coagulation.

The surgeon floods the femoral triangle with 1% lidocaine to relax the arterial wall (Figure 4-39). The artery dilates greatly as spasm is overcome. This relaxation is obtained in only 1 or 2 minutes.

The surgeon applies the vascular clamp to occlude the femoral artery and positions it with the tips projecting just beneath and beyond the artery (Figure 4-40). Before clamping the artery, the surgeon spaces the tips wide apart. The proximal portion of the artery is occluded first. The Louisville clamp has pegs to which stay sutures may be attached; several similar models are available that can be used instead. A smooth forceps is ideal for opening the jaws of the clamp. The surgeon positions the clamp and places a thin strip of latex, previously taken from the glove, beneath the clamp and artery. This serves as

a mat to partition the deeper structures. The clamp can also be placed in the opposite direction. The surgeon uses straight or curved scissors to divide the artery midway between the jaws but not at the origin of the deep femoral trunk (Figure 4-41). The ends of the artery retract at this point. Using jeweler's forceps, the surgeon stretches the adventitia over the end of each vessel (Figure 4-42) and sharply excises the adventitia (Figure 4-43).

Using an insulin syringe with a 27-gauge needle, the surgeon carefully irrigates the arterial lumen with one drop of heparin dissolved in lactated Ringer's solution (Figure 4-44). This removes all blood from the lumen. The surgeon does not grasp the arterial wall, but rather its adventitia. The surgeon then dilates the lumen of each arterial segment with jeweler's forceps (Figure 4-45). This is done only once, and care must be taken to avoid overstretching the artery.

With a smooth forceps, the surgeon brings the tips of the clamp closer together so that the ends of the segments are in proximity but not touching (Figure 4-46). The space separating the two ends should be about one-half

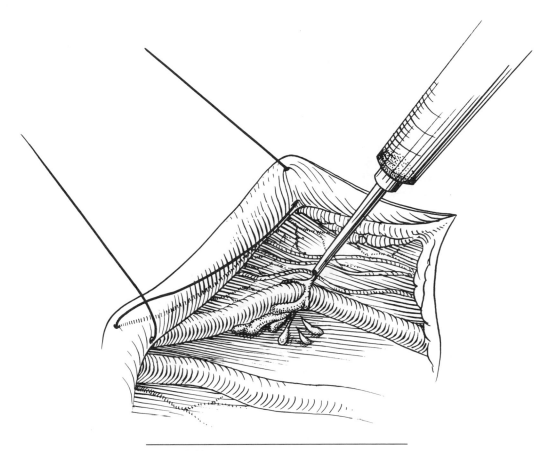

Figure 4-39
The femoral triangle is flooded with 1% lidocaine.

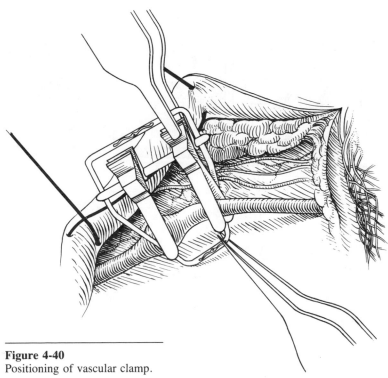

Figure 4-40
Positioning of vascular clamp.

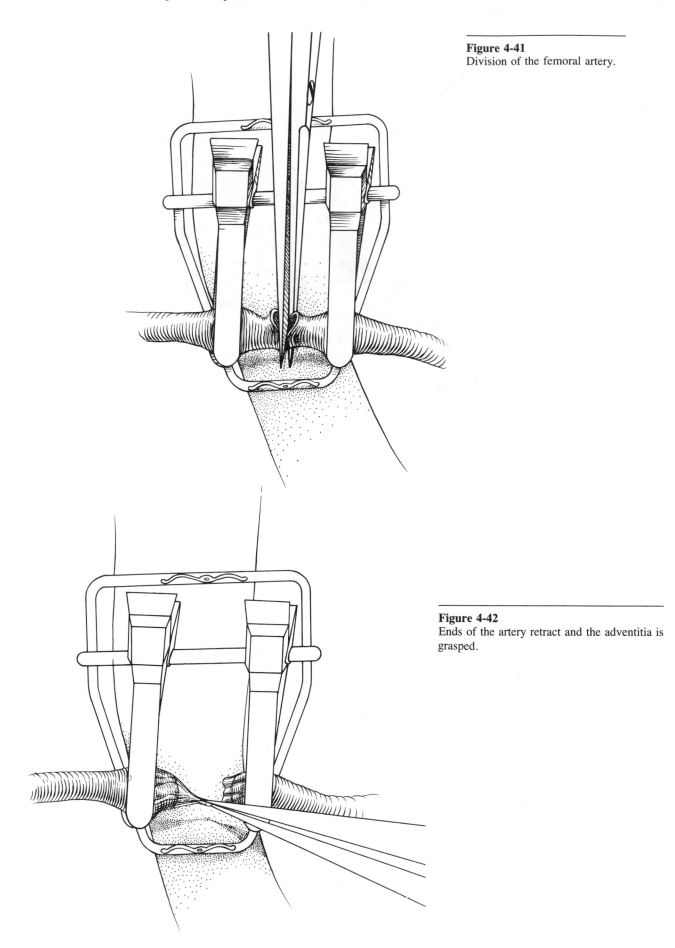

Figure 4-41
Division of the femoral artery.

Figure 4-42
Ends of the artery retract and the adventitia is grasped.

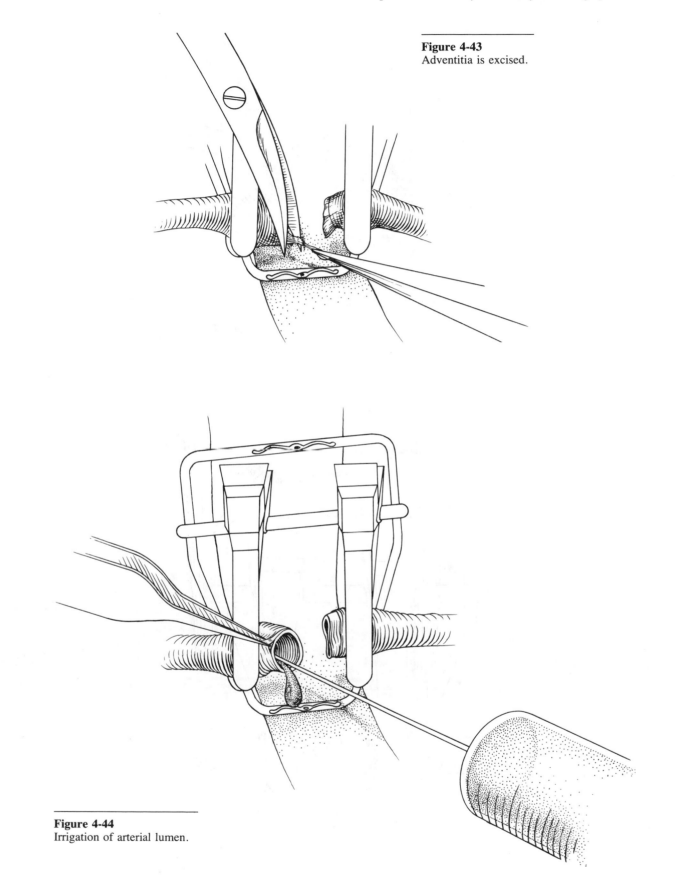

Figure 4-43
Adventitia is excised.

Figure 4-44
Irrigation of arterial lumen.

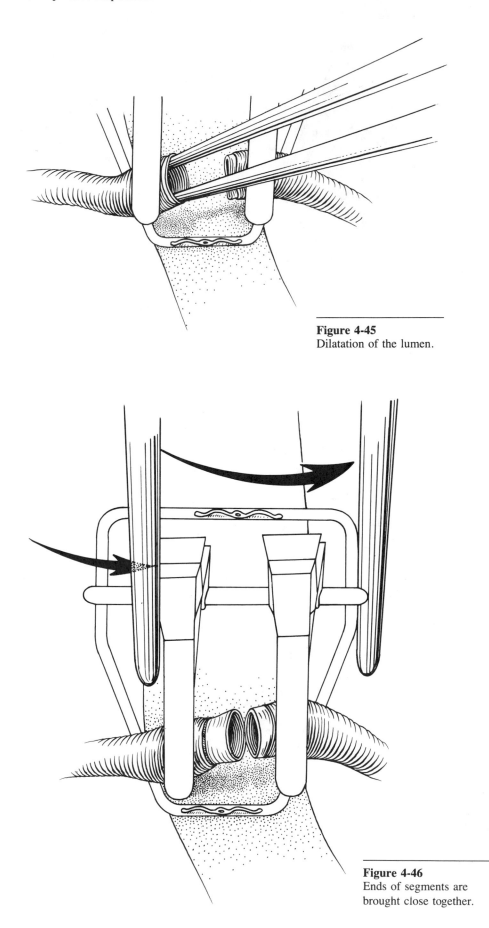

Figure 4-45
Dilatation of the lumen.

Figure 4-46
Ends of segments are
brought close together.

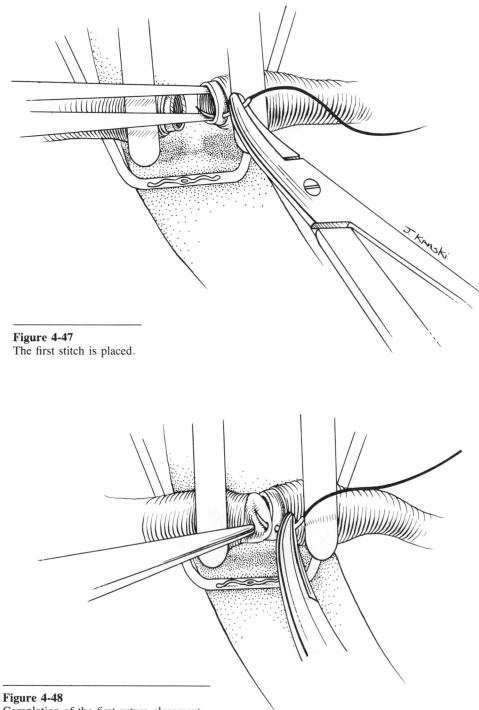

Figure 4-47
The first stitch is placed.

Figure 4-48
Completion of the first suture placement.

the diameter of the artery. With 10-0 nylon on a 75-μ tapered needle, the surgeon places the first stitch (Figure 4-47). With the needle grasped at or shortly back of the midpoint, the surgeon inserts the needle through the wall of the artery, using the tip of the jeweler's forceps to stabilize the arterial wall. Employing counterpressure technique, the surgeon places the needle through the ar-

terial wall of the opposite segment and completes the knot (Figure 4-48). This may be done in one or two passes. The suture is placed under high magnification but tied under low magnification. One end of the suture is left long and the other end is placed around the nearby peg on the frame (Figure 4-49). This serves as one of the stay sutures.

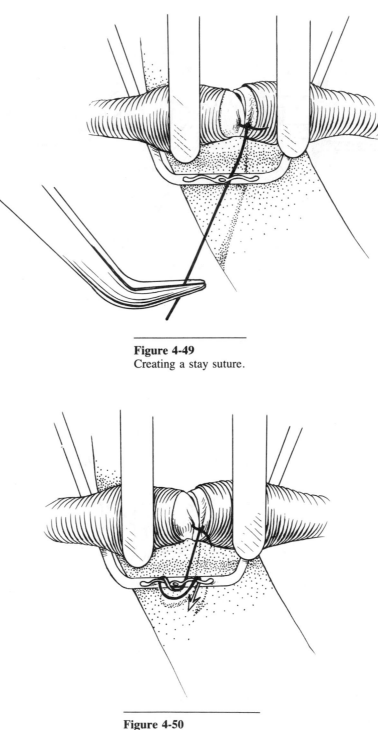

Figure 4-49
Creating a stay suture.

Figure 4-50
Completion of the suture.

The suture is wound around the peg several times and the end is cut (Figure 4-50). The second suture is placed in a similar manner, approximately 120 degrees around the vessel from the first suture (Figure 4-51). This is critical because the posterior wall of the artery will not fall away if they are placed at 180 degrees. The surgeon completes the suture using counterpressure (Figure 4-52), ties the second knot (Figure 4-53), and places the long end around the nearest peg. The short end of this stitch will be used for traction in placing the subsequent stitch. Using the short end of the first suture for traction, the surgeon places and ties the third stitch, leaving one end long (Figure 4-54), and then cuts back the short end of the first suture (Figure 4-55). The fourth suture is

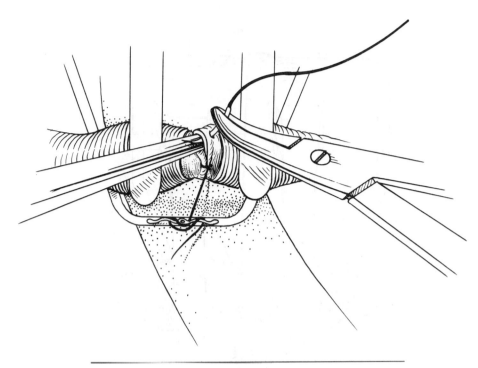

Figure 4-51
The second suture is placed at 120 degrees from the first suture.

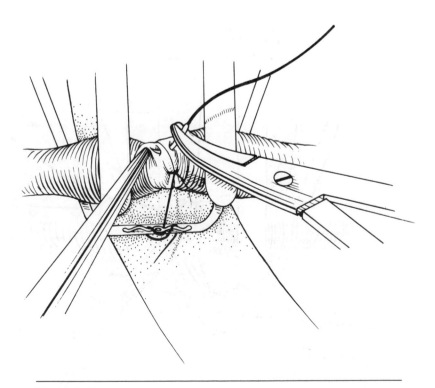

Figure 4-52
The second suture is completed. Note that the arterial wall is not grasped.

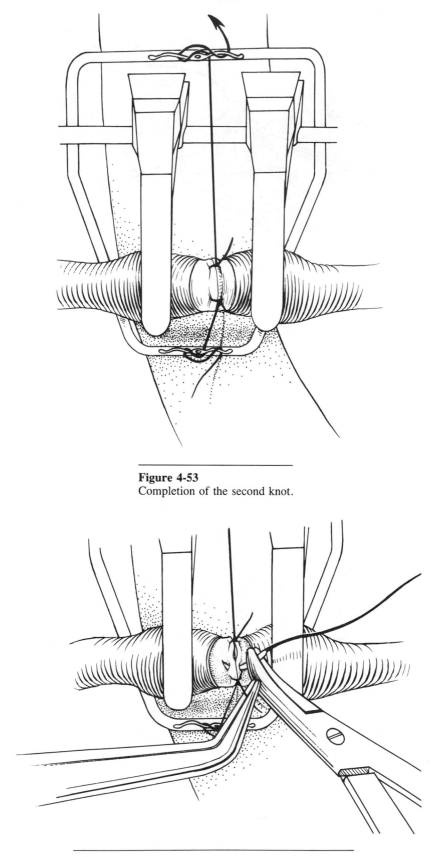

Figure 4-53
Completion of the second knot.

Figure 4-54
The third suture is placed and tied; one end is left long.

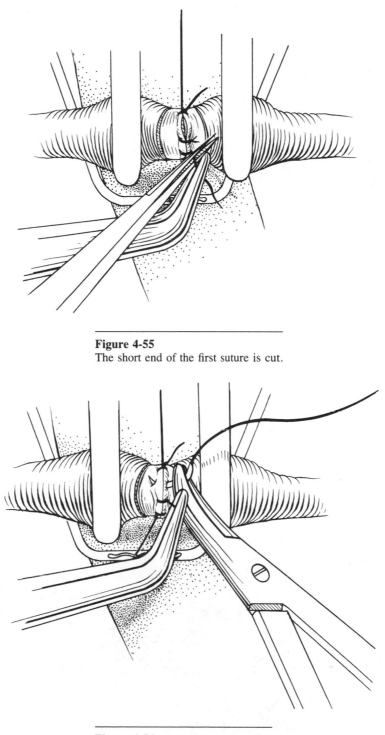

Figure 4-55
The short end of the first suture is cut.

Figure 4-56
The fourth suture is placed and tied.

placed and tied in the same manner (Figure 4-56). This technique is possible because the posterior wall of the artery has dropped away because of 120-degree placement of the first and second sutures. The surgeon cuts all short ends (Figure 4-57), and suturing of the anterior wall of the artery is now complete (Figure 4-58).

The surgeon then turns the clamp over to expose the posterior arterial wall (Figure 4-59). Because the artery is held with the tip of the jaws, the clamp can be turned easily. The surgeon tucks the frame of the retractor beneath the abdominal wall muscles to keep it as flat as possible. Having turned over the clamp and positioned

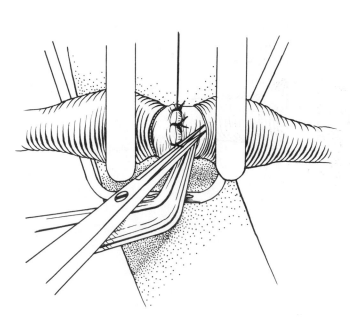

Figure 4-57
All short ends are cut.

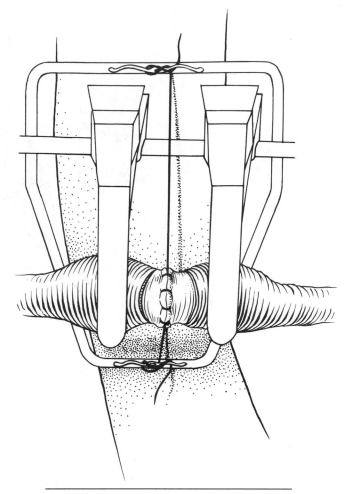

Figure 4-58
Suturing of the anterior arterial wall is complete.

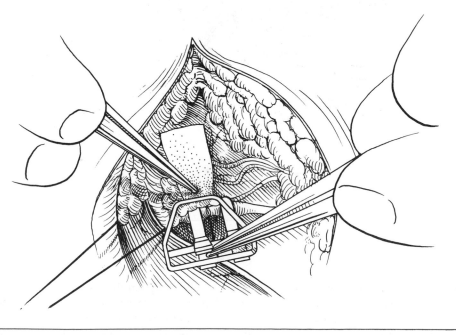

Figure 4-59
The clamp is turned over to expose the posterior arterial wall; the mat is adjusted beneath the clamp.

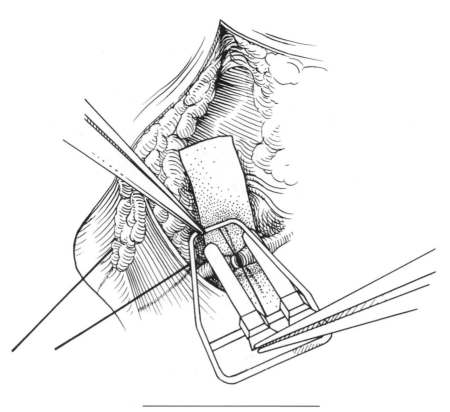

Figure 4-60
Closure of the posterior wall begins.

the mat, the surgeon is ready to begin closing the opposite wall (Figure 4-60).

The first stitch is placed near the opposite stay suture (Figure 4-61). Using traction on the long end of this suture, the surgeon is able to rotate the arterial wall and place the second stitch very close to the angle suture (Figure 4-62). This is a common site for leakage, and meticulous care must be taken in placing the stitch very close to the adjacent stay suture. The third stitch is placed on the near side of the first stitch (Figure 4-63) and the appropriate numbers of stitches are placed in a similar manner to complete the posterior wall anastomosis (Figure 4-64).

All posterior wall sutures are placed and neatly cut (Figure 4-65). The surgeon turns the clamp back over, and removes the clamp, first releasing the distal blade. Before removing the clamp, stay sutures are cut, leaving them long.

The anastomosis invariably leaks when the clamp is removed. To correct this, the surgeon should wrap the anastomosis with a small strip of abdominal wall muscle, harvested just before removing the clamp. If bleeding is too profuse, the surgeon may temporarily reapply the clamp, irrigate the blood from within the vessel, and place one or two additional sutures through the site of leakage. If bleeding resumes after removal of the clamp,

it may be necessary to sacrifice the femoral artery with bipolar coagulation. The rat will usually recover without loss of function because of its rich collateral circulation.

The surgeon checks patency by lifting the artery gently with a closed jeweler's forceps to observe the "flicker sign," the pulsatile flow over the tips of the forceps (Figure 4-66). After hemostasis is obtained and patency checked, the wound is carefully irrigated. The muscle strip is left in place. The monofilament 3-0 traction suture is removed, and this same suture is used to close the skin in a single layer. The suture is placed in a running, nonlocking manner, incorporating the skin and subcutaneous layer. The rat will remove this suture several days later with its teeth. Alternatively, the surgeon may place a subcuticular stitch.

These techniques may be used in performing a femoral vein anastomosis. Because of its low pressure, the vein does not require sutures being placed so close together, and significant leakage is unusual. The only difference in technique is that the distal venous segment is clamped first and released last.

Rat uterine horn

The rat uterine horn is an excellent advanced learning aid. It is appropriate for performing end-to-end anasto-

Text cont'd on p. 68.

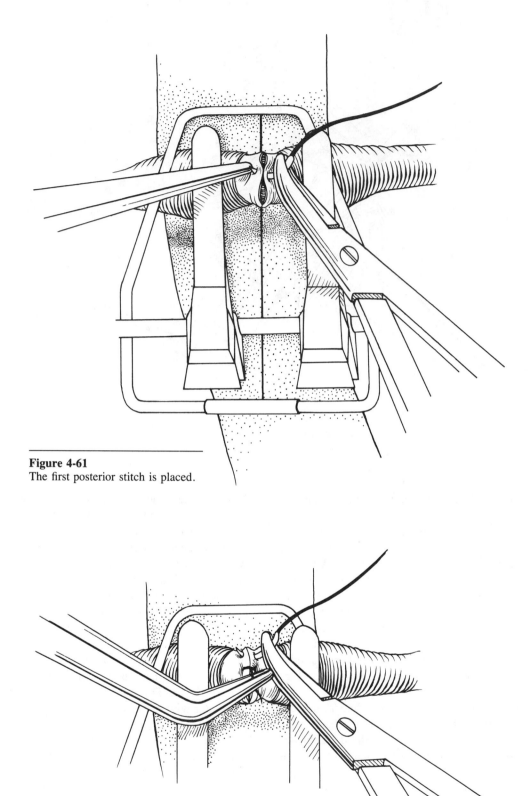

Figure 4-61
The first posterior stitch is placed.

Figure 4-62
The second posterior stitch is placed.

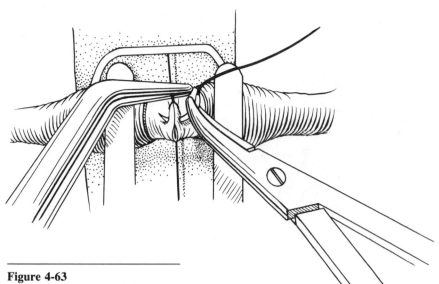

Figure 4-63
The third posterior stitch is placed.

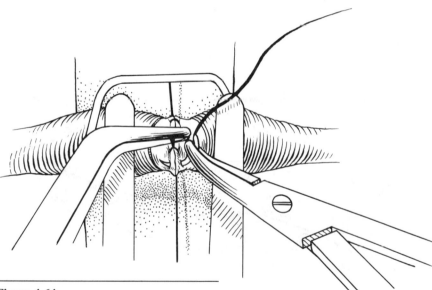

Figure 4-64
The remaining posterior stitches are placed.

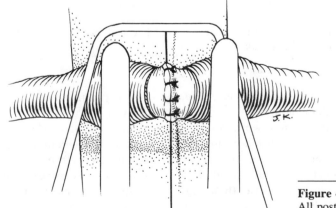

Figure 4-65
All posterior sutures are neatly cut.

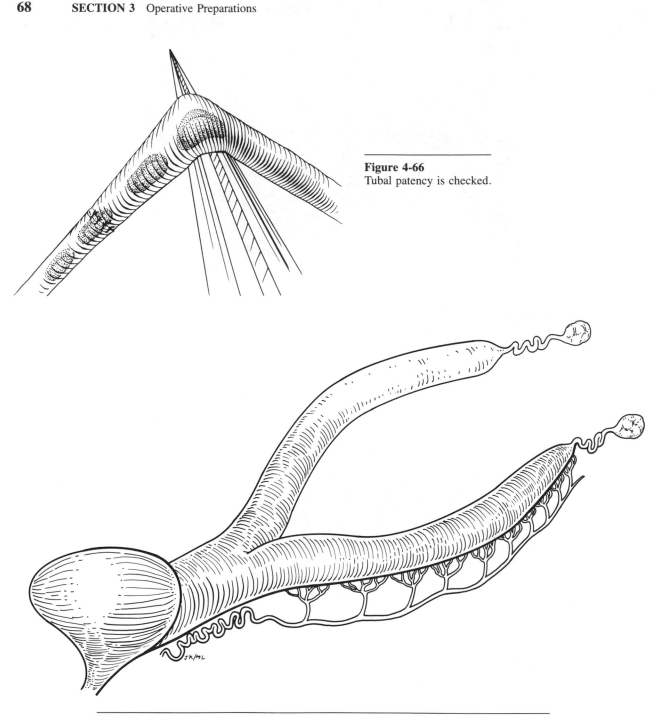

Figure 4-66
Tubal patency is checked.

Figure 4-67
Rat genital anatomy. Note that the oviduct is a highly coiled, narrow organ that is much too small for microsurgical manipulation.

mosis after simple transection or segmental resection, salpingostomy, and lateral salpingotomy.

In the rat, the uterus is divided into two horns. The bifurcation lies posterior to the urinary bladder with both horns extending laterally. After one locates the uterine horns, which are dense, tubular, red, well-vascularized structures supported by individual mesenteries (broad ligaments), both horns should be brought to the exterior by grasping them between the thumb and index fingers and applying upward traction. An avascular, fat-free window of mesentery should be positioned beneath each horn and pierced with a toothpick or similar object. This will prevent the uterus from retracting into the abdominal cavity. The abdomen may be surgically draped or left uncovered. At this point and intermittently throughout the ensuing procedure, one should moisten all exposed tissue by irrigation with saline, Ringer's, or other suitable solution. The rat is then placed beneath the objective of the operating microscope, which is focused on one of the exposed, stabilized uterine horns.

Each uterine horn receives its blood supply from a division of the uterine artery that branches repeatedly in the mesentery and undergoes further arborization before entering the horn (Figure 4-67). The horn is composed of an outer serosal layer, a middle muscular layer, and in inner mucosal layer. The serosa is attached directly to the muscularis with only sparse intervening connective tissue separating them. The serosa, being the outermost layer covering the entire external aspect of the horn, is the easiest layer to identify. The muscularis, analogous to the myosalpinx, is a dense but thin translucent layer of tissue that appears under magnification to be relatively avascular. Because of its toughness and intimate covering of the serosa, the muscularis offers great resistance to passage of the needle. The mucosa, analogous to the endosalpinx, is a soft, thick layer of tissue that lacks the extensive pattern of folds characteristic of the endosalpinx. Under magnification, it appears pulpy and exhibits an extensively branched pattern of fine blood vessels. This layer offers little resistance to passage of the needle and hence may inadvertently be deeply penetrated by a carelessly positioned needle.

PROCEDURES
End-to-end anastomosis

Under microscopic visualization, a relatively avascular area should be selected between major branches of the uterine artery supplying the segment of uterine horn to be transected. Although it is possible to cut between these major vessels, it is necessary to use the bipolar cautery to coagulate the terminal arborization of small vessels that insert into the horn. To do this, the power should be adjusted to a low setting and its effect tested on vessels of comparable size in nongenital tissue, such as the fat in the mesentery or the omentum.

The correct technique of bipolar coagulation is to grasp the tissue without bringing the two electrodes into direct contact. What is desired is a flow of current from one electrode to the other through the intervening space containing the tissue to be coagulated. If the electrodes are squeezed together, tissue will be crushed and extruded, causing the current to bypass it, since the current will flow higher up on the forceps where the electrodes touch. Such torn and crushed noncoagulated vessels will bleed when the forceps are released. Instead, the tissue to be coagulated should be gently grasped, making sure the electrodes are separated, and the foot pedal depressed. The power should be such that the tissue heats up from passage of the current and gradually coagulates. High-power settings should be avoided, since they instanta-

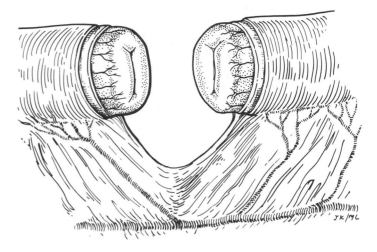

Figure 4-68
Appearance of the rat uterine horn after simple transection. The horn has been completely severed, with the incision carefully placed to avoid adjacent major branches of the uterine artery.

neously carbonize the tissue, welding it to the electrodes and causing bleeding when the forceps are disengaged. The greater the distance between electrodes, the higher the setting required to get a flow of current; similarly, the drier the tissue, the less conductive it is. Therefore one must be sure (1) not to grasp an excessive amount of tissue and (2) that the tissue is moist. If it is necessary to coagulate blood vessels close to tissue that must be protected from thermal trauma, the tissue should be irrigated while the vessels are coagulated. The flow of cool liquid will act as a heat sink. One should be aware, however, that it is possible to form a pool of boiling liquid that will damage a wide area of tissue if a flow of irrigating solution sufficient to carry away the excess heat is not maintained. Also, too copious irrigation may prevent coagulation of the tissue by keeping the tissue cool.

After one has selected an area for transection and coagulation of blood vessels on the mesenteric border, one should transect the horn under low magnification. The horn should be held between the thumb and index finger or grasped gently with forceps and, with fine iris scissors, be cut perpendicular to its long axis, continuing the incision into the mesentery until the horn has been completely severed (Figure 4-68). This procedure must be meticulously performed without chopping or sawing away at the tissue. Instead, the surgeon should try for a clean, continuous cut in a single plane, avoiding excessive dissection and the creation of a large defect in the mesentery. If brisk bleeding from the cut edge of the uterine horn occurs and does not arrest spontaneously, precise, pinpoint, low-power coagulation should be used to achieve hemostasis. If the area is covered with blood,

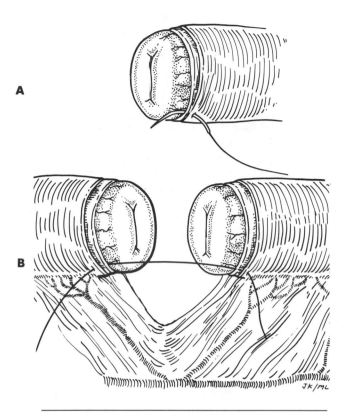

Figure 4-69

A, Placement of initial suture on the mesenteric aspect of the uterine horn. Passage of the needle includes the full thickness of the serosa and muscularis with emergence at the interface between mucosa and muscularis. **B,** Placement is completed and the suture is ready for tying.

making visualization of point bleeders difficult or impossible, the area should be irrigated and each source of bleeding located, grasped with the bipolar forceps, and have current applied. Absolute hemostasis is not necessary. Capillary oozing of the cut edges is consistent with living tissue, and no steps to control it need be taken. Such bleeding arrests spontaneously or ceases when the cut edges of the horn are apposed after anastomosis. If a large defect has been created in the mesentery, one or several sutures should be placed through the cut edges to reapproximate the ends of the uterine horn before beginning the anastomosis.

Next, the transected uterine horn should be examined at high power and the serosa, muscularis, and mucosa in cross section identified. If blood has been allowed to accumulate and clot on the cut surface, it should be irrigated and lifted off with the forceps so the anatomy can be visualized. All three tissue layers must be identified before the anastomosis proceeds. Blindly passing the needle without regard for tubal anatomy invalidates the use of the microscope and propels the surgeon back to the realm of macrosurgery.

Because the rat uterus is a seromuscular organ with little intervening connective tissue between the serosa and muscularis, these layers are both included in the suture as a single unit. The suture will, however, specifically avoid including the mucosa. The first suture placed is positioned at approximately the 6 o'clock position and includes the serosa, continuous with the medial surface of the mesentery, and the muscularis. In a young animal or one that is nulliparous, the muscularis is approximately the same thickness as a 130-μ diameter needle and the full thickness of the muscularis should be included. The needle will thus enter the serosa, penetrate into the muscularis, and exit the tissue at the interface between the mucosa and muscularis (Figure 4-69). Because of the distance between the cut edges of the left and right segments of uterine horn, it is necessary to pass the needle completely through the right-hand segment, regrasp it in the needle holder, and pass it through the left-hand segment.

The detailed sequence for suture placement is as follows. The needle is grasped as in the glove rubber exercise. Under high power, the cut edges of the serosa, muscularis, and mucosa of the right-hand segment of uterine horn are identified. The intended point of entry of the needle (about three needle widths back from the cut edge of the serosa) is selected, with the needle being oriented perpendicular to the long axis of the uterine horn, and the serosa and muscularis are penetrated. The forceps held in the left hand is used to supply counterpressure. The tissue should not be grasped. Instead, the forceps, with the tips kept separated, should be positioned to run across the cut edge of the tissue, bracketing the intended point of exit of the needle. Once the serosa and muscularis are penetrated, the orientation of the needle should be gradually changed so that it is parallel to the long axis of the uterine horn. Depth of penetration may be controlled by simultaneously decreasing the angle of penetration and visually confirming the path of the needle through the semitransparent tissue. The needle should exit at the juncture of the mucosa and muscularis. The microscope is then changed to a lower magnification and the needle is pulled through, using the needle holder and taking care not to damage the point of the needle. The needle is repositioned in the needle holder and the magnification is returned to high power.

A point should be selected on the left stump of the uterine horn that anatomically corresponds to the point of exit of the suture on the right side. This will be the point of entry of the needle into the left side and should be at the point of contact of the mucosa and the muscularis. The needle, held parallel to the long axis of the uterine horn, is driven into the tissue. One should strive to get equal and symmetric bites of tissue on both stumps. With counterpressure applied on the serosal surface around the intended point of needle emergence, the path

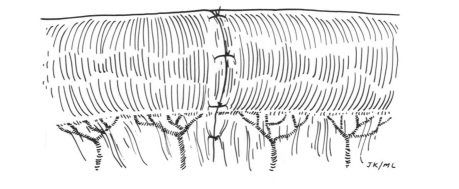

Figure 4-70
Completed end-to-end anastomosis of rat uterine horn after transection. Note the small defect in the mesentery and its repair with a single interrupted suture. When evenly and symmetrically placed, a minimum number of sutures produces excellent coaptation of cut edges.

of the needle should be adjusted so that it is perpendicular to the long axis of the horn when it emerges. The needle is then pulled out, the microscope is changed to low magnification, and the suture is tied. To overcome the tension separating the two uterine stumps, the first part of the knot should be a double throw to prevent the stumps from pulling apart before the knot is completed.

All sutures are placed in this fashion. The second knot is usually placed at the 12 o'clock or antimesenteric position. If each knot is placed symmetrically, the anatomy will be accurately restored. A sufficient number of sutures should be placed to coapt the edges smoothly around the entire circumference without any large gaps. Excessive mechanical manipulation and trauma sufficient to macerate and obliterate the normal anatomy should be strictly avoided. The completed anastomosis should be free of petechial hemorrhages or any obvious signs of trauma. Apart from the presence of a series of circumferentially positioned sutures defining the line of transection, the uterine horn should appear essentially undisturbed (Figure 4-70). Several anastomoses may be performed in this manner.

If suitable holding facilities are available, the laparotomy incision may be closed (using interrupted sutures of 2-0 nylon, silk, etc., placed through all layers or, alternatively, using metal wound clips) and examined several days or weeks later. Rats rarely become infected. Surgery performed under clean conditions requires no antibiotic prophylaxis. The animal is simply returned to its cage and kept warm and free from drafts. If keeping the animal is not feasible, several milliliters of anesthetic should be administered directly into the heart to produce death.

To evaluate the results of surgery, whether immediately on completion or following a period of healing, it is useful to examine the surgical site. The uterine horn should be cut open lengthwise along the antimesenteric border across the anastomosis (or anastomoses) and the internal configuration examined. There should be no obvious constrictions and the mucosa should not be bunched together in the area of anastomosis. A few drops of dilute methylene blue or indigo carmine spread over the exposed mucosa, allowed to stand for 30 seconds, and then irrigated with saline, will place the surface in relief and aid in evaluation of the technical adequacy of the microsurgery. If the examination is made several days after surgery, in addition to the above evaluation, the anastomosis should be examined for the presence of adhesions.

Segmental resection

End-to-end anastomosis following segmental resection furnishes the opportunity to undertake a more ambitious and technically demanding type of procedure. Under low magnification, one selects for resection a length of uterine horn perfused by a well-defined vascular tree consisting of a major branch of the uterine artery and its terminal arborization perfusing the segment (Figure 4-71). The segment is isolated by tying off the blood supply in the mesentery or with bipolar coagulation. The segment of uterine horn is resected and an end-to-end anastomosis performed as above. The length of the resected segment can be varied simply by varying the number of blood vessel branches that are ligated or coagulated.

Salpingostomy

The rat uterine horn may be used as a model for performing terminal salpingostomy. Following transection, a series of interrupted sutures is placed around the circumference of the cut edge. The sutures are placed through the serosa and muscularis and back out through

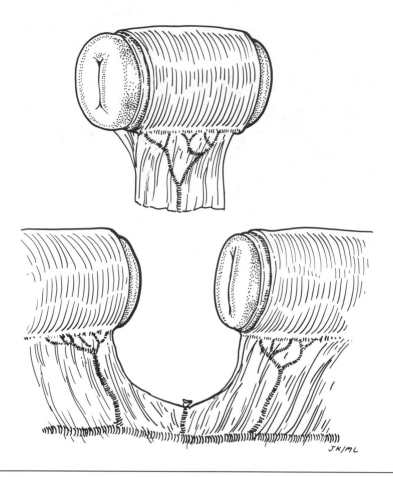

Figure 4-71
Technique of segmental resection in the rat uterine horn. The resected segment has been isolated from its major vascular supply before resection.

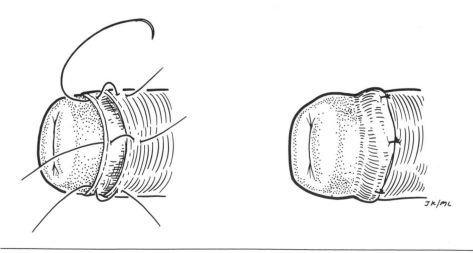

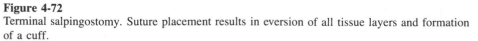

Figure 4-72
Terminal salpingostomy. Suture placement results in eversion of all tissue layers and formation of a cuff.

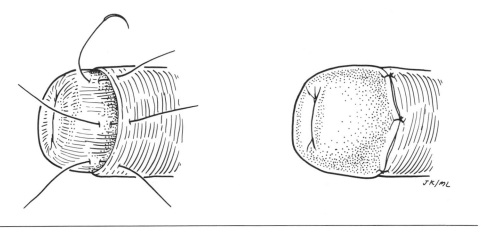

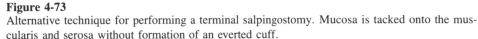

Figure 4-73
Alternative technique for performing a terminal salpingostomy. Mucosa is tacked onto the muscularis and serosa without formation of an everted cuff.

the serosa 1 to 2 mm from the transected end of the horn. The same suture is then placed through the serosa and muscularis, and emerges from the cut end of the stump (Figure 4-72). Tying the suture everts the muscle and forms a cuff to prevent postsurgical occlusion.

Alternatively, the mucosa itself may be everted. This is done by placing a series of interrupted sutures through the serosa and muscularis at the cut edge in a fashion similar to and end-to-end anastomosis, but with the suture placed into the mucosa without penetrating the lumen. When all the sutures are tied, the mucosa is everted and tacked onto the muscularis and serosa (Figure 4-73).

Linear salpingotomy

The rising frequency of ectopic pregnancy and the increasing opportunity, provided by timely diagnosis, to manage the condition conservatively before tubal rupture have generated the need to perform linear salpingotomy so as to remove the products of conception while salvaging the tube. Linear salpingotomy may be performed in the rat uterine horn model. The ideal model is the rat in early pregnancy in which the uterus can actually be incised and the early conceptus and placenta removed. Alternatively, the nonpregnant uterus may incised down to the endometrial cavity and then repaired, this simulating removal of an ectopic gestation.

An incision is made under low magnification into the uterine horn on the antimesenteric border. In an early pregnant uterus, an area over an implantation site should be selected. Such areas are obvious and present as equally spaced spherical swellings along the length of the uterine horn. The incision may be made with a scalpel, scissors, or a unipolar microcautery needle. If unipolar cautery is to be used, it is necessary to shave the back of the animal, spread conductive gel on the skin, and establish good electrical connection with the ground plate. If sharp dis-

section is used, the incision should be made parallel to the long axis of the uterine horn into the endometrial cavity, producing a straight, clean cut. Bipolar cautery is used to control point bleeders. In using unipolar electrocautery, the power settings should be adjusted so that, when blended current is applied, the tissue will be incised and any bleeders coagulated. It is imperative that the lowest-power settings consistent with desired result be used and that the electrode be moved in a steady fashion. This will help minimize the lateral spread of thermal trauma. The tissue should be kept moist. If allowed to dry or become desiccated by an electrode remaining in one place too long, the electrode will adhere to tissue and will not cut.

After the endometrial cavity is opened, the conceptus and attached placenta should be shelled out. The implantation site should then be irrigated to identify point bleeders and bipolar cautery or unipolar cautery in coagulation mode used to achieve hemostasis. The uterine defect is then closed with interrupted suture placed through the serosa and muscularis (Figure 4-74).

HUMAN OVIDUCT

Working with inanimate objects allows one to master the purely mechanical aspects of microsurgery. Progressing to living tissue adds the important dimensions of recognition and manipulation of anatomic features, achievement of hemostasis, and avoidance of unnecessary iatrogenic trauma. Blood vessel anastomosis provides the opportunity to apply microsurgical skills in a technically demanding procedure that furnishes instant positive feedback regarding quality and success once the vascular clamps are removed.

An important final exercise is that undertaken with the fresh or frozen excised human oviduct. Although such

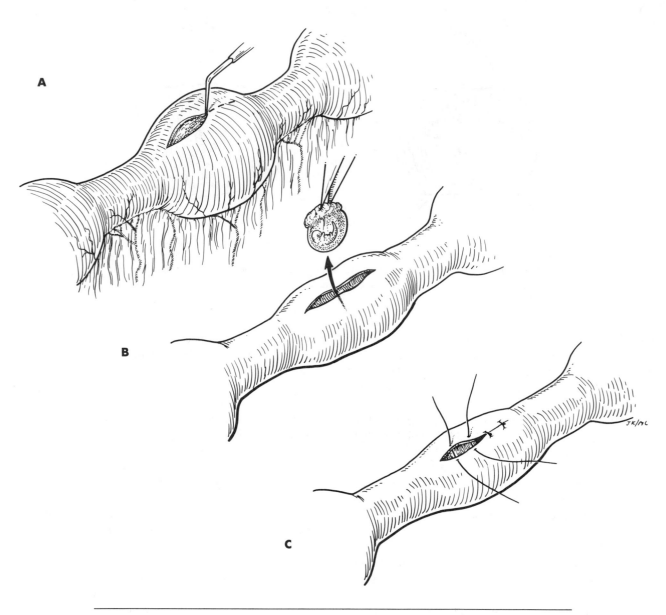

Figure 4-74
Linear salpingotomy performed on a pregnant uterine horn. **A,** The incision is made on the anti-mesenteric border above an implantation site with sharp or electrosurgical dissection (unipolar). **B,** The fetus and placenta are bluntly dissected and removed. Bleeding points are identified with irrigation and cauterized with bipolar forceps. **C,** Repair with interrupted sutures placed through the serosa and muscularis.

specimens do not have a functional blood supply, they nevertheless provide the opportunity to become familiar with tubal anatomy, spatial relationships, and regional differences observed through the perspective of the surgical microscope.

Preparation and storage

Freshly excised specimens should be immersed in a physiologic solution. They should not be placed in fixative, since this will radically alter their physical characteris-

tics, bleaching out the color differences between tissue layers and solidifying the tissue into a stiff, rubbery mass.

After the specimen is released by the pathologist, it should be removed from the physiologic solution to prevent it from becoming water-logged and macerated. If the tissue is to be used within hours or days, it may be covered with a saline-soaked 4 × 4 gauze pad, wrapped in aluminum foil, and refrigerated until used. When needed, tubes can be removed from storage and thawed by leaving them wrapped at room temperature or by immersing them in warm water. Specimens should never be thawed and refrozen, since this renders the tissue gelatinous and unsuitable for use.

The specimen should be placed on a block of Styrofoam, cork, or similar material. With the tissue kept moist at all times, the entire gross specimen should be examined and the segments of oviduct that are present identified. About two-thirds of the oviduct is ampulla, with the remaining length isthmus. The distal ampulla is easily identified by virtue of the attached fimbriae. Middle or proximal segments of oviduct without the fimbriae or uterus attached are difficult to identify grossly. If the gross specimen is a piece of oviduct with no obvious anatomic landmarks on either end, the particular oviductal segment from which the specimen comes must be identified. The myosalpinx should be palpated through the serosa. If the specimen was taken from the ampulla, it will not be possible to discern the myosalpinx easily. In contrast, if the specimen is from the isthmus, the myosalpinx will appear a tough, cordlike mass extending lengthwise in the middle of the specimen.

The specimen should be pinned to the board at the ends through the mesosalpinx, with care taken to avoid the myosalpinx and lumen. The specimen is then transected with a small iris scissors perpendicular to its long axis from the antimesosalpingeal border, completely severing the oviduct. The mesosalpinx should be left as intact as possible to help stabilize the specimen during anastomosis. With the specimen placed under the objective lens of the surgical microscope, the transection site should be examined under low and high magnification. The entire cross section of the oviduct, including the entire circumference of the myosalpinx, should be identified.

At the level of the ampulla, the oviduct in cross section will have a wide lumen loosely filled with a highly branched and folded endosalpinx. If the tissue has undergone autolysis, the endosalpinx may be highly attenuated or even absent, leaving a gaping lumen. Ideally, the intact endosalpinx will render the lumen a virtual space. It may evert spontaneously when the tube is transected and flow out of the lumen. The relatively thin myosalpinx should be identified and the demarcation between it and the endosalpinx noted—a well-defined line easily seen at high magnification. The surrounding intervening thin layer of connective tissue between the serosa and myosalpinx should also be noted.

At the level of the isthmus, the oviduct in cross section will be much smaller than the ampulla and will have a narrow lumen exhibiting a cruciform or stellate cross section created by four or more discrete, sparsely branched folds of endosalpinx. The myosalpinx will be thick and prominent with a clear demarcation between both the endosalpinx and the large mass of connective tissue separating it from the serosa. The subserosal connective tissue, particularly in the mesosalpingeal aspect

of the tube, may contain one or more large arteries, which in cross section may appear quite similar to the isthmus. It is not rare for the beginner to attempt an arterial anastomosis thinking it to be an isthmic-isthmic anastomosis—all because of failure to identify and distinguish properly between tubal and vascular anatomy. Sufficient tubal specimens should be obtained to allow practice of isthmic-isthmic, ampullary-ampullary, and isthmic-ampullary anastomoses.

Isthmic-isthmic anastomosis

All types of tubal anastomosis are performed as two-layer procedures with the myosalpinx and serosa closed as separate layers. The myosalpinx is approximated first with a series of interrupted sutures placed through the muscle only, specifically avoiding the endosalpinx. The first suture is placed at the 6 o'clock position, followed by the second at 12 o'clock. As always, sutures are placed with the aid of counterpressure supplied by the forceps. Equal, symmetric bites are taken. Because of the prominent myosalpinx and narrow lumen of the tubal isthmus, four sutures placed at the so-called cardinal points of 6, 12, 3, and 9 o'clock are often sufficient to join the myosalpinx, particularly at the level of the proximal isthmus. If the anastomosis is farther out toward the ampulla, several additional sutures may be needed. Because a water-tight seal is not necessary, the minimum number of sutures needed to create an anastomosis without gaps should be used (Figure 4-75).

After the myosalpinx is closed, the anastomosis should be reperitonealized by joining the cut edges of the serosa with interrupted sutures. Alternatively, a continuous suture may be used to reperitonealize, beginning at the base of the mesosalpinx on the lateral aspect and continuing to the antimesosalpingeal border. The suture should be tied at this point and a new continuous suture, extending down the medial aspect of the mesosalpinx, begun.

After completion of the procedure the pins should be removed and the patency of the anastomosis tested by slowly introducing several milliliters of dilute methylene blue or indigo carmine into the lumen through a blunt-ended hypodermic needle attached to a syringe and inserted intraluminally into the cut end of the specimen. To check the anastomosis visually, it should be excised and opened up longitudinally with microscissors, and the exposed luminal surface examined (Figure 4-76).

Ampullary-ampullary anastomosis

Anastomosis of the ampullary-ampullary segment of the oviduct requires more sutures because of the larger lumen. Accurate placement of sutures to exclude the endosalpinx is more demanding because the myosalpinx is thin in this segment of the oviduct. The initial suture is placed at the 6 o'clock position. Each additional suture

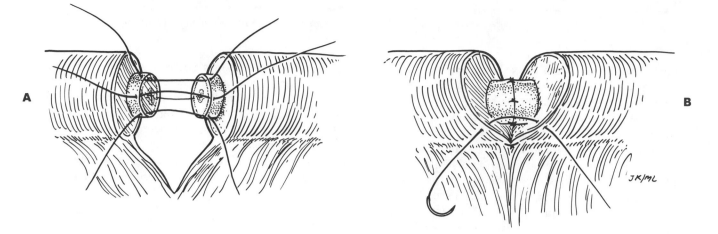

Figure 4-75
Isthmic-isthmic anastomosis of excised human oviduct. **A,** Sutures are placed through the myosalpinx, specifically avoiding the endosalpinx. **B,** Placement of a continuous suture through serosa to reperitonealize the anastomosis.

Figure 4-76
Evaluation of a completed anastomosis performed in an excised human oviduct. **A,** Transluminal passage of dye using a blunt-tipped needle introduced into the lumen. Note absence of leakage around the anastomosis and free spill of dye from the lumen at the distal end of the specimen. **B,** Specimen after longitudinal opening with scissors after the dye test has been performed. The alignment of all tissue layers and technical adequacy of the anastomosis are easily evaluated.

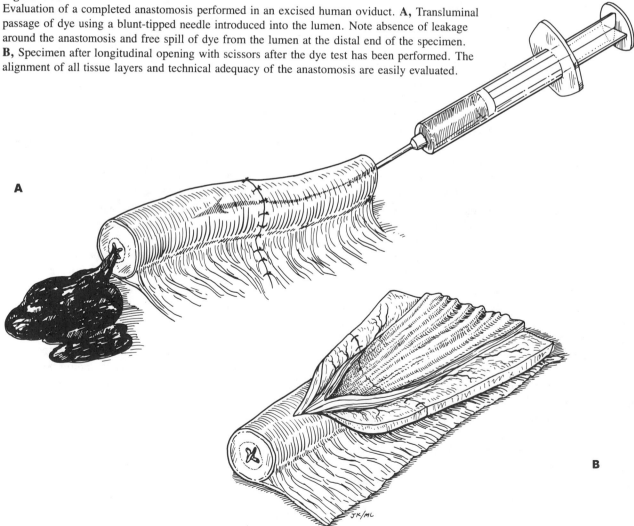

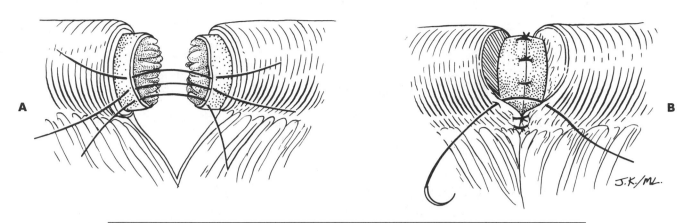

Figure 4-77
Ampullary-ampullary anastomosis of excised human oviduct. **A,** Closely spaced interrupted sutures are placed through the myosalpinx only. Great care must be taken to achieve an undistorted anastomosis with all endosalpinx returned to the lumen, not ensnared in the sutures, and incorporated into the wall of the myosalpinx. **B,** Reperitonealization with interrupted sutures.

must be placed with care to ensure that the anatomy is not distorted and that corresponding points on the left and right segments are joined (Figure 4-77). As the anastomosis proceeds, the endosalpinx, which everts spontaneously and flows out of the lumen, must be systematically pushed into the lumen. After the anastomosis is complete, patency should be tested and morphologic configuration evaluated as was done after isthmic anastomosis.

Isthmic-ampullary anastomosis

Isthmic-ampullary anastomosis entails the management of significant disparity in luminal diameters and reflects the absence of considerable intervening tissue in which the ampulla and isthmus are normally in gradual transition. Such a procedure is common in reversing elective midtubal sterilization. Most surgeons, when performing this type of tubal surgery, prefer to avoid the creation of luminal disparity by not resecting the blind stump of the ampullary segment. Instead, they surgically establish an opening the diameter of which approximates that of the isthmic segment. When it is not possible to establish such an opening surgically, several techniques of anastomosis are available (Figure 4-78):

1. The isthmus may be cut at an angle to increase its apparent luminal diameter.
2. The isthmus may be bivalved or fishmouthed to achieve the same goal.
3. Sutures may be placed at similar locations in the isthmus and ampulla so that, when tied, the ampulla will be pleated and will therefore be reduced to the approximate diameter of the isthmus.

4. The isthmus may be sutured to the ampulla using sutures that join its perimeter to the corresponding lower portion of the ampulla. The upper redundant portion of the ampulla not sutured to the isthmus is closed on itself by using several interrupted sutures.

To simulate ampullary-isthmic anastomosis, a 2- to 3-cm length of midoviduct should be resected so as to produce a marked luminal disparity and anastomosis performed using the above techniques. After the anastomosis is completed, patency and free flow of dye should be checked, and the internal morphology examined as previously described.

Other techniques

Linear salpingotomies may be performed at the level of the isthmus and ampulla, using both sharp and electrosurgical dissection. Terminal salpingostomy may also be performed with these same segments of the oviduct.

CONCLUSION

The skills acquired through successful completion of the exercises described in this chapter will furnish the basis for improved surgical precision and, with suitable clinical integration, should enable the surgeon to undertake virtually any type of meticulous tuboplastic procedure. Should there not be opportunity to use microsurgical skills clinically at least once every 7 or 10 days, several hours should be set aside regularly each week for laboratory practice to maintain the fine motor skills and spatial relationships required for gynecologic microsurgery.

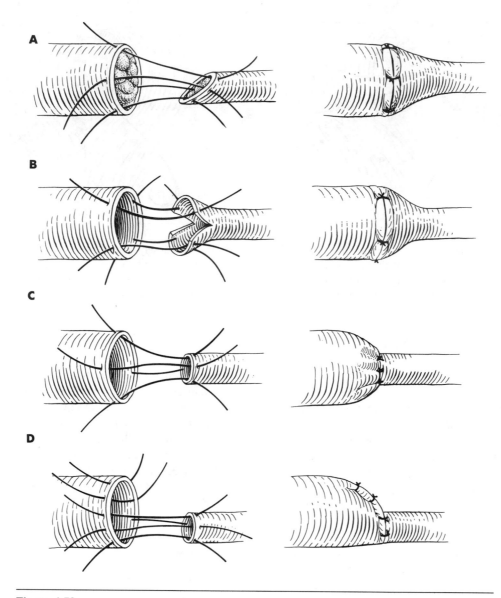

Figure 4-78
Isthmic-ampullary anastomosis technique. **A,** Isthmic lumen is cut obliquely. **B,** Isthmus is bivalved. **C,** Ampulla is squeezed together to conform to much narrower isthmus. **D,** Redundant ampulla closes on itself after anastomosis of the isthmus to the lower ampulla.

SELECTED READING

Acland RD: *Microsurgery practice manual,* St. Louis, 1980, C.V. Mosby.

Bunke HJ et al: *The manual of micro-vascular surgery,* San Francisco, 1975, Ralph L. Davies Medical Center.

Crosignani PG and Rubin BL (eds): *Microsurgery in female infertility,* New York, 1980, Grune & Stratton.

Patkin M: Ergonomics in microsurgery, *Aust NZ J Obstet Gynaecol* 21:134-136, 1981.

Reyniak JV and Lauerson NH (eds): *Principles of microsurgical techniques in infertility,* New York, 1982, Plenum Press.

Serafin D et al: *A laboratory manual of micro-vascular surgery,* Durham, NC, 1978, Duke University Medical Center.

Winston RML: Evaluating instrumentation for gynecologic microsurgery, *Contemp Obstet Gynecol* 15:153-166, 1980.

5

Surgical Microscope and Loupes

MICHAEL ALAN BERMANT

RAYMOND E. SHIVELY

Magnification for the surgeon is available in various formats and costs. The choice is confusing at best. Two formats are available. The loupe, French for magnifier, is the conventional name for a head-worn device. Its design is compact and light-weight. The microscope is usually mounted on a stand and has its own light supply. This larger system is heavier, more complicated, more suited for higher magnification, and has accessories to add special features.

Magnification is the result of the manipulation of light by lenses. Figure 5-1 demonstrates the simple lens, a compound lens, a simple telescope (Galilean), and the wide-field telescope or Kepler prism loupe. Figure 5-2 depicts two formats for the surgical microscope. The most simple is the fixed Galilean system. Variable magnification is provided by either a rotating drum or a zoom mechanism.

DEFINITIONS

The lens is a device that bends the rays of light. A simple lens has a single component; several lenses are grouped to form a compound lens. Each color of light bends at a different angle through a simple lens. Cheaper units manifest this aberration as a rainbow halo about points of light. Compound lenses compensate for this effect.

Focal length

Magnification systems have a point of focus at which the image perceived by the eye is sharpest. The length from the lens to that point is called the focal length. This distance is important to the surgeon, since it translates into working distance. The human lens compensates to some degree by changing the point of focus. Prolonged compensation by the eye's lens is uncomfortable and a frequent source of headache. Relaxing the ciliary muscles by keeping the eyes focused at infinity minimizes discomfort.

Depth of field

Depth of field is the distance through which an object stays in focus without compensation of the user's eye. When including the eye's compensation, the range of focus is called depth of vision. Depth of vision decreases with eye fatigue. Higher magnifications have a narrow depth of field. The head's natural motion during surgery is enough to exceed the depth of field of moderate-magnification loupes (3.5×4.5). High-power loupes (over $4.5 \times$) are difficult to keep in focus. A microscope's rigid mounting helps maintain focus.

Angle of convergence

Angle of convergence is the angular difference between the visual axis and the median line. From birth, the brain is oriented to a specific set of values for each working distance. Most microscope manufacturers have chosen to retain this natural angle, using a popular focal length for the calculation. Microscopes with unusual convergent angles may possibly be uncomfortable for the surgeon who is already familiar with other systems. Loupes are manufactured or adjustable to the appropriate angle.

Stereoscopic vision

Stereoscopic vision is important in surgery for accurate hand-to-eye coordination. Magnification for surgery uses a system for each eye to provide this vision. The brain is presented with two images, each from a different angle, to add depth perception. The two images must be carefully aligned to prevent double vision. The external eye muscles may compensate but over time will fatigue, giving the surgeon a headache. Each lens system must be viewed through its optical axis. This necessitates an alignment method to compensate for interpupillary distance. Each manufacturer has its own arrangement to accomplish this.

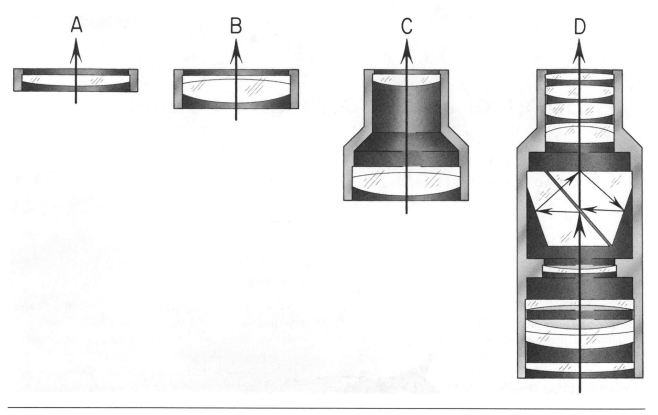

Figure 5-1
Loupe designs. **A**, Simple lens; **B**, compound lens; **C**, simple Galilean telescope; **D**, Kepler
prism telescope.

Field of view

Field of view is the extent of the magnified area seen.
As magnification increases, the field of view diminishes.
Larger fields of view help the surgeon by giving a better
sense of the surrounding area.

Exit pupil

Exit pupil size determines how critical eye placement
must be in relation to the eyepiece to obtain full width
of field. Optical systems with larger exit pupils are easier
to use.

Lens quality

Certain values measure the quality of a lens system.
Resolution is the ability to differentiate between points.
This translates into how sharp the image is for the surgeon. Distortion is the twisting of the image out of its
natural shape. Less expensive systems have curvilinear
edge distortion where the image at the edge of the field
is bent. Light transmission (or brightness) is how much
light passes through the system. Contrast is the difference
between light and dark. Better optical systems with multiple lenses must defeat internal reflections that rob the

surgeon of light and contrast. An antireflective lens coat-
ing improves transmission.

THE LOUPE

There are two ways to mount magnifications on the head.
The most common is the one in which the loupes are
mounted on or through the normal eyeglass lenses. The
surgeon's corrective prescription must be incorporated
into the loupes in the latter method. Eyeglasses or loupes
incorporating prescriptive lenses individualize the unit so
that another surgeon with different eye corrections cannot
wear it. Bifocal prescriptions can be incorporated into
many loupe frames. Some prefer the headband, which
is worn alone or over existing eyeglasses, enabling several individuals to use the same loupes regardless of
whether they wear eyeglasses. In a teaching program
where residents have not yet purchased a magnification
system, this is an ideal investment. Some surgeons require a coaxial light source with their magnification. Illuminated fiberoptic systems, which can be purchased
separately for eyeglass units or as part of the headband-
mounted loupe, are available (Figure 5-3).

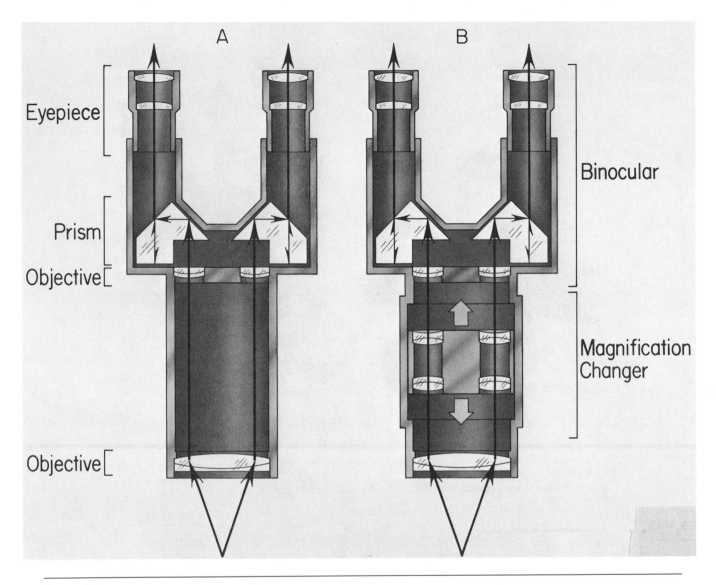

Figure 5-2
Galilean microscopes. **A**, Fixed magnification; **B**, drum or zoom magnification.

Simple magnifier loupe

The simple magnifier is a one-lens unit that is by far the least expensive. The low-magnification headband (Figure 5-4) is an example. Magnification of $2\times$ or greater requires unacceptably close working distances; this is the major shortcoming of a simple lens.

Galilean telescope

The Galilean telescope lens system offers improvements. Multiple lenses combine to provide a longer working distance. Various designs are available (Figure 5-5), all better than the simple lens magnifier. The useful range of magnification is $1.5\times$ to $3.5\times$. Higher magnification with the Galilean system severely restricts the field of view unless the lens system is very close to the eye. Even

so, the field of view is limited over $3\times$. Simple lenses added to this system for greater magnification shorten the working distance, which is not practical for the operating room.

Kepler prism telescope

A quantum step in both quality and price occurs with the Kepler prism telescope (Figure 5-6). It is the most complex of the formats shown in Figure 5-1. The prism functions as a longer optical pathway, allowing for the designs that are otherwise too long for head mounting. The results are a wider field of view, a sharper image, and more light at higher magnification.

Magnifications range from $2.5\times$ to $8\times$ (Figure 5-7). Various focal lengths are available, with some companies

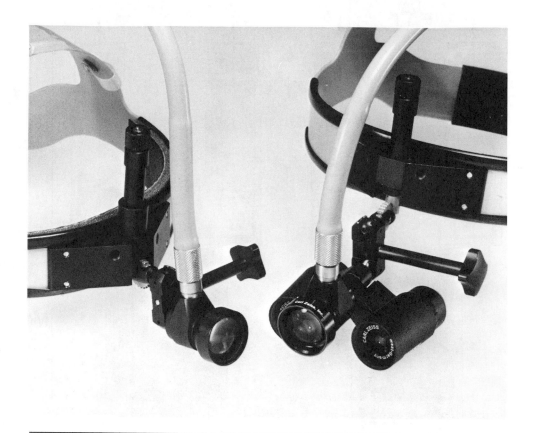

Figure 5-3
Zeiss headband with coaxial illumination **A**, alone; **B**, with loupes.

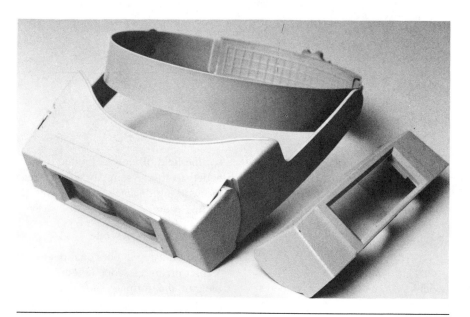

Figure 5-4
Low-magnification headband.

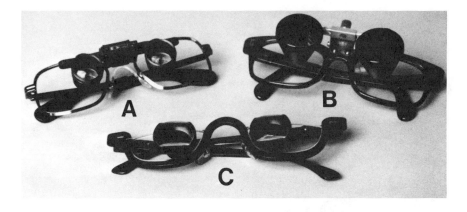

Figure 5-5
Various Galilean telescopes. **A**, Keeler; **B**, Occulus; **C**, Designs for Vision.

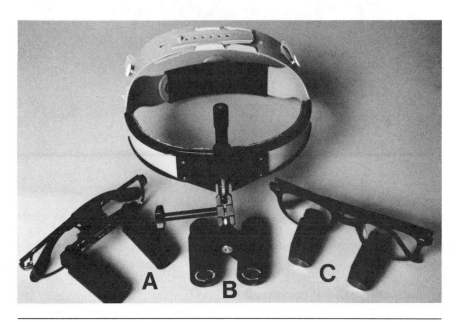

Figure 5-6
Kepler prism telescopes. **A,** Keeler; **B,** Zeiss; **C,** Designs for Vision.

offering greater choice than others. Resolution and light transmission are improved because of higher-quality optical designs. At magnifications greater than 5×, many prefer to use a microscope because loupe weight is burdensome. A limited depth of field makes focusing difficult, and head motion produces a bouncing field.

Mounting systems

There are two types of loupe mounts: permanent factory-fitted and user-adjusted. Each has its own advantages. Nonadjustable designs are crafted for the individual surgeon. With no adjustments to change, the loupes are ready to use when needed and can easily be removed

and replaced during surgery. Through-the-lens design mounts the loupes closer to the eyes, increasing the width of field. To remove magnification, the surgeon must either turn and look through the periphery of the glasses or have someone remove the loupes. Focal length (operating distance), interpupillary distance, magnification, eyeglass correction, and frame size must be fitted by a factory representative. Changes must be made by the manufacturer.

Adjustable designs allow the surgeon to adapt the loupes. Most permit changes of interpupillary distance and for the loupes to be flipped up out of the line of vision. Some adjust vertical positioning, distance away

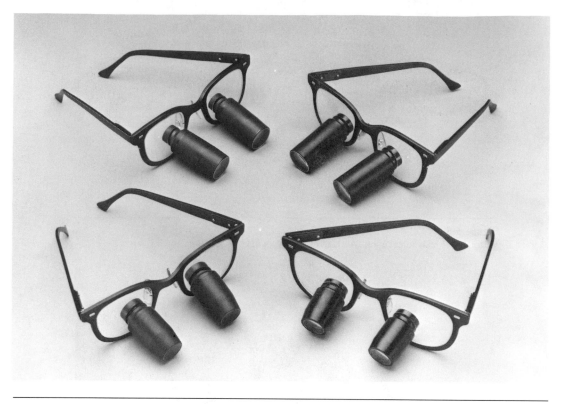

Figure 5-7
Various power Kepler prism telescopes by Designs for Vision (2.5X to 6X).

from glasses, convergence angle, and tilt. Although there are locks on most adjustments, slippage occurs, requiring readjustments. Some need fitting before each use. A few adjustments are interdependent and can be difficult to set. Slight misalignments that seem correct at first may result in a headache after prolonged use. Instead of sending the loupes back to the factory, a local optometrist can change the prescriptive lenses. Magnification, focal length, and frame size are chosen when ordering. Such designs can be worn by different surgeons when used without prescriptive lenses.

Eyeglass mounts tend to orient themselves more reliably than headband mounts (Figure 5-6). Because of variable headband positioning, preoperative adjustments are inevitable. Loupes are heavy and some prefer the headband mount to a painful nose. Headbands also can be worn by surgeons who do and do not wear eyeglasses. Such mounts are well suited for situations in which many persons must wear a single pair of loupes (extra set for an operating room or training programs whose members have not yet purchased loupes).

Protective side shielding may help lessen the chance of blood exposure. Several manufacturers have attachments that connect to the eye frames (Figure 5-8). Clear face mask extensions or visors may offer better protection but are cumbersome to wear with the longer loupes.

Choosing loupes

There is no simple answer to which loupe an individual should buy. Each surgeon must assess his or her own needs. For example, suture size and desired anatomic detail determine the magnification and quality resolution. If magnification greater than $3 \times$ is required, the wide-field prism is best. The higher price is offset by the expanded field's greater surgical ease and flexibility.

The following should be considered in determining the mounting system: number of persons who will use the loupes, that is, one individual or several; whether the surgeon prefers to remove the loupes or have them flip out of the way; and the nuisance factor of readjusting the loupes.

Each surgeon must use the loupes to decide a personal preference for working distance. A longer distance of 350 to 450 mm (14 to 18 inches) allows the head to remain comfortably upright. Focal lengths under 300 mm (12 inches) are impractical since the surgeon must bend the neck while performing surgery, which focuses the head too close to the wound.

The individual manufacturer is also important. It is best to deal with someone who lets the surgeon use the loupes for several procedures in the operating room. Most will permit changes in magnification and focal length at no charge, if within a reasonable time from purchase.

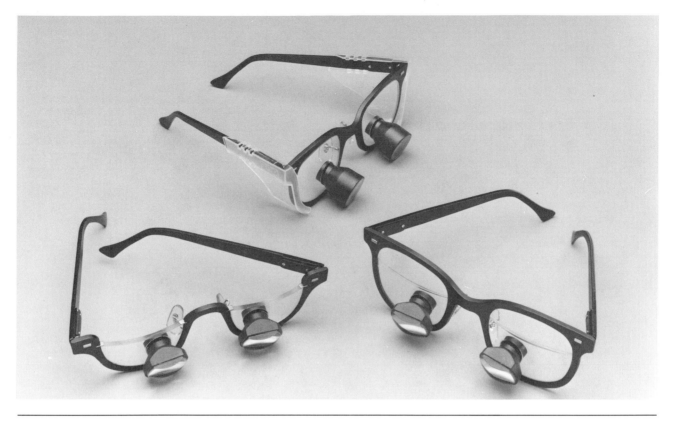

Figure 5-8
Protective shielding for the Designs for Vision.

MICROSCOPE

The surgical microscope has several subsystems, including magnification, light supply, mounting, accessories, and manufacturer support. Two formats are available. The system approach maintains independence of each subsystem, permitting interchange, modification, updating, and simple customizing. The microscope is then easily altered for a variety of procedures. The factory-preassembled unit allows only limited change within various subsystems. The manufacturer customizes each microscope for the particular features required by the surgeon. Modifications that are easily accomplished within the system format require a technician for the factory preassembled instrument. This benefits the individual who does not want anyone else using the microscope. Updating and modifying these units, however, results in major expense and inconvenience.

Magnification subsystem

Most manufacturers use the Galilean telescope design for their microscopes, including eyepieces, binocular tubes, magnification changer, and objective. A separate optical assembly for each eye maintains depth perception. For changes in magnification, some incorporate a drum that introduces various lens combinations into the optical pathway. Others alter the magnifications by moving optical assemblies along a track, thus varying the distance between lenses. Drum systems have several distinct magnifications while zoom systems permit a continuous change between minimum and maximum. Although drum configurations are usually manual, both designs can be motorized for remote operation.

Each manufacturer has several eyepieces. The different powers change the magnification range of the microscope. With the eye placed at a specific distance from the eyepiece, the observer sees the entire field of view. High-eye-point eyepieces allow eyeglass wearers enough distance between eyes and microscope. Eyepieces that are not so designed require the surgeon who wears eyeglasses to press firmly against the microscope to see the entire width of field. A rubber cushion adjusts on the eyepiece to let either eyeglasses or the orbital rim stabilize against the microscope.

The binocular assembly (Figure 5-9) corrects interpupillary distance. Here rotating prisms allow the eyepieces to be moved closer or farther apart. The eyes should be totally relaxed when making this adjustment. If the external eye muscles must compensate for an incorrectly adjusted interpupillary distance, headache often results. Several manufacturers offer various angles of

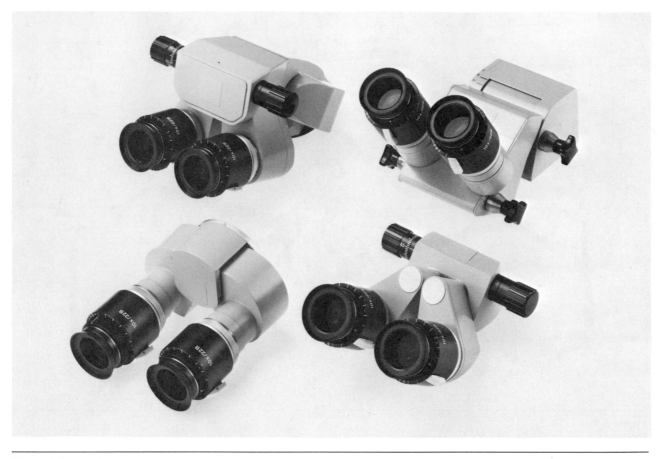

Figure 5-9
Various binocular assemblies show interpupillary adjustment. Viewing angle not adjustable. Adjustable viewing angle.

inclination for the binocular assembly. This feature increases the surgeon's comfort in different operating positions. Adjustable-angled assemblies (Figure 5-10) let the surgeon choose the best angle. Ideally, the surgeon should sit upright, with a straight back, and the head in a relaxed vertical position. Body weight then transmits down through the skeleton instead of being supported by muscle action. The variable tilting binocular tube used with an adjustable chair encourages good posture and thus comfort for long procedures.

The magnification changer increases or decreases the total magnification of the objective lens. Magnification powers ($6\times$, $10\times$, $16\times$, $25\times$, and $40\times$) printed on a microscope are only accurate for a certain combination of binocular tube focal length, objective focal length, and eyepiece power. The magnification factor is a coefficient used to determine the final magnification factor on the microscope instead of the power.

The objective lens establishes the focal length or working distance of the surgical microscope. In the factory-preassembled instrument, the entire head assembly,

which costs many thousands of dollars, must be changed to vary this distance. The system approach allows this change by simply substituting the single objective lens. The Ziess OPMI CS microscope has modules for its body. One module has internal lens adjustment of the focal length, permitting intraoperative changes. Varying focal lengths intraoperatively permits positioning the microscope at one distance from the patient and focusing on different depths in the patient. Procedures that require work both superficially and deeply will benefit.

Final magnification is a function of eyepiece power, binocular tube length, drum or zoom magnification factor, and objective lens focal length. The formula is as follows:

$$Mf = \frac{f\ tube}{f\ objective} \times M\ eyepiece \times M\ changer$$

where the Mf is the final magnification; $f\ tube$ is the focal length of the binocular tube (a number that can be supplied by the manufacturer and is often stamped directly on the binocular assembly); $f\ objective$ is the focal length of the objective (this translates into the working distance under the microscope); *M eyepiece* is the magnification of the eyepiece; and *M changer* is the zoom magnification factor.

An example using a binocular focal length of 125 mm, objective of 200 mm, and 20× eyepieces would be:

$$Mf = \frac{125 \text{ mm}}{200 \text{ mm}} \times 20 \times M \text{ changer}$$

or

$$Mf = 12.5 \times M \text{ changer}$$

Thus to obtain the magnification for this combination of optics, multiply each changer factor by 12.5.

Magnification factor: 0.4   0.6   1.0 1.6 2.5
Final magnification: 5× 7.5× 12.5× 20× 31×

The well-designed microscope will maintain its focus as the drum or zoom changes magnification. This is called parfocality. A microscope that is not parfocal requires adjustment of the focus when changing magnifications. Since the higher powers have less depth of field, loss of focus also can occur when moving from low to high power. Therefore one must focus under the highest magnifications where the depth of field is narrow, so that when moving to the lower magnifications that have greater depth of field, the image will be in focus. When this is not so, the microscope may not be parfocal.

Most eyepieces have an adjustable diopter setting that alters the focus for each eye independently. A lock on this adjustment prevents unwanted movement. When calibrating the microscope, the zero-diopter setting shows where to set the eyepiece for parfocality.

To establish parfocality, set the eyepiece of the dominant eye to zero and firmly seat it in the binocular assembly. An eyepiece slightly withdrawn from the binocular tube is no longer parfocal at the printed zero mark. Using high magnification, focus on a flat piece of paper with print. Being careful not to change the microscope position or focus, zoom the magnification to the lowest setting. Adjust the diopter ring for the nondominant eye. The dominant eye should be in focus. If it is not, the microscope representative may have to adjust the microscope, or the surgeon is not wearing normal corrective lenses. Surgeons who use both diopter adjustments off the zero mark to compensate for removed eyeglasses often lose parfocality. Although any eyepiece equipped with a diopter scale can be preset to a known correction, it is best visually to verify that both eyes are in focus before beginning the procedure.

Working with an assistant

Several formats have evolved to enable more than one surgeon to see the magnified field and add accessories.

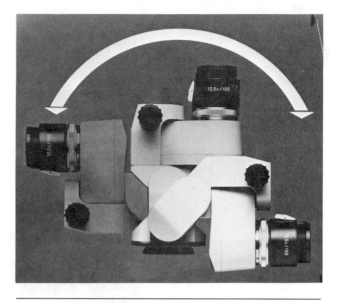

Figure 5-10
Adjustable-angle binocular assembly shows variety of positions.

The following points should be considered in the evaluation of each format:

1. Is stereoscopic vision preserved for the observer, or do the optics use only one set of lenses from the microscope's body? Even a binocular head will not give stereoscopic vision when it is limited by a single set of the body's lens system.
2. Can the surgeon and assistant choose independent magnifications, and is the changing system manual or remote? This choice allows the surgeon to optimize magnification for each task, which can be different from what the assistant is performing. With independent action, acclimatization is often awkward for those trained on systems with no choice.
3. Is there adequate light for each? The more accessories that take light from the field, the less light there is for the surgeon.
4. What are the relative positions of the surgeon and the assistant; can they be changed? The 90-degree position, so well suited for neurosurgery, is awkward for the assistant in tuboplasties.
5. Does the surgeon see the same field as the assistant? Separate microscope bodies allow independent magnifications, but there can be alignment problems in seeing the same field. In addition, a different angle of view can block the assistant's view into a cavity or recess in the surgical field.

A beam splitter is a prism lens system that divides each optical path in two, one path continuing in the original direction and a second usually at right angles (Figure 5-11). Two systems are included in each simple beam splitter, one dividing the left and the other dividing

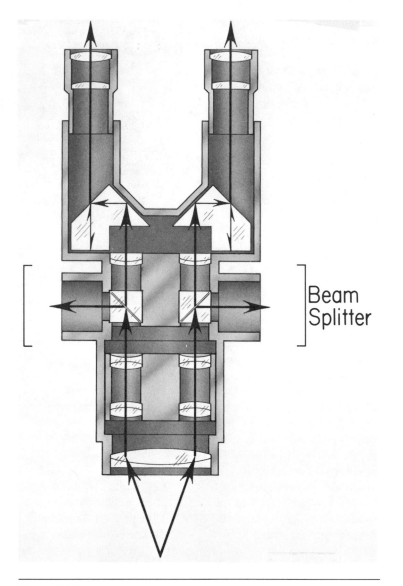

Figure 5-11
Diagram of microscope with beam splitter.

the right optical pathway. Each accessory or observer then "sees" through only one set of the body's dual lens system. The beam splitter takes a certain percentage of light away from the original path. The 50/50 beam splitter divides the light equally between the surgeon and the accessory parts. A 60/40 unit sends 60% to the surgeon and 40% to the other pathway. The choice of percentage depends on the amount of available light and the light needs of the accessories. One microscope has so much available light that it uses a 20/80 beam splitter where only 20% of the light goes on to the surgeon. The beam splitter can be an accessory in the system microscope design or a built-in option. The lack of stereoscopic vision limits the simple beam splitter to an observer or camera accessory.

The dual viewing adapter is an advanced beam splitter that sends light from each of the body's lens systems to each surgeon (Figure 5-12). Both have the same view, equal light, and stereoscopic vision. Present designs limit the positioning of each surgeon to 180 degrees apart. The magnification changer and objective lens are shared by both surgeons. Each has the same magnification except when using different-powered eyepieces. This is not as flexible as an independent choice of magnification provided by separate bodies. Light for cameras and other observer accessories can come from a second beam splitter, a beam splitter incorporated into the microscope or dual viewing adaptor, or a separate set of optics in the microscope.

Microscopes designed for one surgeon can be converted for dual use with an adapter (Figure 5-13). Models are available for the Zeiss OPMI 1, 6, MD, CS, Storz Urban, and Wild microscopes. They often have one or more nonstereoscopic ports for accessories. Limitations of older designs include height, lighting demands, and tunnel vision effect for the assistant.

Another method mounts two complete microscopes together (Figure 5-14). Here both surgeons choose individual magnifications as needed. Each microscope has its own zoom magnification changing system. Lighting is a problem at times. A beam splitter for accessories built into only one microscope head changes the amount of light that a particular surgeon receives. Adjusting the light level for both surgeons can therefore be difficult. Two separate angles of observation make glare reduction a problem. When glare is reduced for one surgeon, the other is often at an angle of increased glare. Overlapping field and different angles of view also are problems when partners assume they are seeing the same thing. Fields that are not level result in different distances to each microscope unless the scope is tilted parallel to that plane. Different distances leave one surgeon out of focus in an otherwise correctly adjusted microscope. Trying to compensate with the assistant's eyepieces by moving both off the zero setting destroys parfocality. These difficulties must be weighed against the major advantage of independent magnification.

The final method is a clip-on second microscope attached to the body of the main unit. Here again, each surgeon has completely separate optics. Available units are manual or have a single magnification. Overlapping fields and a different angle of vision also present problems.

Lighting

For surgery deep in cavities, the light must be directed close to the optical axis (Figure 5-15). In other words, when viewing into a hole, light coming from an angle far away from the line of sight will not illuminate the bottom. Illumination near the optical axis is called coaxial lighting. Since many surgical fields are not necessarily deep in cavities, some manufacturers mount the light farther off the optical axis (Figure 5-16). Shadows occur, but glare is reduced. Coaxial light reflects off wet and metallic surfaces; light at 45 degrees to the optical axis gives less glare but cannot illuminate deep cavities. There is thus a trade-off between deep cavity illumination and glare reduction.

Light needs increase with higher magnifications, long focal lengths, and beam splitters. There will not be sufficient light if enough of these factors are present, and the system will have to be changed or augmented. Also, extremely powerful lights warm and dry the surgical field. The light systems include a light supply, trans-

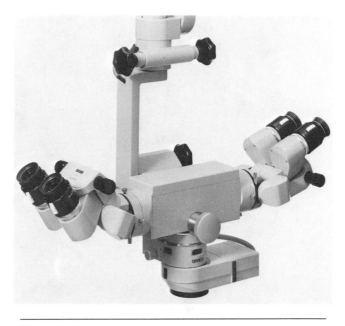

Figure 5-12
Dual viewing adapter.

mission guide, and focusing lens. Complete units are offered both by microscope manufacturers and other sources.

The light supply is mounted in the microscope body or in a remote location. A high-intensity bulb generates a good deal of heat. Making enough light for all surgical conditions and for light-stealing accessories was a problem until fiberoptic cables made remote lighting possible. Now most manufacturers mount a bright tungsten-halogen bulb in a remote fan-cooled assembly. The tungsten-halogen bulb offers almost constant intensity and color throughout its life. Light intensity is adjustable. For microscopes needing intense light, an accessory metal halide light source offers higher output (Figure 5-17). Their brighter light has a color closer to true daylight. These bulbs are expensive but have a long life that brings their cost per hour close to that of the halogen bulbs. The light output dims as the bulb ages. A time is mounted on some of these bulbs to permit a preoperative check because changing them intraoperatively is difficult. Extra transmission cables and fewer accessories also improve the amount of light. Too much light, however, causes a headache during long procedures. Since bulbs will burn out, it is important to make sure the lamps work and that a spare lamp or lamp module is nearby before starting any procedure. Better light sources have built-in spare bulbs; all should be functional before a procedure is begun.

The light transmission guide can be a series of lenses as in a microscope-continued light supply, or a fiberoptic cable. Some microscopes have internal lenses, mirrors, and prisms that bend light onto the surgical field (Figure 5-18). A fiberoptic transmission cable is composed of

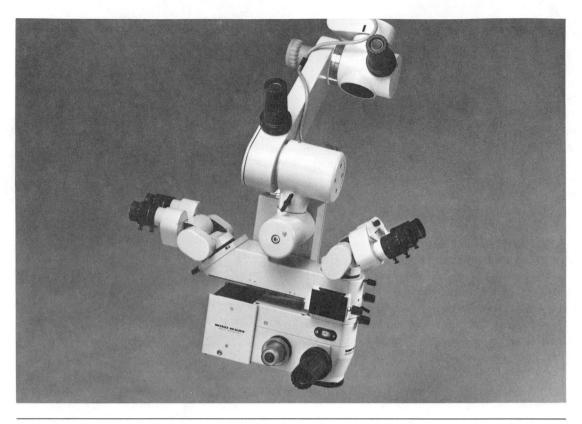

Figure 5-13
Microscope converted for two surgeons; each has stereoscopic vision.

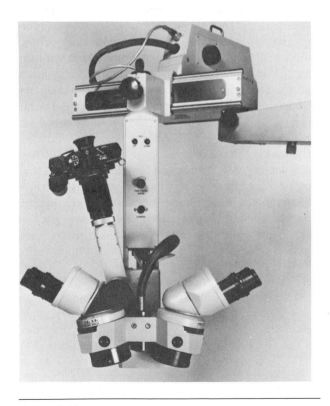

Figure 5-14
Weck Kleinert microscope (discontinued).

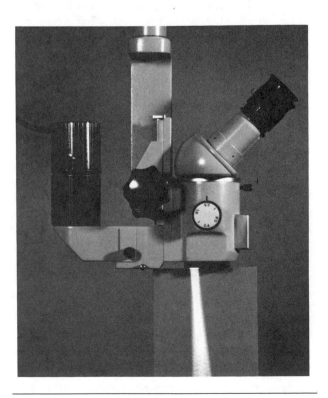

Figure 5-15
Coaxial internal light source.

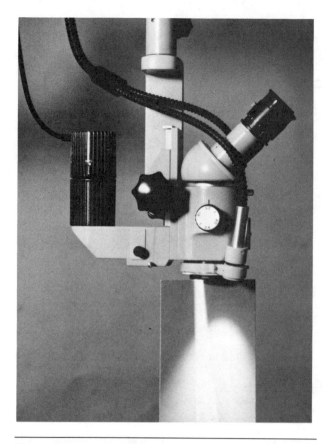

Figure 5-16
External mounted light source in addition to internal source.

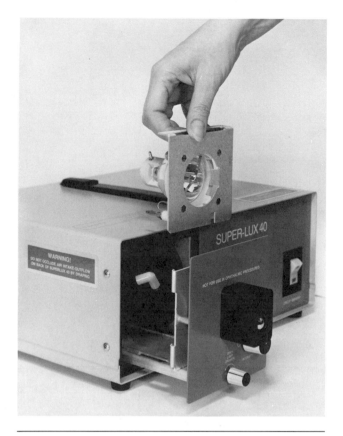

Figure 5-17
Zeiss Superlux vapor arc light source.

many individual glass fibers randomly arranged and encased in a protective sheath. These fibers conduct light with only some loss. Careless trauma or overbending of the cable will cause individual fibers to break, diminishing the light-carrying capacity. The ends are metal encased and polished. They should be kept clean to maintain light transmission.

The light exiting from an internal lighting system or a fiberoptic cable must be concentrated onto the field of view. Concentration is either by the microscope's objective lens (for coaxial lighting systems) or through an accessory outlying lens. Some units allow adjustment to fill the field of view of different objective lenses. Internally lighted units already compensate for different objectives, since the light passes through and is concentrated by the objective. Some manufacturers meet the greater lighting demands of higher magnification by concentrating the beam into the smaller field of view. As magnification changes, a lens inside the body shifts, optimizing light for the width needed.

Mounting systems

The mounting system varies in complexity and features as much as the microscope body does. Better systems improve handling of the microscope and minimize unwanted motion. The mount should position the microscope body both vertically and laterally over the surgical field. Movement to a new location should be easy. Vertical position must allow for coarse adjustment and fine focus. Using only the fine focus over a long distance wastes valuable time. Coarse focus alone is inadequate for the narrow depth of vision found with higher magnifications. The lack of fine focus can cause headaches when the eyes must compensate for poor focusing.

Motorized adjustments offer remote control, thus freeing the surgeon's hands and reducing surgery time. The common foot control must be positioned for the surgeon's comfort and ease of use. Most are not waterproof and are best protected with a plastic bag. Hand-operated controls require either the surgeon or the assistant to stop for adjustment, interrupting the flow of the procedure. Voice-operated controls are available from some manufacturers, but early designs have been hard to use.

Adjustments should lock or provide frictional resistance. Manufacturers have diverse tightening mechanisms. A well-designed manual lock applies a variable restraining friction to the pivot. The surgeon thus adjusts

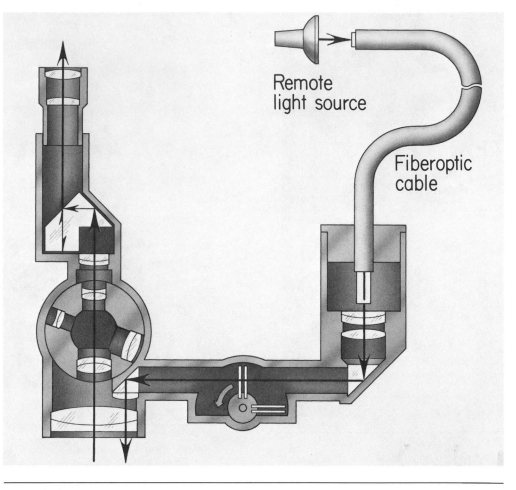

Figure 5-18
Internal lighting system.

the force required to move the microscope's position. The mechanism also should lock the arm tightly. A long arm or series of arms beyond the lock, however, acts as a lever, causing motion even in the best of locks. Locks tend to wear excessively when abused, forcing motion on a locked arm. Several manufacturers offer a soft metal bearing to absorb wear, and this eventually must be replaced. A better design uses large sleeve bearings that compress to provide the necessary friction. An alternative design has concentric controls, one to provide friction, the other to lock the arm. The surgeon must not try to apply friction with the locking control because it will easily wear out.

Most manufacturers use the rotating arm design (Figure 5-19) in which a series of arms rotating about the horizontal plane position the scope over the field. Height is adjusted along a vertical pole. Most units offer a second vertical control that acts as fine focus located near or in the body of the microscope. This is commonly a vertical linear gear controlled either by hand or motor. If necessary, the vertical height control of the stand itself,

driven with a slow-moving motor, converts into a fine focus. A separate gross height adjustment is easier to use.

The cantilever design counterbalances the weight of the microscope and springs (Figure 5-20) or weights. The arms extend the microscope over the field and permit easy horizontal and vertical movement. Unless height and vertical motion locks are provided, the easy movement presents a problem with drift from head to eyepiece contact. The variable friction lock is useful here. Most stand adjustments are done manually, requiring either sterilized knobs or draping. Fine focus can be motorized. A knob that varies tension on internal springs counterbalances the arm and permits adjustment for the variable weights of accessories. Certain stands (Figure 5-21) electromagnetically hold the position of the microscope. An electrical switch releases the locks on this counterbalanced stand, allowing the microscope to be moved freely to any new location. Releasing the switch relocks the position. The Mitaka stand for Wild microscopes will keep the microscope aimed at the same point as the sur-

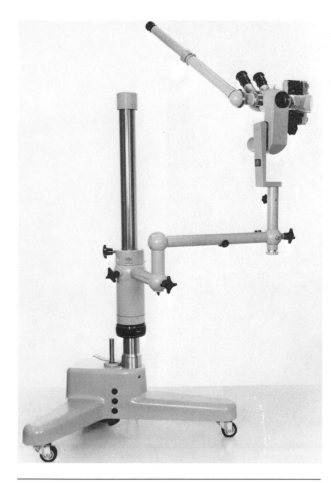

Figure 5-19
Rotational arm microscope stand configured for colposcopy.
Taller designs also can be used for intraabdominal work.

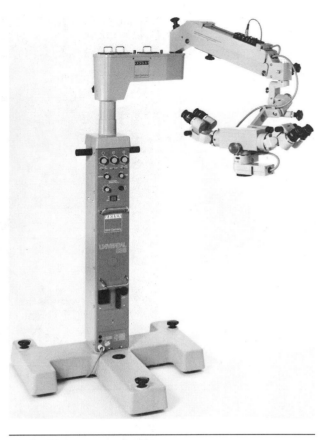

Figure 5-20
Cantilever microscope stand.

geon moves the microscope to a new angle of view. Originally designed for neurosurgery, electromagnetic stands are extremely expensive and have massive bases. They are not easy to use without investing some time to learn their operation.

Hand-free movement over the X-Y plane expedites some procedures. Just as motorized focusing and zoom magnification free the surgeon from interruption, so does a foot-operated lateral motion device. Reconstructive microsurgery frequently calls for back-and-forth changes between two sites. The required range is usually greater than the 2 cm available in standard accessories designed for ophthalmology. At present there are no X-Y adaptors with greater range.

Other accessories extend the microscope body farther away from the stand or tilt the body to view fields that are otherwise inaccessible. The surgeon must make sure that the microscope will reach the field desired. What is suitable for surgery of the hand may not reach far enough

to work in the abdomen. The tilt device is essential for access to many sites. Interrupting the procedure to reposition or redrape the patient adds unnecessarily to surgery time.

The base of the mounting system can be free standing or attached to a ceiling or wall. A track mount permits movement across the ceiling. A computer module can provide positional memory to bring the mount away from the wall back to the patient. Maneuverability and stability are of concern in the free-standing units. The ceiling and wall mounts are expensive and are restricted to one or two rooms. They offer exceptionally fast set-up time and minimize floor clutter.

Although mobile units can be brought from room to room, they are a problem to bring into the crowded operating room. A heavy stand does not roll easily over wires and tubing lying on the floor. Stands with larger-diameter wheels are easier to move over these obstructions. Wheels pick up floor debris, and thus periodic cleaning is necessary to optimize free motion. Planning before surgery minimizes microscope set-up time.

Stability problems increase with the use of heavy accessories and long extension of the microscope away

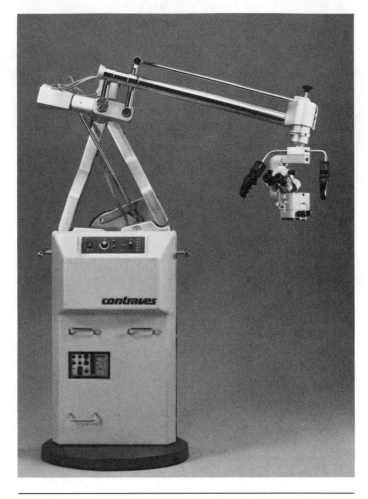

Figure 5-21
Contravus microscope stand.

from the base. Each stand has certain directions of increased and decreased stability. When testing for stability, one must evaluate all directions to prevent surprises in the middle of the procedure. Some companies limit rotation of the central extension arm to the range of stability. In setting up the microscope, the desired position must be in the center of this range for maximum flexibility later in the procedure. Most companies offer add-on weights to increase base stability and have heavy-duty models that accommodate greater weight and extension. Wider-based stands are more stable but are more difficult to move about.

Accessories

Observer tubes attach to a beam splitter or internal microscope optics and give monocular vision even with a binocular head. Students and scrub nurses need not have a stereoscopic view. An internal prism rotates the visual field for proper orientation.

A television camera is a valuable accessory, especially in long microsurgical procedures when the operating room staff wants to see what is going on. With video available, scrub nurses and students can participate, and video tapes can document procedures. To see 10-0 sutures and other details, high-resolution cameras are necessary. Television, 35mm, and movie cameras connect to the beam splitter and photographic adapters.

Maintenance and manufacturer support

Microscopes must be cared for. Expensive high-resolution systems cannot perform when coated with dust, fingerprints, and blood. Dust even creeps into the body itself, although the better systems have good protection. Covering the microscope optics with a lint-free cloth or plastic bag during storage helps, as does keeping the microscope assembled to minimize dust entry points. Accessories should be stored in dust-proof containers and handled carefully to prevent fingerprints and scratches.

When dirty, optics must be cared for like expensive photographic equipment. First, dust is dislodged with compressed air. Then the lens is cleaned with lens paper moistened in approved cleaner. The optics themselves must never be moistened because the fluid gets into the fittings. Xylene, alcohol, and other solvents destroy the lens coatings and cements. When internal optics such as zoom or drum systems become dirty, cleaning should be done by experienced personnel.

Here manufacturer support is essential: cleaning, periodic maintenance, and emergency service must be available; parts require dealer checking, lubrication, and replacement; if an item wears excessively, other pieces also may be destroyed. The surgeon must choose a dealer carefully, checking with others who have purchased similar units. It is also wise to investigate accessibility of loaner items when parts must be repaired. Depending on speed of service, one might consider purchasing a service agreement. Good dealers will keep purchasers informed of developments and improvements. Some will help with trade-in price reductions.

6

Electrosurgery

JACQUES E. RIOUX

Electosurgery is the use of electrically operated instruments for cutting or coagulating tissues during surgery. All surgical specialities have used some form of electrical current to perform or simplify their techniques during the past 50 years. Few, however, have relied on it as much as gynecologists have done in the past decade. In the early 1970s, laparoscopic electrocoagulation of the fallopian tubes became the most popular method of female sterilization. After three deaths from bowel injury and delayed peritonitis occurred with unipolar techniques in 1978 and 1979,[1] it became evident that these indispensable electrical systems were dangerous: they would have to be mastered or banned.

Electricity is no mystery.[2] It can be and should be understood by everyone using it, above all when it is used on the human body with the possibility of fatal complications. Obviously, laparoscopists cannot be expected also to be electrical engineers, nor is this necessary; however, we feel that a basic knowledge of terms, the workings of a generator, a few principles by which systems function, and finally, of the different types of instruments is mandatory.

TERMS

Only the terms most frequently used and absolutely necessary for adequate comprehension are defined and explained. They are compared with a simple hydraulic system for better integration.

Electric current: a stream of electrons flowing through a conducting body. "A stream of electrons" should make one think of quantities of particles that are so small as to exist only in the atomic world, yet so real as to produce reactions that are quite tangible. "Flowing through" evokes the notion of motion with penetration of matter. "A conducting body" confirms without defining if the flow is through a transmitting system (wires) or any type of matter (the human body) that will allow such a molecular movement.

Watt (James Watt, Scottish engineer, 1736–1819): the prac

tical unit of electrical power. It is defined as the rate of work represented by a current of one ampere under a pressure of one volt. It takes 746 watts of electricity to perform the work equivalent to that done by a motor of one horsepower.

Volt (Alessandro Volta, Italian physicist, 1745–1819): the unit of electromotive force, which, when steadily applied to a conductor whose resistance is one ohm, will produce a current of one ampere. The volt is a measure of electrical pressure, just as pounds per square inch is a measure of pressure in a hydraulic system.

Ampere (Andre M. Ampere, French physicist, 1775–1836): the practical unit of electric current strength. An ampere is defined as the steady current produced by one volt applied across a resistance of one ohm. It is a measure of the rate at which current flows. It corresponds to the unit gallons per minute in a liquid system, or to the number of quantities of electrons.

Ohm (Georg Simon Ohm, German physicist, 1787–1854): the electric resistance equal to the resistance of a circuit in which a potential difference of one volt produces a current of one ampere. An ohm is therefore the measure of resistance of

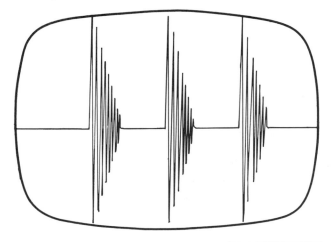

Figure 6-1
Oscilloscopic pattern of a highly damped or *coagulating current*. Bursts of rapidly decreasing current separated by gaps when no current passes.

a material to the flow of electric current through it. Resistances of tissues within the human body vary between 100 and 1000 ohms.

To summarize and to establish the analogy between an electrical system and a hydraulic system, we can picture that: the height of the reservoir represents the voltage or pressure; the diameter of the conduit represents the amperage or flow; the resistance offered by the turbines corresponds to the ohms; and the rate of work represents the wattage produced in the system.

Hertz (Heinrich Hertz, German physicist, 1857–1894): a unit of electromagnetic wave frequency equal to one cycle per second. It is abbreviated Hz.

High frequency: to be used efficiently in the human body, an electrical current must be delivered at a frequency high enough to avoid stimulating nerves and muscle; lower frequencies stimulate involuntary movements that cannot be prevented, even by deep anesthesia. Therefore we need electrogenerators capable of transforming the low-frequency current that flows in our electrical system (60 Hz or 60 cycles per second) to a high-frequency range that can be tolerated by the human body. The frequencies must be higher than 10,000 cycles per second.

ELECTROSURGICAL GENERATORS

In 1928 Harvey Cushing, an American neurosurgeon, introduced the concept of using electric current in surgery by publishing a series of 500 procedures in which brain tumor removal was facilitated by electrocoagulation. The unit producing the necessary high-frequency current had been designed by WT Bovie; the name Bovie has become a generic term for electrosurgical units.

These first generators were crude spark-gap units that consisted of a transformer to boost the voltage and high-voltage capacitors discharging through a certain number of gaps of fixed spacing.[3] Through them the current sparks or jumps at a very high frequency, thus producing a pulsating type of output. These gaps had to be compensated for to maintain an original setting regardless of temperature variations. They generated a highly damped current that was mostly hemostatic without cutting effect. For that reason, they were called coagulators. A survivor of that type is the Hyfrecator (Birtcher), which is commonly used in gynecologists' offices for electrodesiccation of condylomata. Such a unit has no place in endoscopy.

To add a smoother cutting current while making the generators more dependable (that is less likely to undergo variations secondary to temperature and relative humidity changes), the vacuum tube units were introduced. These generators have oscillators that are tuned at a radio frequency and that operate within a vacuum. They produce an undamped current that, when pure, delivers a cutting effect with very little coagulation.

During the past decade, the generators produced have been completely transistorized and for this reason are called solid state. They seem to be more versatile than earlier generators; they are smaller, yet they can generate the same types of currents or a combination.

As we have seen, two basic types of currents, or a combination thereof, can be used surgically. They differ in their physical effects in the body and can be identified by the wave patterns they display on an oscilloscope.

Coagulating current is highly damped and causes cellular dehydration: its effect is mainly hemostatic. Its the only type of current that could be produced by the spark-gap generators. As has been noted, this type of current has very little cutting effect and chars the tissue completely when applied over a long time. On the oscilloscope, it is characterized by bursts of rapidly decreasing current, separated by gaps when no current passes (Figure 6-1).

Cutting current is undamped and produces its cutting effect primarily by "exploding" cells, an effect secondary to the intense heat generated within the tissue itself. It is the typical current produced by the vacuum tube generators: very little hemostasis is produced and bleeding may occur when it is used in its pure form. On the oscilloscope, it is characterized by a constant flow of oscillations of equal amplitude and a frequency between 300,000 and 5,000,000 oscillations per second (Figure 6-2).

Blended current is by definition, a blend of the two types of waves discussed above and results in a combined cutting-coagulating effect. On the oscilloscope, it is characterized by a wavy but continuous type of current, without gaps (Figure 6-3). The newer generators can achieve a smooth and efficacious blended current by adding to the basic cutting as much hemostasis as desired.

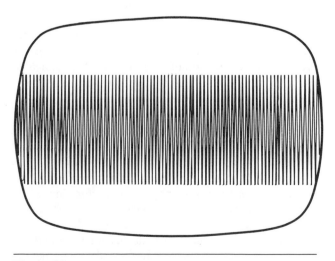

Figure 6-2
Oscilloscopic pattern of an undamped or *cutting* current. A constant flow of oscillations of equal amplitude at a very high frequency.

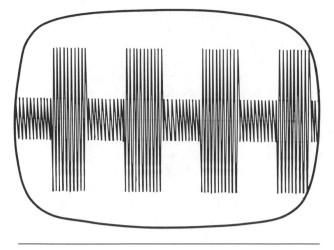

Figure 6-3
Oscilloscopic pattern of a blended *cutting—coagulating* current; a wavy but continuous type of current without gaps.

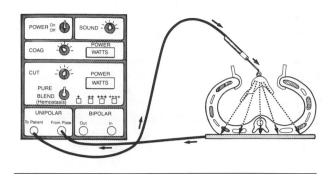

Figure 6-4
The unipolar system. The high-frequency current is applied at the site of the active electrode that being small concentrates the current to obtain the desired effect. From that point the current must return to the generator via the return electrode, which is large enough to prevent tissue destruction.

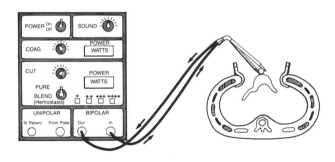

Figure 6-5
The bipolar system. The active and the return electrodes are both small; being in close approximation the current has a very short path and does not have to travel through the body to complete the circuit.

To conclude this section on electrosurgical units, let us say that they should be high in frequency, low in power, and preferably isolated.

It has been noted that the waveform frequency should be higher than 10,000 per second to avoid stimulating the neuromuscular junction. The newer generators use frequencies between 300 kHz and 1000 MHz, which is more than needed. Clinically there seems to be no difference, and no scientific medical research has ever determined the superiority of one frequency over another within this range.

It is important to stress the fact that in gynecologic endoscopy, using fine instruments in a dry field, a great deal of power is not necessary. When discussing the power of a generator, it is difficult to decide if one should use its voltage or its wattage output. Voltage being the measure of pressure under which current is delivered, it is dangerous and should be limited. For example, some generators can produce up to 9000 V (peak-to-peak open circuit) while others do not go above 300 V. Wattage is also important, since it takes resistance of tissues into consideration. For example, knowing that the resistance of a normal fallopian tube is approximately 500 ohms, under routine conditions, 60 W are quite adequate to coagulate it. Some generators can produce up to 700 W, which may be necessary for a urologist removing large segments of prostate under water. If the gynecologist has to share a generator with physicians performing other procedures, however, a wide range may be necessary, and great care will have to be exercised with its use.

It has been mentioned that the generator should be isolated. This concept has been introduced with the newer solid-state generators and should represent an improvement. In the grounded system, the conventional one until recently, the active electrode delivers the therapeutic current to the site at which it is required in the patient, and a ground plate collects the current as it leaves the patient's body. The plate here is a true ground, and the current thus collected is truly ground seeking and must be retrieved or it will find another path of escape, which could be dangerous. In the isolated (floating) output system, the patient plate is not a ground. Here also the current deposited into the patient must return to the generator by way of the return plate, which is not ground seeking. With the patient forming part of the circuit, a complete loop of current results, which is also isolated from the ground and the generating current. Such a unit will not function if the return electrode is placed improperly or is not connected, thus adding an element of safety to the system.

ELECTROSURGICAL SYSTEMS

The **unipolar system** is the most effective electrosurgical system, being used since the introduction of the ground plate. Indeed, a high-frequency current is presented at the site of the active electrode, which, being small, concentrates and thus achieves a high-density current, which can cut or coagulate tissues or both, according to the setting on the generator (Figure 6-4). From the point at which it is applied, the current must return to the generator by way of the ground plate, where the density must be low (since the electrode is large) so as to prevent a second site of tissue destruction. The integrity of the circuit is essential, since if the ground plate is not connected properly, the current would by necessity search out another avenue or route of escape. Thus any point at which the patient's body happened to be grounded would suffice, for example, through electrocardiogram electrodes, where skin burns would occur at the point of contact. This, however, could not happen with an isolated unit, since here the patient plate is not a ground. Indeed, here also the current deposited into the patient must return to the generator, but this time it is by way of the return plate and the current is not ground seeking.

In the **bipolar system,** the return electrode is not dispersive but acts as a return by being placed in close approximation to the active electrode. The current therefore does not have to travel through the entire body of the patient to complete the circuit, but only through the very small area interposed between the electrodes, destroying the tissue or coagulating the vessels (Figure 6-5). The area of destruction is strictly limited to the space between the forceps, and injury to the surrounding areas is impossible unless the tissues are grasped inadvertently. This is the greatest advantage of the use of bipolar systems in endoscopy, since it eliminates the danger of intraabdominal sparking and unrecognized bowel burns.

INSTRUMENTS

To review every instrument available on the market would be obviously impossible. In the light of what has been discussed, fairly good comprehension of their workings can be achieved by dividing them in three categories: the unipolar instruments, bipolar instruments, and others, which although they work by electricity, do not use it with the same principles. Also, the discussion is limited to electrical instruments; light sources and optical systems are not included unless some mention becomes mandatory.[4,5]

Unipolar instruments

Unipolar instruments have a few characteristics in common:

1. They carry only the active electrode.
2. Therefore they should always be used with a ground plate or a return electrode, otherwise they can be dangerous.
3. They should be well isolated to prevent accidental burns to patient and doctor (this is less dangerous when an isolated generator is used).
4. They have a wide range of sizes, shapes, and functions: (a) probes for aspiration and coagulation; (b) needles for destruction of endometrial implants; (c) needles for aspiration and coagulation; (d) hooks; (e) scissors of all shapes and forms; (f) graspers; (g) biopsy punches; and (h) the Palmer biopsy drill forceps or one of its modification, which is the most versatile instrument of them all.

These instruments can be used with a secondary trocar in the two-entry technique of surgical laparoscopy. They can also be used within the channel of a surgical laparoscope, but here a serious word of caution is mandatory. When using a unipolar electrosurgical instrument through a surgical laparoscope, the trocar sleeve should be made of metal so as to disperse within the abdominal wall the electricity that could be stored within the laparoscope acting as a capacitor. Indeed, when high-frequency current passes within a hollow metallic tube, and in spite of isolation of the instrument and within the conduit, the current jumps in the tubing, in this case the surgical laparoscope. It will either be dispersed without undue effect if the trocar sleeve is metallic, or be stored within the scope if no escape is possible when an isolated sleeve is used. We are convinced that many bowel burns have been caused by a "charged" laparoscope, the gynecologist being unaware of it because the scope does not receive any current at all. It is to be noted that this phenomenon does not occur when a bipolar forceps is used because of a canceling out of the waveforms coming in and out through the same channel.

With the advent of surgical hysteroscopy, a whole new line of unipolar instruments must be added at this point. They are mostly derived from urologic instruments, and the prototype is the resectoscope and its variations (for example, loops of different shapes, roller-ball electrodes, etc.).

When embarking on resectoscopic surgery, the gynecologist, like the urologist, joins the major league of electrosurgery. The work is done in a wet field; that is, within a liquid medium that must be circulating to maintain good visibility. The resistance of the tissues is greater, much like that of prostatic tissue, and therefore more power is needed, at least 150 W. All this can be done safely if adequate safeguards are respected.

Bipolar instruments

The bipolar instruments (1) carry both the active and the return electrodes; for this reason, (2) they either have two plugs or one combining the entry and the exit; with them therefore, (3) a ground plate or return electrode is

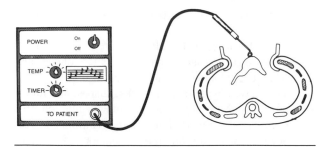

Figure 6-6

Thermocoagulation. Heat is the working agent. It is not diathermy, since high-frequency current is not used to cause an electric burn. Low-voltage current heats the tip of the instrument, which works by causing a thermal burn.

not necessary and should not be used; (4) they should be well isolated to function properly; and (5) they do not present a wide range of functions because they were designed primarily for coagulation in tubal sterilization.[6]

Fine bipolar coagulating forceps have been used for years by neurosurgeons and plastic surgeons because of the limited area of coagulation without spread along the vessels to deeper tissues. This application to gynecologic endoscopy was made in March of 1973, when the first bipolar instrument was developed for laparoscopic tubal sterilization.[7,8] The first prototype was a Palmer-type forceps that had been bipolarized by isolating the two prongs and connecting one to the active electrode and the other to the return or ground socket. Many prototypes were made and the final one was never commercially produced because of government roadblocks. This, however, did not stop private companies from going ahead and developing their own. Presently, bipolar tubal coagulation is the most popular form of interval female sterilization in North America. It is also the safest way to use electricity in gynecologic endoscopy. Indeed, with a bipolar system, the patient is not part of the circuit; only the tissue grasped between the two prongs is used to complete the circuit. Therefore the path of the current is limited to the space between the uninsulated forceps surfaces. The burn or coagulation is strictly limited to the area between the prongs and therefore has no spread.

Unfortunately, the choice of instruments is limited, and the bipolar forceps, because of their own nature, do not grasp tissues well and are sometimes awkward when one tries to use them for other uses than sterilization, for example, to coagulate adhesions before section or to coagulate endometrial implants for therapeutic purposes.

THERMOCOAGULATION

Thermocoagulation is a procedure that is based on none of the principles discussed. The instrument uses heat as its working agent and not electricity itself, although electricity is necessary to produce the heat. The instrument consists of an insulated holder that has at its tip a wire that is heated by a low-voltage current produced by a step-down transformer or simply, batteries. The heat is transferred directly to the tissue from the heated tip and no current at all flows through the patient.

The main application is the endocoagulator devised by Semm.[9] The transformer (Figure 6-6) has two main dials: one to preset the temperature and a timer that controls the heating cycle for the number of seconds. The instruments available are varied and can be used for tubal sterilization, lysis of adhesions, coagulation of myomas, and so on. It is less dangerous than diathermy because only a small amount of current is necessary to heat the element, which causes a thermal burn, not an electrical one.

SUMMARY

A few recommendations are in order. The gynecologist should:

1. Know the generator; it should be high-frequency, low-power, and preferably isolated.
2. Know what to expect from the generator and should not increase the output when the results are not within expectations.
3. Know all other instruments, how they function, how they should be cleaned, and how to put them together.
4. Know the people who will be handling the instruments and make sure they treat all equipment with the greatest care.
5. Use common sense.

REFERENCES

1. Peterson HB et al: Deaths associated with laparoscopic sterilization by unipolar electrocoagulating devices, 1978 and 1979, *Am J Obstet Gynecol* 139:141-143, 1981.
2. Rioux JE and Yuzpe AA: Electrosurgery untangled, *Contemp Obstet Gynecol* 4:118-124, 1974.
3. Rioux JE and Yuzpe AA: Know thy generator, *Contemp Obstet Gynecol* 6:52, 1975.
4. Phillips JM (ed): *Laparoscopy,* Baltimore, 1977, Williams & Wilkins.
5. Phillips JM (ed): *Endoscopy in gynecology,* Proceedings of the third International Congress of Gynecologic Endoscopy. Downey, Calif, 1978, American Association of Gynecologic Laparoscopists.
6. Rioux JE and Yuzpe AA: Evaluation of female sterilization procedures, *Curr Probl Obstet Gynecol* 2(9):1-43, 1979.
7. Rioux JE and Cloutier D: Laparoscopic tubal sterilization: sparking and its control, *Vie Med Can Franc* 2:760-765, 1973.
8. Rioux JE and Coutier DA: A new bipolar instrument for laparoscopic tubal sterilization, *Am J Obstet Gynecol* 119:737-739, 1974.
9. Semm K: *Atlas of gynecologic laparoscopy and hysteroscopy,* Philadelphia, 1977, WB Saunders.

7

Laser Basics and Safety

DAN C. MARTIN

Power density and absorption are major predictors of the surgical effect of a laser. At low power density, the specific effects of lasers are noted, whereas at high power density, all lasers vaporize tissue. Absorption is tissue dependent,[1] and the power density needed to vaporize tissue with the neodymium:yttrium-aluminum-garnet (Nd:YAG) laser may be less than that needed for water vaporization, since the coefficient of absorption is higher in tissue than in water. The difference in vaporization coefficients between tissue and water are even greater for the argon and 532-nm potassium-titanyl-phosphate (KTP) lasers. These two lasers have almost no absorption by water and are selectively absorbed by hemoglobin.

HISTORY

Surgical lasers have been used since the 1960s. Early reviewers[2,3] concluded that, with the exception of photocoagulation of the retina, the disadvantages of its use outweighed any advantages. The equipment at that time was bulky, and concepts of safety were ill defined. By 1971[4] the surgical carbon dioxide (CO_2) laser had been used to perform partial hepatectomy with minimal hemorrhage, no bile leakage, sound healing, and no late complications.

Development continued, and the CO_2 laser was first used in gynecology in the treatment of cervical disease in 1973.[5] Its use subsequently was reported in gynecologic malignancy[6] and in reconstructive pelvic surgery.[7] Single-puncture CO_2 laser laparoscopic equipment was developed[8] and second-puncture applications were presented.[9] Daniell et al introduced laparoscopic use in the United States of CO_2 laser[10] and KTP laser.[11] Others concentrated on the argon laser[12] and the Nd:YAG laser.[13]

LASER BASICS

Laser energy is generated by manipulation of the atomic structure of molecules in a laser tube. The laser is named for the types of molecules within the tube (resonating chamber). The CO_2, argon, and helium-neon (HeNe) laser tubes contain the gas that is their name. The KTP and Nd:YAG lasers contain modified YAG crystals.

Lasers have some common characteristic with respect to energy. The beams are monochromatic, coherent, and collimated. Coherent photons (light units) vibrate together. Monochromatic beams have a specific color (wavelength). Collimated beams are in an energy bundle that is more compact than a spotlight. Some characteristics, however, vary from one laser to another (Table 7-1). These include color (wavelength), penetration, absorption, and scatter. The color can be visible (argon, HeNe, KTP), infrared (CO_2, Nd:YAG), or ultraviolet (Excimer), and the tunable free electron laser can produce the range from x-ray (far ultraviolet) through visible color to far infrared.[1]

ENERGY CONVERSION

Absorption converts the light energy into thermal energy. At low power density, the slow heating results in warming, desiccation, or slow vaporization. Table 7-2 is specific for the CO_2 laser, but similar tables can be created for the other lasers. As noted above, lasers with greater penetration need higher power densities for sufficient absorption to produce vaporization. Very low power densities are used to unwind the collagen in an attempt to promote welding[1] (Table 7-3). High power density produces rapid heating and vaporization or sublimation. There is no precise distinction between low and high power densities. This is a concept that is dependent on the purpose of laser use and the experience of the operator.

High power density produces rapid vaporization while decreasing the extent of thermal necrosis (Figure 7-1). At high power density, thermal necrosis is generally less than 300 μ for all lasers and is directly related to the length of time the laser takes to make the incision, which in turn is related to power density. Although this thermal

Table 7-1 General laser characteristics

Laser	Color	Wavelength (nm)	Tissue penetration (mm)	Absorption	Scatter
CO_2	Infrared	10,600	0.1	Water	Minimal
Argon	Blue-green	488-515	0.4	Hemoglobin	Minor
KTP	Green	532	0.4	Hemoglobin	Minor
Nd:YAG	Infrared	1064	4.2	Tissue	Great

Table 7-2 Power densities for CO_2 laser tissue effect

W/cm²	Tissue effect
0-50	Warming
5-200	Superficial desiccation and contraction
400-4000	Slow, wide vaporization and sublimation
>1200	Rapid, narrow vaporization and sublimation

Table 7-3 The effect of heating tissue

Temperature		Effect
°C	°F	
37.0	98.6	Euthermic
38.0	100.4	Febrile symptoms
42.5	108.4	Death of malignant cells
44.0	111.2	Death of normal cells
60.0	140.0	Collagen helix uncoils
65.0	149.0	Coagulation of protein
100.0	212.0	Vaporization of water
3652.0	6605.6	Sublimation of carbon

necrosis is related to the penetration of the laser, the conduction of heat from the vaporization of water (100° C) and the sublimation of tissue (including carbon at 3652° C) appear to be the most important factors.

Proper parfocusing of the microscope and laser lenses is necessary to focus the laser correctly and to predict the tissue effect. By adjusting the focal distance at the highest power and the oculars at the lowest power, magnification can be changed without changing the focus. Unless this is done, the laser can be out of focus when the microscope is in focus.

CO_2 laser

The CO_2 laser is a high-intensity source of infrared light. As this light contacts various material, it can be transmitted, reflected, absorbed, or scattered (Figure 7-2). The CO_2 laser is transmitted through air and zinc arsenic lenses. It is reflected off polished surfaces but absorbed by water, water-containing tissue, glass, plastic, and many other materials.

With high power density, the CO_2 laser is a "what you see is what you get" laser, with thermal necrosis generally limited to 0.04[14] to 0.5 mm.[15] This is used in a no-touch technique, with the extent of surgery controlled by the setting on the panel. This combination allows the surgeon to work at a distance with no tissue resistance. With incision, however, traction on the tissue produces a cleaner cut and less tissue vaporization and smoke.

The beam of the laser as it exits the port is 10 to 2 mm for many clinical lasers. At 20 W output, this port beam has a power density of 25 to 637 W/cm². These power densities are useful for surface coagulation or large area vaporization. Lens systems are used to focus the CO_2 laser to smaller spot sizes and higher power densities (Figure 7-3). A defocused zone distal to the focal point has low power density that can be used for coagulation and for surface contraction.

Argon and KTP lasers

Argon and KTP lasers are absorbed by hemoglobin and pass through water and the clear portions of the eye. This property makes the argon an excellent laser at low power density for retinal surgery. In addition, it has been used on endometriosis because of the hemoglobin concentration in many lesions.[12,16] The KTP is a frequency-doubled Nd:YAG laser that has the tissue effect of argon and has only one primary frequency rather than the range of frequencies of argon.

Small fibers (0.3 and 0.6 mm) and artificial sapphire tips are used to produce high power density and create effects similar to those of the CO_2 laser but with increased hemostasis. This is useful in clinical situations where hemostasis is a major problem. Also, surgeons may desire a touch technique. In addition, they may experience problems with CO_2 laser alignment, and thus often find fibers more acceptable than the CO_2 laser port.

The power density for a fiber (Figure 7-4) is greatest as it exits the fiber. In the immediate vicinity of the fiber, the power density can be high enough for vaporization.

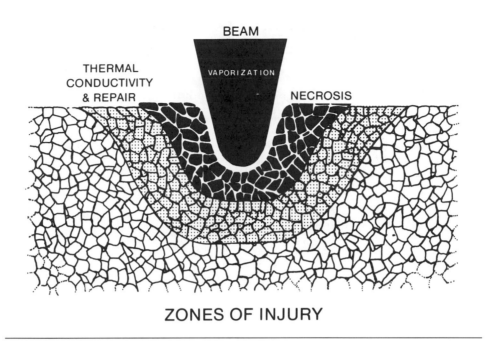

ZONES OF INJURY

Figure 7-1
Zones of thermal injury are related to both the intrinsic penetration of the laser and the thermal of heat at the base of the crater. From Martin DC (ed): *Techniques and safety in intra abdomi-nal laser surgery* (slide set), 1984.

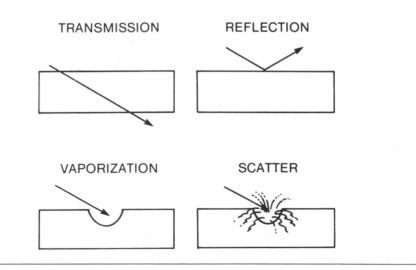

Figure 7-2
Laser interaction with tissue is dependent on the specific laser. From Martin DC (ed): *Techniques and safety in intra-abdominal laser surgery* (slide set), 1984.

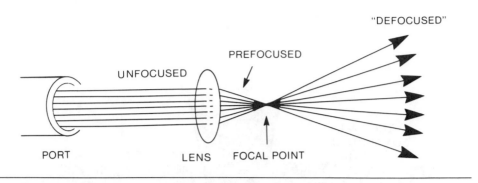

Figure 7-3
Laser beams can be focused using a lens system. This is the general method when using the CO_2 laser but can also be used with other lasers. From Martin DC (ed): *Techniques and safety in intra-abdominal laser surgery* (slide set), 1984.

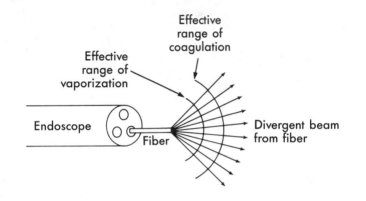

Figure 7-4
Fiber-directed lasers diverge rapidly from the end of the fiber. With a high enough power density, the initial zone is vaporization. At a distance from this is coagulation, and past this point there is only heating. From Martin DC (ed): *Intra-abdominal Laser Surgery*, ed 2 (in preparation).

Within a few centimeters, it decreases to the point at which it will coagulate. Past a certain level, the power density decreases to such a low level that energy transfer results in heating with no long-term biologic effect.

Nd:YAG laser

The low-power-density Nd:YAG laser has a great deal of penetration in tissue and in water and can be used to photocoagulate the vessels in a hemorrhagic ulcer or in the endometrium. It also has a great deal of scatter and may be redirected through the optics of an endoscope, damaging the surgeon's eye. Specific filters and lenses are necessary to prevent this from occurring.

Although the major uses of Nd:YAG lasers have been in gastrointestinal hemostasis and gynecologic uterine endometrial ablation, these instruments are also helpful in endometriosis.[13,17] With small sapphire tips the power can be concentrated and used for vaporization.

Developmental lasers

Krypton, gold vapor, and tunable dye lasers are used to activate hematoporphyrin derivatives in the palliative therapy of cancer and to treat endometriosis in animal models.[18] Excimer (excited dimer) lasers have a unique tissue effect with little thermal component. This lack of thermal heating may be useful where laser-induced hemostasis is not important.

LASER SAFETY

Lasers are potentially dangerous devices because they concentrate large amounts of energy into very small beams. Their use has been associated with skin rashes, skin burns, retinal swelling, pneumothorax, ocular hemorrhage, emergency laparotomies, colostomies, pulmonary explosions, blindness, and death.[19-22] To maintain a safe record, all surgeons must have the greatest regard for careful application of this equipment. Initial education in safety techniques must be followed by reeducation as more sophisticated lasers become available. Specific areas of concern include burns from the equipment, damage to auxiliary equipment, mutagenicity of the vapor smoke, carcinogenicity of the remnant tissue, and the possible spread of disease.

Standards for the operating room

The American National Standards Institute (ANSI) published the following standards for the use of class IV lasers[23,24]:

1. Direct supervision is required.
2. Access by spectators requires approval. Use safety latches or interlocks to prevent unexpected entry of personnel into laser controlled areas.
3. Appropriate warning signs are posted:
    a. "DANGER" should be on signs and labels associated with the laser.
    b. "Laser Radiation: Avoid eye or skin exposure to direct or scattered radiation" should be displayed prominently.
    c. "Invisible" should be included in the sign when using wavelengths that cannot be seen.
4. Any potentially hazardous beam should be terminated in a beam stop.
5. The beam stop should be highly absorbent, non-reflecting, and fire resistant.
6. Use diffusely reflective materials, such as dull-surfaced instruments, in or near the beam path.
7. All windows in areas with levels above the ocular maximum permissible exposure are covered or restricted.

Equipment hazards

Although control with the microscope is great, it has been responsible for the most damage to surgeons' hands. Because of the long depth of field, the invisible beam can easily cut when microsurgeons roll their hands through the surgical field. No-touch surgery must be mastered to avoid this complication.[25]

The mechanical shutters are kept closed until the laser is ready for use, while the shutter of the aiming beam is kept open. The site of the laser is kept in mind at all times. The use of pedals other than the laser is avoided unless it is absolutely necessary. This is to prevent unintended activation of the laser.

High voltages are stored inside the main power box of the laser and remain even after the equipment is unplugged.[26,27] Panels protecting this area should be removed only by a skilled technician because the voltages in this box may exceed 15,000 V and can cause pain, burns, ventricular fibrillation, and death.[28]

Surgical drapes can be ignited by the laser, by cautery, or by high-intensity photographic lights.[26,29,30] These should be fire retardant and, when feasible, wet. A fire extinguisher is kept in the room or nearby.

Alcohol, ether, and combustible anesthetic gases may be ignited and can cause burns. Vaporization of solutions creates a plume containing the chemical remnants of the solutions. The plume from vaporizing chlorhexidine can cause a rash.[19]

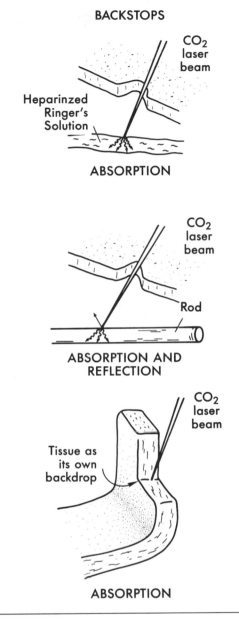

BACKSTOPS

Figure 7-5
The CO_2 laser is generally stopped by solutions, rods, or the tissue itself. Solutions and tissue absorb the beam in its entirety. Rods both absorb and reflect the beam. From Martin DC (ed): *Intra-abdominal laser surgery*, ed 2 (in preparation).

Backstops

Glass, Pyrex, and quartz rods have been used as backstops, but they shatter since they do not disperse heat well. Other materials, such as water solutions, soaked sponges, soaked Telfa pads, and etched rods, are currently substituted to avoid this danger (Figure 7-5). Polished metal mirrors have replaced rhodium front-surfaced glass to redirect the beam in the deep pelvis (Figure 7-6).

INCISION OF SUBOVARIAN ADHESIONS

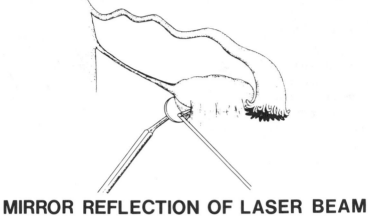

MIRROR REFLECTION OF LASER BEAM

Figure 7-6
Mirror reflection techniques are used to incise beneath the ovary at microsurgery. From Martin DC (ed): *Techniques and safety in intra-abdominal laser surgery* (slide set), 1984.

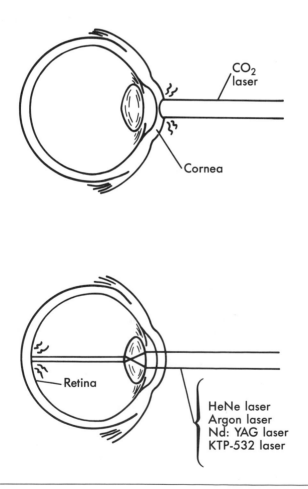

Figure 7-7
Eye damage can occur with any type laser. In general, the CO_2 laser damages the cornea the other lasers damage the retina. From Martin DC (ed): *Intra-abdominal laser surgery*, ed 2 (in preparation).

The use of solution in the pelvis as a backstop can be easier to control than rods. In addition, retroperitoneal injection of solution is recommended to move the peritoneum away from structures such as ureter, bladder, bowel, and vessels.[31] This technique is useful for the surgeon who does not wish to dissect and isolate these areas.

Teflon-coated rods commonly used for tissue manipulation in regular surgical cases should not be used as a backstop during laser surgery. When Teflon is vaporized, it produces a toxic vapor.

Eye protection

Eye protection is necessary to shield the surgeon, operating room personnel, and patient from inadvertent damage. For microscopic intraabdominal procedures, the equipment itself is never aimed at the patient's head, and this provides sufficient protection. The same is true of laparoscopic procedures. Eye wear for operating room personnel should be sufficient to protect from a specific laser. Although any type of eye wear will stop a CO_2 laser, other lasers require specific lens characteristics. Glasses that may be useful for one laser may not be with another.

Because of the differential absorption by tissue types, the damage from a CO_2 laser is on the surface while that from other lasers generally is on the retina (Figure 7-7). The retinal damage can be significant because the eye may focus the laser to a small spot size.

Nd:YAG cooling

The Nd:YAG laser tips can become very hot and may represent a biologic hazard with unintentional contact with unaffected tissues. In addition, four instances of fracture of the sapphire tip occurred in 38 patients but with no loss of any or all of the tip.[32] Both air and liquid cooling systems have been used to cool the tip. Saline solutions at 30 drops per minute rapidly cool the tip but also cause frosting. Water cooling appears safer for the patient than air cooling.

The air-cooled Nd:YAG laser, when used for hysteroscopy, has been associated with massive air embolus. This has resulted in several deaths and an alert from the Food and Drug Administration (FDA). The equipment can be changed over to water or liquid cooling by most operating rooms without modification of the equipment.[33,34]

Carcinogenicity

The particulate concentration in an operating room after vaporizing 1 g of canine tissue was 52 times higher than regulated environmental standards. It was found that 77% of these particles were of small enough size to be deposited in the alveoli. These particles demonstrated mutagenic activity in *Salmonella typhi* similar to activity noted with cigarette smoke and other particulate smoke.[35,36] This was less mutagenic than smoke from an electrical coagulator.[37] Suctioning within 1 cm of the target reduced the particulate concentration by 98.6%.

Fibroblasts exposed to the carbon dioxide laser showed no increased frequency of malignant transformation.[38] Studies of RNA, DNA, and cytology indicate that the vapor plume is biologically inactive and contains no viable particulate matter when using a continuous CO_2 laser.[39,40] There was no evidence of spread, recurrence, or metastasis related to the CO_2 laser when used in surgery on the Cloudman S-91 melanoma.[41] This is in contrast to the dissemination of tumor cells with a pulsed Nd:YAG laser,[42] the dissemination of bacteriophage with a pulsed erbium:YAG laser,[43] and the finding of intact viral DNA of papillomavirus in the vapor of laser-treated verrucae.[44]

Pulmonary hazards

Bronchitis and pneumonitis have occurred when the smoke-evacuation systems were inadequate during research or hands-on teaching in the laboratory. This acute response to an accumulation of smoke is worrisome. The chance that extended exposure to this smoke may be as dangerous as cigarette smoke was noted above.[35-37] In addition, the possibility of disseminating viral, malignant, and other particles has become of increasing importance, with worries regarding the dissemination of human immunodeficiency virus (HIV).[45]

The two main approaches to protection have been the use of high-flow smoke evacuator systems and mask filters. High-flow evacuation systems must be kept close to the surgical site for effective evacuation.[46] Distances of greater than 1 cm[35,37] to 2 inches[46] were likely to result in exposure to high concentrations both near the laser interaction site and throughout the room.

Most surgical masks do not filter out the 0.10-μ to 0.80-μ particles that are found in the plume of cigarette smoke.[47] Because of this, the filter systems themselves must be capable of filtering out these particles. Using a system of an inner position of a cartridge filter plus an ultralow-penetration air filter to trap 0.1-μ particles, pulmonary lesions were not noted in a rat model.[48]

SUMMARY

The choice of a laser in surgery is often made on the basis of what is available. Thus it is good that manipulation of the laser beam can result in overlapping tissue effects. For physicians who have access to or who will be ordering new lasers, understanding the tissue effects and methods by which they are produced may influence their choice.

It should be expected that, when the laser is used with skill, discretion, and common sense, an excellent record of safety can be maintained. Taking short cuts and disregarding these principles can result in harm to the physician, operating room personnel, and the patient.

REFERENCES

1. Harris DM and Werkhaven JA: Biophysics and applications of medical lasers, *Adv Otolaryngol Head Neck Surg* 3:91-123, 1989.
2. Ketcham AS, Hoye RC, and Riggle GC: A surgeon's appraisal of the laser, *Surg Clin North Am* 47:1249-1263, 1967.
3. Fox JL: The use of laser radiation as a surgical "light knife," *J Surg Res* 9:199-205, 1969.
4. Hall RR, Beach AD, and Hill DW: Partial hepatectomy using a carbon dioxide laser, *Br J Surg* 60:141-143, 1973.
5. Kaplan I, Goldman JM, and Ger R: The treatment of erosions of the uterine cervix by means of the CO_2 laser, *Obstet Gynecol* 41:795-796, 1973.
6. Bellina JH: Gynecology and the laser, *Contemp Obstet Gynecol* 4:24-34, 1974.
7. Bellina JH: Carbon dioxide laser in gynecology, *Obstet Gynecol Ann* 6:371-391, 1977.
8. Bruhat MA, Mage G, and Manhes M: Use of the CO_2 laser by laparoscopy. In Kaplan I (ed): *Proceedings of the third International Congress for Laser Surgery*, Tel Aviv, 1979, Ot-Paz.
9. Tadir Y et al: Laparoscopic applications of the CO_2 laser. In Atsumi K and Nimsakul N (eds): *Proceedings of the fourth congress of the International Society for Laser Surgery*, Tokyo, 1981, Japanese Society for Laser Medicine.
10. Daniell JF and Pittaway DE: Use of the CO_2 laser laparoscope in laparoscopic surgery: initial experience with the second puncture technique, *Infertility* 5:15-23, 1982.
11. Daniell JF, Miller W, and Tosh R: Initial evaluation of the use of the potassium-titanyl-phosphate (KTP/532) laser in gynecologic laparoscopy, *Fertil Steril* 46:373-377, 1986.
12. Keye WR and Dixon J: Photocoagulation of endometriosis with the argon laser through the laparoscope, *Obstet Gynecol* 62:383-386, 1983.
13. Lomano JM: Laparoscopic ablation of endometriosis with the YAG laser, *Lasers Surg Med* 3:179, 1983.
14. Luciano AA et al: A comparison of thermal injury, healing patterns, and postoperative adhesion formation following CO_2 laser and electromicrosurgery, *Fertil Steril* 48:1025-1029, 1987.
15. Taylor MV et al: Effect of power density and carbonization on residual tissue coagulation using the continuous wave carbon dioxide laser, *Colposc Gynecol Laser Surg* 2:169-175, 1986.
16. Keye WR et al: Argon laser therapy of endometriosis: a review of 92 consecutive patients, *Fertil Steril* 47:208-212, 1987.
17. Kojima E et al: Nd:YAG laser endoscopy, *J Reprod Med* 33:907-911, 1988.
18. Petrucco OM et al: Ablation of endometriotic implants in rabbits by hematoporphyrin derivative photoradiation therapy using the gold vapor laser, *Lasers Surg Med* 10:344-348, 1990.
19. Baggish MS: Complications associated with carbon dioxide laser surgery in gynecology, *Am J Obstet Gynecol* 139:568-574, 1981.
20. Rogers P, Schellhas HF, and Moss E: Hazards associated with the use of surgical lasers. In Rockwell J (ed): *Laser safety in surgery and medicine*, ed 4, Cincinnati, 1983, Rockwell Associates.
21. Martin DC and Diamond MP: Operative laparoscopy: comparison of lasers with other techniques, *Curr Probl Obstet Gynecol Fertil* 9:563-617, 1986.
22. Wulwick R and Brenner SH: Pneumothorax in association with laseroscopy, *Colposc Gynecol Laser Surg* 3:221-223, 1987.
23. American National Standards Institute, Inc: *American national standard for the safe use of lasers* (ANSI Z136.1 - 1986), New York, 1986, American National Standards Institute.
24. American National Standards Institute, Inc: *American national standard for the safe use of lasers in health care facilities* (ANSI Z136.3 - 1988), New York, 1988, American National Standards Institute.
25. Daniell JF: CO_2 laser in infertility surgery, *J Reprod Med* 28:265-268, 1983.
26. Schellhas HF: Safety aspects for carbon dioxide laser surgery. In Bellina JH (ed): *Gynecologic laser surgery*, New York, 1981, Plenum Press.
27. Tsuzuki M: System approach for safety assurance in laser surgery. In Atsumi K, Nimsakul N (ed): *Proceedings of the fourth congress of the International Society of Laser Surgery*, Tokyo, 1981, Japanese Society for Laser Medicine.
28. Rogers P, Schellhas HF, and Moss E: Hazards associated with the use of surgical lasers. In Rockwell J (ed): *Laser safety in surgery and medicine*, ed 4, Cincinnati, 1983, Rockwell Associates.
29. Fisher JC: CO_2 lasers for gynecologic surgery: how safe are they? *Contemp Obstet Gynecol* 21:39-54, 1983.
30. Patel KF and Hicks JN: Prevention of fire hazards associated with the use of carbon dioxide laser, *Anesth Analg* 60:885-888, 1981.
31. Nezhat C and Nezhat F: Safe laser endoscopic excision or vaporization of peritoneal endometriosis, *Fertil Steril* 52:149-151, 1989.
32. Shirk GJ: Use of the Nd:YAG laser for the treatment of endometriosis, *Am J Obstet Gynecol* 160:1344-1351, 1989.
33. Baggish MS and Daniell JF: Death caused by air embolism associated with neodymium:yttrium-aluminum-garnet laser surgery and artificial sapphire tips, *Am J Obstet Gynecol* 161:877-878, 1989.
34. Baggish MS and Daniell JF: Catastrophic injury secondary to the use of coaxial gas-cooled fiber and artificial sapphire tips for intrauterine surgery, *Lasers Surg Med* 9:581-585, 1989.
35. Mihashi S et al: Some problems about condensates induced by CO_2 laser irradiation. In Atsumi K and Nimsakul N (eds): *Proceedings of the fourth congress of the International Society for Laser Surgery*, Tokyo, 1981, Japanese Society for Laser Medicine.
36. Baggish MS and Elbakry M: The effects of laser smoke on the lungs of rats, *Am J Obstet Gynecol* 156:1260-1265, 1987.
37. Tomita Y et al: Mutagenicity of smoke condensates induced by CO_2 laser irradiation and electrocauterization, *Mutation Res* 89:145-149, 1981.
38. Apfelberg DB, Mittelman H, and Chabi B: Carcinogenic potential of in vitro carbon dioxide laser exposure of fibroblasts, *Obstet Gynecol* 61:403-496, 1983.
39. Bellina JH, Sterjernholm RL, and Kurpel JE: Analysis of plume emissions after papovavirus irradiation with carbon dioxide laser, *J Reprod Med* 27:268-270, 1982.
40. Mihashi S et al: Laser surgery in otolaryngology: interaction of CO_2 laser in soft tissue, *Ann NY Acad Sci* 267:263-294, 1976.
41. Oosterhuis JW, Verschueren RCJ, and Oldhof J: Experimental surgery on the Cloudman S91 melanoma with the carbon dioxide laser, *Acta Chir Belg* 4:422-429, 1975.
42. Hoye RC, Ketcham AS, and Riggle GC: The airborne dissemination of viable tumor by high energy neodymium laser, *Life Sci* 6:119, 1967.
43. Ediger MN and Matchette LS: In vitro production of a viable bacteriophage in a laser plume, *Lasers Surg Med* 9:296-299, 1989.
44. Garden JM et al: Papillomavirus in the vapor of carbon dioxide laser-treated verrucae, *JAMA* 259:1199-1202, 1988.
45. Jako GJ: CO_2 laser in surgery for prophylaxis of HIV infection (letter), *Lasers Surg Med* 8:139, 1988.
46. Smith JP et al: Evaluation of a smoke evacuator used for laser surgery, *Lasers Surg Med* 9:276-281, 1989.
47. Nezhat C et al: Smoke from laser surgery: is there a health hazard? *Lasers Surg Med* 7:376-382, 1987.
48. Baggish MS, Baltoyannis P, and Sze E: Protection of the rat lung from the harmful effects of laser smoke, *Lasers Surg Med* 8:248-253, 1988.

8

Clinical Use of Lasers

DAN C. MARTIN

Surgical lasers have been used for more than 25 years. The history of their development is reviewed in Chapter 7 on laser basics and safety. This chapter addresses laboratory and clinical studies on the surgical use of lasers.

LABORATORY STUDIES
Tissue response

Studies suggest that a sharp knife and the Shaw scalpel cause less initial damage than either the electrosurgical unit or laser. Although the laser created a greater scar width than the electrosurgical unit in skin incisions in an initial study,[1] the same degree of damage occurred when electrosurgery was used at high speed.[2,3] The zone of thermal necrosis is related to the power density and the speed of the incision. The narrow zone of thermal damage noted with high-power-density lasers[4] is also noted with high-power-density electrosurgery.[5,6]

Delay in healing of skin incisions, but not abdominal wall incisions, was noted when laser or electrosurgical units were compared with a knife.[7] The residual damage in peritoneal incisions caused by the laser was minimal compared with that of the electrosurgical unit.[8] Laser incisions healed more slowly than electrosurgical incisions.[2,9,10] However, decreased resistance to bacterial infection has been demonstrated.[1,2]

Thermal spread and thermal necrosis are decreased when using several short-duration impulses of the carbon dioxide (CO_2) and neodymium:yttrium-aluminum-garnet (Nd:YAG) lasers, compared with continuous use for the same depth of penetration.[11-13] These short impulses can be generated by short-duration (pulse) activation of the shutter or by multiple electronic stimulations (superpulse, ultrapulse) of the laser. These two techniques can maintain high power density while lowering average power density. This combination can be used to decrease thermal damage and increase the control of the laser unit.

This increased control also increases the time required for surgery.

At a low power density of 30 W/cm^2, the zone of thermal necrosis was 2.7 mm with a CO_2 laser,[13] whereas with low-power-density, noncontact Nd:YAG, the zone was 4.2 mm.[14] These similar zones were the result of two different types of thermal transfer. For the CO_2 laser, thermal transfer was related to extended time and to exposure to the vaporization of water at 100° C and the sublimation of carbon at 3652° C. This type of transfer decreases with increased power density.[13] The result with the Nd:YAG laser was due to penetration by the laser beam with conversion of laser energy into heat. This type of thermal necrosis increases with increased power density when using noncontact techniques.[14] As discussed in Chapter 7, the Nd:YAG laser is poorly absorbed by tissue or water and penetrates deeper than the CO_2 laser. The argon and potassium-titanyl-phosphate (KTP) lasers are not absorbed by water to any appreciable extent and are absorbed greatly by hemoglobin, melanin, and other pigmented tissue.[15]

At high power density, CO_2 laser thermal necrosis can be as low as 60 μm.[14] The zone that appears to offer a useful combination of hemostasis with a clean incision is 100 to 500 μm.[13]

Tubal anastomosis

Welding and low-power-density techniques do more harm than good. An 18% overall success rate was seen using welding techniques.[16] Subsequent low success rates were noted in implantation and anastomosis,[17] welding, and suturing techniques at low power densities,[18] and low-power-density incisions with subsequent welding and anastomosis.[19]

Low-power-density (1000 W/cm^2) incisions followed by immediate anastomosis of rat uterine horns[20] produced 75% stenosis with hydrometra and hydrosalpinx formation (Figure 8-1). Similar problems have been seen in

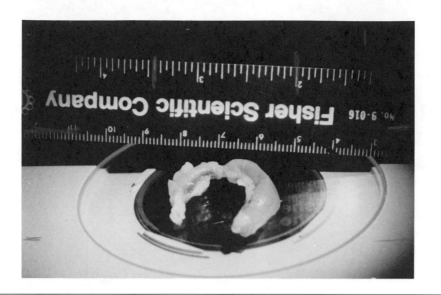

Figure 8-1
Low-power-density laser incision was associated with stenosis at the anastomotic site and hydrometra distal to the ligation. From Martin DC (ed): Tissue effects of lasers, *Semin Reprod Endocrinol* 9(2):127-137, 1991.

human surgery (see below). High power density (11,000 W/cm^2) produced no stenosis. Power density of 11,000 W/cm^2 appears to offer a good compromise of speed, control, hemostasis, and healing.[8,20]

Cuff salpingostomy

Neofimbriae were induced in rabbits by excising the fimbriae and performing a cuff salpingostomy on the remnant tube.[21] Pregnancy occurred in 72% of these animals when opened with the laser compared with 50% when opened by standard microsurgery.

Adhesions

The CO_2 laser decreases intraperitoneal adhesions when compared with microsurgery. In rabbits, no peritoneal adhesions were demonstrated with the laser, whereas 30% of animals had adhesion formation with nonlaser microcautery.[22] Similar peritoneal findings were published in a second study.[8] Both laser and microsurgery groups formed ovarian adhesions in 30% of animals.[22] However, ovarian adhesions may be more related to the closure or lack of closure than to the incisional equipment. Sutures have long been known to increase peritoneal adhesions.[23-25] Two studies[26,27] showed similar results in the ovary. The same or fewer adhesions were noted with no closure compared with microsurgery. The ability of the laser to make a hemostatic incision appears to result in less suturing and a subsequent decrease in adhesions in ovarian surgery. This is discussed in the clinical section, since there is a lack of stage relationships in laparoscopic endometriosis surgery when sutures are not used.[28-30]

Adhesions were surgically induced and subsequently lysed with laser and with electrosurgery. At a third operation, 85% of laser-treated animals and 61% of electrosurgically treated animals had decreased adhesions.[31] A combination of laser and hydrocortisone gave the best results when compared with other combinations of laser or microelectrode with hydrocortisone or Hartman's solution.[32]

MICROSURGERY

Both general and specific considerations are essential for proper use of laser microsurgery. Determining the relative advantages of various surgical techniques is highly subjective and remains largely a matter of opinion.[33] Furthermore, equipment is not a replacement for surgical skill. Requirements include lecture and laboratory experience, proper temperament and motivation, continuing statistical studies, surveys of opinion differences, options in equipment, and a forum for long-term education and standards.[34] Suggestions for training and credentialling criteria have also been published.[35]

Lasers can be used with microsurgery to decrease blood loss, tissue manipulation, surgical difficulty, and surgery time.[36-38] In comparative studies with microsurgery and laser surgery for adhesiolysis, salpingostomy, and anastomosis, no differences were noted in the clinical results.[39-41]

Studies comparing electrosurgery and CO_2 laser techniques for cuff salpingostomy resulted in term pregnancy rates of 17% and 24%, respectively.[40] Cuff salpingostomy was performed with a laser using an initial incision

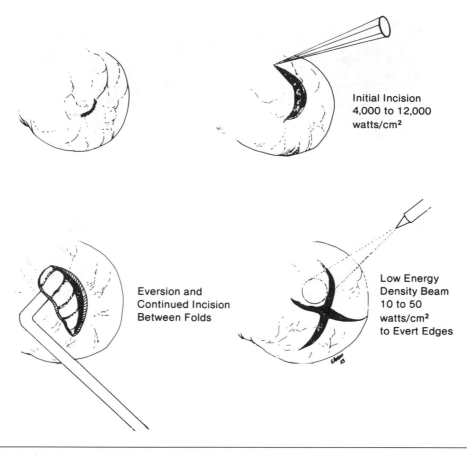

Initial Incision
4,000 to 12,000
watts/cm²

Eversion and
Continued Incision
Between Folds

Low Energy
Density Beam
10 to 50
watts/cm²
to Evert Edges

Figure 8-2
Cuff salpingostomy is performed by making an initial incision into the tube. This is followed by
a series of radial incisions and then by low-power-density coagulation of the tubal serosa. This
low-power-density coagulation everts the edges. From Martin DC (ed): *Techniques and safety in
intra-abdominal laser surgery* (slide set), 1984.

to the lumen at 4000 to 12,000 W/cm² (Figure 8-2).
After the initial incision, the folds were turned back and
the incision was continued between them in a stellate
fashion. The laser beam was then used in a defocused
fashion to cause a surface contraction of the serosa. This
serosal contraction everts the edges and avoids suturing.
Patency with this technique is reported at 85%[39] to 91%.[40]

In reversal of previous sterilizations, 60% to 84% term
pregnancy rates were reported.[37,39,42] Bellina used a low-
power-density laser for the serosa and adhesions but not
for the tubal incision.[36] Scissors were used for this incision. This low-power-density serosal technique has
been associated with loss of the mesosalpinx and tubal
stenosis (Figure 8-3). It would appear that most reports
and most surgeons have better results with sharp incision
than with laser techniques.[43]

In a mixed group of 61 patients undergoing reconstructive pelvic surgery using the CO_2 laser, 8 (13%) had
intrauterine pregnancies and 2 (3%) tubal pregnancies at
initial follow-up.[36] When this was corrected for danazol
and other medications, 8 (24%) of 33 patients had intrauterine pregnancies. A subsequent study reporting 230

of 910 women with 91 (40%) conceptions, including 81
(38%) conceptions in 216 patients who underwent surgery for adhesive pathology.[37] These patients had 2 years
of follow-up. A more recent summary disclosed pregnancy rates of 84% after tubotubal anastomosis, 32%
overall after salpingostomy, and 54% with adhesiolysis
or fimbrioplasty.[42] The results after salpingostomy were
time dependent, and at 5 years the overall rate was 39%
with a 29% term pregnancy rate.

LAPAROSCOPY

The laser laparoscope was developed in France by Bruhat
et al[44] and in Israel by Tadir et al[45,46] and was introduced
to the United States by Daniell.[47-49] Parallel development
of pelviscopy by Semm[50] and videolaseroscopy by Nezhat et al[30] have aided in the clinical use of all laparoscopic procedures.

Lasers may be directed into the pelvis through single-
puncture surgical laparoscopes, second-puncture probes,
wave guides, or fibers. Second-puncture probes and wave
guides that can be used through the second puncture or

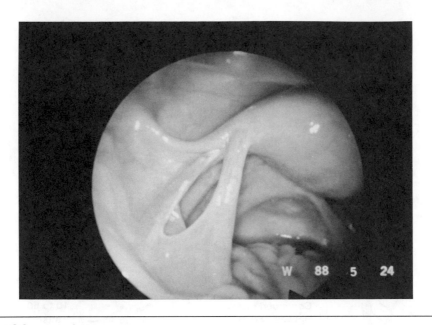

Figure 8-3
Loss of the mesosalpinx has been noted after laser microsurgery. This appears related to inadvertent coagulation and devascularization of the mesosalpinx. The clean appearance is similar to that seen after bipolar or thermal coagulation of tubes. From Martin DC (ed): Tissue effects of lasers, *Semin Reprod Endocrin* 9(2):127-137, 1991.

through the surgical laparoscope can be equipped with backstops to limit penetration of the CO_2 laser. These are flat, and there is no reflection from these into the pelvis. Open-ended probes are more useful when vaporizing deep lesions but require backstops to limit the depth when a CO_2 laser is used. Fiber-directed lasers have a rapid divergence and do not generally require as close attention to the use of backstops.

For therapeutic laparoscopy, a second-puncture probe is placed higher than commonly used for laparoscopic sterilization. If the location is too low (Figure 8-4), the cul-de-sac may not be accessible. Before placing the second-puncture probe, pressure should be exerted on the abdominal wall. When viewed through the laparoscope, this pressure will be seen to push the abdominal wall between the uterus and the laparoscope, and the position should be correct for an angle into the cul-de-sac (Figure 8-5).

Surgical techniques are generally chosen based on the size and type of tissue. Small lesions and the base of adhesions can be coagulated or vaporized. Larger lesions are more generally excised (Figure 8-6). The decisions regarding this are generally made based on the findings at surgery and depend on the equipment used, the smoke evacuators available, and other considerations at the time of treatment.

Tubal surgery

Of 5 (18%) of 28 patients pregnant at 6 to 20 months of follow-up after laparoscopic cuff salpingostomy, 1 miscarried, 1 had an ectopic pregnancy, and 3 had term

pregnancies.[49] Ten (63%) of 16 patients were pregnant after adhesiolysis, and 3 (30%) of 10 patients were pregnant after fimbrioplasties with the CO_2 laser at 1 year of follow-up.[51]

Endometriosis

In an initial report of therapy of endometriosis, the CO_2 laser laparoscope was used to treat three patients with stage I and 7 patients with stage II disease.[52] Of these 10 patients, 3 (30%) had continuing pregnancies and 3 had aborted at 6 months of follow-up.

A summary of 12 series with 1536 patients revealed a 56% overall pregnancy rate and a 68% rate when patients had only endometriosis.[53]

Studies of the argon laser in the photocoagulation of endometriosis are being performed. The argon laser is selectively absorbed by deeply pigmented and hemoglobin-containing material such as endometriosis. This technique was reported in 5 patients at laparoscopy and 15 at laparotomy. One patient with rectal endometriosis was treated through a flexible sigmoidoscope, with relief of rectal bleeding and painful defecation.[54,55] When corrected for length of fertility, the pregnancy rates were similar to those with the CO_2 laser.[56,57] The KTP laser also has been used in gynecologic laparoscopy.[58]

An interesting finding regarding severe endometriosis is that three life table analyses showed the same or better results comparing laparoscopic laser series with laparotomy series.[28-30] In addition, 159 of the 1536 patients reviewed had severe endometriosis as an isolated finding

PLACEMENT OF SECOND
PUNCTURE LASER PROBE

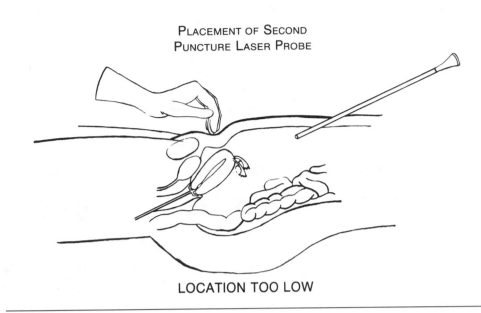

LOCATION TOO LOW

Figure 8-4
If the second puncture is placed over the uterine fundus, it may lacerate the fundus. In addition, the probe may be kept out of the cul-de-sac with the fundus in the way. (From Martin DC (ed): *Techniques and safety in intra-abdominal laser surgery* (slide set), 1984.

PLACEMENT OF SECOND
PUNCTURE LASER PROBE

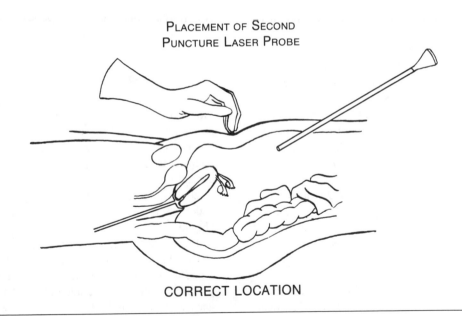

CORRECT LOCATION

Figure 8-5
The second probe is placed between the first puncture and the uterine fundus. In this position, the angle is correct for insertion into the cul-de-sac and is far enough away from the laparoscope that it will not interfere with the primary puncture. From Martin DC (ed): *Techniques and safety in intra-abdominal laser surgery* (slide set), 1984.

Surgical Technique

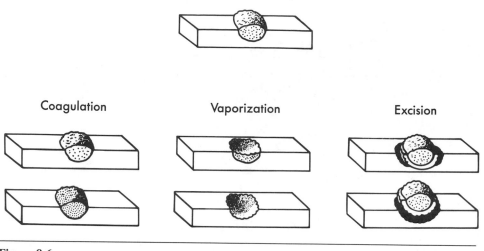

Coagulation   Vaporization   Excision

Figure 8-6
Coagulation is denaturing and desiccating tissue without removing it. Vaporization implies turning the entire lesion into a plume of smoke, which is evacuated. Excision is the surgical removal of tissue so that it can undergo pathologic examinations. From Martin DC (ed): *Intra-abdominal laser surgery*, ed 2 (in preparation).

associated with infertility.[53] This group had a pregnancy rate of 65%. It has been suggested that the limited surgery done at laparoscopy compared with laparotomy, and the decreased use of suturing, retraction, and drying of tissue may be responsible for this high pregnancy rate in patients with severe endometriosis.

The Nd:YAG laser was adapted for use through a laparoscope.[59] In treating 22 patients, photocoagulation was continued until blanching was noted. No cavity was formed, and there was no penetration. Deep penetration of the laser was used to destroy deep tissue with no surface disruption. This technique might decrease the potential for adhesion formation, since there was no surface exudate. Subsequent studies documented the usefulness of the modality using artificial sapphire tips.[60-63]

Uterine nerve ablation

The incisional capabilities of the CO_2 laser were used to approximate the Doyle procedure of paracervical denervation.[51,64] This was subsequently studied as a laparoscopic uterine nerve ablation (LUNA). In this technique the paracervical plexus is transected to relieve dysmenorrhea by making a small incision at the uterine origin of the uterosacral ligament. The depth and width are controlled, since the descending branch of the uterine artery is in close proximity and the ureter is only slightly lateral to this. With this procedure, 23 (64%) of 36 patients with endometriosis and 7 (50%) of 14 patients with primary dysmenorrhea experienced resolution of pain.[51]

A controlled study demonstrated 91% relief at 3 months and 45% at 1 year.[65] The control group reported no pain relief.

General concerns

Although there is significant controversy over the removal of large ovarian cysts at laparoscopy, the consensus is that removal of small cysts is reasonable. In the process of removal, dermoid cysts will invariably be opened. If this occurs, the patient should be moved into a head-up position, since the cul-de-sac has a capacity of 20 to 80 ml, and fluid will rapidly move into the upper abdomen if the Trendelenburg position is maintained (Figure 8-7).

Tadir et al[45,46] described and followed up on the use of CO_2 laser for sterilization in women. Of 12 patients, 1 had a subsequent pregnancy and 5 undergoing hysterosalpingograms had occluded tubes. The authors no longer use these techniques.

SUMMARY

Although lasers are more predictable for certain applications than other equipment, predictability is not always an indication for its use. Continued development and increased understanding of specific indications will determine if this expensive, high-intensity equipment is cost effective and should continue to play a prominent role in intraabdominal surgery.

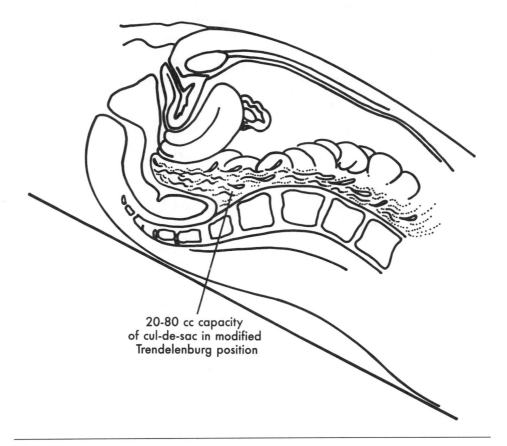

Figure 8-7
When performing laparoscopic procedures that may contaminate the pelvis, the patient should be taken out of Trendelenburg position. Irrigation with as little as 20 cc of fluid may push pelvic material into the upper abdomen. From Martin DC (ed): *Intra-abdominal laser surgery*, ed 2 (in preparation).

REFERENCES

1. Masterson BJ, Nealon N, and Sowas D: Tissue effects of lasers on wound healing (abstr), *Lasers Surg Med* 3:153, 1983.
2. Madden JE et al: Studies in the management of contaminated wound: persistence to infection of surgical wounds made by knife, electrosurgery and laser, *Am J Surg* 119:222-224, 1970.
3. Nishimura M et al: Comparative study of CO_2 laser scalpel with electroscalpel. In Atsumi K and Nimsakul N (eds): *Proceedings of the fourth congress of the International Society for Laser Surgery*, Tokyo, 1981, Japanese Society for Laser Medicine.
4. Mage G, Pouly JL, and Bruhat MA: Laser microsurgery of the oviducts. In Baggish MS (ed): *Basic and advanced laser surgery in gynecology*, Norwalk, Conn, 1985, Appleton-Century-Crofts.
5. Luciano AA et al: A comparison of thermal injury, healing patterns, and postoperative adhesion formation following CO_2 laser and electromicrosurgery, *Fertil Steril* 48:1025-1029, 1987.
6. Filmar S et al: A comparative histologic study on the healing process after tissue transection. I. Carbon dioxide laser and electromicrosurgery, *Am J Obstet Gynecol* 160:1062-1067, 1989.
7. Hall RR, Beach AD, and Hill DW: Partial hepatectomy using a carbon dioxide laser, *Br J Surg* 60:141-143, 1973.
8. Bellina JH et al: Carbon dioxide laser in electrosurgical wound study with an animal model: a comparison of tissue damage and healing patterns in peritoneal tissue, *Am J Obstet Gynecol* 148:327-334, 1984.
9. Fox JL: The use of laser radiation as a surgical "light knife," *J Surg Res* 9:199-205, 1969.
10. Hall RR: The healing of tissues excised by carbon dioxide laser, *Br J Surg* 58:222-225, 1971.
11. Oshiro T, Itoh E, and Kato Y: Multi and one shot laser therapy: which is better in clinical use? In Atsumi K and Nimsakul N (eds): *Proceedings of the fourth congress of the International Society for Laser Surgery*, Tokyo, 1981, Japanese Society for Laser Medicine.
12. Yamamoto T, Fukomoto I, and Satio M: Dynamic characteristics of the light reflected from the living tissue under laser irradiation. In Atsumi K and Nimsakul N (eds): *Proceedings of the fourth congress of the International Society for Laser Surgery*, Tokyo, 1981, Japanese Society for Laser Medicine.
13. Taylor MV et al: Effect of power density and carbonization on residual tissue coagulation using the continuous wave carbon dioxide laser, *Colposc Gynecol Laser Surg* 2:169-175, 1986.
14. Joffe SN et al: Resection of the liver with the Nd:YAG laser, *Surg Gynecol Obstet* pp 437-442, 1986.
15. Harris DM and Werkhaven JA: Biophysics and applications of medical lasers, *Adv Otolaryngol Head Neck Surg* 3:91-123, 1989.
16. Klink F et al: Animal in vivo studies and in vitro experiments with human tubes for end to end anastomotic operations by CO_2 laser technique, *Fertil Steril* 30:100-102, 1978.
17. Grosspietzsch R et al: Experiments on operative treatment of tubular sterility by CO_2 laser technique. In Kaplan I (ed): *Proceedings of the third international congress for laser surgery*, Tel Aviv, 1979, Ot-Paz.
18. Baggish MS and Chong AP: Carbon dioxide laser microsurgery of uterine tube, *Obstet Gynecol* 58:111-116, 1981.
19. Fayez JA, McComb JS, and Harper MA: Comparison of tubal surgery with CO_2 laser and unipolar electrode, *Fertil Steril* 40:476-480, 1983.

20. Martin DC, McCoy TD, and Poston WM: *Reanastomosis of the rat uterine horn following sharp and laser microincisions.* Presented at the world congress of tubal surgery, West Palm Beach, Fla, May 1983.

21. Inoue M et al: *Microsurgery of the rabbit oviduct by a CO_2 laser technique.* In Atsumi K and Nimsakul N (eds): Proceedings of the fourth congress of the International Society for Laser Surgery, Tokyo, 1981, Japanese Society for Laser Medicine.

22. Pittaway DE, Maxsom WS, and Daniell JF: A comparison of the CO_2 laser and electrocautery on postoperative intraperitoneal adhesion formation in rabbits, *Fertil Steril* 3:366-368, 1983.

23. Ellis H: Internal overhealing: the problem of intraperitoneal adhesions, *World J Surg* 4:303-306, 1980.

24. Ellis H: The aetiology of post-operative abdominal adhesions: an experimental study, *Br J Surg* 50:10-16, 1962.

25. Elkins TE et al: A histologic evaluation of peritoneal injury and repair: implications for adhesion formation, *Obstet Gynecol* 70:225-228, 1987.

26. Brumsted JR et al: Postoperative adhesion formation after ovarian wedge resection with and without ovarian reconstruction in the rabbit, *Fertil Steril* 53:723-726, 1990.

27. DeLeon FD, Edwards M, and Heine MW: A comparison of microsurgery and laser surgery for ovarian wedge resections, *Int J Fertil* 35:177-179, 1990.

28. Olive DL and Martin DC: Treatment of endometriosis-associated infertility with CO_2 laser laparoscopy: the use of one- and two-parameter exponential models, *Fertil Steril* 48:18-23, 1987.

29. Adamson GD, Lu J, and Suback LL: Laparoscopic CO_2 laser vaporization of endometriosis compared with traditional treatments, *Fertil Steril* 50:704-710, 1988.

30. Nezhat C, Crowgey SR, and Nezhat F: Videolaseroscopy for the treatment of endometriosis associated with infertility, *Fertil Steril* 51:237-240, 1989.

31. Scheidel P, Wallwiener G, and Hepp H: CO_2 laser in treatment of pelvic adhesions—experimental results. In Kaplan I (ed): *Proceedings of the third international congress for laser surgery,* Tel Aviv, 1979, Ot-Paz.

32. Tadir Y et al: Intraperitoneal adhesiolysis by CO_2 laser microsurgery. In Atsumi K and Nimsakul N (eds): *Proceedings of the fourth congress of the International Society for Laser Surgery,* Tokyo, 1981, Japanese Society for Laser Medicine.

33. Wood C: Microsurgical controversies: oviductal function and fertility, *Aust NZ J Obstet Gynaecol* 21:137-140, 1981.

34. Phillips JM and Winchester WJ: Teaching microsurgery to gynecologists, *J Microsurg* 1:120-130, 1979.

35. American National Standards Institute, Inc: *American national standard for the safe use of lasers in health care facilities* (ANSIZ136.3 - 1988), New York, 1988, American National Standards Institute.

36. Bellina JH: Reconstructive microsurgery of the fallopian tube with the carbon dioxide laser. In Bellina JH (ed): *Gynecologic surgery,* New York, 1981, Plenum Press.

37. Bellina JH: Microsurgery of the fallopian tube with the carbon dioxide laser: analysis of 230 cases with 2-year follow-up, *Lasers Surg Med* 3:255-260, 1983.

38. Bruhat MA, Mage G, and Pouly JL: The use of the CO_2 laser in neosalpingostomy. In Kaplan I (ed): *Proceedings of the third international congress for laser surgery,* Tel Aviv, 1979, Ot-Paz.

39. Kelly RW and Roberts DK: Experience with the carbon dioxide laser in gynecologic microsurgery, *Am J Obstet Gynecol* 146:585-588, 1983.

40. Mage G and Bruhat MA: Pregnancy following salpingostomy: comparison between CO_2 laser and electrosurgical procedures, *Fertil Steril* 40:472-475, 1983.

41. Taylor SN: Carbon dioxide laser in the practice of infertility. Presented at the Ortho Symposium luncheon, thirty-ninth annual meeting of the American Fertility Society, San Francisco, Calif, 1983.

42. Kelly RW: Laser surgery of the fallopian tube. In Keye WR (ed): *Laser surgery in gynecology and obstetrics,* ed 2, Chicago, 1990, Year Book Medical Publishers.

43. Martin DC: Tubal microsurgery. In Martin DC (ed): *Intra-abdominal laser surgery,* Memphis, 1986, Resurge Press.

44. Bruhat MA, Mage G, and Manhes M: Use of the CO_2 laser via laparoscopy. In Kaplan I (ed): *Proceedings of the third international congress for laser surgery,* Tel Aviv, 1979, Ot-Paz.

45. Tadir Y et al: Laparoscopic CO_2 laser sterilization. In Semm K and Mettler L (eds): *Human reproduction,* Amsterdam, 1981, Excerpta Medica.

46. Tadir Y et al: Laparoscopic application of CO_2 laser. In Atsumi K and Nimsakul N (eds): *Proceedings of the fourth congress of the international society for laser surgery,* Tokyo, 1981, Japanese Society for Laser Medicine.

47. Daniell JF and Pittaway DE: Use of the CO_2 laser in laparoscopic surgery: initial experience with the second puncture technique, *Infertility* 5:13-15, 1982.

48. Daniell JF: The CO_2 laser in infertility surgery, *J Reprod Med* 28:265-268, 1983.

49. Daniell JF: Laparoscopic salpingostomy: early clinical results (abstract), *Lasers Surg Med* 3:161, 1983.

50. Semm K: Course of endoscopic abdominal surgery. In Semm K and Frederich ER (eds): *Operative manual for endoscopic abdominal surgery,* Chicago, 1987, Year Book Medical Publishers.

51. Feste JR: Laser laparoscopy: a new modality (abstract), *Lasers Surg Med* 3:170, 1983.

52. Kelly RW and Roberts DK: CO_2 laser laparoscopy: a potential alternative to danazol in the treatment of stage I and II endometriosis, *J Reprod Med* 28:639-640, 1983.

53. Martin DC (ed): *Laparoscopic appearance of endometriosis,* Memphis, 1990, Resurge Press.

54. Keye WR, Matson GA, and Dixon J: The use of the argon laser in the treatment of experimental endometriosis, *Fertil Steril* 39:26-29, 1983.

55. Keye WR and Dixon J: Photocoagulation of endometriosis with the argon laser through the laparoscope, *Obstet Gynecol* 62:383-386, 1983.

56. Keye WR et al: Argon laser therapy of endometriosis: a review of 92 consecutive patients, *Fertil Steril* 47:208-212, 1987.

57. Keye WR and McArthur GR: Laser laparoscopy: argon. In Keye WR (ed): *Laser surgery in gynecology and obstetrics,* ed 2, Chicago, 1990, Year Book Medical Publishers.

58. Daniell JF, Miller W, and Tosh R: Initial evaluation of the use of the potassium-titanyl-phosphate (KTP/532) laser in gynecologic laparoscopy, *Fertil Steril* 46:373-377, 1986.

59. Lomano JN: Laparoscopic ablation of endometriosis with the YAG laser (abstract), *Lasers Surg Med* 3:179, 1983.

60. Kojima E et al: Nd:YAG laser endoscopy, *J Reprod Med* 33:907-911, 1988.

61. Kojima E et al: Nd:YAG laser laparoscopy for ovarian endometriomas, *J Reprod Med* 35:592-596, 1990.

62. Corson SL et al: Laparoscopic laser treatment of endometriosis with the Nd:YAG sapphire probe, *Am J Obstet Gynecol* 160:718-723, 1989.

63. Shirk GJ: Use of the Nd:YAG laser for the treatment of endometriosis, *Am J Obstet Gynecol* 160:1344-1351, 1989.

64. Doyle JB: Paracervical uterine denervation by transection of the cervical plexus for the relief of dysmenorrhea, *Am J Obstet Gynecol* 70:1-16, 1955.

65. Lichten EM and Bombard J: Surgical treatment of primary dysmenorrhea with laparoscopic uterine nerve ablation, *J Reprod Med* 32(3):37, 1987.

9

Pelvic Preparation and Choice of Incision

ROBERT B. HUNT

HUGO A. ACUNA

Preparation of the patient for microsurgery begins with the selection of an effective, smoothly working operating room team. The surgeon should assemble physician- and nurse-assistants whose primary interest is fertility surgery. The personnel should also be temperamentally disposed to working in a calm, unhurried atmosphere. Microsurgical fertility procedures are exacting and time consuming, and their outcome is of crucial importance to the patient and her partner. Impatience and disinterest on the part of any team member will not ensure optimal results.

The surgeon should arrive 30 minutes before the scheduled starting time to be available for consultation and to go over the patient's history briefly with the operating room team. Included in this discussion should be details of the proposed procedure and the expected outcome.

The first assistant need not be a gynecologist. For example, a general surgeon trained in vascular surgery will be familiar with microsurgical techniques. A physician's assistant can also be trained to be a superb first surgical assistant.

It is helpful for at least one or two members of the team to be present at all microsurgical procedures performed by any one surgeon. Given the sophistication of equipment used in these procedures, such familiarity with the surgeon's personal technique will lead to coordinated, efficient work.

Both the surgeon and the first assistant should make certain their practices are covered during surgery so that they are not distracted. Ample time must be allotted for the procedure. Since a surgeon performs more procedures, it will become easier to estimate the precise amount of time needed. During the initial few surgeries, at least 2 hours extra should be allowed to deal with unforseen problems.

OPERATING ROOM SET-UP

It is advisable to use the same operating room for each microsurgical case, since the team becomes accustomed to arranging the equipment in this particular room. For example, a constant problem is that of too few electrical outlets; as many as a dozen can be used during a procedure. Connecting additional electric cords can be done swiftly if team members are able always to make such accommodations in the same room.

With the fiscal restraints applied to hospitals, the surgeon most likely will have to use the operating room table already available. The table should be heavy and stable to prevent it from tilting over. If the surgeon plans to sit during surgery, the patient must be placed so that her pelvis is off center from the pedestal. Another method is to reverse the table after placing an extension at its foot (Figure 9-1). A disadvantage to this is that the controls are at the opposite end of the table from the anesthetist and must be adjusted by the circulating nurse.

If a laparoscopy is to be performed immediately before laparotomy, it is best done on a separate table. The patient can be transferred and then prepared for the microsurgical procedure.

Either general or regional anesthesia such as spinal or epidural block may be used. The surgeon should discuss this with the anesthesiologist and patient beforehand and make the choice with them.

The patient is positioned on the modified operating room table so that she rests comfortably with no undue pressure points. When she has been anesthetized and after appropriate monitoring equipment has been attached, the surgeon places her in the "frog leg" position to prepare the perineum. A separate table containing equipment for this purpose should be set up (Figure 9-2).

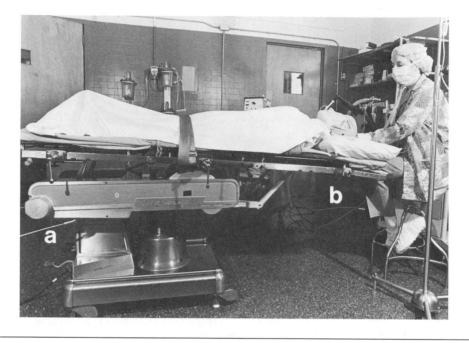

Figure 9-1

A mock-up demonstrating the patient positioned on the reversed table. Controls are located as shown *(a)*. The patient's head must be positioned as far up on the extension *(b)* as possible.

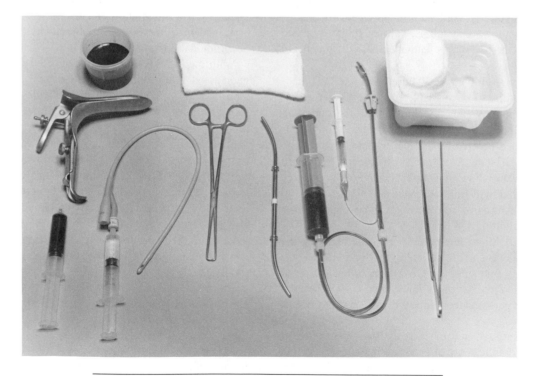

Figure 9-2

Set-up for vaginal preparation. Note the Betadine drawn up for urethral irrigation; dilute indigo carmine drawn up and connected to an intrauterine catheter (available from ZSI); and saturated Kerlix gauze for vaginal packing.

If an intrauterine catheter is to be used for lavage purposes, the surgeon may use either a no. 8 pediatric Foley or a special intrauterine catheter such as that offered by ZSI. Intrauterine placement of the catheter has the advantages of allowing lavage to be done during the surgery in a "no-touch" manner and has the theoretical disadvantage of introducing bacteria into the uterine cavity at the time of placement.

To place the preferred catheter properly, a bivalved speculum with one side open, such as used in laparoscopy, is placed in the vagina and opened widely. A tenaculum is placed on the anterior lip of the cervix and a small dilator is inserted in the uterine cavity to determine the direction of the cervical canal. The catheter is then placed and the balloon inflated with air.

A Foley catheter is inserted into the urinary bladder after the urethral meatus has been irrigated with povidone-iodine (Betadine).

The surgeon places the vaginal pack if this is to be used. The pack has the advantage of elevating the uterus into the field. Some surgeons believe this advantage is offset by increasing vascular congestion in the pelvis and also taking up valuable space in the pelvis. The vaginal pack is recommended except in the case of a retroflexed, fixed uterus, as occurs in a patient with endometriosis.

To place the pack properly, the gauze is soaked in lactated Ringer's solution (Kerlex gauze is ideal). The surgeon places the nondominate hand in the vagina and depresses posteriorly. Using dressing forceps, the tip of the gauze is placed beneath the cervix and approximately three folds of gauze inserted directly beneath the cervix. The remaining gauze is then placed inside the surgeon's glove to prevent moisture from soiling the adjacent sheets. It is important to place the packing just beneath the cervix and not to pack the vagina (Figure 9-3).

The surgeon then straightens the patient's legs and the appropriate abdominal skin is shaved. Doing this in the operating room takes only a moment and minimizes the chance of skin infections. It also avoids patient discomfort.

A ground plate is placed and the patient is draped. After the four initial towels are placed on the wound site, the intrauterine catheter tubing is connected to sterile tubing from the surgical field by the circulating nurse. A plastic sheet can be placed over the final abdominal drape after the skin incision has been marked. This seals off the wound to prevent instruments and sponges getting lost beneath the sheets.

After the Trendelenburg position is attained, the nurse moves in the instrument stand and table, and the procedure is ready to begin.

INCISIONS

Since Pfannenstiel's original description in 1900, the incision named for him has gained an established place in

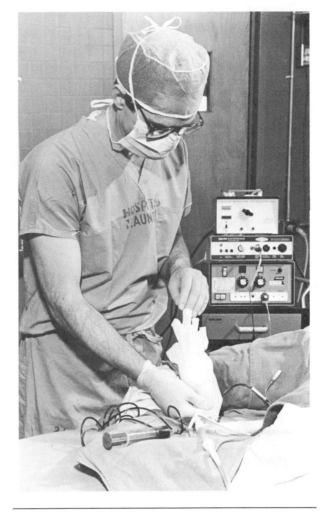

Figure 9-3
Preparation of the perineum is complete. The surgeon's left glove is turned inside out to contain excess wet gauze. When draping the patient, the surgeon passes off sterile tubing filled with indigo carmine from the surgical field; this is then connected to the intrauterine catheter tubing by the circulating nurse. This allows the surgeon to control tubal lavage from the surgical field.

pelvic surgery.[1] If performed properly, it provides the surgeon ample room to carry out most pelvic procedures. Its advantages are apparent; the incision is cosmetic, very strong, and causes the patient relatively little discomfort.

The Hunt—Acuna incision is an alternative that offers the following advantages:

1. It is more cosmetic, as significant lateral subcutaneous tissue and vasculature are spared, maintaining a more natural contour.
2. Less numbness and paresthesias occur superior to the incision since there is much less dissection, thus sparing perforating vessels and accompanying sensory nerves.

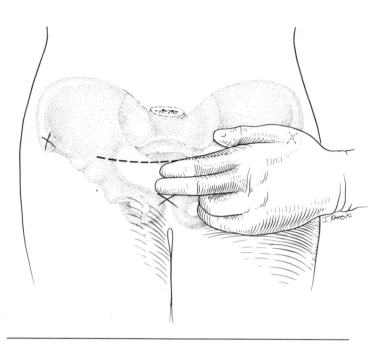

Figure 9-4
The incision is marked out.

3. There is no danger to major nerve trunks in the abdominal wall, especially the ilioinguinal nerves.
4. Greater exposure to pelvic structures is achieved as the anterior fascia is opened to the symphysis, thus removing resistance.
5. There is less discomfort postoperatively; subjectively, patients walk much straighter and complain of less discomfort, apparently because of less dissection and trauma to abdominal wall tissue.
6. There is less damage to rectus muscles from the lateral retractor blades because the muscles are protected by the anterior fascia.
7. If the patient has had a previous Pfannenstiel incision, the Hunt—Acuna incision is much easier to effect than a repeat Pfannenstiel, since most dissection is made in unscarred tissue.

There are a few disadvantages to the Hunt—Acuna incision. Theoretically, it is associated with an increased frequency of hernia formation because the fascia is opened vertically. Careful hemostasis and wound closure using newer synthetic absorbable sutures make this a strong incision, however. It takes approximately 5 minutes longer to perform and 3 minutes longer to close than the low midline incision. Finally, the Hunt–Acuna incision does not offer as much upper abdominal exposure as the low midline incision because of resistance of the upper wound flap.

An illustrated description of the two incisions follows.

The Pfannenstiel incision

The surgeon carefully marks out the incision using the anterior superior iliac spine, umbilicus, and symphysis pubis as landmarks (Figure 9-4). The incision should be a straight line made approximately two fingerbreadths superior to the symphysis pubis. If it is curved, the extreme ends of the scar will "smile" out of bathing suits or underwear.[2] Failure to mark out the incision, preferably immediately after the initial four towels are symmetrically placed, will lead to a less than ideal incision.

When draping is completed and the scrub nurse, surgeon, and assistant have carefully washed their gloves in sterile water, the surgeon makes the incision half way through the dermis (Figure 9-5). Electrosurgery is used to complete the incision through the dermis.

The surgeon lifts each vessel with DeBakey vascular forceps and coagulates and divides it electrosurgically. Since no clamps are used, this technique is quick and leaves an unencumbered surgical field. Cutting current is much more efficient and chars less than coagulating current.

With fatty tissue retracted superiorly and inferiorly, fibrous strands are divided with cutting current (Figure 9-6), preserving fat lobules where possible. Keeping tissues under tension when dividing them eliminates excessive thermal damage. The fascia is opened carefully on either side of the midline using electrosurgery (Figure 9-7). The fascial incision is curved superiorly (Figure 9-8) to avoid damaging the ilioinguinal nerves and to give a wider fascial opening. The incision is extended to the lateral borders of the rectus muscles.[3,4] The surgeon must elevate the fascia off the muscles with a Kelly clamp to avoid cutting muscle fibers. There must be no contact with the cautery, clamp, and skin.

Text cont'd on p. 123.

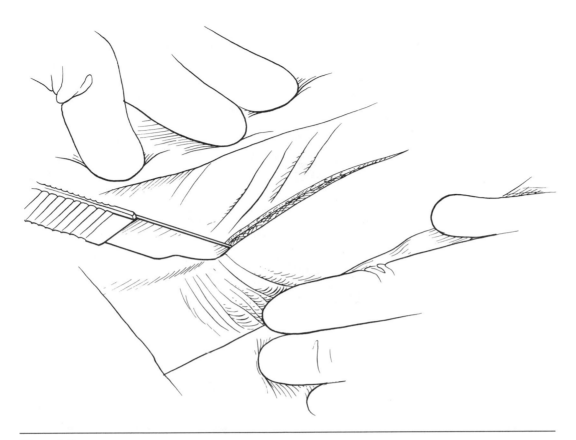

Figure 9-5
The Pfannenstiel incision is made half way through the dermis.

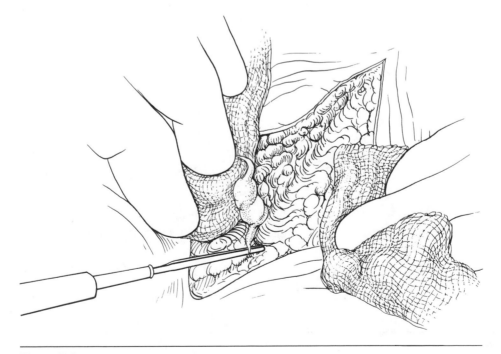

Figure 9-6
Fatty tissue is retracted and fibrous strands are divided.

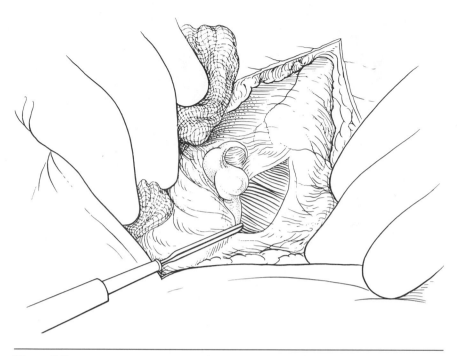

Figure 9-7
The fascia is opened electrosurgically.

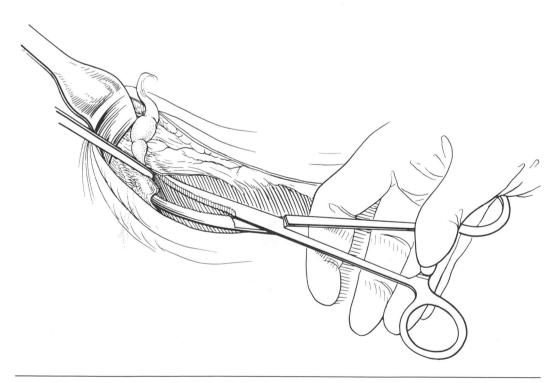

Figure 9-8
The curved fascial incision is designed to avoid causing damage to the ilioinguinal nerve.

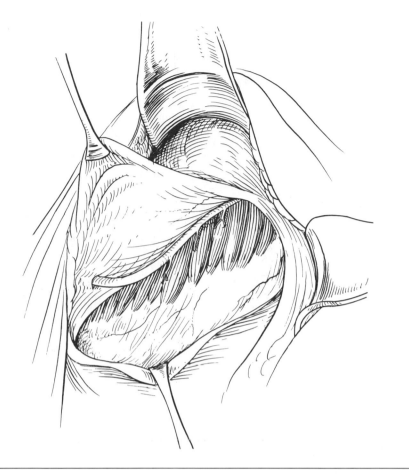

Figure 9-9
Ilioinguinal nerve. Note its exit through the external oblique aponeurosis.

The ilioinguinal nerves lie between the internal oblique muscle and the external oblique aponeurosis at this level (Figure 9-9). These nerves are susceptible to damage that can cause either numbness or burning in the groin.

Using three Kocher clamps and DeBakey vascular forceps, the surgeon elevates the fascia off the rectus muscles and individually coagulates the perforating vessels with cutting current, developing an adequate space beneath the fascia (Figure 9-10). Since iliohypogastric nerves accompany perforating vessels, the surgeon should dissect near the midline and divide the minimal number of vessels to avoid excessive numbness of the abdominal wall. The surgeon should warn the patient of this numbness before surgery, since a certain amount is unavoidable.

The inferior leaf of fascia is dissected off the rectus muscles. The surgeon elevates the pyramidalis muscles with the fascia where feasible (Figure 9-11A). At this point, the incision can be converted to a Chernez incision (Figure 9-11B). After separating the rectus muscles sharply, the surgeon elevates each rectus muscle off the

peritoneum (Figure 9-12). This allows wider retraction and better exposure. This must be done gently to avoid causing bleeding from deep epigastric vessels. The scrub nurse irrigates tissues at this point.

The scrubbed surgical team members again wash their gloves. The surgeon opens the peritoneum in the area of the urachus as this is consistently located superior to the urinary bladder. The nurse instills approximately 50 ml of warm heparinized lactated Ringer's solution (5000 U per liter) into the abdomen (Figure 9-13). This prevents small blood clots and thus diminishes adhesion formation. After extending the peritoneal incision superiorly, the surgeon identifies the urinary bladder and opens the peritoneum on either side of the bladder in the direction of the origin of the deep epigastric vessels (Figure 9-14). The peritoneum is elastic and need not be opened to an extreme degree. The abdominal muscles are stretched laterally to break up any fibrous bands. The abdomen is then carefully explored in a systematic manner, with assessment of at least the liver, diaphragm, kidneys, gallbladder, pancreas, appendix, cecum, and rectosigmoid.

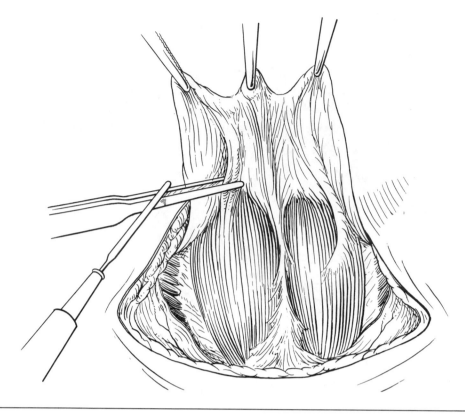

Figure 9-10
The fascia is elevated off the rectus muscles. Perforating vessels are coagulated using DeBakey forceps and cutting current.

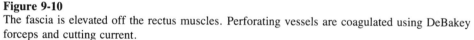

A wound protector is placed carefully so that bowel is not trapped. This minimizes drying of tissues in the abdominal wall and prevents blood running into the abdomen. A 5-inch wound protector is appropriate for the Pfannenstiel incision.

The surgeon positions an abdominal retractor, taking exceeding care to keep bowel away from the blades. When using the Kirschner retractor, the two medium blades are placed laterally and two small ones inferiorly and superiorly (Figure 9-15). If a patient is overweight, a large blade is placed superiorly, two medium blades laterally, and a small blade inferiorly. Alternatively, large blades may be placed superiorly and laterally and a medium blade inferiorly. When ordering this retractor, the surgeon should ask for three large curved blades in addition to the four standard blades. After the retractor is positioned, pressure points must be padded, particularly the anterior and superior iliac spine. The intraabdominal portion of the procedure can now proceed.

Wound closure

Once the pelvic procedure is complete, the surgeon removes all packing and places the rectosigmoid into the posterior cul-de-sac.

The peritoneum is closed, beginning inferiorly, with the wound protector left in place to prevent serosanguineous fluid from the abdominal wall from running into the abdomen (Figure 9-16). After approximating the peritoneum for approximately one-third its length, the surgeon ties and holds the suture; 0 or no. 1 synthetic absorbable material is used. Care must be taken to avoid damaging the deep epigastric vessels and urinary bladder.

The surgeon continues closure of the peritoneum beginning superiorly (Figure 9-17). The wound protector is removed and adjunctive agents are placed in the abdomen. Alternatively, the peritoneum may be closed around a large catheter, the agents instilled through the catheter, and the catheter withdrawn, tightening the peritoneal suture to close the defect where the catheter had been. The rectus muscles are loosely approximated by suturing them superficially with three interrupted sutures (Figure 9-18). If necessary, the pyramidalis is reattached to the rectus muscles. If a Chernez incision is used, the distal rectus tendons are attached to the posterior surface of the inferior fascial leaf with 0 or no. 1 synthetic absorbable material. The surgeon must obtain careful hemostasis at this point. The retractor frequently tamponades bleeders, and a careful search for bleeders must be made when the retractor is removed.

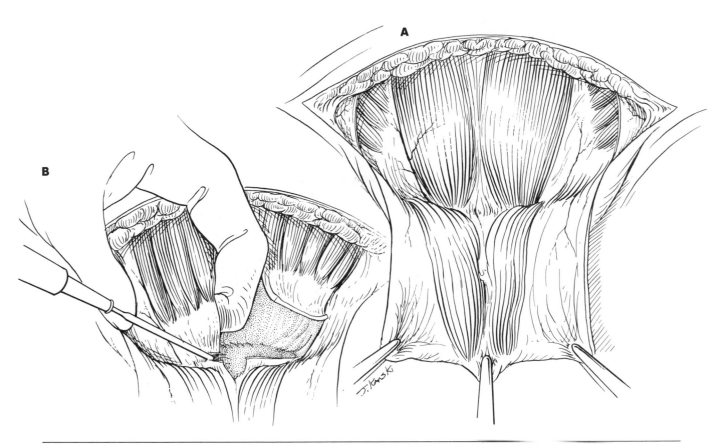

Figure 9-11
A, The inferior leaf of fascia is dissected off the rectus muscles. **B,** The incision is converted to a Chernez incision.

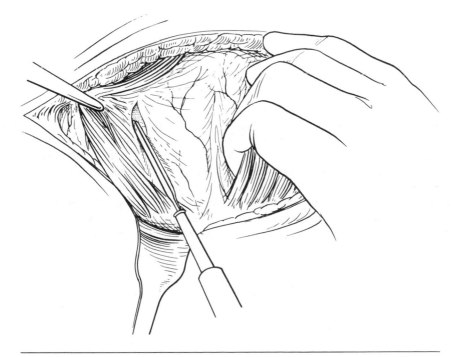

Figure 9-12
The rectus muscles are separated and elevated off the peritoneum.

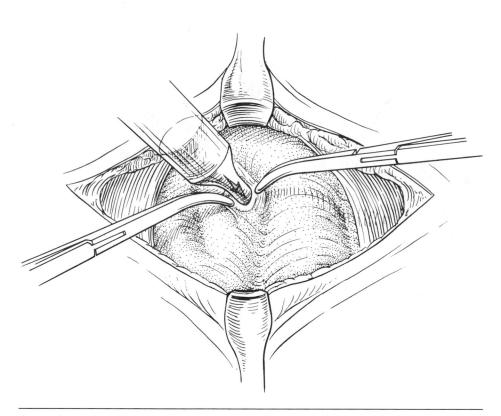

Figure 9-13
The peritoneum is opened in the area of the urachus and heparinized lactated Ringer's solution is instilled.

Angle sutures are placed to avoid entrapping the ilioinguinal nerves (Figure 9-19). After a midline suture is placed (Figure 9-20), the fascia is closed with a continuous suture of 0 or no. 1 synthetic absorbable material (Figure 9-21 and 9-22). The surgeon must avoid going greater than 0.5 cm from the fascial incision so as to minimize the risk of nerve entrapment.

Before the skin is closed, Scarpa's fascia is approximated with interrupted sutures of 3-0 synthetic absorbable material. When skin clips are applied, the skin edges must be carefully everted; alternatively, interrupted skin sutures or a subcuticular closure may be used (Figure 9-23). Sutures or clips may be removed on the fifth postoperative day and Steri-Strips are applied for reinforcement. The patient removes these 7 to 14 days after discharge.

If a subfascial drain is placed, the surgeon should use a closed system and bring this through an opening in the midline 1 cm inferior to the skin incision. The drain is sutured in place and removed in 24 to 48 hours.

At the conclusion of the procedure, the surgical team must make certain all vaginal appliances are removed, except the Foley catheter for bladder drainage, and inspected for missing parts.

Text cont'd on p. 133.

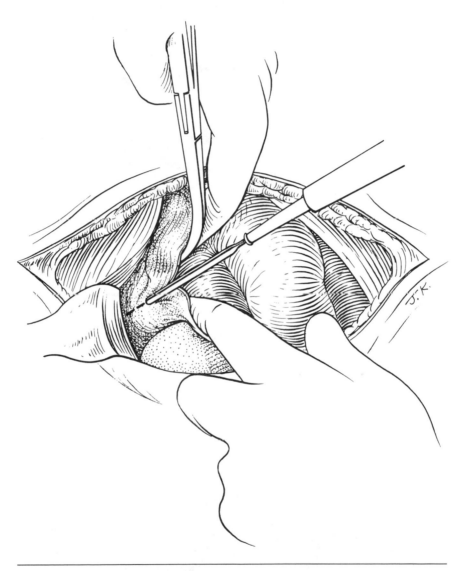

Figure 9-14
The peritoneum is opened on either side of the urinary bladder.

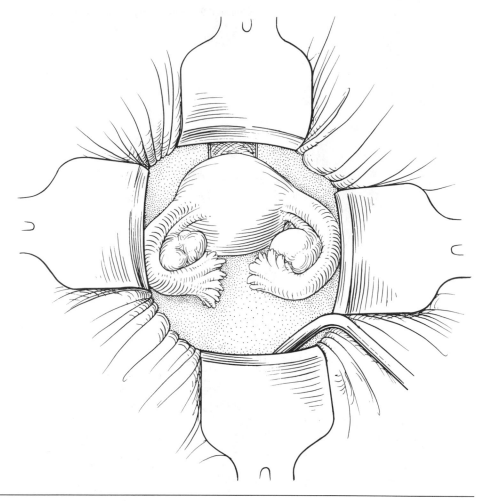

Figure 9-15
Placement of Kirschner retractor and exposure of the pelvis are completed. Note the wound protector and sump drain.

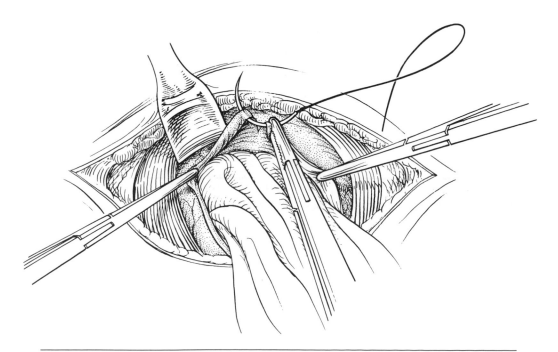

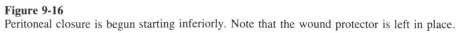

Figure 9-16
Peritoneal closure is begun starting inferiorly. Note that the wound protector is left in place.

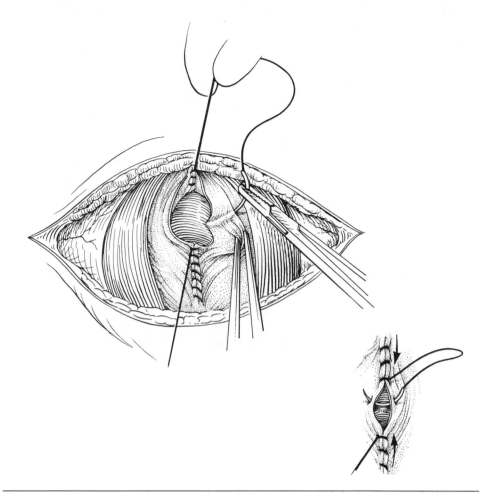

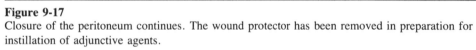

Figure 9-17
Closure of the peritoneum continues. The wound protector has been removed in preparation for instillation of adjunctive agents.

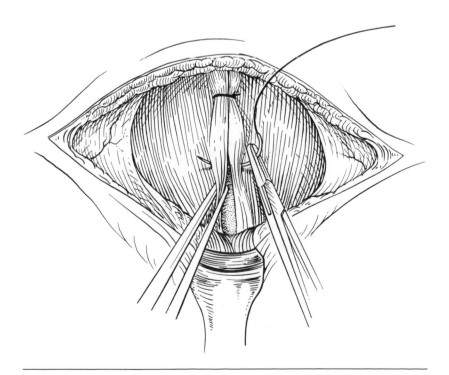

Figure 9-18
Rectus muscles are loosely approximated.

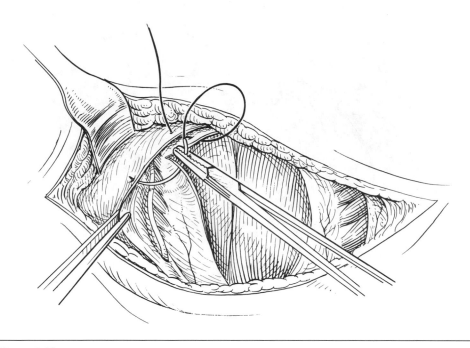

Figure 9-19
Angle placement of sutures, taking care to avoid the ilioinguinal nerves.

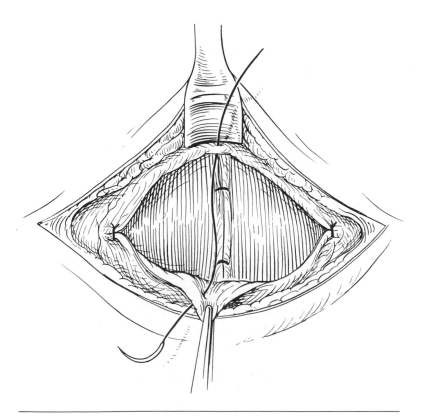

Figure 9-20
Midline fascial suture.

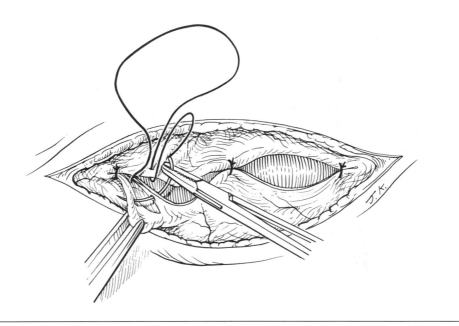

Figure 9-21
The fascia is closed with a continuous suture, taking care to incorporate all fascial layers.

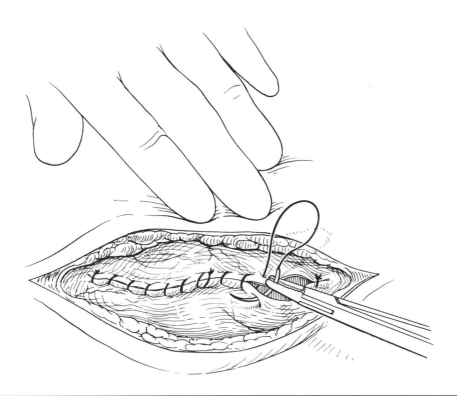

Figure 9-22
Fascial closure is being completed. Four additional interrupted fascial sutures are placed for reinforcement.

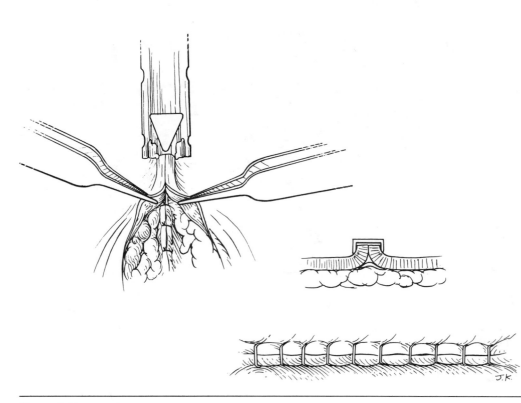

Figure 9-23
Placement of skin clips.

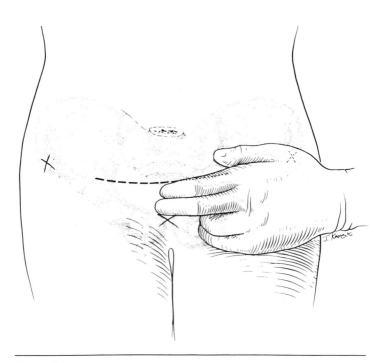

Figure 9-24
The Hunt—Acuna skin incision is marked out (see Figure 9-4).

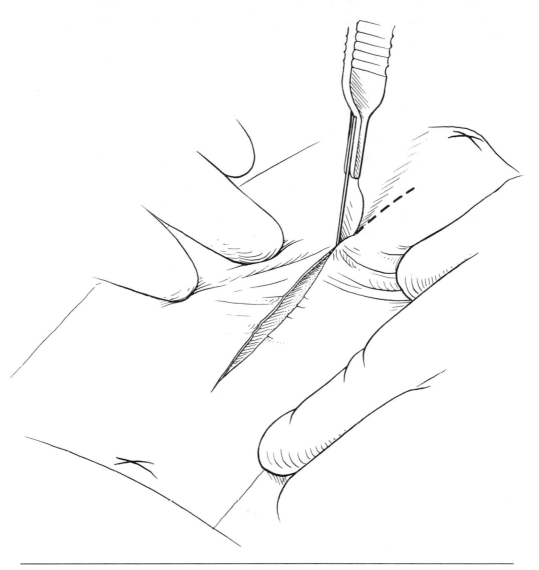

Figure 9-25
The Hunt—Acuna incision is made halfway through the dermis.

The Hunt—Acuna incision

The concept of the Hunt—Acuna incision was shown in two drawings and explained briefly by TeLinde and Mattingly.[5] The details of opening and closing the incision have been worked out to maximize its advantages and avoid its potential complications.

Results of the first 100 consecutive Hunt—Acuna incisions are as follows:

Hernia	0
Wound abscess	0
Wound disruption	0
Hematoma	0
Seroma	4 (1 infected)
Hygroma	1
Persistent pain	0
Cosmetic complaint	0
Paresthesia or numbness	1
Inadequate exposure	0

Two seromas occurred in our first 30 cases. At that time, we began using a subcutaneous closed drainage system (⅛-inch Hemovac). Of the four total, two were aspirated through the incision and two resolved spontaneously.

The single subcutaneous hygroma occurred secondary to Hyskon. Although several patients weighed in the area of 200 pounds, we achieved adequate exposure in all of them.

We have had no experience using this incision in cesarian sections. It would appear to offer more exposure than the Pfannenstiel, however. We now use the Hunt—Acuna exclusively, unless the patient has had a previous low midline incision.

An incision similar to the Pfannenstiel is marked out using the same landmarks (Figure 9-24; see Figure 9-4). The skin is opened half way through the dermis with a scalpel and the incision is completed using cutting current with a small amount of blend (Figures 9-25 and 9-26).

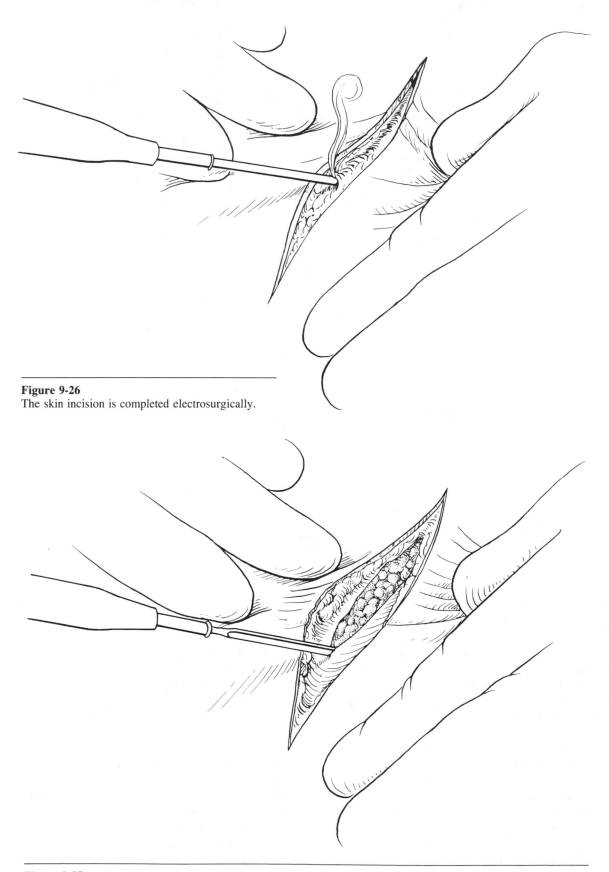

Figure 9-26
The skin incision is completed electrosurgically.

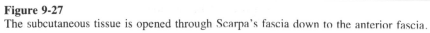

Figure 9-27
The subcutaneous tissue is opened through Scarpa's fascia down to the anterior fascia.

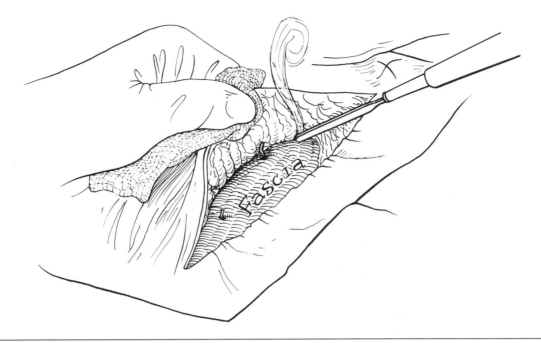

Figure 9-28
Dissection of subcutaneous tissue superiorly.

The subcutaneous tissue is opened through Scarpa's fascia down to the anterior fascia (Figure 9-27). Except in an obese patient, the superficial epigastric vessels may be preserved, and the subcutaneous incision is not carried far laterally as in the Pfannenstiel. Preserving subcutaneous tissue laterally as well as vasculature and nerve branches improves the body contour postoperatively and diminishes the likelihood of the patient developing paresthesias.

The superior wound flap is grasped in the midline with a sponge and lifted anteriorly. Using curved Mayo scissors with tips pointed posteriorly or the electrosurgical scalpel, the subcutaneous tissue is dissected off the anterior fascia superiorly in the midline (Figure 9-28). If the patient has had a previous Pfannenstiel incision, the scar tissue where the subcutaneous tissue joins the fascia laterally will have to be freed from the anterior fascia to give greater exposure. Perforating vessels are grasped with a long DeBakey forceps and coagulated with the cutting current (Figure 9-29). The dissection is not carried laterally but stays close to the midline to preserve perforating vessels and accompanying nerve bundles. As the dissection is continued superiorly, progressively larger retractors are used to retract the abdominal wall anteriorly. The dissection is carried approximately two-thirds the distance to the navel from the symphysis. A

headlamp is extremely useful in aiding the surgeon to visualize the surgical site.

The inferior wound flap is grasped in the midline, and with Mayo scissors, the subcutaneous tissue dissected off the anterior fascia to the symphysis pubis. Alternatively, the electrosurgical knife may be used (Figure 9-30). This is usually a very short distance. After the wound is irrigated, the anterior fascia is grasped in the midline with toothed forceps and is opened in the midline with a scalpel (Figure 9-31). The surgeon inserts a forefinger between the rectus muscles and the anterior fascia and dissects the muscle away from the fascia in the midline superiorly (Figure 9-32). The fascia is then opened in the midline superiorly, with a medium Kelly retractor facilitating exposure (Figure 9-33). Having found the midline, the surgeon opens the thin membrane between the rectus muscles and the plane between them and the urinary bladder is dissected down to the symphysis (Figure 9-34).

If the patient has previously had surgery in the space of Retzius or has had this space opened in the past, care must be taken as the bladder will frequently seal to the undersurface of the rectus muscles and a cystotomy will result during this dissection. In this case, the surgeon is advised not to open this space but to open the peritoneum

Text cont'd on p. 143.

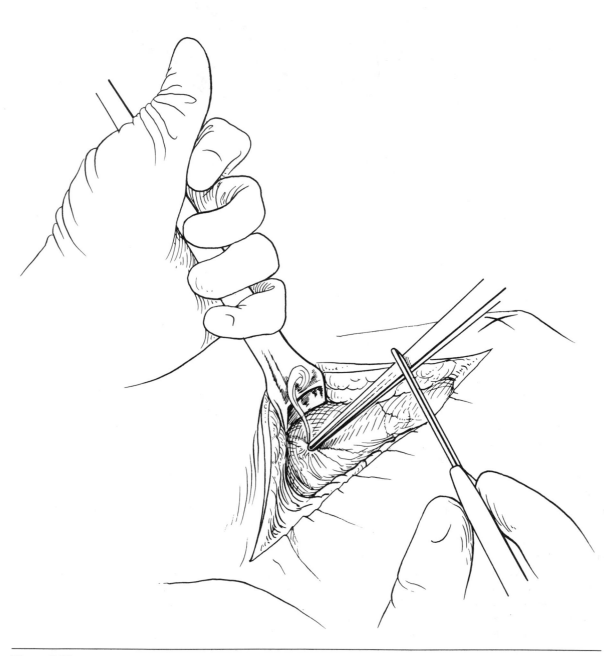

Figure 9-29
Coagulation of perforating vessels with DeBakey forceps and cutting current.

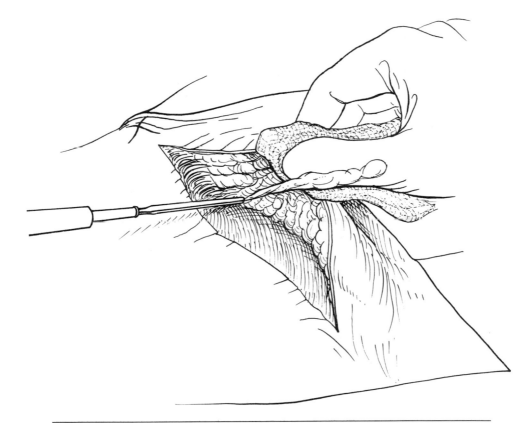

Figure 9-30
Subcutaneous tissue is dissected off the anterior fascia to the symphysis pubis.

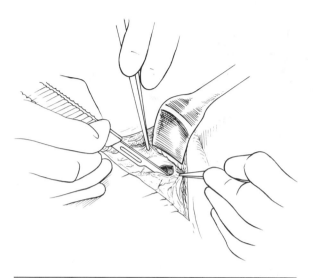

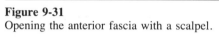

Figure 9-31
Opening the anterior fascia with a scalpel.

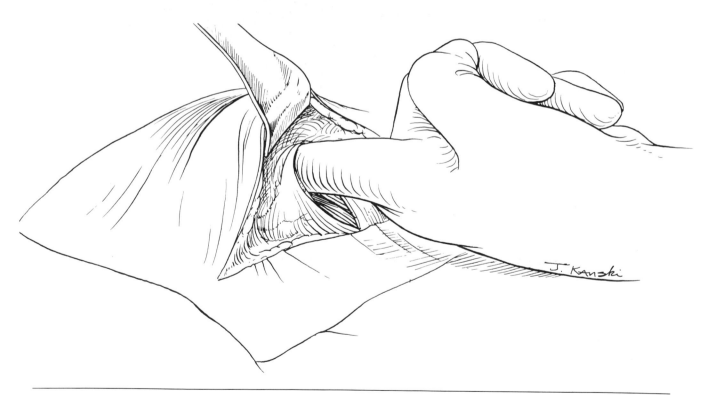

Figure 9-32
Rectus muscles are dissected away from the fascia by forefinger dissection.

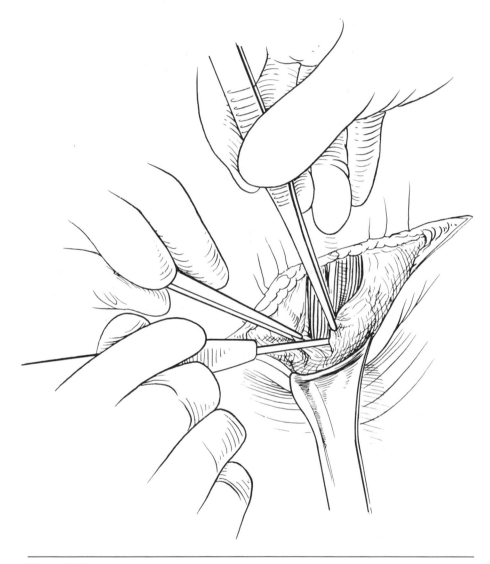

Figure 9-33
The fascia is opened in the midline.

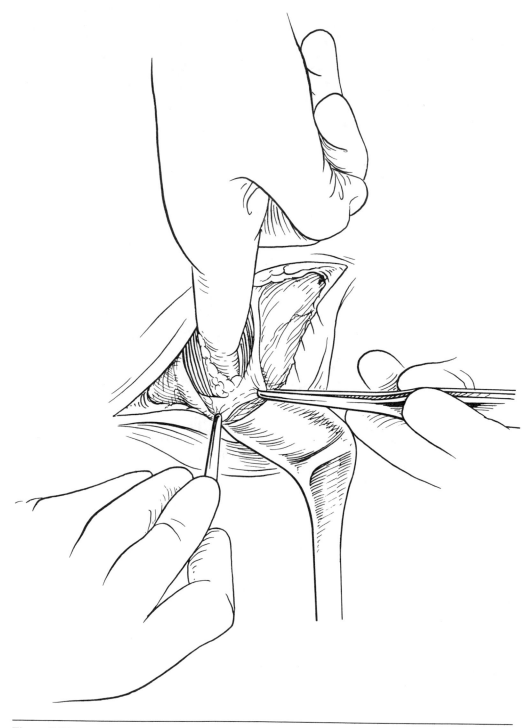

Figure 9-34
The plane between the rectus muscles and the urinary bladder is opened down to the symphysis by careful dissection with the forefinger.

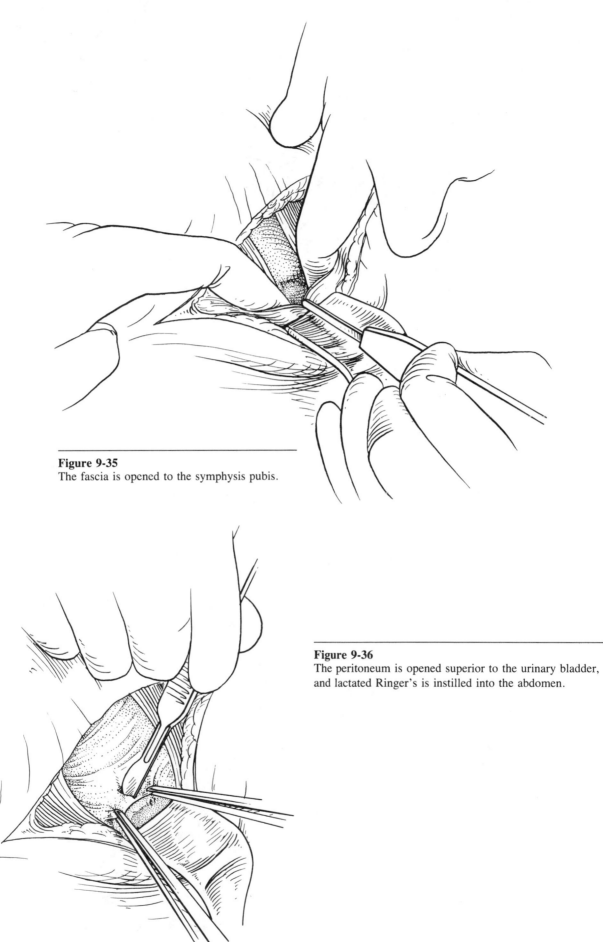

Figure 9-35
The fascia is opened to the symphysis pubis.

Figure 9-36
The peritoneum is opened superior to the urinary bladder, and lactated Ringer's is instilled into the abdomen.

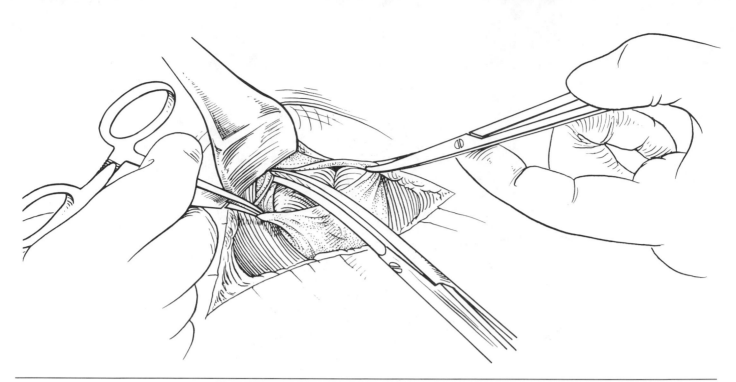

Figure 9-37
The peritoneum is opened superiorly using scissor dissection.

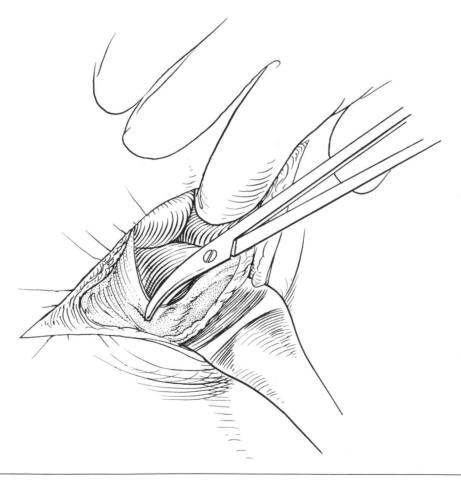

Figure 9-38
The peritoneum is opened inferiorly on either side of the urinary bladder. This may be done electrosurgically or with scissor dissection.

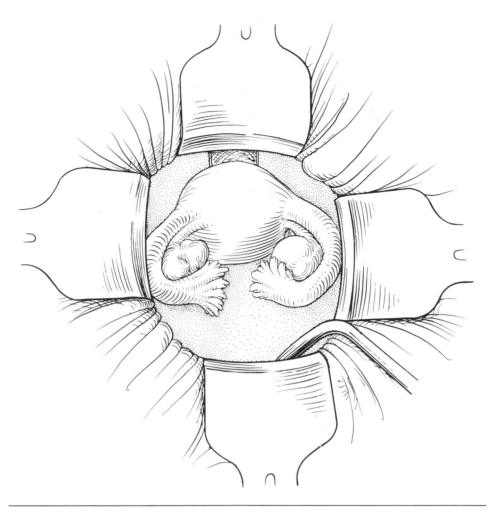

Figure 9-39
Placement of the wound protector and Kirschner retractor, and exposure of the pelvis are
completed.

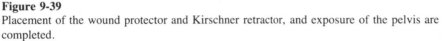

lateral to the bladder with the bladder viewed from the
peritoneal side. The surgeon and assistant place their
forefingers beneath the fascia, which is opened to the
symphysis pubis (Figure 9-35). Care must be taken to
keep the bladder reflected posteriorly. The peritoneum is
now opened superior to the urinary bladder (Figure 9-
36). Heparinized lactated Ringer's solution is placed in
the abdomen at this point to prevent blood from clotting.
The peritoneum is opened superiorly with scissors dissection (Figure 9-37). Using scissors dissection, the surgeon opens the peritoneum inferiorly, staying lateral to
the urinary bladder (Figure 9-38). After abdominal exploration is complete and the wound protector and
Kirschner retractor are positioned (Figure 9-39), the surgery proceeds. In the obese patient, a large blade should
be used superiorly, two medium blades laterally, and a
small blade inferiorly or large blades superiorly and laterally and a medium blade inferiorly. This is similar to

the arrangement of the retractor blades in an obese patient
having a Pfannenstiel incision.

Wound closure

When the intraabdominal portion of the surgery is complete, the abdomen is ready for closure. The inferior
portion of the incision is closed carefully to avoid damage
to the urinary bladder and deep epigastric vessels. This
closure is carried to approximately one-third the length
of the incision, at which time the suture is tied and held
with a Kelly clamp (Figure 9-40).

The superior closure is begun as follows. With careful
retraction superiorly, the surgeon identifies the anterior
fascia and the peritoneum. The first suture incorporates
the apex of the fascial incision and the apex of the peritoneal incision (Figure 9-41). Incorporating the fascia at
the beginning of the superior suture simplifies closure of

Text cont'd on p. 146.

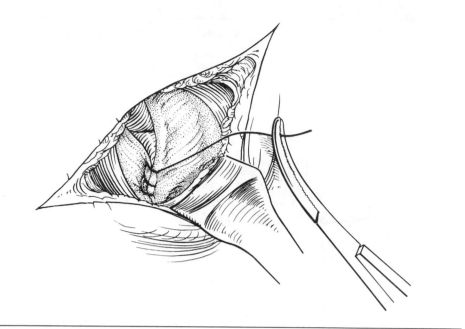

Figure 9-40
Closure of the inferior one-third of the peritoneum. The wound protector may be left in place until peritoneal closure is almost completed.

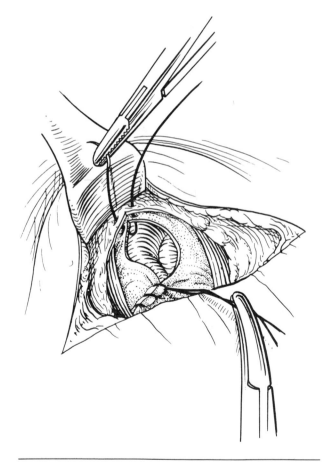

Figure 9-41
The suture of the superior peritoneal closure incorporates the apices of the fascial and peritoneal incisions. Including the fascia is extremely important in preventing hernia formation and in assisting in placement of the continuous superior fascial suture.

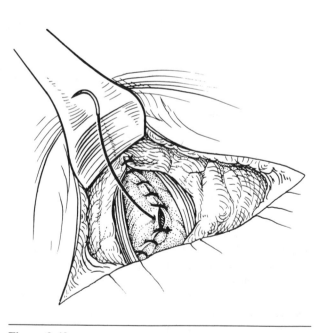

Figure 9-42
Peritoneal closure is completed. The wound protector has been removed. Adjunctive agents are added.

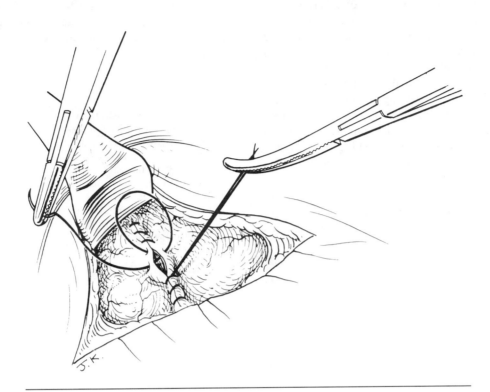

Figure 9-43
Fascial closure is completed with a running suture.

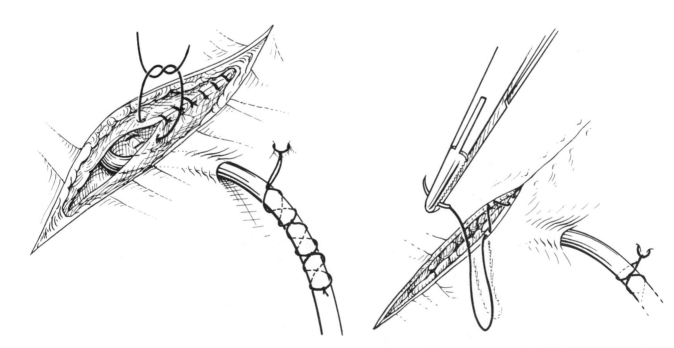

Figure 9-44
Placement of Hemovac drain and closure of Scarpa's fascia. Care must be taken to avoid suturing the drain with the sutures in Scarpa's fascia.

Figure 9-45
Subcuticular closure is completed. Steri-Strips will be applied to support the closure and will be removed by the patient several days later.

the fascia and minimizes the danger of a hernia developing at the apex of the fascial incision. It also serves as a guide when the surgeon begins the fascial closure. When the first suture is tied, peritoneal closure is continued down to the inferior peritoneal suture (Figure 9-42) and the second suture is tied, thus completing closure of the peritoneum. Adjunctive agents are placed intraabdominally just before peritoneal closure is completed.

Fascial closure is effected with running sutures of 0 or no. 1 synthetic absorbable material (Figure 9-43). Four additional interrupted sutures are placed along the fascial closure for reinforcement.

After hemostasis has been checked carefully, a Hemovac drain is placed in the subcutaneous space, brought out in the midline, 1 cm inferior to the incision, and tied in with a 3-0 suture (Figure 9-44). Scarpa's fascia is closed with interrupted sutures of 3-0 absorbable material.

Subcuticular closure with 4-0 synthetic material is performed and Steri-Strips are applied (Figure 9-45). The surgeon may elect to close the skin with clips or interrupted sutures.

REFERENCES

1. Pfannenstiel F: Abdominal and vaginal celiotomy; a comparative study of the value and effectiveness of both operations, with notes on their indications and technic, *Am J Obstet* 58:277-282, 1908.
2. Taylor HC: Pfannenstiel's incision in gynecology, *Surg Gynecol Obstet* 2:538-540, 1906.
3. Maguire DL Jr: The Pfannenstiel incision, *J South Carolina Med Assoc* 43:356-359, 1947.
4. Tovey DW: The Pfannenstiel incision, *Am Med* 40:289-290, 1934.
5. TeLinde RW and Mattingly RF: *Operative gynecology*, ed 4, Philadelphia, 1970, JB Lippincott.

10

Equipment, Instruments, and Sutures

··

ROBERT B. HUNT

The surgeon will need to try many types of instruments and pieces of equipment as well as needles and sutures before deciding on the best set-up. This chapter discusses certain important characteristics of these items. It is meant as a starting place and is not designed to sway a surgeon toward any particular instrument, equipment, company, or supplier.

OPERATING ROOM EQUIPMENT

The surgeon should use a comfortable chair, preferably padded, that can be adjusted to individual requirements. A back is a welcome addition. These chairs can be borrowed from ophthalmologic colleagues (Figure 10-1).

Microscope

Several excellent microscopes are available. If the hospital does not have a suitable microscope, the surgeon should try several different makes and designs to select a preferable model. Several features are very worthwhile. First, the stand should be heavy and stable. This prevents the microscope from tilting over and also dampens vibrations transmitted to the microscope head. These vibrations tend to blur intraoperative photographs if they are taken and tire the surgeon's eyes.

An extension on the horizontal arm of the microscope allows the microscope stand to be remote from the microscope head. This reduces crowding in the area of surgery and also helps sterility to be maintained more easily (Figure 10-2). An X-Y axis is useful, since it permits the surgeon to move the microscope head short distances without having to grasp it. This minimizes erratic movements of the microscope head. Inclinable binoculars are helpful (Figure 10-3) so that each surgeon can adjust the angle of the eyepieces. Eyepieces sometimes have adjustable cups. These are usually extended when the surgeon does not wear eyeglasses and are turned down when glasses are used (Figure 10-4). Eyepieces should be selected in conjunction with the lens to give a wide range of magnification. We use a 10 × eyepiece; which, in conjunction with a 250mm lens, gives 5 × to 20 × range of magnification (Figure 10-5). A beam splitter is necessary if one plans to photograph through the microscope or use a video camera. A beam splitter may reduce light delivered to the surgeon's eyes by greater than 50% (Figure 10-5). The surgeon should compensate for this by having a proper light source. The microscope company representative can advise the staff in this regard.

The decision as to whether microscopic drapes should be used should be made jointly by the surgeon, the nurses, and the operating room supervisor, as well as the infection control officer (Figure 10-6). Microsurgical teams elect to use them either most of the time or almost never. Infections are rare with and without drapes. When used, they are changed for each procedure. When a surgical case is completed, the drapes can be left on as a dust cover; they are replaced with sterile ones when the microscope is used next. If drapes are not used, autoclavable handles are placed on the microscope controls so that the surgeon may touch these during the case for various adjustments. When the surgeon is ready for the microscope and is not using drapes, the head of the microscope is moved over the field with a sterile towel.

The microscope can be positioned between the lower extremities if a split table is used or the patient's legs are placed in surgical stirrups. We position it at the head of the table (Figure 10-7).

When checking the microscope for adjustment, the surgeon will wish to make certain the eyepieces are at the proper diopter setting, the cups on the eyepieces are positioned appropriately, the correct lens is positioned securely, and the focus and zoom controls function (Figures 10-8, 10-9, and 10-10). If still photographs are to be taken through the microscope, the surgeon should check the microscope camera for film and proper adjustment and function (Figure 10-11). A video camera, if used, should be in position and functional. Blank tape

Text cont'd on p. 153.

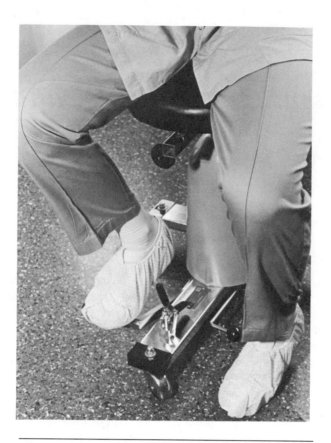

Figure 10-1
Controls of an ophthalmologic surgical chair.

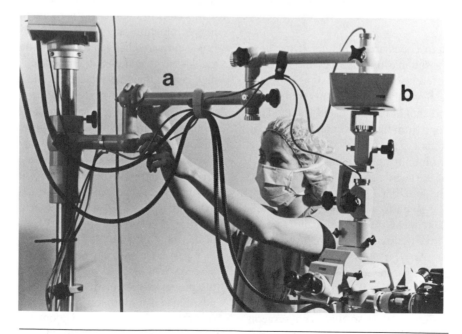

Figure 10-2
Adjustments are made on the horizontal arm of the microscope. Note *(a)* the extension and *(b)* the X-Y axis.

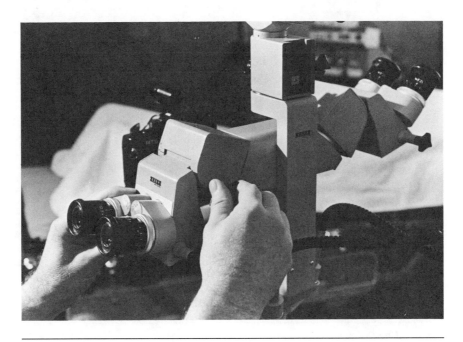

Figure 10-3
The inclinable binoculars are adjusted.

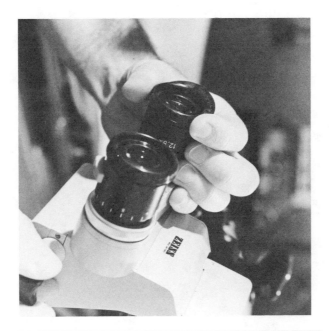

Figure 10-4
Eye cups can be folded down to accommodate eyeglasses.

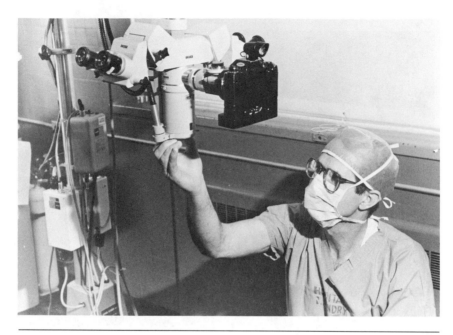

Figure 10-5
The surgeon installs a 250mm lens. Note the beam splitter to
which the camera is attached.

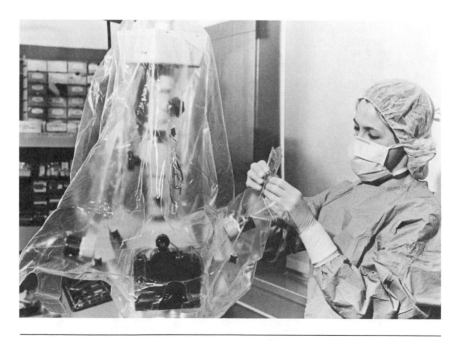

Figure 10-6
The nurse positions the microscope drape (available as order
no. 89-0004, microlaser pack, Cunningham Woodland; and
Xomed, Inc.).

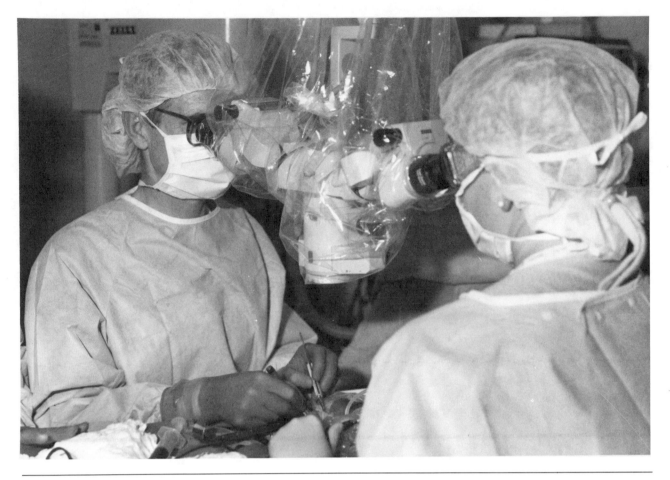

Figure 10-7
A microsurgical procedure in progress.

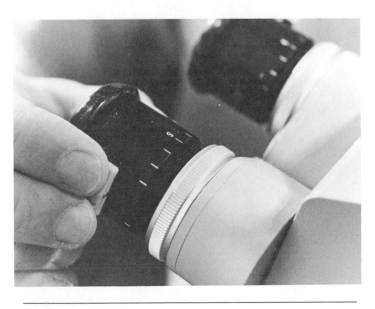

Figure 10-8
The eyepieces are set to the correct diopter setting before
draping the microscope. (See Chapter 4.)

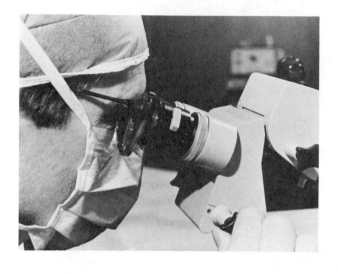

Figure 10-9
Interpupillary distance is adjusted.

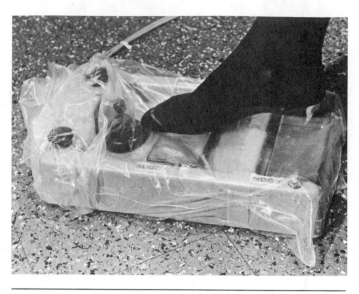

Figure 10-10
The surgeon checks the focus and zoom controls. Performing surgery in stocking feet allows precise control. Note the foot pedal is covered with plastic. Dust or fluids may result in malfunction.

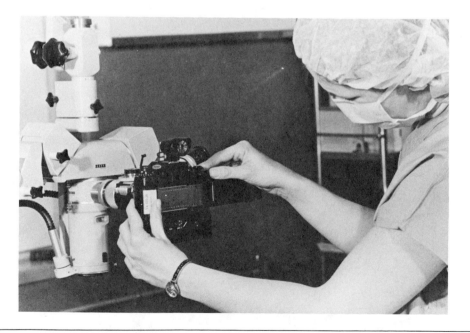

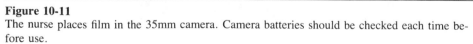

Figure 10-11
The nurse places film in the 35mm camera. Camera batteries should be checked each time before use.

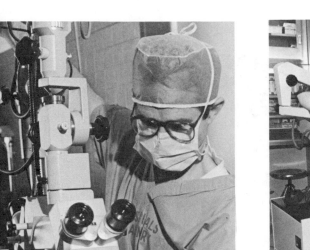

Figure 10-12
The surgeon checks light intensity. Spare bulbs are kept in the operating room suite.

should be installed. The proper consent for photography must be signed by the patient. The light on the microscope must be checked; it should always be activated while it is at its lowest setting and its intensity increased to maximum to prevent overloading the bulb (Figure 10-12). Replacement bulbs must be readily available. The surgeon places the base of the microscope in the proper position to allow easy positioning of the microscope head over the field.

If the carbon dioxide laser is used, appropriate checks must be made on the unit and the articulating arm draped if appropriate (Figure 10-13).

The "fogging" problem

Condensation on the surgeon's glasses can be frustrating. There are several steps to take to lessen this problem.

The operating room supervisor may order special masks with a plastic or foam liner on the superior border.

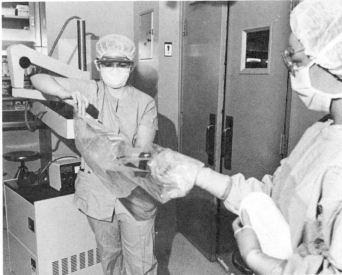

Figure 10-13
Nurses drape the CO_2 laser articulating arm (available through Xomed, Inc.). Note safety glasses.

These are molded to fit the surgeon's face (Figure 10-14). When putting on the mask, the inferior strings should be tied so that the mask fits loosely. This prevents heat build-up (Figures 10-15 and 10-16).

Antifogging solutions can be applied to eyeglasses before starting the procedure. These are usually available through an optometrist.

Electrosurgical units

Electrosurgical units must be selected very carefully. The patient should be grounded with a large, well-lubricated ground plate to prevent "hot spots." Optimally, the electrosurgical unit providing unipolar energy for the conventional as well as microsurgical aspects of the procedure should have both a standard and a low-power output. The latter is used for the microsurgical electrodes. Too much wattage will both deform the microelectrode tip and produce excessive tissue damage.

Although many of these electrosurgical units have a bipolar as well as a unipolar component, we find it best to have a separate unit for bipolar coagulation (Figure 10-17). Many combined units require the circulating nurse to switch the unit when going from one component to the other. In performing microsurgery, we frequently use both components simultaneously, and to have the circulating nurse try to keep up with the two is an unworkable situation. Some newer units are designed to allow simultaneous use of unipolar and bipolar modes. We have the first assistant operate the bipolar coagulator while the surgeon operates the unipolar electrode. This allows the procedure to progress promptly.

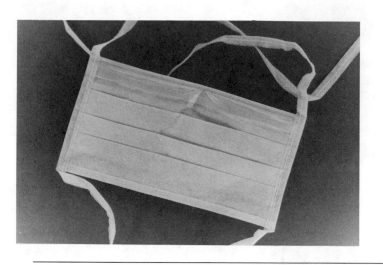

Figure 10-14
Mask with a plastic insert (available as order no. 4238, Surgikos, Inc.; and order no. 3322, Precept).

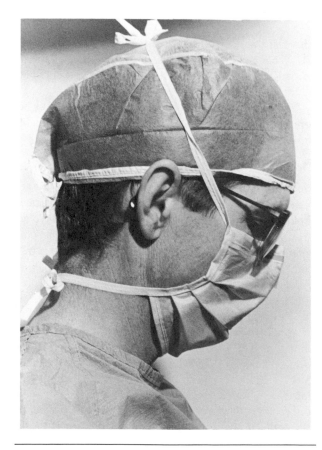

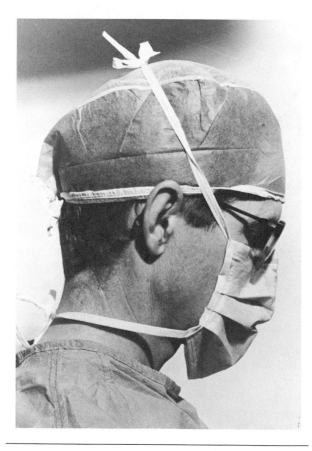

Figure 10-15
The lower border of the mask is fastened too snugly.

Figure 10-16
The lower border of the mask is fastened loosely, thus preventing heat build-up.

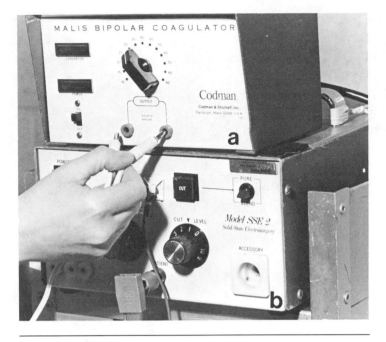

Figure 10-17
The nurse carefully connects electrical cords to bipolar unit
(a). Notice the separate unipolar unit *(b)*. (Bipolar unit available from Codman and Shurtleff and the unipolar unit from Valleylab, Inc.).

Operating room accessories

Many accessories are available to the surgical team to allow better organization of equipment and instruments. A plastic holder is very useful. This device has pockets in which instruments may be placed to minimize the chance of their being dropped to the floor (Figure 10-18).

A mat for cleaning conventional coagulation tips is helpful. This is placed on the operating room drapes and used throughout the procedure (Figure 10-19). The nurse may use a cloth for cleaning microsurgical instruments.

A demagnetizer is indispensable. Microsurgical instruments become magnetized and this must be corrected to allow effective handling of delicate sutures (Figure 10-20).

Bone wax and foam, which the suture is packed in, are excellent microsurgical needle holders. A magnetic needle holder should be avoided, since this magnetizes the needles.

Photography

A 35mm camera designed for operating room use is of great value. We photograph almost every case before and after the reparative work has been done. At the conclusion of each case we photograph the patient's name plate for identification. One copy of the slides is sent to the patient, one copy to the referring gynecologist, and one set retained for the patient's records. Our equipment includes a Nikon 35mm model F camera with 55mm lens equipped with a ring light and battery box (Figure 10-21). This eliminates the need for one more electrical outlet. The settings were worked out in our initial cases. This equipment gives consistently excellent slides. We use Kodak Ektachrome film, daylight, ASA 100.

A silicone mat may be used and provides an excellent background for photography as well as a smooth surface on which to work (Figure 10-22).

INSTRUMENTS AND INTRAOPERATIVE ACCESSORIES
Abdominal retractor

The surgeon should select an abdominal retractor that is low-profile, gives excellent exposure, and avoids the risk of damage to the pelvic nerves such as the femoral nerve. An excellent choice is the Kirschner retractor (Figure 10-23). When purchasing it, one should obtain three additional large, curved blades for overweight patients. When positioning the retractor, the surgeon ordinarily places the two medium blades laterally and the two small blades in the midline, retracting inferiorly and superiorly. One large blade is used superiorly, two medium blades laterally, and one small blade inferiorly or a medium blade inferiorly, and large blades laterally and superiorly when a transverse incision is used in the overweight patient.

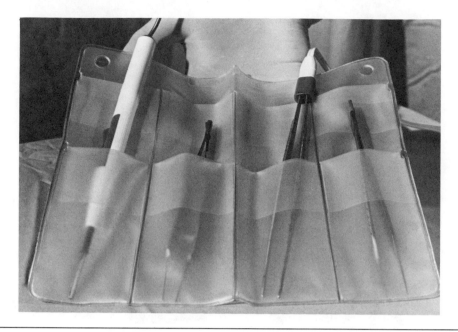

Figure 10-18
A useful instrument holder (Eight-Pocket Surgi-Kit, order No. SK-100, Ethox Corp.).

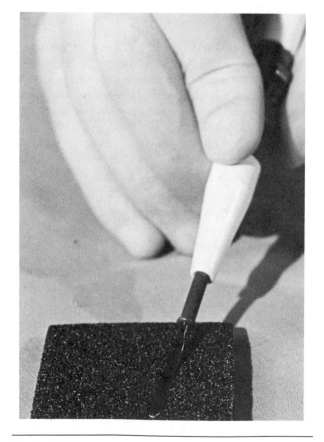

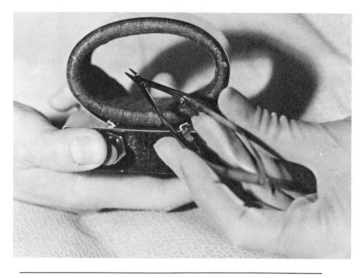

Figure 10-20
A needle carrier is demagnetized. The surgeon passes the instrument through the center of the coil and slowly withdraws it as the circulating nurse activates the demagnetizer. Sterility is maintained (Available through ASSI, model AD19-202).

Figure 10-19
A standard scalpel electrode is cleaned. (Electrosurgical Tip Cleaner, reorder no. 4315, Surgikos, Inc.).

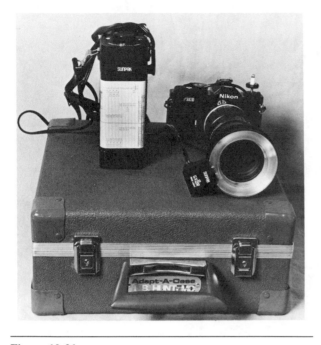

Figure 10-21
Nikon photographic equipment. I use a 105mm Micro-Nikkor lens with a ring light.

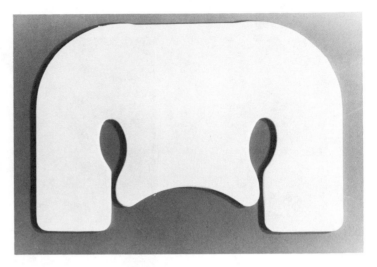

Figure 10-22
The silicone mat gives an ideal background on which to perform surgery and photograph (order no. SP-1015, ASSI; order no. FM-220-15-V, Downs Surgical, Inc.; order no. 297-260, ZSI, order no. 32-998-01, Martin).

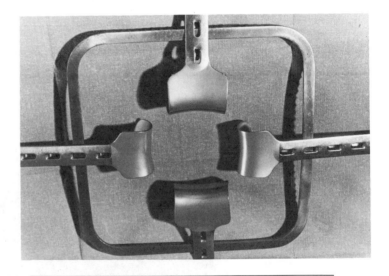

Figure 10-23
Kirschner retractor. The standard two small and two medium blades are shown. The surgeon should have available three additional large, curved blades for overweight patients. Note the low-profile and shallow blades. (Available through Downs Surgical, Inc., order no. BG-245-00-C; Elmed, Inc., order no. 15300-00; Martin, order no. 15-884-00; and ZSI, order no. 51-125.)

Wound protector

A plastic wound protector is very helpful (Figure 10-24). The ring is placed within the abdominal cavity in such a manner that bowel is not entrapped. The retractor is then placed over this and the plastic sheathing folded beneath the retractor frame to give the surgeon additional forearm support and reduce pressure on the patient's body.

Suction

A sump drain should be available to place in the cul-de-sac to keep the pelvis suctioned during the procedure. We pack the cul-de-sac with Kerlex guaze over the drain. We find the Jackson-Pratt catheter to be an excellent instrument (Figure 10-25). In addition, conventional suction is needed with small and regular tips available.

Irrigation

An irrigator is a necessity. One may elect to use 30-ml syringes with plastic cannulas. They are inexpensive and readily available; however, they require constant refilling by the already busy scrub nurse. An alternative, which works exceptionally well, is the Gomel irrigator with an 18-gauge plastic catheter (Figure 10-26). It is connected to a liter intravenous bag of warm heparinized lactated Ringer's solution and irrigation is accomplished by gravity. The solution must be replaced as needed to keep the irrigant at a warm temperature.

Lighting

A headlamp is absolutely essential for adequately visualizing areas deep in the pelvis. The surgeon uses this

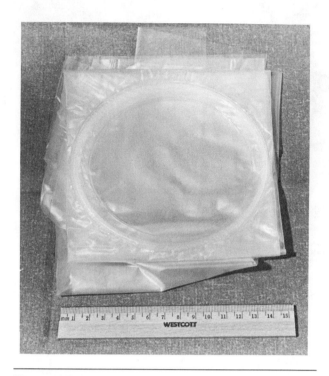

Figure 10-24
The 5-inch wound protector pictured is suitable for most pelvic operations. If a large vertical incision is used, a 7-inch size is better. (The 5-inch protector available as reorder no. 1062-1, Deseret medical.)

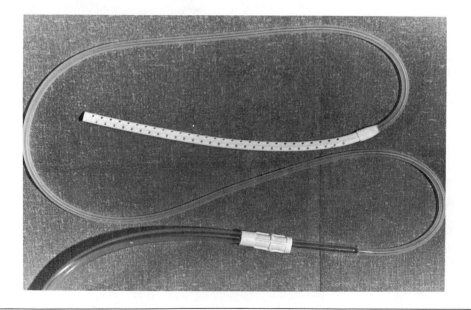

Figure 10-25
A 7-mm Jackson-Pratt catheter. Note the medicine dropper (pictured). Either a medicine dropper or a Christmas tree adaptor may be used to join the catheter to standard wall-suction tubing. (Catheter available as order no. SU 130-1310 [flat] and order no. SU 130-1325 [round], Baxter V. Mueller; the medicine dropper as order no. 12550, Baxter Healthcare.)

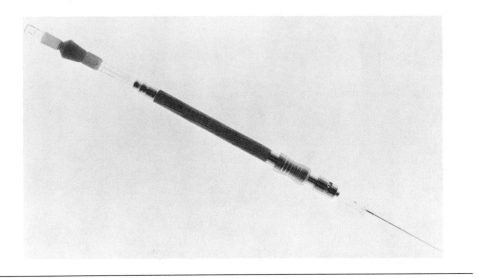

Figure 10-26
Gomel irrigator (order no. 18200-01, Elmed, Inc.; and order no. 18-530-01, Martin). An 18-gauge plastic cannula should be used as the tip.

in the initial stages while setting up the procedure and for closing (Figure 10-27). The only time the headlight is not used is while the microscope is being used.

Loupes

Surgical loupes are extremely useful during fertility operations. They are helpful in performing ovarian surgery, lysing adhesions, ferreting out endometrial implants, and repairing distal tubal disease. Some surgeons use loupes for distal tube work such as fimbrioplasty and salpingostomy. Loupes have the advantage of being quick to position, which is helpful when the site of surgery must be changed rapidly, such as when working from the dome of the uterus to the depth of the pelvis. Loupes have the disadvantage of causing fatigue of the surgeon's neck muscles when 4.0 power or greater is used. I prefer a magnification factor of 2.5 (Figure 10-28).

Bakes dilators

We calibrate the fimbriated ends of fallopian tubes with nos. 3, 4, and 5 French Bakes dilators. Most fallopian tubes will accept a 4-mm or 5-mm dilator easily (Figure 10-29).

Retrograde lavage

A set of lavage cannulas designed by Stangel is available (Figure 10-30).

Bipolar instruments

A long bipolar instrument is of great advantage for coagulating structures deep in the pelvis such as adhesions and small implants of endometriosis (Figure 10-31). These are usually obtainable from the neurosurgical service and are approximately 18 cm long. The short bipolar instrument should have a fine tip. Flat handles are acceptable and a stabilizing pin is an advantage. An additional short bipolar forceps with a medium tip is helpful (Figure 10-31).

Microelectrodes

The handle of the microelectrode should have an extender for work deep in the pelvis (Figure 10-32). When working on the fallopian tubes and ovaries, a standard-length handle is used; this should be hand operated. The microelectrode should be insulated to prevent damage should a contiguous structure such as the fallopian tube drop onto it. The surgeon must remember to turn the power down to a low level when using the microelectrode.

It is helpful to have a larger needle electrode available for dividing dense adhesions and opening the ovarian cortex (Figure 10-33).

Dissecting rods

Dissecting rods are extraordinarily valuable in dissecting adhesions and in performing distal tubal work such as salpingostomy. These are available in glass and Teflon coated (Figure 10-34). Glass rods may break but are less expensive. If laser is to be used, special dissecting rods such as quartz should be purchased. Dissecting rods should be of varying lengths as well as have a variety of tip shapes.

Scissors

Microscissors should have rounded handles and stabilizing pins. Those with rounded tips allow less traumatic

Text cont'd on p. 164.

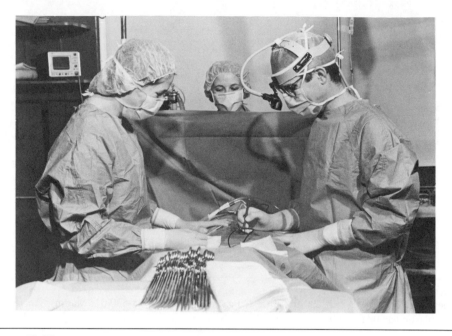

Figure 10-27
The surgeon works with the aid of a headlight. (Available from Applied Fiberoptics, Inc., Cuda Products Corp., Designs for Vision, Keeler Instruments, Inc.; Lutex Corp, Carl Zeiss, Inc.; and ZSI.) is now available through Luxtec Corp.)

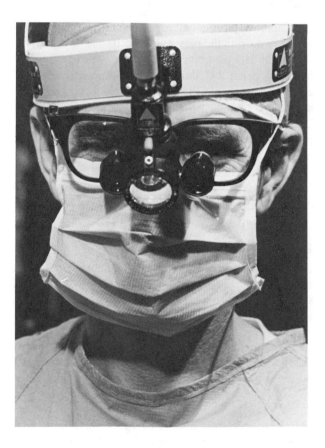

Figure 10-28
The surgeon may prefer loupes with added illumination of headlight for certain steps of the procedure. (Available from Designs for Vision; Elmed; Keeler Instruments, Inc.; and Carl Zeiss, Inc.)

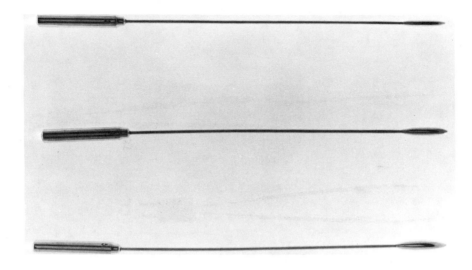

Figure 10-29
Bakes dilators, 3 mm, 4 mm, and 5 mm (order nos. 25-4006, 25-4007, and 25-4008 respectively, Codman and Shurtleff).

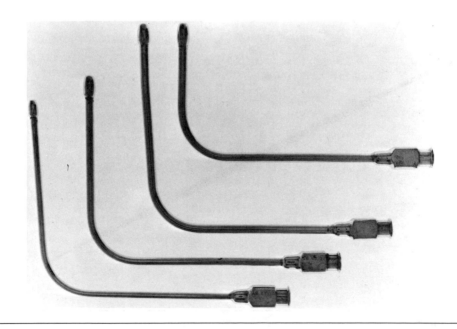

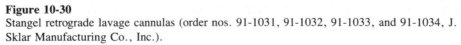

Figure 10-30
Stangel retrograde lavage cannulas (order nos. 91-1031, 91-1032, 91-1033, and 91-1034, J. Sklar Manufacturing Co., Inc.).

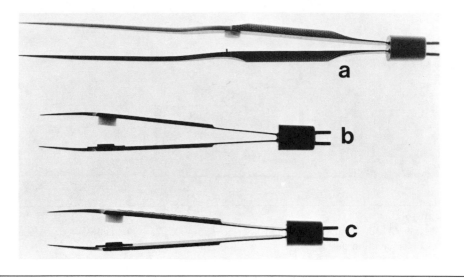

Figure 10-31
The three titanium bipolar forceps described in the text are shown. (Available as *(a)* long rhoton bayonet forceps, order no. 80-1708; *(b)* E-Series bipolar forceps, 1-mm tip, order no. 80-6012; and *(c)* 0.25-mm tip, order no. 80-6011, Codman and Shurtleff. Stainless steel bipolar forceps are available through Elmed, ZSI, Martin, and Cameron-Miller, Inc.)

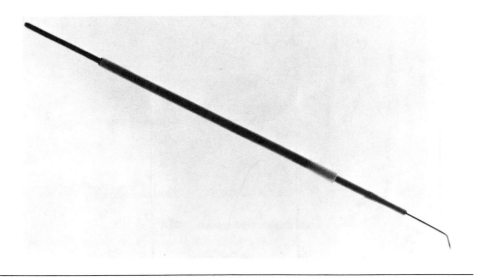

Figure 10-32
Needle electrode with an extender (model E 1502, ³/₃₂″ shaft, 3¼″ insulation, Valleylab. An insulated extension is also available, order no. 5107, Elmed.)

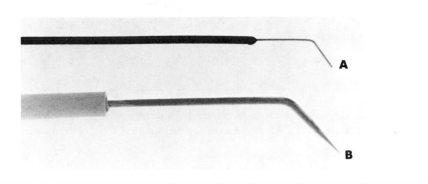

Figure 10-33
An angulated insulated microelectrode **A,** and angulated needle electrode **B,** Excellent micro-electrodes are also available from Cameron-Miller, Inc., Elmed, Inc., Martin, and ZSI.

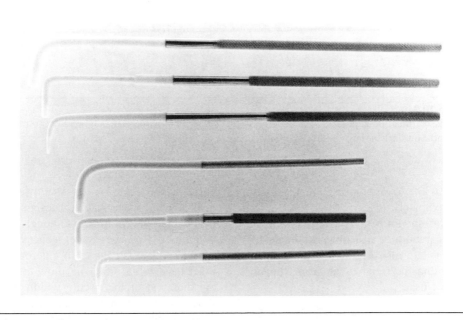

Figure 10-34
An assortment of Teflon-coated dissecting rods of various lengths, tip, and shapes (Elmed, Inc., Martin USA, Inc., and ZSI). (Glass rods available as order no. GP 3 glass probes, ASSI—Accurate Surgical and Scientific Instruments, Inc.; and order nos. FM-220-52-C and FM-220-54-G, Downs Surgical.)

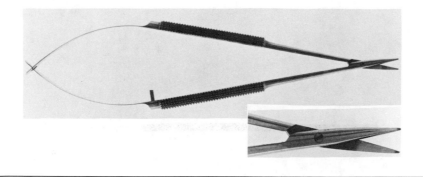

Figure 10-35
Microscissors. Note rounded handles and *(Inset)* tips with rounded points. (order no. 11501, Elmed, Inc., and no. 11-757 Martin. Additional microsurgical scissors are available from ASSI and ZSI.)

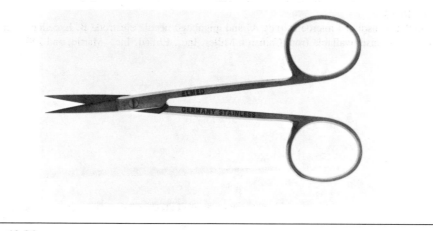

Figure 10-36
Iris scissors must be kept sharp and used only for cutting tubal tissue (order no. 54-6500, Codman and Shurtleff; order no. 11502, Elmed, Inc.; or order no. 11-622-10, Martin).

dissection (Figure 10-35). An appropriate length of scissors would be approximately 12 cm.

A sharp iris scissors should be available to divide the fallopian tube in preparation for anastomosis (Figure 10-36). Serrated scissors are also available and have the advantage of preventing the tubal tissue from slipping when the blades are closed.

Needle carriers

The surgeon must select a needle carrier carefully and should try many types before making a final choice. Several characteristics should be looked for. The needle carrier should be approximately 12 to 15 cm long. The jaws may be straight or curved but should be heavy enough to hold the microneedle securely. The jaws should not be too broad, however, since this tends to flatten the needle. If they are of a concave-convex design, the surgeon must make certain the curves within the jaws correspond to the curve of the needle being used. If the

curve is too acute or too shallow, it will deform the needle. The concave-convex design is excellent because it holds the needle firmly, although only at right angles (Figure 10-37). The convex-concave shape can also be used to replace the curve in a deformed needle. On the other hand, a flat jaw will allow the surgeon to change the direction of the needle within the jaws to accommodate different angles as needed.

The handles on the needle carrier should be round. This allows the surgeon to rotate the needle carrier between the fingers in a smooth manner (Figure 10-38). A "locking" needle carrier should probably be avoided, since a locking and unlocking motion tends to jerk the needle and damage the tissue. An exception is the needle carrier designed to lock when passing the suture to the nurse and is not used while suturing.

The surgeon should never use a microneedle carrier on a suture larger than 8-0, since the larger needle that is required will damage the jaws. A small plastic needle

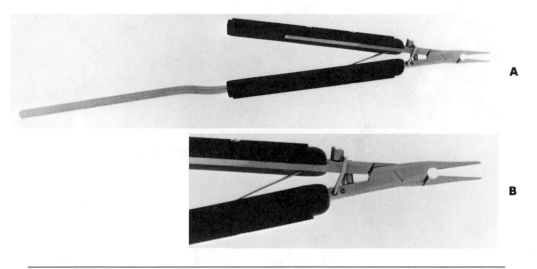

Figure 10-37
A, Vickers-Owens needle carrier. **B,** The tips are sturdy and of concave-convex configuration. The lock is used only to transport the needle to and from the surgical field (Available from Elmed, Inc., Keeler Instruments, Inc., and Martin). When ordering, it is important to provide specific information to the company such as whether the surgeon is right- or left-handed and whether a straight or curved tip is desired. Keeler Instruments, Inc. offers a long version in addition to the standard one.

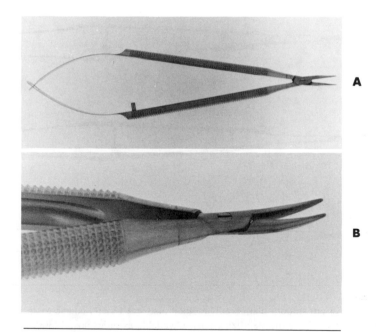

Figure 10-38
A, A curved needle carrier of conventional design. **B,** The sturdy curved tip is apparent. Superb needle carriers are available through ASSI, Elmed, Inc., Martin, and ZSI.

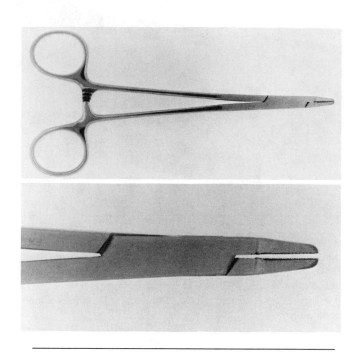

Figure 10-39
A plastic needle carrier of a bulldog design is excellent for
5-0 and 6-0 sutures (available from Weck).

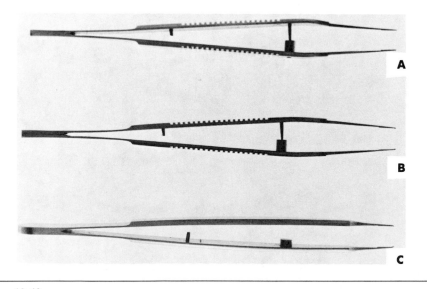

Figure 10-40
A, Pictured are 14-cm smooth platform **B,** toothed platform **C,** and coarse-tooth platform forceps for heavy work. Note the stabilizing pins. (Available as order nos. 12300, 12301, and
12302, respectively, Elmed, Inc.; and order nos. 12-158, 12-159, and 12-385 respectively, Martin.) Excellent forceps are also available through ASSI and ZSI.

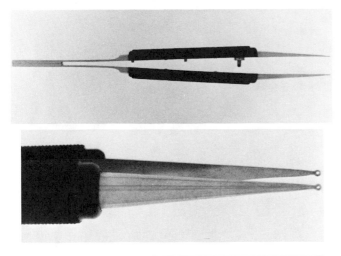

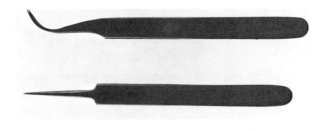

Figure 10-41
Ring forceps. The rings are fragile and must be protected with rubber or plastic tip covers when not in use. The forceps are available as order no. 12303, Elmed, Inc., order no. 12-154, Martin, as well as from Keeler Instruments, Inc.

Figure 10-42
Curved and straight jeweler's forceps. Note the delicate tips. (Available as order nos. ST-JFC 7 curved, and ST-JFS3 straight, ASSI Inc.; order nos. 12-85-11 curved, and 2-84-11 straight, Elmed, Inc.; order nos. 297-227 curved, and 297-225 straight, ZSI, Inc.; and order nos. FM-220-36-E curved, and FM-220-32-V straight, Downs Surgical.)

carrier is used to handle larger needles, such as that accompanying a 6-0 suture (Figure 10-39). A fine vascular needle carrier is an excellent alternative when a larger instrument is required.

It is useful to have a long microneedle carrier (18 cm) available when performing surgery on an overweight patient.

Forceps

Platform forceps are often used for tying and grasping tissues. They have the advantage of allowing the surgeon to pick up the sutures easily for tying and have the disadvantage of crushing tissue when it is pressed between the platforms. They are excellent forceps, however, and are preferred by many microsurgeons (Figure 10-40).

Toothed forceps are essential. A heavy toothed forceps is used in grasping segments of fallopian tube to be excised and thick adhesions to be removed (Figure 10-40C). A lighter pair should be available for finer work. The surgeon must avoid picking up tissue that is to be left behind with the toothed forceps, since the forceps may inflict significant damage to the structure.

A ring forceps has many advantages. It allows the surgeon to pick up tissue with minimal trauma and minimal pressure. The rings act as superb platforms in tying and aid in grasping the tip of the needle when the needle exits from the tissue to allow easy retrieval of the needle (Figure 10-41). The surgeon should try both the platform and the ring forceps before choosing one or the other. They both serve the purpose quite well.

A very fine jeweler's forceps should be available for gently dilating the tubal lumen before anastomosis (Figure 10-42).

Special scalpel blades

In performing a cornual resection, a curved cornual blade designed by Gomel may be used. Also, a disposable ophthalmic blade works very well for this technique. The surgeon may also elect to use a no. 67 Beaver blade, which is available in most operating rooms (Figure 10-43).

A stent should be on hand for use in cornual anastomosis. A polyethylene stent is available, but a 0 or no. 1 nylon suture or polypropylene works quite well (Figure 10-44).

Uterine clamp

A uterine clamp should be available for tubal lavage even if a transcervical lavage apparatus is used. Sometimes the transcervical apparatus does not function properly and has to be removed during the case. The uterine clamp will provide a back-up lavage mechanism (Figure 10-45).

Cork bore

A 1-cm reamer is necessary for tubal implantation procedures. These are available commercially (Figure 10-46).

Ovarian vascular clamp

A modified pediatric vascular clamp designed by Cohen is especially useful in ovarian surgery. The instrument is gently closed just enough to control the arterial blood supply in the mesovarium. This technique allows the surgeon to perform almost bloodless surgery on the ovary with no damage to the blood supply by the atraumatic clamp (Figure 10-47).

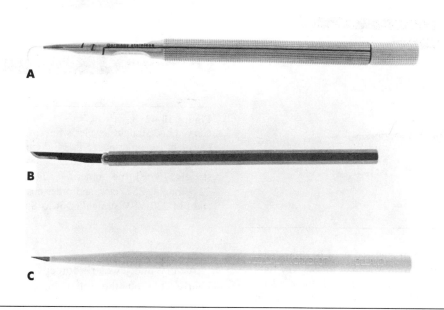

Figure 10-43
Three cornual scalpels. **A,** Gomel scalpel **B,** Beaver blade and **C,** a disposable ophthalmic scalpel. (Gomel handle available as order no. 10300, Elmed, Inc.; order no. BHS-12, ASSI; and order no. 10-094, Martin.) Right and left cornual blades should be ordered in addition to the handle. (Beaver handle available as order no. 3H-4″-OP7-2, Baxter V Mueller.) Two excellent disposable ophthalmic scalpels are the Super Blade 15 (shown, and available through Medical Workshop) and order no. 92-1501 through Sharpoint, Inc.

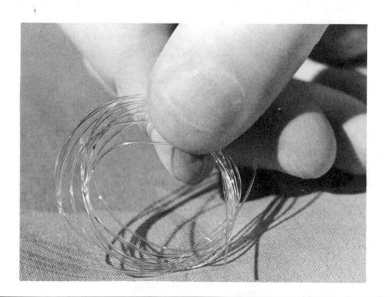

Figure 10-44
Polyethylene splint material (order no. SM-45, Accurate Surgical and Scientific Instruments Corp., Springer and Tritt; also available as order no. FM-220-95-W, Downs Surgical; order no. 32-999-00, Martin USA, Inc.; and order no. 32301-00, Elmed, Inc.).

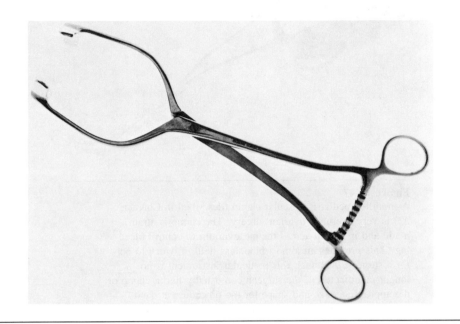

Figure 10-45
Uterine clamp. (order no. 91-4010, J. Sklar Manufacturing Co., Inc.; and order No. FM-220-12-P, Downs Surgical; several other vendors offer this instrument, including ZSI).

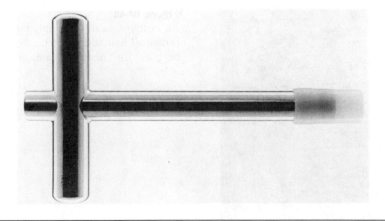

Figure 10-46
A 1-cm Cohen reamer for implantation procedures. This instrument must be protected at all times when not in use to maintain its sharpness. (Available as order no. 392-210, ZSI.)

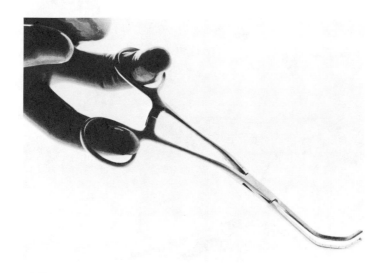

Figure 10-47
A modified pediatric vascular clamp (described in Chapter 22) is very useful in ovarian surgery. The clamp is atraumatic and is placed across the mesovarium to control bleeding. This provides an almost bloodless field in which to perform surgery. Although this particular instrument is no longer manufactured, the surgeon can usually find a clamp of the appropriate size and shape for the procedure at hand from the assortment available in most operating rooms.

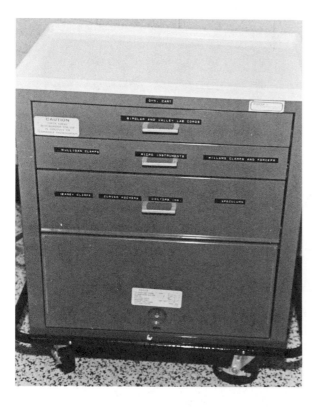

Figure 10-48
An instrument cart for storing infertility instruments. Make certain all four wheels rotate. Available through Sears Roebuck and Co., and most hardware stores.

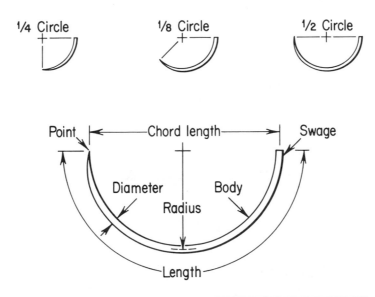

Figure 10-49
The anatomy of a needle. (Courtesy of ETHICON, Inc.)

Instrument cart

The operating room supervisor should make a cart available exclusively to store instruments used for infertility surgery (Figure 10-48). This saves enormously in time and frustration. All four wheels should rotate to ensure easy maneuverability.

Needles and sutures

The surgeon must be familiar with the terminology used to describe the different parts and dimensions of a needle (Figure 10-49). There are basically three microneedles available. The spatula needle is a cutting tool designed for ophthalmic surgery and is not used in gynecology. It produces too large a defect in tissue, which results in bleeding and tissue damage.

The tapered needle is useful in serosa such as the second layer of a double-layer anastomosis and in performing a salpingostomy. A new-generation tapered needle with a cutting tip is now available and is extraordinarily useful in performing an anastomosis (Figure 10-50).

The surgeon will need to decide what curve the needle should have. I prefer a 105-degree curve, since it allows precision placement of the needle during an anastomosis.

Microsuture materials are nonabsorbable (polypropylene and nylon), as well as absorbable (polyglycolic acid, polyglactin, and polydioxanone). These are all excellent materials, with no one offering a decided advantage. Favorable characteristics to be looked for are increased color contrast, stiffness of the suture, and suture "memory." Sutures with each of these characteristics will tie easily.

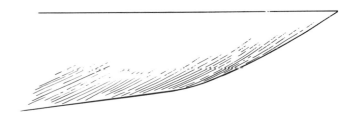

Figure 10-50
Drawing of a tapered needle with cutting tip. (Courtesy of Xomed, Inc.)

The size of the suture used is generally 8-0, although I prefer 9-0 on the inner layer of a tubal anastomosis. Permanent 6-0 sutures are excellent for stay sutures during an anastomosis, since they relieve tension on the anastomotic site.

SUMMARY

When purchasing instruments, the surgeon should consider the feel. Also, research has shown closing pressure should not exceed 50 gm for fine work,[1] since tremor develops when greater force is required to close the instruments.

Instruments usually are made of either stainless steel or titanium. Titanium is lighter, has a blue color that eliminates glare, and is very strong. It also resists rust and does not magnetize readily. The disadvantages of titanium instruments are that they are expensive and are not manufactured by most instrument companies. The

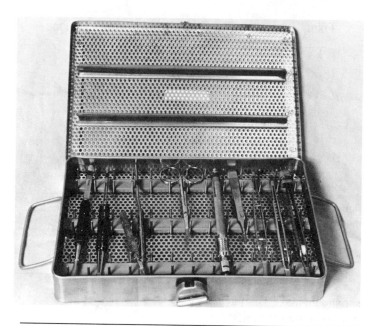

Figure 10-51
A sturdy microsurgical instrument box is a necessity. Note the transverse ridges to stabilize instruments. (Available as order no. 42-347, ZSI. Also available as order no. 55-107-26, Elmed, Inc.; order no. ICFM-2326, ASSI; and order no. 55-396-00, Martin.)

surgeon should try both types of instruments. The overriding consideration should not be the material but rather the ease with which one can work with the instruments.

Proper care will enable instruments of either titanium or stainless steel to have a long life.[1,2] When a new instrument arrives, it must be checked carefully under the microscope. If any flaw exists, it is returned to the manufacturer. Should a defect develop in a used instrument, it is returned to the manufacturer for repair.

Instruments must be handled with extreme care at all times. After each procedure they should be hand washed in distilled water, never saline, after box locks have been opened for more complete cleaning. It is advisable to use the detergent recommended by the instrument manufacturer. If the instruments are titanium or stainless steel, the ultrasonic cleaner is helpful, but the instruments must be kept separated from each other to avoid damage. After all detergent is removed, the instruments should be dried and have plastic or rubber tips applied for protection before they are stored in their case (Figure 10-51). These precautions will pay rich dividends in providing a long and useful life to the microsurgical instruments.

In addition to the materials discussed, there are many other superb instruments, sutures, and set-ups produced by companies throughout the world. The ideas and considerations presented here should give the microsurgeon some idea of features that will be helpful in making choices from the variety of tools available.

REFERENCES

1. Patkin M. Selection and care of microsurgical instruments, *Adv Ophthalmol* 37:23-33, 1978.
2. The care and handling of surgical instruments. Brochure. Randolph MA, Codman, and Shurtleff, 1981.

HYSTEROSALPINGOGRAPHY AND ENDOSCOPY

11

Hysterosalpingography

ALVIN M. SIEGLER

Hysterosalpingography (HSG) is one of the basic procedures to perform before undertaking surgical correction of pelvic causes of infertility. Although this examination does not define the extent of certain conditions, such as endometriosis and periadnexal adhesions, it does reveal the shape of the uterine cavity and characteristics of the tubal lumina, besides their patency. With the advent of modern diagnostic gynecologic techniques, including laparoscopy, endoscopy, ultrasonography, and magnetic resonance imaging, why continue to use the HSG? The HSG remains a nonsurgical, simple, relatively painless screening procedure. Three recent books devoted primarily to this subject have been published and represent comprehensive discussions.[1-3]

This chapter reviews the fundamentals for performing a proper HSG and describes abnormalities encountered. Careful interpretation is essential so that the findings can be compared with those of endoscopic studies. Indeed, when the hysterogram is normal, it is unusual to find any significant intrauterine lesions at hysteroscopy. With normal fill and spill from both fallopian tubes, it is uncommon to find significant tubal disease. Salpingography has limitations, however, principally its inability to detect periadnexal adhesions or significant endometriosis. Abnormal shadows must be interpreted in association with the history and physical examination.

INSTRUMENTS

Various cannulas have been used but the simplest and preferred is the Jarcho type with an adjustable steel collar and rubber acorn (Figure 11-1). The acorn is fixed securely by means of a set screw in the metal collar located about 0.5 cm from the perforated end of the cannula.

The test requires image intensification with spot films taken during television fluoroscopy for proper monitoring at propitious intervals. Indeed, four exposures can be recorded on one 10 × 12 film (Figure 11-2).

Media

All media used for HSGs contain iodine, some being soluble in water and others in oil. Both types have certain advantages and disadvantages, and it is important for the physician to be aware of these characteristics, since they influence the technique of the examination and the interpretation of the films. Water-soluble media pass through the uterus and tubes more quickly than oily media, and greater amounts of it are needed. Only with water-soluble media can the healthy rugal folds, evidenced by longitudinal dark lines, be detected (Figure 11-3). In distally obstructed tubes, a dark line often is visible clearly when the endosalpinx is not damaged severely. An oily medium will not mix with the fluid in a hydrosalpinx, so that pearly cluster formations form in it.

TECHNIQUE

Although the technique, media, and instruments for HSG have improved, too many studies still cannot be interpreted, principally because of failure to attend to the relatively simple details of proper performance.

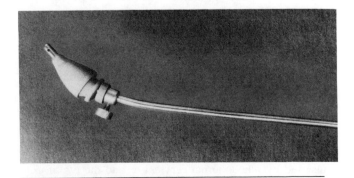

Figure 11-1
Properly positioned rubber acorn is noted on a Jarcho cannula.

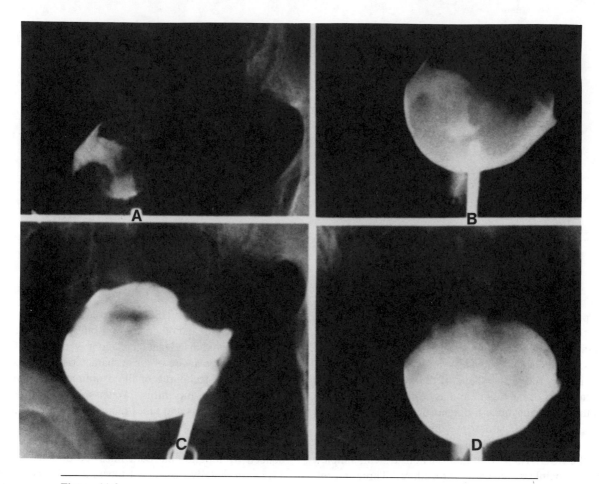

Figure 11-2
A-D, sequential radiographs show stages of filling of a uterine cavity that contains a submucous myoma. No tubal opacification is noted either because of tubal obstruction or the use of an insufficient quantity of contrast agent.

One can elicit the best pictures with fewest complications by gaining the confidence and cooperation of the patient and by attempting gentle pelvic manipulation of the instruments. A tranquilizer may be used for an apprehensive patient. Tubal occlusion caused by uterotubal spasm can result from stress or from irritation caused by the contrast material. Certain medications are reported to cause relaxation of the uterine musculature that envelops the interstitial tubal segment.

The time chosen for the HSG varies according to the patient's clinical condition, although most procedures are done in the first week after menses. The search for an incompetent isthmus probably should be done premenstrually, however, when physiologic contraction of the lower uterine segment is greatest. The cannula is filled with contrast material to flush out the air. After a tenaculum is fixed on the anterior cervical lip, the cannula is inserted into the external cervical os and the two instruments are held together. Some pressure should be maintained on the fluid-filled syringe, but the study should be terminated if the patient complains of increasing abdom-

inal pain during the injection. Excessive contrast material exposes the patient needlessly to risk of mucosal or peritoneal irritation and prevents proper interpretation of the films. Insufficient fluid results in an incomplete study.

A follow-up or drainage film is essential to observe the dispersion of the liquid medium. It should be taken about 30 minutes after removal of the instruments from the cervix if a water-soluble material is used. With oil-based substances, it is advisable to delay the drainage film until the next day because these media do not disperse as rapidly in the peritoneal cavity.

Drainage or follow-up film

Peritoneal spill from a normal HSG is identified easily. The dispersion of the agent in the pelvis depends on the type and amount of fluid used, the degree of tubal patency, and the presence or extent of significant periadnexal adhesions. Such adhesions can be discerned as a collection of medium in the lateral pelvis and should not be mistaken for centrally placed fluid retained within the uterine canal or vagina (Figures 11-4 and 11-5). Inter-

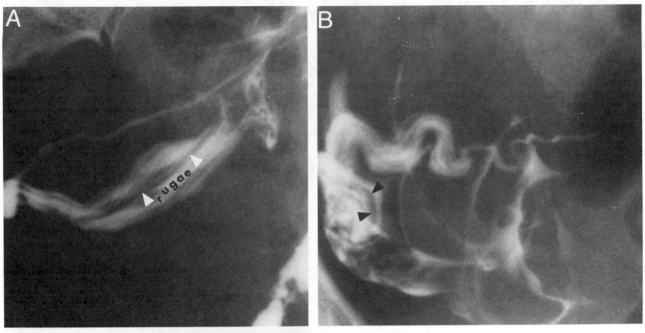

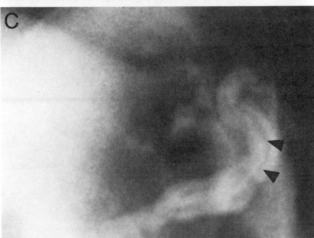

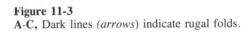

Figure 11-3
A-C, Dark lines *(arrows)* indicate rugal folds.

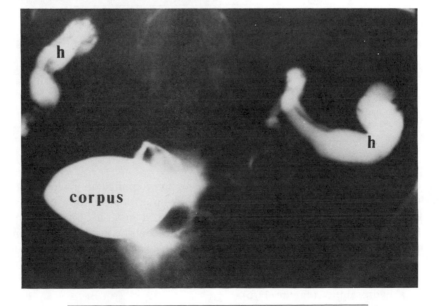

Figure 11-4
Bilateral hydrosalpinges (h) are present with moderate distal
dilation (degree III).

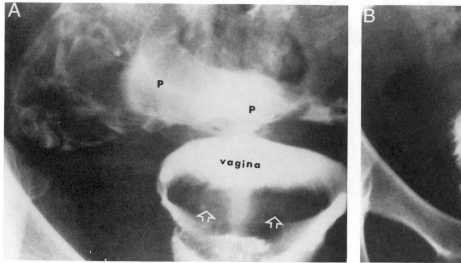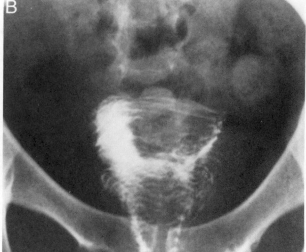

Figure 11-5
A, Triangular midline shadow is caused by contrast fluid in the vagina *(arrows)*. Contrast is also noted in the pelvis (p).
B, Note transverse lines, which indicate vaginal mucous membrane.

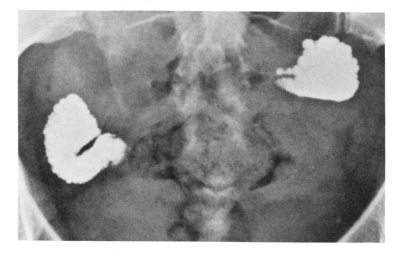

Figure 11-6
This 24-hour delayed study, using oil-soluble contrast medium, clearly outlines the distal tube obstructions in this patient with proved bilateral hydrosalpinges. Note the pearly drops of medium. From Bateman BG et al: Utility of the 24-hour delay hysterosalpingogram film, *Fertil Steril* 47:613, 1987.

preting small, localized pelvic collections of contrast material caused by significant peritubal adhesions, fimbrial phimosis, or even hydrosalpinges can be difficult. Contrast material coming from one patent tube may obscure the configuration of the contralateral oviduct. When an oily material is used, it may be difficult to be certain whether the pearly clusters are in the cul-de-sac fluid or if they are enclosed in a hydrosalpinx (Figure 11-6).

Some tubal configurations look normal initially, but the follow-up or drainage film may disclose localization of the contrast material. Sharply defined borders suggest that the contrast medium is confined within the tube, whereas a halo configuration indicates periadnexal adhesions that allows some of the fluid to surround and outline the tubal wall (Figure 11-7).

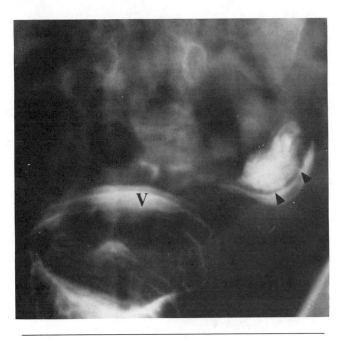

Figure 11-7
Halo *(arrowheads)* resulted from peritubal adhesions
and fimbrial phimosis. Contrast material is seen in the
vagina (v).

Some adverse effects from HSG have been caused by
faulty selection of patients and poor technique, but
morbidity and sequelae occasionally result despite
careful use.

INTERPRETATION OF RESULTS
The uterine cavity

Evaluation of the HSG always begins with viewing the
endocervical canal. Its serrated borders (Figure 11-8) are
caused by normal anatomic plicae palmatae. Abnormalities of the endocervical canal detectable by the HSG
include polyps and adhesions, which cause filling defects. The normal lower uterine segment has parallel
borders that are usually regular. This segment may be
unusually wide—greater than 1 cm in an incompetent
os. Diverticula may be congenital outpouchings or iatrogenic from a previous cesarean surgery (Figure 11-9).

The normal uterine cavity has a triangular appearance
with smooth borders. Physiologic alterations may cause
various indentations along the lateral borders of the uterine shadow, but their persistence on sequential films suggests an organic defect rather than a contraction. The
upper border, the fundus, may be convex or saddle
shaped, and the cornua are generally pointed.

Congenital malformations

Uterine anomalies have been classified into several
groups, each having particular characteristics and clinical
sequelae. They represent heterogeneous malformations

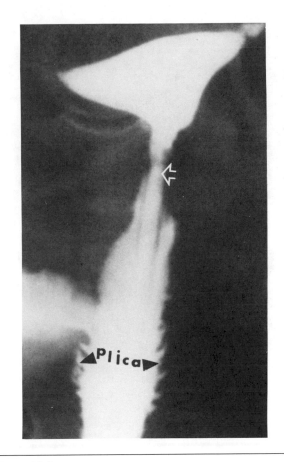

Figure 11-8
The cannula tip *(arrow)* almost reaches into the uterine cavity. Endocervical markings *(arrowheads)* are clearly seen.

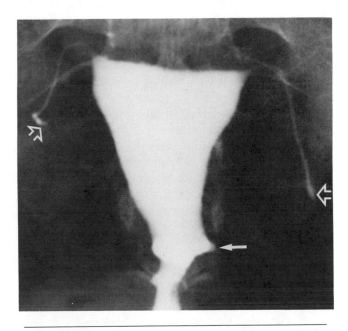

Figure 11-9
The small outpouching *(arrow)* in the lower uterine segment
represents a cesarean scar. The patient also has a tubal ligation *(open arrows)*.

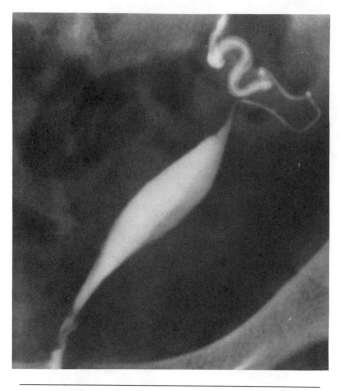

Figure 11-10
Typical HSG of an oval-shaped unicornuate uterus with a
normally opacified tube originating from the upper pole.

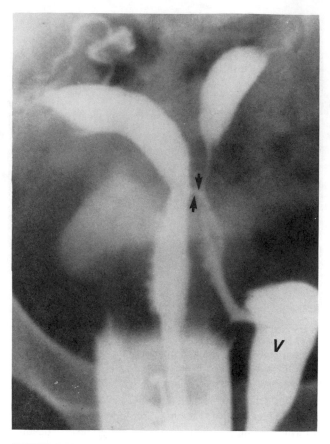

Figure 11-11
This HSG shows a double uterus (didelphys) connected the
lower uterine segment *(arrows)*. The left uterus empties into
a blind vaginal pouch (v).

that result from arrested development, abnormal formations, or incomplete fusion of the mullerian ducts. Some
malformations cause complications at menarche, during
pregnancy, or in labor. Although malformed uteri do not
prevent implantation or nidation, and most pregnancies
proceed to term without difficulty, anomalies do increase
the frequency of obstetric complications. A classification
proposed by the American Fertility Society seems flexible
enough to fit most possibilities. The HSG is a screening
procedure that gives the surgeon the initial clue to the
possibility of a uterine anomaly. Ultrasonography (US)
and magnetic resonance imaging (MRI) also have been
used to evaluate several types of uterine anomalies.

On the HSG a true unicornuate uterus usually is displaced laterally (Figure 11-10). Since 80% of these
women do not have a kidney on the contralateral side,
an intravenous pyelogram is essential in their evaluation.
The condition should be suspected whenever the uterus
is displaced, pointing either to the left or right, with a
poorly developed lateral fornix. This type of uterus must
be differentiated from an incompletely filled cavity, an
intense spasm of one horn, and blockage by severe synechiae that prevent access to the opposite horn. A lateral
film and uterine manipulation help to rule out the possibility of uterine spasm or an artifact caused by uterine

torsion. Hysteroscopy and laparoscopy can substantiate
the diagnosis and detect the presence of a rudimentary
horn.

The so-called double uterus can be bicornuate or didelphic, the latter having two cervices, with or without
a vaginal partition (Figure 11-11). The HSGs of the
didelphic uterus show two entirely separate uteri; the
horns appear flexed toward each other or in opposite
directions. Duplications of the uterus and vagina are
caused by complete failure of the mullerian ducts to fuse.
Independent study of each horn will show the characteristic shadow of the unicornuate uterus. In such cases
the Foley uterine catheter technique has an advantage,
since the vaginal canal sometimes cannot accommodate
two sets of instruments (i.e., cannulae and tenacula).

The bicornuate uterus cannot be differentiated from
the septate uterus by the HSG or hysteroscopy because
the crucial diagnostic point lies in the configuration of
the serosal surface (Figures 11-12 and 11-13). The division may be complete to the cervix or partial, and the

external surface reflects the character of this division. Imperfect absorption of the median partition results in paired uterine horns. The septate uterus is either completely or partially divided by a longitudinal central septum. The length and width of the septum cause different shadows on the HSG and, if complete, two separate, usually symmetric cavities are formed. A cannula inserted beyond the internal os can prevent adequate observation of one of the horns. Data suggest that women with a septate uterus are about twice as likely to abort as those with a bicornuate uterus. Both conditions must be differentiated from a fundal submucous myoma.

The arcuate uterus is a minor malformation in which the fundus appears concave, although the depth of the depression is less than 1.5 cm (Figure 11-14). The uterine cavity has smooth contours and symmetric horns. The hysterographic appearance can be verified hysteroscopically.

Another type of congenital uterine malformation has been described in some women who were exposed to diethylstilbestrol in utero. The uterus appears hypoplastic and T shaped, with indentations on its lateral borders (Figure 11-15). On hysteroscopic examination these radiologic changes can be explained by structural alterations within the myometrium that resemble submucous myomas. Bulbous cornual extensions often arise from the upper end of the uterine cavity.

Intrauterine adhesions

The HSG is the initial diagnostic test used to detect intrauterine synechiae. The defects can be single or multiple, variable in size and shape, central or marginal, and tend to persist on sequential films. Too much contrast material tends to obliterate these abnormal shadows. Intravasation associated with multiple filling defects and a distorted but not enlarged uterine shadow in a patient with a history of repeated early abortion and postabortal curettage followed by hypomenorrhea, is diagnostic of intrauterine adhesions. Amenorrhea is associated with a distorted uterine shadow revealing numerous intracavitary defects. Intrauterine adhesions cause filling defects that are usually sharply defined. Extensive or severe adhesions produce a distorted shadow associated with tubal occlusion or vascular intravasation (Figure 11-16). The defects must be differentiated from those caused by polyps, myomata, septa, and artifacts caused by air bubbles. With hysteroscopy the surgeon can ascertain the size and location of the adhesions and evaluate the surrounding endometrium. The HSG tends to overdiagnose rather than miss the presence of intrauterine adhesions.

Uterine tumors

When polyps are suspected, the medium should be instilled in fractional, small amounts so as not to overfill the cavity. Endometrial polyps may be large or small,

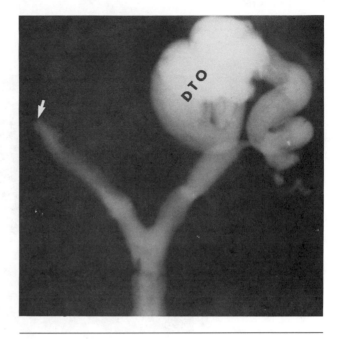

Figure 11-12
Bicornuate uterus with an associated left distal tubal obstruction (DTO) and right proximal tubal obstruction *(arrow).*

single or multiple, pedunculated or sessile. A single polyp does not distort the triangular shape of the cavity, but multiple polyps producing larger defects cause some loss of the normal uterine outline (Figure 11-17). Disclosure of a polyp radiographically indicates the need to confirm it and then a polypectomy under hysteroscopic control.

Submucosal and intramural myomata often enlarge and distort the shape of the uterine cavity and cause filling defects not easily obliterated by increments of the medium (Figure 11-18). A myoma may occlude the tubal ostia and cause abnormal uterine bleeding and spontaneous abortion. The HSG can detect these tumors and test tubal patency, but the x-ray picture cannot show the size of the growth or its precise location. Hysteroscopy is advisable so that the gross characteristics of the myoma can be ascertained and a decision can be made concerning its possible resection hysteroscopically.

Submucous tumors, endometrial tuberculosis, and intrauterine adhesions are among the predisposing causes of vascular intravasation. It may also be iatrogenic (Figure 11-19). The patient's menstrual history and previous fertility furnish clues and aid in the differential diagnosis.

The fallopian tubes

In the search for tubal patency, the end point of the HSG is either tubal fill and spill or increasing abdominal pain.

Text cont'd on p. 184.

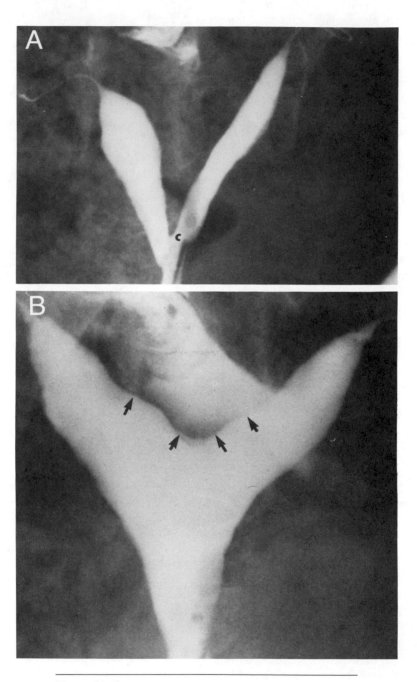

Figure 11-13
Sequential films. **A,** These unequal-sized horns of a septate
uterus create an almost 45-degree angle with each other, and
they have a common cervix. The cannula tip (c) is easily
seen. **B,** After hysteroscopic metroplasty was performed, the
fundal defect *(arrows)* is significantly smaller.

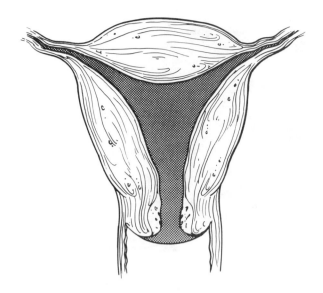

Figure 11-14
This saddle-shaped, smooth fundus *(arrows)* with widely separated horns is an arcuate uterus.

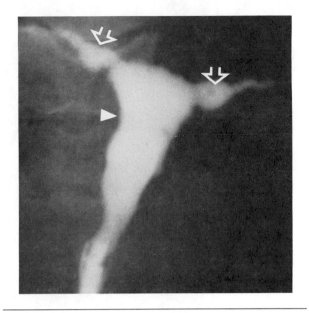

Figure 11-15
Bulbous horns *(open arrows)* in this uterine cavity and the irregularities along the lateral borders *(arrowhead)* are typical of diethylstilbestrol exposure.

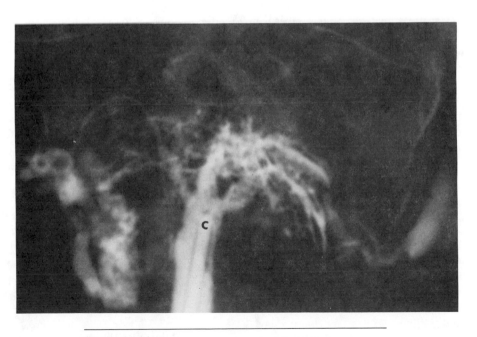

Figure 11-16
Severe intrauterine adhesions. Note the cannula tip (c) and bizarre uterine shadows with evidence of intravascular intravasation.

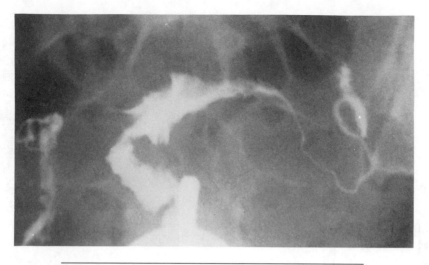

Figure 11-17
This irregularly shaped uterine cavity contained numerous endometrial polyps.

If the tubes are not opacified on the HSG, it is important to know if the cervix was occluded adequately, the amount of contrast agent used, and the reason for discontinuation of the procedure before tubal filling. To differentiate spasm from organic disease, the intramural segment should appear filled, that is, pointed rather than rounded, since it is uncommon to see proximal tubal obstruction caused by organic disease in the intramural segment. It may be difficult to differentiate isthmic from intramural obstruction on HSG, since the myometrial width cannot be discerned radiographically. It may be helpful to remember the so-called thumb sign; if the thumb is placed at the cornu, its width will approximate that of the myometrium, the tubal shadow underneath the thumb representing the intramural segment (Figure 11-20).

Proximal tubal obstruction

Luminal fibrosis and salpingitis isthmica nodosa are the most common causes of proximal tubal obstruction. A prior tubal ligation, chronic salpingitis, tubal tuberculosis, or intraluminal debris also can result in that condition. The differential diagnosis can be made by observing the intramural and isthmic segments carefully to search for diverticula, filling defects, and luminal continuity. Salpingitis isthmica nodosa has a characteristic honeycombed appearance (Figure 11-21). Tuberculous salpingitis also affects the distal part of the tube, causing it to have a rigid pipe-stem appearance with terminal strictures (Figure 11-22).

Ostial salpingography is a technique used in patients who have proximal tubal obstruction diagnosed from a properly performed and adequately interpreted HSG and a confirmatory laparoscopy during which several attempts to overcome the obstruction by chromopertubation are made. This interventional radiographic procedure is advisable before an attempt at tubocornual anastomosis. Under fluoroscopic control a 5.5 French catheter is wedged into the cornu with a J guidewire. After withdrawing the guidewire, 2 to 5 ml of a water-soluble contrast material is inserted through the catheter and into the uterotubal ostium. Indications for stopping the procedure are increasing abdominal pain, intravasation, and tubal fill and spill. If the obstruction persists, an attempt is made at recanalization with a guidewire passed through a 3 French nylon catheter. Once the wire is thought to pass into the isthmic segment, the catheter is advanced over it and the wire removed. About 2 to 3 ml of contrast medium is injected to test for tubal patency (see Chapter 12).

Tubal polyps create oval shadows in the intramural segment as the contrast fluid flows in a thin line above or below them (Figure 11-23). The remainder of the tube is normally patent in most women, and it is doubtful that these tumors cause infertility. Sometimes they are seen at hysteroscopy; some are excised at laparotomy through a small tubal incision. In most instances the diagnosis is made on the HSG in the course of an infertility study.

Distal tubal obstruction

Ampullary opacification indicates that the proximal tube is patent although not necessarily normal. Although distally obstructed, tubes sometimes have small, club-shaped ends, or they can reach as much as 4 to 5 cm in diameter, accommodating large amounts of fluid (Figure 11-24). Linear dark shadows seen within the lumen obtained with water-soluble medium are formed by the rugae, and their presence portends a better prognosis after

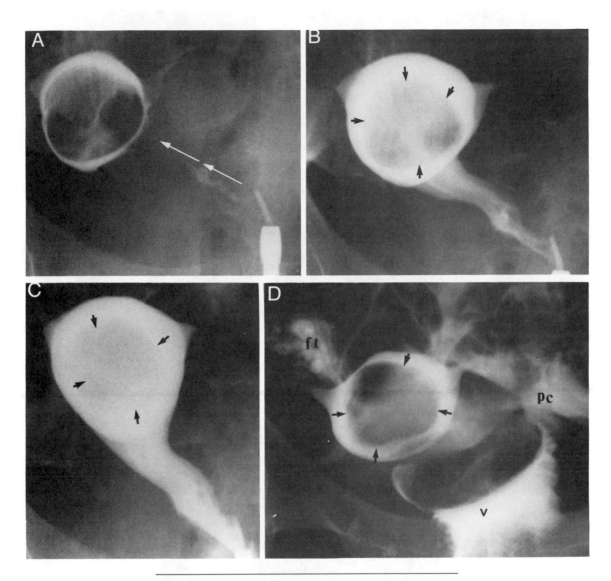

Figure 11-18

Sequential films of a submucous myoma. **A,** Only 1 ml of contrast outlines the tumor *(arrows).* **B,** Additional medium opacifies the lower uterine segment and one fallopian tube. Note the filling defect persists. **C,** As more contrast is added, the enlarged uterine cavity remains outlined, but the definition of the myoma *(arrows)* is diminished. **D,** On the postdrainage film the filling defect *(arrows)* is again readily apparent. Contrast is also present in the vagina (v), the peritoneal cavity (pc), and one fallopian tube (ft).

neosalpingostomy than if they are not evident. Distal tubal obstructions have been classified into four groups based on the HSG findings, varying from degree I, fimbrial phimosis, to degree IV, occlusion with ampullary diameter greater than 25 mm (Figures 11-25 and 11-26).

One of the prognostic factors after neosalpingostomy besides thickness of the tubal wall, the percentage of ciliated cells, and the morphologic condition of the tube is the degree of ampullary dilatation ascertained with HSG.

Text cont'd on p. 188.

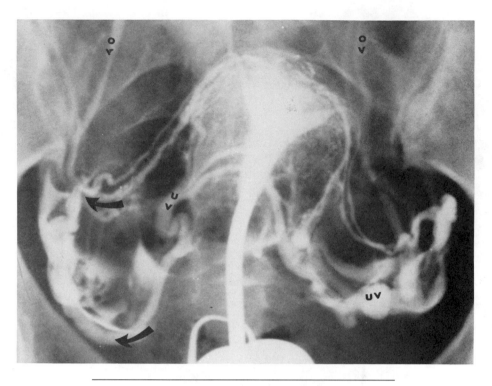

Figure 11-19
Although the tip of the cannula cannot be seen clearly, it
seems to have penetrated the left lateral uterine wall, resulting in this characteristic picture of both ovarian (ov) and
uterine (uv) vessels. Arrows show direction of contrast
agent. (Courtesy Dan C. Martin, M.D., Memphis, TN.)

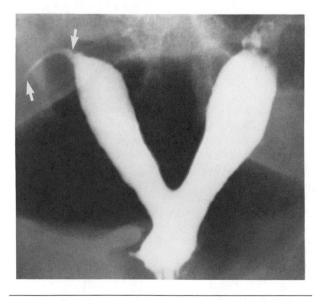

Figure 11-20
Tubal segment between the arrows represents the intramural
section. It is actually the width of the myometrium.

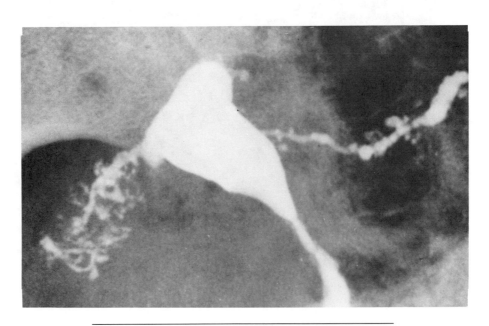

Figure 11-21
Tubal diverticulosis of this type could result from salpingitis isthmica nodosa, tubal tuberculosis, or endometriosis.

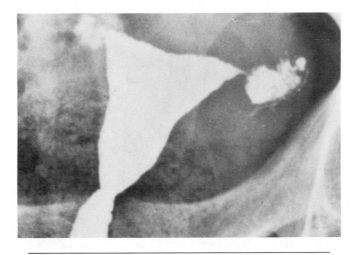

Figure 11-22
Bilateral proximal occlusions in a patient with documented tubal tuberculosis. From Bateman BG et al: Genital tuberculosis in reproductive-age women, *J Reprod Med* 31:287, 1986.

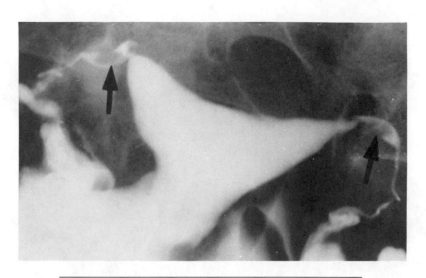

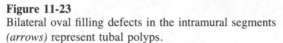

Figure 11-23
Bilateral oval filling defects in the intramural segments *(arrows)* represent tubal polyps.

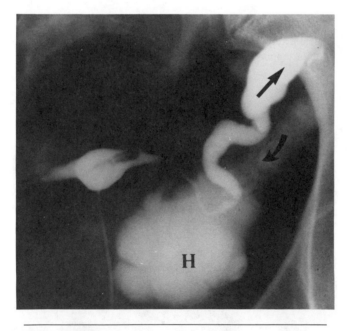

Figure 11-24
Right isthmic tubal obstruction and huge hydrosalpinx (H) are apparent. Arrows indicate the direction of flow.

SUMMARY

Despite the continued use of hysterosalpingography, there remains a need for its review with amplification and clarification of abnormal findings. Many HSGs are technically unsatisfactory or poorly interpreted. Therefore offering suggestions to improve skills in performance and interpretation seems justified.

REFERENCES

1. Hunt RB and Siegler AM: *Hysterosalpingography: techniques and interpretation*, Chicago, 1990, Mosby–Year Book.
2. Winfield AC and Wentz AC, eds: *Diagnostic imaging of infertility*, Baltimore, 1987, Williams & Wilkins.
3. Yoder IC: *Hysterosalpingography and pelvic ultrasound in infertility and gynecology*, Boston, 1988, Little, Brown & Co.

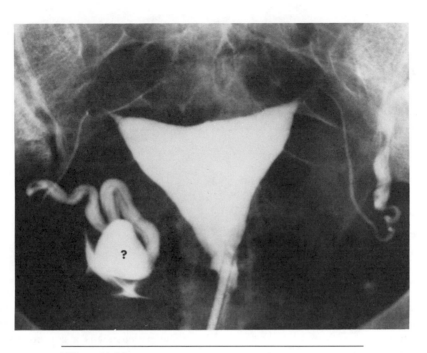

Figure 11-25
Excellent mucosal folds with minimal tubal dilation and possible spill into the peritoneal cavity. In the absence of a drainage film, patency cannot be determined (degree I).

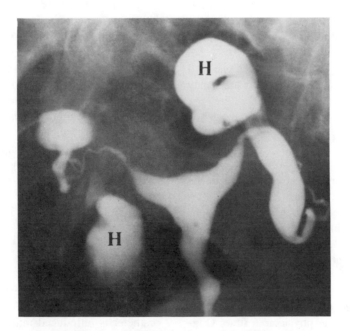

Figure 11-26
Severe (degree IV) bilateral distal tubal obstruction with hydrosalpinges (H) is present.

12

Fluoroscopic Fallopian Tube Catheterization

AMY S. THURMOND

Fallopian tube catheterization is an extension of hysterosalpingography and angiographic techniques. It is a nonsurgical treatment for infertility caused by proximal tubal obstruction.

The causes of apparent proximal tubal obstruction include cornual spasm, fibrosis, and intratubal debris.[1] Before introduction of fluoroscopically guided fallopian tube catheterizations, treatment was often laparotomy with segmental tubal resection and microsurgical reanastomosis, or in vitro fertilization to bypass the obstructed tubes altogether. The introduction of this technique has resulted in more efficient and less invasive care for many patients with proximal tubal obstruction.[2]

The technique illustrated in this chapter is the one used by our department. Alternatively, the fallopian tubes may be catheterized hysteroscopically.

PREFERRED APPROACH
Timing

Fallopian tube catheterization is best performed in the follicular phase of the cycle, at least 2 to 3 days after the cessation of menstrual bleeding but before ovulation. This is to avoid flushing blood clots into the tubes or peritoneal cavity, since the endometrium is less engorged at this time, and to ensure that the patient is not pregnant.

Patient preparation

The procedure is scheduled on an outpatient basis, allowing 30 to 45 minutes of the physician's time. Optimally, patients receive 5 days of doxycycline antibiotic, 100 mg orally twice a day starting 2 days before the procedure. Patients who are studied without advance notice receive 200 mg of doxycycline orally just before the procedure and continue taking 100 mg orally twice a day for 5 days. Patients are advised to have someone transport them to and from the appointment so that sedatives can be given. They generally go home without having to recover in the radiology department.

The patient signs a consent form, which includes a description of the complication of uterine or tubal perforation. She is also advised that an ectopic pregnancy may result from opening the tube, a condition that can be life-threatening and may require surgical treatment.

An intravenous line is started, and 1 mg midazolam is given before the procedure. This small dose is usually adequate sedation, since the procedure is often more stressful than painful. If necessary, midazolam can be given approximately every 15 minutes in 1-mg doses, and fentanyl in 25-μg doses may be added.

The patient is positioned on the fluoroscopic table with her knees flexed over triangular cushions and her heels together in the lithotomy position. The hips are elevated approximately 5 inches from the table using folded towels placed under the buttocks. The legs and perineum are draped to maintain sterility. The cervix is exposed using a bivalved speculum, and the cervix and vagina are copiously swabbed with an antiseptic. Vital signs are recorded. The cervix is then dried with a sterile gauze.

Equipment

The equipment described is available from Cook Ob/ Gyn (see Appendix B.) The diameter of Hysterocath is chosen to match the cervical size. The Tuohy-Borst adaptor is placed on the 9 French sheath, the 5.5 French catheter is introduced into the 9 French sheath, and together they are introduced into the Hysterocath so that their tips just barely extend out the acorn tip of the Hysterocath. The adaptor is tightened to stabilize the catheters within the Hysterocath. The catheter is filled with half-strength water-soluble contrast medium. Half-strength contrast agent is chosen, since it does not impede

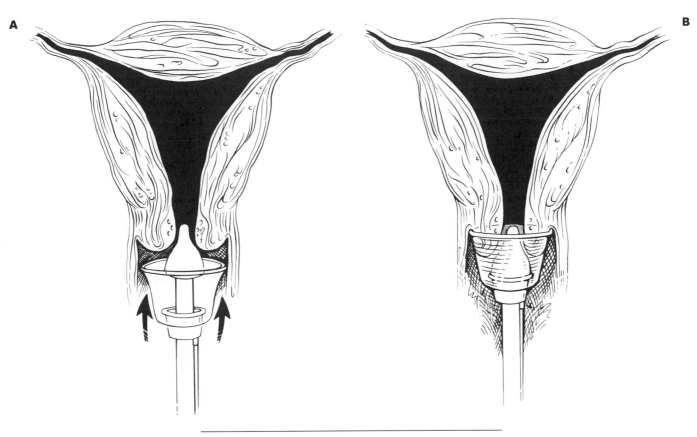

Figure 12-1
A, The acorn tip of the hysterocath is extended to engage the cervical os. **B,** The cup is advanced over the external cervix.

subsequent visualization of the catheters; full-strength contrast material is used when injecting directly into the fallopian tube for better visualization. Extension tubing is attached to the vacuum line of the Hysterocath, and the entire assembly is transferred from the sterile preparation table to the fluoroscopy table for placement in the patient.

Placing the Hysterocath

The Hysterocath allows traction to be placed on the uterus by the vacuum cup and provides a sterile conduit through which catheters can be advanced.[3] To obtain the best fit on the cervix, the central shaft containing the acorn tip is advanced all the way out. By maneuvering the speculum so that one has a bull's-eye view of the external cervical os, the acorn tip is placed in the external os (Figure 12-1 *A* through *C*). Next, the cup is slid over the cervix, and a vacuum equivalent to 10 in. Hg is applied (vacuum pump available from Mityvac, Neward Enterprises, or Cook Ob/Gyn: See Appendix B). If the acorn tip is well seated in the cervical os, the tissue of the cervix can be visualized through the translucent cup as it is pulled symmetrically around the acorn and into the cup by the vacuum. At this time the speculum and

folded towels can be removed, providing more comfort for the patient and resulting in better-quality radiographs.

Initial hysterosalpingogram

To avoid unnecessary irradiation, the x-ray tube is correctly positioned over the pelvis. Using fluoroscopic guidance, contrast agent is injected. If there is significant resistance to injection and no contrast agent exits the Hysterocath, the acorn tip probably is not in the cervical os and should be repositioned or replaced. If the injected contrast medium seems to go in the uterus but is pulled back into the cup or out into the vagina, the acorn tip must be advanced farther into the cervical canal to improve the cervical seal.

Films are taken to document tubal obstruction. Occasionally, one or both tubes that were thought to be blocked will be open on the initial hysterosalpingogram. Such blockage probably was due to technical factors or cornual spasm. Also, a true blockage may have resolved spontaneously.

Selective salpingography

If a tubal obstruction is encountered, the next step is to advance the 5.5 French catheter into the tubal ostium

C

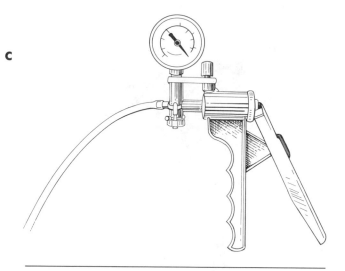

Figure 12-1, cont'd
C, The vacuum line from the cup is attached to the vacuum pump, and a vacuum equivalent to 10 in. Hg is applied.

(Figure 12-1 *D* through *F*). This is accomplished using the 0.035-inch J guidewire initially to maneuver the catheter into the cornual portion of the uterus. Once this is accomplished, the 0.035-inch straight LT guidewire is used to lodge the catheter directly in the tubal ostium. The 9 French catheter is advanced over the 5.5 French catheter into the miduterus. This stabilizes the system. Proper placement of the 5.5 French catheter tip into the tubal ostium is crucial, since embedding the catheter in the myometrium results in painful intravasation and obscures anatomy. Successful placement in the tubal ostium makes the remainder of the procedure straightforward. Most patients have some cramping and sharp pain when the uterus is stretched with contrast medium or when the catheters are manipulated. Probing in the fallopian tube itself is rarely uncomfortable.

With the 5.5 French catheter successfully wedged in the ostium of the fallopian tube, full-strength contrast medium is injected (Figure 12-1 *G*). Approximately 20% of the time this direct injection will open the tube. If it does not, it will often indicate the direction of the proximal portion of the tube and the exact site of the obstruction, which is usually 1 to 3 cm from the tubal ostium.

Fallopian tube recanalization

Initially the 3 French Teflon catheter and 0.015-inch platinum-tipped guidewire are advanced together through the 5.5 French catheter and into the fallopian tube with the guidewire extended approximately 5 mm beyond the catheter tip (Figure 12-1 *H*). When resistance is encountered at the site of obstruction, short probing motions

with the guidewire are used to try to overcome the obstruction. If this is unsuccessful, if the obstruction is located more distally, or if there is a bend in the fallopian tube that must be traversed, the small catheter and wire are exchanged for a softer, tapered system consisting of a Tracker 18 catheter and Taper guidewire available from Target Therapeutics.[4] With either system, once recanalization is accomplished with the guidewire, the catheter is advanced over the guidewire to dilate the tube, the guidewire is removed, and full-strength contrast medium is injected into the tube (Figure 12-1 *I*). Films are taken to document the anatomy of the distal tube. The small catheter is withdrawn, and contrast medium is injected directly into the fallopian tube through the 5.5 French catheter to demonstrate the proximal portion in the region of the recanalization.

If the contralateral tube is also blocked, the 5.5 French catheter is pulled back into the uterine cavity, the J guidewire reinserted, and the process repeated (Figures 12-1 *J* and 12-2).

Postprocedure hysterosalpingogram

After recanalization of one or both fallopian tubes, the 5.5 French catheter is withdrawn into the uterine cavity and contrast material injected to confirm tubal patency. In cases of bilateral recanalization, sometimes the first side that has recanalized does not fill on the postprocedure hysterosalpingogram, probably because of less resistance and easier flow through the more recently dilated tube. The patient is advised to have a hysterosalpingogram at 3 to 6 months if she has not conceived.

FOLLOW-UP

The patient is told that she may have vaginal spotting for up to 3 days. Many patients return to work the same day, although most prefer to wait for 1 day. We see no reason why intercourse should be postponed, and in fact, many patients have conceived within a week of the procedure and have delivered healthy infants.

The patient is instructed to contact her physician as soon as she misses a period. We advise close monitoring with quantitative measurement of human chorionic gonadotropin levels and pelvic ultrasound to confirm the presence of an intrauterine pregnancy.

CONTRAINDICATIONS

Fallopian tube catheterization should not be performed in a patient with active pelvic infection. In a woman with allergy to iodinated contrast agents, the same considerations and precautions are taken as with any other radiologic procedure using iodine. The procedure is difficult in patients with uterine fibroids, polyps, or scarring, and in those who have had tubal obstruction after tubal anastomosis.

(Text cont'd on p. 198.)

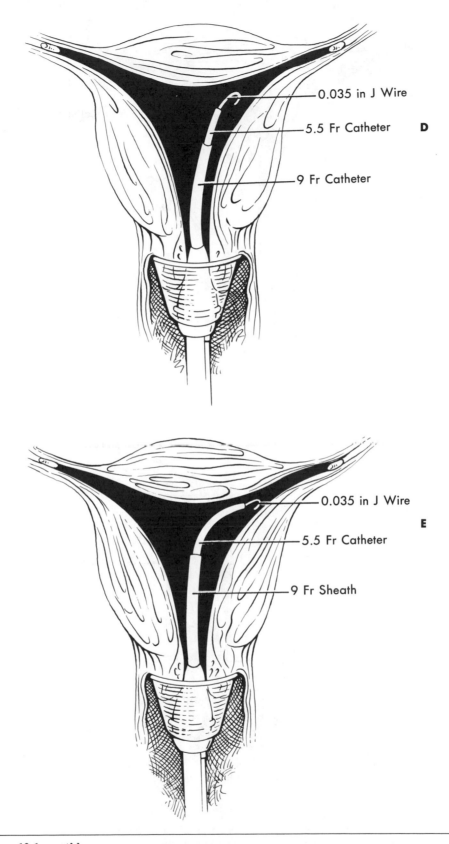

Figure 12-1, cont'd
D, With the help of the larger catheter, the 0.035-inch J guidewire is advanced and directed toward the uterine cornu. The sheath can be advanced to the miduterus to help stabilize the system. **E,** The 5.5 French catheter and J guidewire are advanced to the tubal ostium.

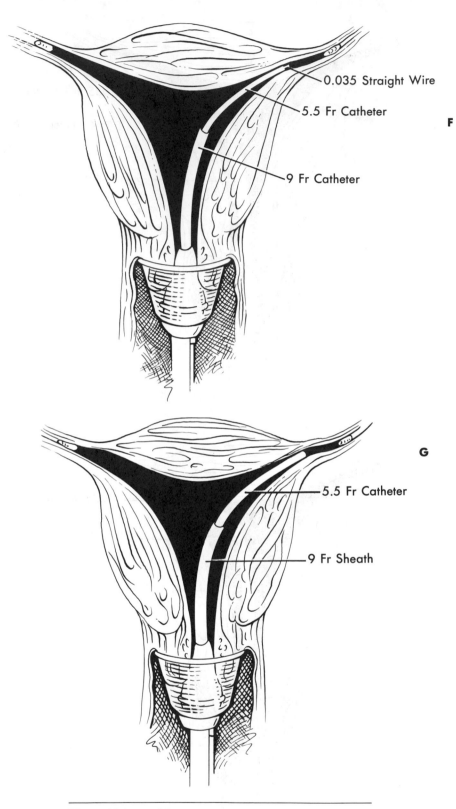

Figure 12-1, cont'd
F, The J guidewire is exchanged for a straight guidewire, which is used to wedge the 5.5 French catheter firmly into the tubal ostium. **G,** The straight wire is then removed and contrast agent is injected.

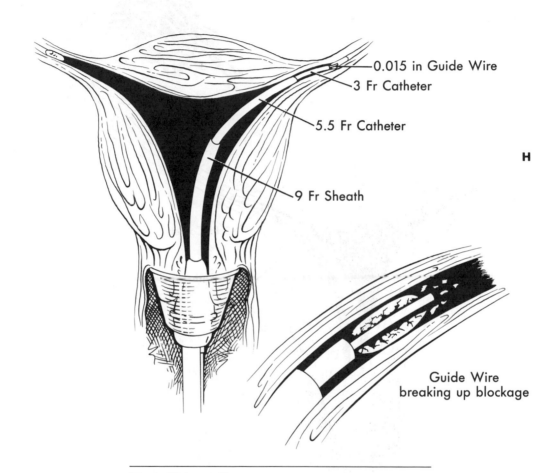

0.015 in Guide Wire

3 Fr Catheter

5.5 Fr Catheter

9 Fr Sheath

H

Guide Wire
breaking up blockage

Figure 12-1, cont'd
H, If the tube fails to open with selective injection directly
into the tubal ostium, a 0.015-inch guidewire and 3 French
catheter are advanced together to the level of the obstruction,
and attempts are made to open the tube with gentle probing
movements of the guidewire *(inset).*

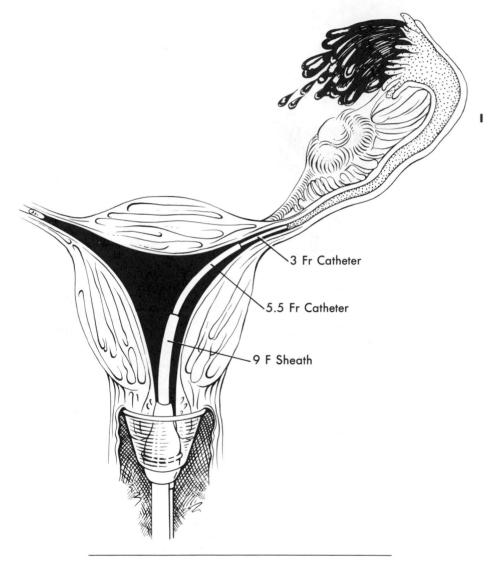

I

3 Fr Catheter

5.5 Fr Catheter

9 F Sheath

Figure 12-1, cont'd
I, The small guidewire is removed, and contrast agent is injected through the 3 French catheter directly into the tube to confirm successful recanalization and to document distal tubal anatomy.

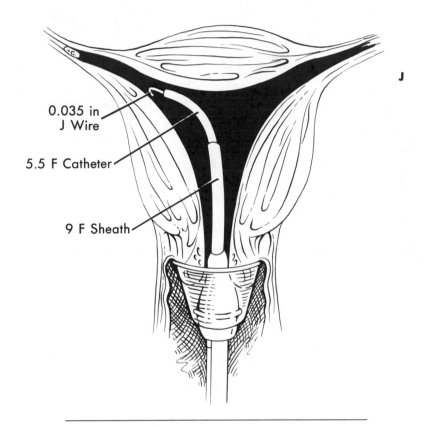

0.035 in
J Wire

5.5 F Catheter

9 F Sheath

J

Figure 12-1, cont'd
J, The procedure can be repeated on the contralateral side by removing the 3 French catheter, retracting the 5.5 French catheter into the uterine fundus, replacing the 0.035-inch J guidewire, and flipping the 5.5 French catheter to the other cornu.

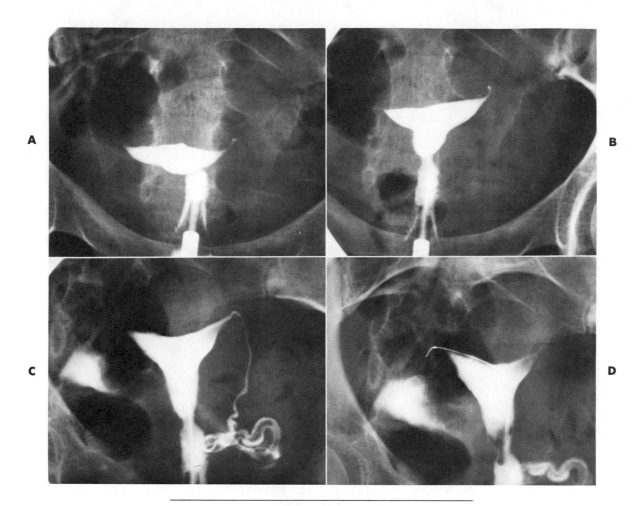

Figure 12-2
Successful bilateral fallopian tube recanalization and selective salpingography in a 26-year-old woman with 5 years of infertility and bilateral proximal tubal obstruction confirmed by two hysterosalpingograms and by laparoscopy. She conceived shortly after this procedure. **A,** Initial HSG confirmed bilateral obstruction. The uterus is flexed. **B,** The vacuum cup allows the uterus to be straightened, which makes catheterization easier. **C,** The 5.5 French catheter was placed in the left tubal ostium using the appropriate guidewires, and selective injection showed the tube to be open. **D,** On the right side, selective injection failed to open the tube, so the 0.015-inch guidewire and a 3 French catheter were advanced to the level of the obstruction, with the tip of the guidewire extended 5 mm beyond the tip of the catheter. The catheter tip is marked with a radiopaque bead.

COMPLICATIONS

The tubal perforation rate is 5%, and has occurred in patients with severe tubal disease such as salpingitis isthmica nodosa, and in women with previous tubal surgery, particularly tubal anastomosis. Thus far no tubal pregnancies have occurred in patients with successful proximal tubal recanalization and no distal tubal disease.[5] In patients who have successful proximal tubal recanalization and a history of distal tubal disease or previous tubal surgery, ectopic pregnancy rate is less than 10%.[2] We have not experienced any other major complication.

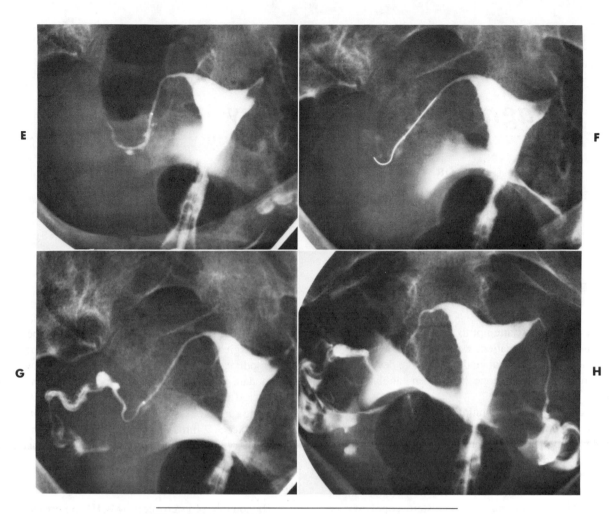

Figure 12-2, cont'd
E, After removal of the guidewire, injection of contrast
agent revealed a second obstruction at the isthmic-ampullary
junction. **F,** The 0.015-inch guidewire was advanced to the
level of the second obstruction, and gentle probing motions
were used until the obstruction was overcome. **G,** Selective
intratubal injection revealed tubal patency. **H,** A postprocedure hysterosalpingogram confirmed bilateral tubal patency.

RESULTS

Using this technique, approximately 90% of fallopian
tubes can be recanalized. The ability of the patient to
conceive depends in part on her age, the condition of the
distal tube, and other fertility factors. In patients with
isolated proximal tubal obstruction and no distal tubal
disease, the pregnancy rate is greater than 50% by 1
year.[2] In those with concurrent distal tubal disease the
rate is slightly lower.

REFERENCES

1. Sulak PJ et al: Histology of proximal tubal occlusion, *Fertil Steril*
   48:437-440, 1987.
2. Thurmond AS: Fallopian tube catheterization: current applications,
   AJR, 1990.
3. Thurmond AS and Rosch J: Device for hysterosalpingography and
   fallopian tube catherization, *Radiology* 174:571-572, 1990.
4. Thurmond AS and Rosch J: Fallopian tubes: improved technique
   for catheterization, *Radiology* 174:572-573, 1990.
5. Thurmond AS and Rosch J: Nonsurgical fallopian tube recanalization for treatment of infertility, *Radiology* 174:371-374, 1990.

13

Diagnostic Hysteroscopy

PATRICK J. TAYLOR

HOWARD A. PATTINSON

JEREMY V. KREDENTSER

The first attempt to visualize the interior of the uterus of a living patient was made by Pantaleoni in 1869. The major historical landmarks in the development of the modern hysteroscope have been tabulated[1] and extensively reviewed.[2]

Two complementary techniques, panoramic and contact, have evolved. Panoramic hysteroscopy is performed after the uterine cavity has been distended with a liquid or gaseous medium. Contact hysteroscopy is achieved without uterine distention; instead, the objective lens of the telescope is held in contact with the structure under scrutiny. The Hamou microcolpohysteroscope may be used with either procedure. It has magnification capabilities of $1\times$, $20\times$, $60\times$, and $150\times$.

INSTRUMENTS

The Hysteroser, a contact hysteroscope that depends on the collection of ambient room light for illumination, has not been used extensively in our unit. Since our experience with this instrument is limited, it is not discussed. The interested reader is referred elsewhere.[3,4]

Panoramic hysteroscope

The conventional panoramic hysteroscope (Figure 13-1) is a modified cystoscope. The viewing system consists of a telescope that is equipped with a stainless steel sheath. Sheaths are available through which are passed both the distention medium and rigid, semirigid, or flexible ancillary instruments. Telescopes range from 4 to 6 mm in diameter and may have a foroblique or 180-degree lens system.

For diagnostic hysteroscopy a calibrated probe is required, since it may be difficult to assess the size of intrauterine lesions. In addition, fine suction-irrigation cannulas, soft tubal probes, biopsy forceps, scissors, and well-insulated electrocautery capability should be available if surgical hysteroscopy is to be undertaken.

A modification of the urologic resectoscope will accommodate a standard hysteroscope.[5] The cutting loop is powered by a transistorized unit and set at 60 to 80 W cutting current. Tissue destruction with this instrument will not exceed 2 mm. The range of telescopes, sheaths, and ancillary instruments has been reviewed extensively.[6]

Hamou microhysteroscope

The Hamou microhysteroscope (MCH) comprises a composite telescope 4 mm in diameter (Figure 13-2) and a sheath 5.2 mm in diameter. Miniature operating instruments are available. The special feature is a system of lenses that, controlled by a switch in the handle, permits magnification of 1, 20, 60, and $150\times$. The direct lens allows observation at $1\times$ if used in a panoramic role and $60\times$ if used in contact. The offset lens allows 20 or $150\times$ views when similarly used. The higher magnifications are of particular value when the instrument is employed as a colposcope and microcolposcope in cases of cervical intraepithelial neoplasia.

A cheaper and less complicated model (Hamou II) has dispensed with the turret lens, and hence the high-magnification system necessary to perform in situ colpomicroscopy. For the physician who wishes simply to perform diagnostic procedures it is an ideal piece of office equipment.

LIGHT SOURCES

For routine use with both the conventional panoramic instruments and the Hamou MCH, a standard 150-W bulb will provide more than adequate illumination. The light is transmitted by a fiberoptic cable, and the light systems

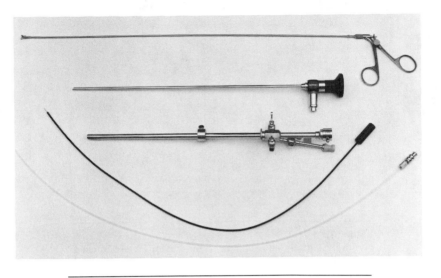

Figure 13-1
Panoramic hysteroscope, sheath, and flexible ancillary instruments. Courtesy R. Laborie. From Hamou J, Taylor PJ: *Panoramic, contact, and microcolpohysteroscopy in gynecologic practice*. In Leventhal JM (ed): *Current problems in obstetrics and gynecology*, vol. 6(2), Chicago, 1982, Year Book Medical Publishers.

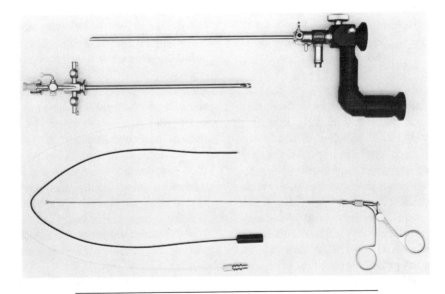

Figure 13-2
The Hamou MCH, sheath, and flexibile ancillary instrument. From Hamou J and Taylor PJ: *Panoramic, contact, and microcolpohysteroscopy in gynecologic practice*. In Leventhal JM (ed): *Current problems in obstetrics and gynecology*, vol 6(2). Chicago, 1982, Year Book Medical Publishers.

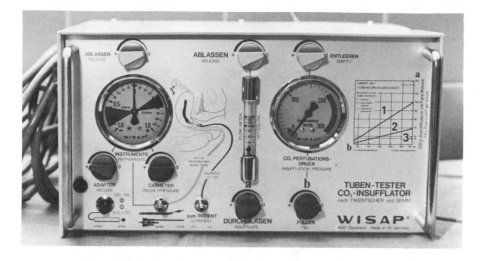

Figure 13-3
Semm hysteroscopic insufflator. From Taylor PJ and Hamou
J: *Hysteroscopy, J Reprod Med* 28:359-387, 1983.

in current use for laparoscopy are ideal. If photography, cinematography, or videotaping is to be undertaken, a xenon light source is necessary.

DISTENTION MEDIA

Whereas carbon dioxide (CO_2) may be used to distend the uterine cavity for both conventional and Hamou MCH hysteroscopy, high-molecular-weight dextran and dextrose can be used only with panoramic instruments.

Carbon dioxide

Special equipment is required if CO_2 is to be used; that is, only instruments specifically designed for hysteroscopy. The Hystero-flator 1000S and Semm insufflator (Figure 13-3) are both excellent machines. When CO_2 is used with conventional panoramic instruments, the cervix must be rendered gas-tight by means of cervical suction cup through which the telescope and sheath are passed. Both of these insufflators have built-in vacuum apparatus for securing this cup. No suction cup is required when the Hamou MCH is used. A flow rate of 40 to 60 ml per minute has proved to be safe if pressures do not exceed 100 mm Hg.[6]

  Carbon dioxide is safe to use. Fifteen hundred cases of panoramic CO_2 hysteroscopy were recorded without complications.[7] The effects on arterial partial pressure of CO_2 (pCO_2) were compared using both a constant pressure/variable gas volume source that required nitrous oxide and a constant volume/variable pressure source that delivered CO_2.[8] Results showed that the pCO_2 did rise in the former group, and one case of cardiovascular collapse occurred. Therefore it would appear that con-

stant volume/variable pressure devices are safer. Furthermore, this study stressed that insufflators designed for laparoscopy must never be used to perform hysteroscopy, since death was reported when 40 to 50 L CO_2 were insufflated.[9]

High-molecular-weight dextran

Initial attempts to use a mixture of polymers of different chain lengths and molecular weights such as polyvinyl-pyrolidine (Luviskol K94%) were unsuccessful, since it is yellow, which obscures the view, and is not biodegradable.[10] Hyskon is a dextran with an average molecular weight of 70,000 made up to a 32% concentration in 10% dextrose.[11] It is electrolyte free, nonconductive, and, of particular importance if surgery is to be performed, immiscible with blood. We have performed over 1000 panoramic hysteroscopies in infertile patients using Hyskon as the distention medium and have found it to be eminently satisfactory. The view is perhaps not quite as sharp as that obtained with CO_2; however, we are rarely troubled with bubbles in the medium or with blood obscuring the field of view, particularly if operative procedures are performed.

  If Hyskon is used as the distention medium, no special equipment is required. Many authorities recommend connecting a 20-ml syringe filled with Hyskon to a plastic tube, which is then connected to one of the inflow channels of the hysteroscope sheath, with infusion maintained by an assistant. We have found that connecting the syringe directly to the hysteroscope is satisfactory, and infusion can be controlled by the surgeon without the need of further assistance. Hyskon will leak around the hysteroscope, but this does not pose any difficulty in visualization. Most evaluations are performed using less than 20 ml of the fluid. Although dextran enters the cul-de-sac in 50% of patients, this does not appear to pose a problem, and indeed, Hyskon has been used as an antiadhesion agent in tubal reparative surgery.[12] In our combined experience we have had one case of anaphylaxis. This occurred early during an attempt to remove an embedded intrauterine contraceptive device, and very large quantities of Hyskon were used.[13] The total volume of Hyskon used should not exceed 300 ml.

Hyskon has the disadvantage of solidifying when it dries, and if the instruments are not thoroughly cleansed with warm water, the moving parts may jam. Should such an event occur, soaking in warm water will relieve the blockage. Stopcocks should not be forced, since they will snap.

Dextrose 5% in water

Dextrose 5% in water (D5W) is particularly useful for outpatient hysteroscopy, since it is inexpensive and readily available. Much larger quantities of D5W are required than of dextran, since D5W runs freely around the instruments. Instillation is achieved by connecting one inflow channel to a 500-mm plastic bag wrapped in a blood pressure cuff inflated to between 80 and 120 mm Hg. Approximately 150 ml is used in 10 minutes. Unfortunately, D5W does mix with blood and mucus, and these must be removed from the uterine cavity or visualization will be difficult. To remove debris, a fine polyethylene catheter introduced through one of the operating channels permits the injection of D5W at higher pressures than are obtainable with the gravity feed system and results in flushing of mucus and blood from the uterine cavity.[14] Net absorption of D5W should not exceed 2000 ml to avoid hyponatremia. Full reviews of distention media and their relative advantages and disadvantages are available elsewhere.[11,15-17]

TECHNIQUES

The basic techniques of conventional panoramic and Hamou MCH hysteroscopy are different. Aspects that are common to both include timing with respect to the patient's menstrual cycle, positioning of the patient, and anesthesia.

The florid endometrium of the luteal phase makes it rather difficult to interpret hysteroscopic findings. The uterus is best visualized in the early follicular phase. Some investigators, and certainly our unit, combine laparoscopy with hysteroscopy. On occasion, this means that hysteroscopy must be performed in the luteal phase, and strategies to deal with this problem are discussed in Diagnostic Hysteroscopy in the Infertile Patient.

Hysteroscopy is performed with the patient in the dorsal lithotomy position. Before examination the patient is instructed to void. A bimanual examination to determine the position of the uterus is mandatory. Hysteroscopy is performed after full aseptic and antiseptic precautions have been taken. The cervix is exposed with a speculum and the anterior lip is grasped with a tenaculum. It is advantageous to place the single-toothed tenaculum vertically if the Hamou MCH hysteroscope is to be used.

Anesthesia, if required, may be local or general. Hamou MCH hysteroscopy is generally performed on the unanesthetized patient. In 959 women in whom this procedure was performed without any anesthesia, 360 experienced little or no pain. Discomfort comparable with that associated with menstruation was felt by 493, and 50 reported greater but acceptable levels of pain. In general, patients believed that the pain was less than that occasioned by hysterosalpingography.[18] The discomfort can be reduced further if a prostaglandin synthetase inhibitor is administered 1 hour preoperatively. Asking the patient to cough just as the tenaculum is applied seems to minimize the pain.

If conventional panoramic hysteroscopy is to be employed as an office procedure, local anesthesia can be achieved with paracervical blockade with 1% mesacaine, 10 ml on each side of the cervix. It takes 10 minutes for the anesthetic to become effective.[14] If major intrauterine surgical procedures are anticipated, many investigators favor general anesthesia, which is also of value if the patient is unduly apprehensive. If laparoscopy is to be combined with hysteroscopy, either as part of the infertility evaluation or so that laparoscopic monitoring of intrauterine surgical manipulations can be performed, general anesthesia is preferred.

Panoramic hysteroscopy

With the patient suitably positioned, draped, and anesthetized, the cervix is sounded to determine the depth of the uterine cavity. The cervix is dilated to size 7 or 8 Hegar depending on the size of the hysteroscope. The cervical occlusion cap is applied if CO_2 is to be the distention medium. If a fluid medium is to be used, the solution of either D5W or Hyskon is attached to one of the inflow channels and the sheath is flushed to exclude air bubbles. Since we have greatest experience with Hyskon, this technique is described in detail.

With the light cable attached, the sheath and telescope are inserted through the external os and fluid medium is gradually injected. The pressure of the distention medium will overcome any residual cervical tightness. The canal can be examined as the instrument advances, and the uterine cavity is entered safely under direct vision. If there is bleeding or a superfluity of mucus, the uterine cavity can be irrigated with D5W introduced through a fine polyethylene catheter. We have rarely found this to be necessary. A systematic examination of the uterine cavity is performed. The central fundus is examined and each tubal ostium in turn is visualized.[19] The remainder

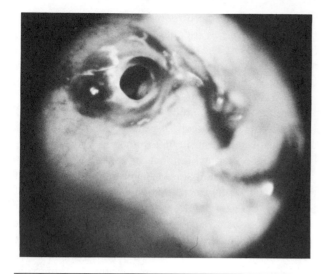

Figure 13-4
Tubal ostium. Note the intratubal polyps. From Taylor PJ and Hamou J: *Hysteroscopy, J Reprod Med* 28:359-397, 1983.

of the uterus is observed, and any lesions are noted and, if necessary, dealt with surgically. At the conclusion of the procedure the hysteroscope is simply removed.

As previously noted, we have preference for combined laparoscopy with hysteroscopy, and we find it of value to carry out simultaneous observation with both endoscopes. This frequently obviates the need for hydrotubation, since the dextran often can be observed dripping from the end of the fallopian tubes, thus confirming tubal patency. If a tube is apparently occluded at the proximal end, selective hydrotubation may be performed by passing a soft polyethylene catheter through the surgical channel into the tubal ostium and injecting methylene blue. Care must be taken to avoid traumatizing the tubal ostium if this technique is employed.

Data are accumulating to suggest that tubal obstruction may be overcome by the passage of a balloon catheter.[20] This approach confirms or refutes the presence of true cornual occlusion and may have some therapeutic benefit. The balloon catheters are expensive. To avoid waste, an attempt should first be made to pass the guidewire of a ureteric catheter through the ostium. Its passage into the isthmus is monitored laparoscopically. If successful entry into the isthmus is confirmed, the guidewire is replaced with the balloon catheter, the balloon inflated, and the catheter gently withdrawn. This technique requires validation in properly controlled studies. (See Chapter 12.)

Hamou MCH hysteroscopy

For fertility studies, the Hamou MCH is best used as a panoramic instrument with CO_2 as the distention medium. No cervical dilation is required. The telescope and sheath are gently inserted into the external os with the magnification set at $20\times$. The CO_2 flow rate is present at a rate of 30 ml per minute or at a pressure of 90 mm Hg, depending on whether the insufflator used has constant flow or constant pressure capability. A tiny cavity is created immediately in front of the hysteroscope by the gas. The instrument is gradually advanced, and at $20\times$ magnification, the endocervical arbor vitae are easily seen. The surgeon can pass the instrument between them without causing trauma and unnecessary bleeding. The length, morphology, and any pathologic features of the cervical canal can readily be identified, and the competence of the isthmus noted. When the uterine cavity is entered, magnification is switched to $1\times$ and a thorough survey performed as described for conventional panoramic hysteroscopy. The Hamou MCH permits detailed observation of the first millimeter of the fallopian tube and small intratubal polyps may be noted (Figure 13-4). It may be helpful occasionally to reduce the gas flow to a rate of 10 ml per minute once the cavity has been entered.

CONTRAINDICATIONS

Although hysteroscopy may be performed during acute bleeding episodes as part of the investigation for abnormal uterine bleeding,[21] it should not be carried out in the menstruating infertile patient. It is unknown whether the procedure would carry a risk of endometriosis, but it would seem wise to avoid even such a risk. Hysteroscopy is absolutely contraindicated if the patient has a recent history or the presence of acute pelvic infection.[14] Great care must be taken in women suspected of suffering from Asherman's syndrome, since their uteri are friable and easily perforated. If there is any suggestion that the patient may have an early pregnancy, hysteroscopy would be avoided unless the instrument is being used specifically as an embryoscope.[22]

COMPLICATIONS

Complications may occur from the anesthetic. The risks of anesthesia in this procedure are not different from those associated with either local or general agents used for any other.

The risks from the distention medium are few. The occurrence of anaphylaxis with the use of Hyskon, already described, is most likely to occur in cases of uterine hypoplasia, tubal occlusion, or recently traumatized uterine cavity.[23] Carbon dioxide should be virtually risk free if used in the appropriate fashion.

The risks of cervical dilation and the performance of hysteroscopy itself are difficult to differentiate. They include cervical laceration, uterine perforation, and reactivation of acute pelvic inflammatory disease (PID). The cervix will be lacerated when there is difficulty dilating it and the tenaculum tears free. Such an event occurred in 4 of 836 women who underwent panoramic hysteroscopy as part of an infertility investigation. In our series, we recorded only those patients who required cervical suturing. Dislodgement of the tenaculum occurs more frequently. Since cervical dilatation plays no part in Hamou MCH hysteroscopy, cervical lacerations are rare.

Uterine perforation may be caused by the uterine sound, the dilator, or the hysteroscope. Perforation caused by sounding or dilation does not differ from that when a routine dilatation and curettage is performed. It is suspected when the instrument passes to a greater depth than anticipated. That such an event has occurred will be instantly apparent if Hyskon is used as a distention medium, since little pressure is required to inject a large volume of the fluid. If the field of vision is cloudy or obscured, the hysteroscope should not be advanced, since it may be in contact with the uterine wall. If the telescope does perforate the uterine wall, abdominal contents will be visualized immediately. This occurred in 2 of the 836 patients described previously. In both instances the instrument was in the hands of a learner under instruction. Perforations occurred in 6 of 5200 hysteroscopies[24] and in 5 of 257 patients.[25] In the latter series, indications for the procedure were not all for infertility, and the perforations occurred in women with severe uterine scarring and cervical stenosis and in one case of postabortal uterus. Only one perforation occurred in a woman with an otherwise normal uterus.

Perforation is extremely rare in Hamou MCH hysteroscopy because of the technique of advancing the instrument under constant visual control. Intrauterine manipulations cause the greatest risk of uterine damage, and probing of the tubal ostia must be extremely gentle because of the risk of creating false passages or perforations at the uterotubal junction.[16]

Uterine perforation does not appear to be a major complication. If it occurs, the instrument should be removed and the patient observed. If there is reason for concern, laparoscopy and, if necessary, laparotomy should be undertaken.

Acute infection does not seem to be a great risk and did not occur at all in our series. In one early study,[26] 1 of 34 infertile women developed a postoperative fever of 101°F. In a series of 1000 Hamou MCH hysteroscopies, 1 severe and 7 mild pelvic infections were identified.[18] The severe infection occurred during removal of a tubal stent after a tuboplasty and should not be regarded as a complication of hysteroscopy. In a subsequent 3000 instances there was not a single episode of infection. However, we would like to add a word of caution. In a study of 195 women with unexplained infertility, 53 underwent diagnostic curettage as part of the investigation and 142 did not.[27] None had an antecedent history suggestive of PID. The frequency of laparoscopically detected chronic pelvic inflammatory changes in the groups was 50.9% and 13.4%, respectively (P<0.001). It was concluded that diagnostic curettage may pose an unrecognized risk in these patients. We have no data to confirm or refute these findings in women with unexplained infertility who undergo hysteroscopy.

There may be some small risk of diagnostic hysteroscopy causing intrauterine adhesion formation. Of 108 women who underwent the procedure, 100 had no evidence of adhesions. At the time of second-look hysteroscopy, only one had developed such lesions.[28] As a general principle, no intrauterine manipulation should be undertaken in the infertile patient without good reason.

In addition to cervical laceration, uterine perforation, and infection, minor complications have been reported with hysteroscopy. The distention medium may cause the formation of a pinhole perforation in a thin-walled hydrosalpinx. Such an event occurred during CO_2 hysteroscopy.[16] We have occasionally noted similar events when Hyskon was used as the distention medium.[22] It would appear, however, that the risks of this procedure are low. Out total complication rate in 836 women so examined was 0.8%.

Sometimes the surgeon may fail to complete the hysteroscopic evaluation, and failure rates in reported series range from 8%[25] to 0%.[14] In our first 100 Hyskon panoramic hysteroscopies we had 4 failures, a rate of 4%. The reasons for failure included two cases of air bubbles in the Hyskon, one case of bleeding, and one of cervical stenosis.[27] In a subsequent 836 patients there were 21 failures, a rate of 2.8%. The reasons for these incompletions included 18 cases of failure to dilate the cervix; one of bleeding that was so excessive as to obscure the view; one of air bubbles in the medium, which occurred in the fifty-eighth patient in the study and has not occurred subsequently; and one instance of inadvertent visualization of early pregnancy. This last event can be regarded both as a failure of the procedure and as a complication. Details of this case were reported elsewhere.[29] It is perhaps worth noting that the patient suffered no ill effects, and although labor commenced somewhat prematurely, she did deliver a healthy infant. Therefore it is clear that the most common cause of failure is inability to dilate the cervix, and this occurs much less frequently when the Hamou MCH is used.

EVALUATION BEFORE HYSTEROSCOPY

Before endoscopy the patient should be examined with regard to two distinct considerations: infertility and investigations that should be performed to ensure maximum safety at the time of hysteroscopy.

Infertility investigation

As previously remarked, invasive procedures should in all instances be carried out as the final step in the work-up of any infertile couple. It is mandatory that evidence of ovulation is confirmed by history, basal body temperature graphing, and, where necessary, measurements of serum progesterone levels and timed endometrial biopsy. At least two properly performed semen analyses should be carried out.[30]

On the basis of these investigations, it would appear reasonable to divide the women into those "infertile, probably anovulatory" and those "infertile, probably ovulatory." The investigation differs for each group. In the former, a proper laboratory search for the underlying cause of anovulation should be sought. It is not productive to carry out investigations of the lower genital tract until at least six courses of successful induction of ovulation have failed to result in a pregnancy. In the event that such a woman requires exogenous gonadotropin therapy, however, we recommend investigation of the lower genital tract before institution of such treatment. Similarly, at this point, it seems reasonable to categorize the male partners as "probably fertile" or "probably infertile" on the basis of their semen analyses.

For couples in whom a male factor is detected, it is realistic either to attempt to overcome this factor or, if such treatment fails or is inappropriate, to try at least six courses of artificial insemination by donor before pelvic assessment. In our experience, only 5% of women who failed to conceive after donor insemination were shown endoscopically to have an intrapelvic cause of infertility.[31] With these simple procedures, it is possible to select a group of patients in whom anovulation and male factors have been excluded as a possible cause of infertility.

Despite extensive literature on such problems as cervical factors, luteal phase defect, and male and female autoantibodies, the role of these entities in the causation of infertility is extremely unclear. One group did nothing further for their patients than determine that each partner had a normal history and physical examination, that the man had a normal semen profile, and that normalcy of ovulation and the lower genital tract were documented in the woman.[32] In 7 years of follow-up with no treatment, 64% of these patients with primary and 79% with secondary infertility achieved successful conception and delivery. We are convinced that additional studies are required in all these areas to determine whether a real causal relationship with infertility exists and, more important, whether treatments currently proposed are more effective than no treatment.

Nevertheless, given the present state of the art, such potential causes of infertility probably should be sought before any invasive investigation of the lower genital tract. While not directly related to hysteroscopy, it is worth remarking that in an earlier laparoscopic study of 81 patients in whom luteal phase defect, hostile cervical mucus, or antisperm antibodies were detected, 49 (61%)

had laparoscopic evidence of intrapelvic disease of sufficient severity to be the major cause of infertility.[33]

Having reached this stage of the investigation, the next logical step is evaluation of the uterine cavity and fallopian tubes. The hysterosalpingogram (HSG) is the initial investigation of choice.

"Advantages of initial hysterosalpingography include (1) identification of uterine anomalies and intrauterine lesions, (2) identification of cornual occlusion and/or cornual lesions, even in the presence of cornual patency, (3) immediate identification of distal tubal occlusion and assessment of intratubal architecture. Endotubal architecture is of prognostic significance and cannot be determined by any endoscopic technique; and (4) there is increasing ability among surgeons to perform corrective laparoscopic surgery for periadnexal adhesive disease."[34]

The detection of either tubal or intrauterine disease by HSG permits scheduling of operating room time if endoscopic surgical correction is to be attempted at the time of confirmatory endoscopy.

We have argued consistently,[19,31] however, that HSG does not provide as accurate an evaluation as laparoscopy, and more recently[22,29] that hysteroscopy is superior in evaluating the uterine cavity. Since this chapter deals specifically with hysteroscopy in the infertile patient, the arguments of laparoscopy versus HSG are not addressed; however, the results of HSG compared with hysteroscopy are described. In 75 infertile women who underwent HSG, the uterine cavities of 71 women were judged to be normal and 4 to be abnormal.[29] In the 71 with normal HSG, hysteroscopy failed in 3, 38 had normal cavities, and 30 had abnormal cavities. Abnormalities included adhesions in 15 patients, polyps in 13, adhesions plus polyps in 1, and a previously unidentified septum in 1. Of the 4 abnormal cavities, hysteroscopy failed in 1, and none of the abnormalities noted on HSG was detected. In all cases these had been reported radiologically as being subseptate uteri.

In 104 patients complaining of infertility, in whom both HSG and hysteroscopy had been performed, 8 hysteroscopies were unsuccessful.[35] The HSG had suggested uterine abnormalities in 19 patients; 2 of these were entirely normal at the time of hysteroscopy. Septa were confirmed in 6, synechiae in 5, and submucous lesions in 2. The significance of surface endometrial petechiae in 3 cavities detected at hysteroscopy was not clear. Some unsuspected uterine pathology was detected in 30 (38.9%) of 77 hysteroscopic examination. Hysteroscopy was normal in 20 (31.7%) of 142 patients, 63 of whom had previously been reported as having an abnormal HSG.[36] When attention was paid specifically to intrauterine adhesions in 55 women who had undergone HSG and Hamou MCH hysteroscopy,[37] the diagnoses by the two methods agreed in 37 (67.2%), disagreed in 12 (17.4%), and were not wholly in accord in another 6 women (10.9%).

Without discussing the significance with respect to infertility of intrauterine lesions noted either by HSG or hysteroscopy, it would appear that direct visualization is the more accurate procedure. It has long been accepted that abnormal tubal appearance on HSG should lead to immediate laparoscopy, whereas 6 months should elapse between a normal HSG and laparoscopy. A similar approach can be undertaken when choosing the optimal time to perform a hysteroscopy.

Laparoscopy and hysteroscopy can be combined in one session to permit a full survey of the uterus and tubes.* Indeed, we support the contention that, "The combination of hysteroscopy and exploratory laparoscopy is especially useful in detecting the cause of infertility in the lower genital tract of the female."[38] Others prefer to reserve hysteroscopy for patients whose work-up has been completed and in whom lesions in the uterine cavity are suspected based on either history or HSG. Adherents to the former philosophy carry out the procedure under general anesthesia. Those of the latter persuasion frequently examine the uterus hysteroscopically under local anesthesia.

Laparoscopy is optimally performed in the luteal phase when it will give evidence with respect to the gross anatomy of the pelvis and also the existing presence or absence of a corpus luteum. If performed early enough in the luteal phase, it can be determined whether the stigma of ovulation is visible. This approach has its drawbacks, however, since the appearance of the endometrium in the florid luteal phase makes hysteroscopic interpretation more difficult. A strategy to overcome this problem is to carry out Hamou MCH hysteroscopy as a simple office procedure in the early follicular phase and laparoscopy in the luteal phase.[40] Minor abnormalities can be detected and dealt with in the office, and if a major lesion is observed, arrangements can be made for surgical hysteroscopy under laparoscopic control.

Investigations to ensure safety

The physician who investigates a woman's infertility must determine her degree of immunity to rubella. The patient who has been investigated and treated and successfully achieves conception only to have the pregnancy terminated because of exposure to rubella is a medical disaster. Although it has been our practice to carry out Veneral Disease Research Laboratory evaluations of both partners, we have not discovered a single positive result in the last 1700 examinations. The cost benefit of this procedure must be challenged.

If general anesthesia is to be administered, the woman's fitness for such a procedure must be evaluated carefully. The hemoglobin and erythrocyte sedimentation rate

should be checked. If a recent Papanicolaou (Pap) smear has not been performed, it should be done before hysteroscopy. Use of the Hamou MCH will permit colposcopy if the smear is abnormal. It has been our practice to take cervical and vaginal cultures for common bacterial contaminants and also for *Chlamydia* and *Mycoplasma* organisms. If an infective agent is cultured, appropriate antibiotic therapy should be instituted. We have found no value in blind administration of prophylactic antibiotics.

Diagnostic hysteroscopy in the infertile patient and in habitual pregnancy wastage

When laparoscopy was first introduced, the practicing gynecologist had little difficulty adapting to this new technique, which was due in large part to the familiarity of the appearance of the healthy woman's pelvis gained at laparotomy. Unfortunately, the hysteroscopic appearance of the uterine cavity is not familiar, and some skill is required in interpreting the findings. Courses in hysteroscopy are available. In addition, we have found examination of recently removed hysterectomy specimens to be helpful. The uterus is clamped at the tubocornual junction and the hysteroscope inserted. The learner can evaluate the findings and immediately effect confirmation by dividing the uterus and examining the cavity with the naked eye.

The frequency of lesions determined hysteroscopically in patients investigated specifically for infertility has ranged from 41.6% to 64.8%. Data in five of the largest series are shown in Table 13-1. The lesions noted most commonly are polyps, adhesions, myomata, and septa.

It must be recognized that the apparent prevalence of hysteroscopically detected lesions are in part a function of the nature of the practice of the reporting physician. Many deal almost exclusively with prescreened patients in whom the detection rate will be high. We reevaluated our data in a largely unscreened population. Eight hundred thirty-seven patients were evaluated using dextran as the distention medium and were compared with 278 patients who were examined with the Hamou instrument using CO_2. Although there was good congruence between the prevalence of septa (1.4% and 3.4%, respectively) and myomata (1.5% and 0.3%, respectively), there was a wide discrepancy in the apparent prevalence of adhesions and polyps. The relative frequency of detection of these lesions is shown in Table 13-2. It was concluded that since cervical dilation is necessary for dextran hysteroscopy, many of the lesions apparently noted represented artifactual dislodgment of strips of endometrium. If these were tethered only at one pole, they were misinterpreted as polyps, and if tethered at both poles, they were misinterpreted as adhesions. It is probable that both of these lesions occur less frequently than previously was thought. If at all possible, histologic evidence of a lesion detected hysteroscopically always should be sought.

---

*References 14, 24, 36, 38, 39.

Table 13-1 Hysteroscopic findings in five series of infertile patients

Findings	Cohen and Dmowski 1977*	Mohr and Lindemann 1977*	Valle 1982*	Taylor et al.†	Hamou and Salat-Baroux 1984††
Number of cases	34	167	142	701	128
Failed	2	0	0	24	0
Normal cavities	20	68	54	419	45
Polyps or polyposis	2	60	34	89	6
Adhesions	4	19	28	155	27
Uterine malformations	2	9	9	9	9
Fibroids	2	11		5	4
Scarred cavity	4	—	—	—	—
Cervical stenosis	—	—	3	—	6
Cesarean section			3		
Scar defect	—		—	—	—
Vascular abnormalities	—		—	—	6
Endometritis	—	—	—	—	10
Bone metaplasia	—	—	—	—	1
Abnormalities (%)	43.7	59.0	62.0	41.6	64.8

*Panoramic hysteroscopy.
†Unpublished data.
††Contact microhysteroscopy.
Adapted from Hamou J and Taylor PJ: Panoramic, contact, and microcolpohysteroscopy in gynecologic
practice. In Leventhal JM (ed): *Current problems in obstetrics and gynecology,* Chicago, 1982, Year Book Medical Publishers.

Table 13-2 The difference in prevalence of adhesions and polyps when dextran or carbon dioxide was used as the distention medium

Lesion	Dextran (N = 837)	Carbon dioxide (N = 278)
Adhesions (%)	22.5	3.5
Polyps (%)	12	0.5

Our most recent data are based on 335 Hamou CO_2 hysteroscopies successfully performed in 160 women complaining of primary infertility, 118 of secondary infertility, and 57 requesting reversal of tubal sterilization. The last group served as potentially fertile controls. These data are discussed in subsequent sections dealing with specific lesions.

When viewed with a panoramic hysteroscope, the normal endometrium is pink or tan and has very few blood vessels in the proliferative phase.[41] The openings of the endometrial glands are defined by punctate, pale whitish areas, and the tubal ostia are easily seen. The secretory endometrium is pink or tan and is velvety in appearance. If panoramic hysteroscopy is performed in the luteal phase, it is common to dislodge fragments of endometrium with the dilator, and these should not be misinterpreted as polyps. Small submucous blood vessels are easily visualized. If Hamou MCH is performed, the appearances are similar at $1 \times$ magnification. It is possible for a trained cytologist to date the endometrium accurately when the Hamou MCH is used at higher magnification and the endometrium is stained with methylene blue. If the MCH is used as a contact hysteroscope, vascular changes are noted. Arterioles intermittently shrink, at which time smaller blood vessels disappear and the color of the endometrium changes from pink to white. The thickness of the endometrium can be assessed with the Hamou MCH by pressing the tip against the uterine wall, which creates a furrow.

Polyps

Although it is not surprising that polyps have been reported in between 9%[42] and 41.6%[25] of patients who undergo hysteroscopy for the symptom of abnormal bleeding, their frequency in the eumenorrheic infertile patient is surprisingly high, ranging from 6.25% in an early series of 35 women[26] to 35.9% in 160 patients.[38] We detected polyps in 2 (1.25%) of 160 women with primary infertility and in none of 118 patients with secondary infertility or 57 requesting reversal of sterilization.

The cause-and-effect relationship between polyps and infertility has not been established. It has been difficult to determine the frequency in a healthy population. We attempted to use women requesting reversal of sterilization as a potentially fertile control group. Based on our data, it is difficult to support a contention that small polyps noted hysteroscopically can exert any significant influence on reproductive performance. That is not to say

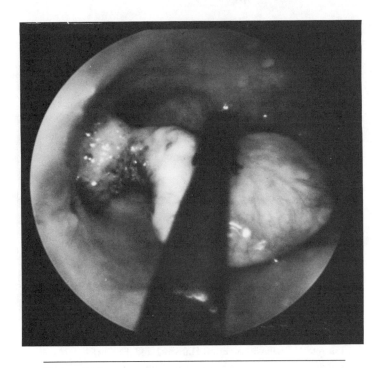

Figure 13-5
Cautery of the base of an endometrial polyp. From Hamou J
and Taylor PJ: *Panoramic, contact, and microcolpohysteroscopy in gynecologic practice*. In Levanthal JM (ed): *Current
problems in obstetrics and gynecology*, vol. 6(2), Chicago,
1982, Year Book Medical Publishers.

that they should not be noted and removed at the time
of hysteroscopy. This can be done simply with a small
hysteroscopic snare or by cauterizing the base (Figure
13-5) if single polyps are present. Multiple polyps are
probably best dealt with by removing the hysteroscope,
performing curettage, and then immediately reevaluating
the patient hysteroscopically to ensure complete removal.

When visualized by panoramic hysteroscopy, polyps
must be differentiated from dislodged strips of endometrium and also from submucous myomata. Myomata
are fixed, whereas polyps undulate with the ebb and flow
of the distention medium. If the panoramic hysteroscope
is used, a final histologic diagnosis of polyps may be
difficult to substantiate. In 7 of 237 examinations carried
out by panoramic means, significant misinterpretations
occurred.[25] This may in part be due to the magnification
effect of the hysteroscope but may also reflect the fact
that after removal, the typical histologic characteristics
of polyps may be lost so that the pathologist is unable
to confirm their presence. The Hamou MCH with its
higher magnification capabilities permits in situ histologic diagnosis to be made.

Adhesions

Intrauterine adhesions (Figure 13-6) occur in from 11%[26]
to 24% of infertile women (Plate 1). It is of interest that

in these series none of the patients suffered from amenorrhea, and it is clear that the original definition of Asherman's syndrome—amenorrhea traumaticum—must
be expanded to include those whose menstrual function
has not been deranged but within whose uterine cavity
fibrous adhesions are detected. In 192 patients with adhesions, 72 were eumenorrheic, 22 had amenorrhea, and
98 complained of a variable degree of hypomenorrhea.[43]
Although this chapter primarily discusses the application
of hysteroscopy in the patient with otherwise unexplained
infertility, it is perhaps appropriate to remark that the
procedure should not be undertaken in an amenorrheic
woman unless there is clear biochemical and pharmacologic evidence that the uterine cavity is compromised.
As a minimum investigation, the patient with amenorrhea
should undergo assessment of follicle-stimulating hormone (FSH), luteinizing hormone (LH), and prolactin
levels; and the uterus should be challenged both with
progestational agents alone and in combination with estrogen. Hysteroscopy should be reserved for the amenorrheic patient who is eugonadotropic and normoprolac-
tinemic, and who fails to demonstrate withdrawal
bleeding both to progestational challenge and combined
estrogen-progesterone challenge.

In 69 patients in whom intrauterine adhesions were
evaluated and managed by MCH hysteroscopy, menstrual

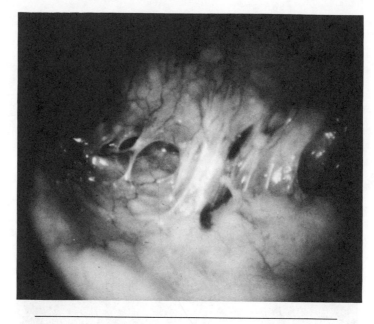

Figure 13-6
Intrauterine adhesions. From Hamou J and Taylor PJ: *Panoramic, contact, and microcolpohysteroscopy in gynecologic practice*. In Levanthal JM (ed): *Current problems in obstetrics and gynecology*, vol. 6(2), Chicago, 1982, Year Book Medical Publishers.

disorders were present in 46 (66.5%), amenorrhea in 21 (30.4%), and hypomenorrhea in 25 (36.2%).[37] Associated dysmenorrhea was present in 7 women (10.2%), but the remaining 23 had normal cyclic menses.

The etiology of these adhesions has not firmly been established. It would appear that their occurrence is rare without a history of either a preceding pregnancy or intrauterine manipulation. It is probable that vascularization and fibrosis in placental fragments after either spontaneous abortion or delivery play an etiologic role.[42,43] In 192 cases the mechanical intervention preceding discovery of adhesions included puerperal curettage, 39; spontaneous abortions, 72; legal abortions, 59; molar abortions, 9; diagnostic curettage, 1; myomectomies, 5; and cesarean sections, 7.[43] The use of an intrauterine contraceptive device may predispose to adhesion formation[36]; it would seem that diagnostic curettage may do so as well. When 76 infertile women who had undergone this procedure were compared with 147 infertile patients who had not, the frequency of hysteroscopically detected adhesions was 37 and 11, respectively (P<0.0005).[44]

The position of the adhesions was described as central and marginal.[43] Histologically, they may be classified as endometrial, myofibrous, or composed of connective tissue.[45] These can be distinguished hysteroscopically by their surface appearance and by the force required to divide them.[43] At 20 × magnification with the Hamou

MCH, the histologic nature of the adhesions is easily discernible. Of the adhesions in 69 patients, 17 were endometrial, 15 myometrial or myofibrous, and 37 fibrous or connective tissue.[37] When such adhesions are detected they may be dealt with by simple pressure with the tip of the hysteroscope in the case of finer and less dense adhesions, or they may require formal dissection.

An innovative technique that has been developed using the MCH is target abrasion (Figure 13-7).[43] This procedure can be performed only with the Hamou MCH. Using 20 × magnification it is possible to determine the most avascular part of the adhesion. The tip of the instrument is angled and slightly sharp. By progressively abrading both ends of the adhesion with the tip of the instrument under direct visual control, complete lysis may be achieved. Target abrasion was successful in 59 of 69 patients. The procedure was done in the office without need of local anesthesia or cervical dilation. Ten patients whose adhesions were more severe or who found abrasion to be painful were treated successfully under general anesthesia.[37]

As with polyps, the exact significance of intrauterine adhesions as a causative factor of infertility is unclear. In our most recent series, adhesions were detected in 4 (2.5%) of 160 women with primary infertility, 5 (4.2%) of 118 with secondary infertility, and 1 (1.75%) of 57 requesting reversal of sterilization. Although the difference in results between patients with secondary infertility and sterilized patients was statistically significant, none was noted between those with primary infertility and those requesting reversal of sterilization. However, we made no attempt to classify the adhesions by severity, which is clearly a flaw. When more dense adhesions were detected,[37,43] accurate diagnosis and removal clearly improved the pregnancy rates. Of 30 infertile patients, 51.3% conceived, and 38% of whom subsequently had uncomplicated deliveries.[37] In 192 patients in whom adhesions were treated by hysteroscopic lysis, 79 (41.2%) became pregnant. Of these, 29 (36.7%) aborted spontaneously, 2 had premature deliveries, and 45 experienced at least one term delivery.[43] Among the 50 term or premature deliveries (some patients delivering more than once), 8 required manual removal of the placenta or postpartum curettage.

It would appear that the hysteroscopic search for intrauterine adhesions in the eumenorrheic or hypomenorrheic infertile patient is justified, and that the more severe the histologic grading, the more likely the lesions are to interfere with the patient's reproductive performance.

Myomata

Submucous fibroids (Figure 13-8) detected hysteroscopically during the infertility investigation have been shown to occur in between 0%[36] and 6.5%[38] of patients. Of 701 patients with infertility, we detected submucous fibroids in only 5. While it is probable that large myomata may interfere with ability to conceive and certainly may play a role in habitual pregnancy loss, it is unlikely that small lesions negatively affect reproductive ability. It is probable that such small lesions are incidental findings only.

On occasion, differentiating polyps from submucous myomata can be difficult (Plate 2). Fibroids tend to bulge into the uterine cavity under a thin endometrium. They are smooth, firm, pale, and rounded, and, of particular importance, do not move as the pressure of the distention medium varies. Polyps invariably are seen to undulate gently in the medium.

Septa

Septa are noted infrequently in infertile patients, with frequency varying from 6.3%[36] to 1.3%. The latter figure represents 9 such findings in 701 patients. It is unlikely that septa cause infertility, although they may certainly be a cause of habitual abortion and obstetric complications (see below). Effective hysteroscopic management of such lesions is now possible.

The appearance of a septum is typical (Plate 3). The paired uterine cornua are readily noted to be divided by a fibrous band. The surface appearance of this fibrous band varies with the stage of the menstrual cycle at which the observation is made. Whereas hysteroscopy is of value in septate and subseptate uteri, it is of little help in patients with a true bicornuate deformity, and inter-

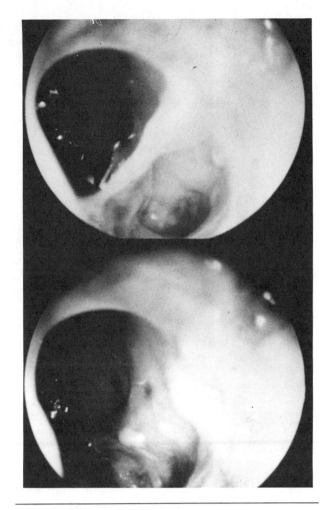

Figure 13-7
Target abrasion of intrauterine adhesions. From Hamou J and Taylor PJ: *Panoramic, contact, and microcolpohysteroscopy in gynecologic practice.* In Levanthal JM (ed): *Current problems in obstetrics and gynecology,* vol. 6(2), Chicago, 1982, Year Book Medical Publishers.

pretation in minor degrees of arcuate and planiform uterine cavities can be difficult in the extreme.

Less common lesions

With improved access to the uterine cavity, particularly at magnification with the Hamou MCH, cervical stenosis, cesarean section scar defects, vascular abnormalities, endometritis, and even radiolucent bony metaplasia[22] have been described in the uterine cavities of infertile women. The appearance of adenomyosis is typical, involving much increased vascularity and dark-appearing blobs on the endometrial surface.

We described 9 cases of heterotopic intrauterine bone formation.[46] The symptoms were secondary infertility in 7, pelvic pain in 1, and passage of bone fragments in 1. Despite apparent removal of all the bony fragments in

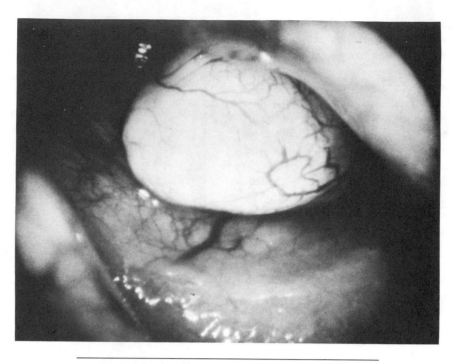

Figure 13-8
Submucous fibroid. From Hamou J and Taylor PJ: *Panoramic, contact, and microcolpohysteroscopy in gynecologic practice.* In Levanthal JM (ed): *Current problems in obstetrics and gynecology,* vol. 6(2), Chicago, 1982, Year Book Medical Publishers.

all patients, recurrence was noted in 4 of 8 in whom follow-up was possible, and required a second removal. This lesion, although rare, appears to occur after pregnancy. Although 4 of the 6 infertile women who were followed conceived, the numbers are too small to allow the conclusion that removing the bony fragments cured the infertility. It is reasonable to suggest if such fragments are detected that they should be removed.

Habitual abortion

Malpas's[47] original studies, which suggested that after three successive abortions a woman had only 27% chance of achieving a term pregnancy, are incorrect. In fact, it was suggested that such a woman has 53% chance of carrying a fourth pregnancy,[48] and some maintained that 68% will have a healthy baby.[49] Chromosomal abnormalities and uterine malformations can clearly be implicated as causes of habitual abortion,[50] but the roles of T mycoplasma[51] and human leukocyte antigen tissue antibodies[52] are still under investigation.

If chromosomal abnormalities have been excluded in both partners, it would seem appropriate in cases of habitual abortion to examine the uterine cavity hysteroscopically to detect the presence of and deal surgically with any uterine septa. It is also possible that intrauterine adhesions may contribute to habitual abortion. An im-

proved live delivery rate was achieved in a group of women in whom such adhesions were diagnosed by HSG.[53] In 51 patients with history of repeated abortion, adhesions were detected and removed hysteroscopically.[43] Eighteen of these patients remained infertile, 12 conceived and aborted, and 19 delivered at term. Premature delivery and stillbirth both occurred in 1 patient. These studies do not permit the conclusion that intrauterine adhesions are indeed a cause of habitual abortion, but a reasonable suspicion has been raised.

COMBINED LAPAROSCOPY AND HYSTEROSCOPY

Our practice has been to combine laparoscopy with hysteroscopy in the investigation of infertility. While reiterating that some hysteroscopic findings may be of little significance, we believe that this combination offers the most complete evaluation of the lower reproductive tract of the woman with otherwise unexplained infertility.

We attempted to correlate hysteroscopic with laparoscopic findings in 497 patients, 285 of whom complained of primary and 212 of secondary infertility. In neither group could any statistically significant relationship be demonstrated between a laparoscopic finding of chronic pelvic inflammatory disease and the hysteroscopic finding of intrauterine adhesions, polyps, fibroids, or septa.

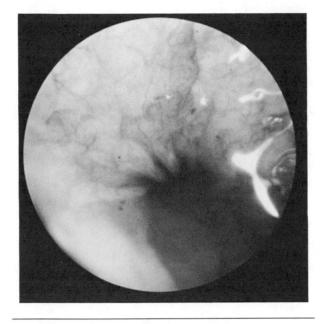

Figure 13-9
Retrograde tuboscopy. From Hamou J and Taylor PJ: *Panoramic, contact, and microcolpohysteroscopy in gynecologic practice.* In Levanthal JM (ed): *Current problems in obstetrics and gynecology*, vol. 6(2), Chicago, 1982, Year Book Medical Publishers.

There was no relationship between laparoscopic findings of endometriosis and such hysteroscopic findings. The only statistical dependency was between secondary infertility and the finding of hysteroscopic adhesions (P<0.01). A similar relationship existed between laparoscopic evidence of chronic pelvic inflammatory disease and secondary infertility (P<0.01).

ANCILLARY TECHNIQUES OF HYSTEROSCOPY IN THE INFERTILE PATIENT

Although hysteroscopy is of primary value in diagnosis and in certain surgical procedures in the infertile patient, other applications have been suggested, including selective hydrotubation, the removal of intratubal stents, extended postcoital testing, and evaluation of women requesting reversal of a previous sterilization. In cases of apparent cornual occlusion detected both at laparoscopy and by HSG, the surgeon is still faced with the dilemma as to whether results truly represent occlusion or if failures of laparoscopic technique are due to uterine spasm during HSG. It has been our misfortune to have performed surgery on three patients in whom cornual occlusion was suspected by both investigations, only to find the tubes were patent at laparotomy. With careful identification of the tubal ostium at the time of hysteroscopy and selective catheterization[23] or cannulation, such events can be avoided. Although hysteroscopic re-

moval of stents placed to facilitate tubal reparative surgery has been described,[22] it is likely that this practice will find little general favor. Results of animal work suggest that rather than being of value, such stents cause damage to the tubal epithelium.[54] Gomel[55] cautioned against the use of these stents.

It is clear that the postcoital test is at best an inaccurate evaluation of sperm transport in the female genital tract. Extended postcoital testing can be performed laparoscopically[56] and tubal fluid can be aspirated hysteroscopically. Twenty percent of patients studied in this fashion did not have sperm in the tubal aspirates despite a normal postcoital test.[57] This procedure must be considered experimental but holds promise for the future.

In view of the pregnancy rates after reversal of sterilization, which are now approaching those seen in the normally fertile population,[23,58] it is difficult to perceive that, in this group of patients, many intrauterine lesions exist that might interfere with fertility. We have argued for performing routine laparoscopy in patients wishing reversal of sterilization[59] and believe that in many such patients, HSG may be required to demonstrate the status of the proximal tubal segment. Selective hydrotubation in these patients, if hysteroscopy is performed at the time of laparoscopy, may obviate the need for HSG.

TUBOSCOPY

Using 20 × magnification, the Hamou MCH permits detailed examination of the first millimeter of the interstitial portion of the fallopian tube. Peristalsis and mucosal folds can be observed. The instrument can also be used at laparotomy for retrograde tubal evaluation. The gas flow is set at 10 ml per minute and the pressure at 40 to 50 mm Hg. The microcavity so created permits gradual and atraumatic advance of the objective lens. Staining of the mucosa with methylene blue permits more accurate observation to be made (Figure 13-9). Whether tuboscopy will be of value in predicting the probable outcome from tubal surgery or to permit dissection of intratubal adhesions and lower the ectopic pregnancy rate in these cases is not yet clear. It does, however, present an interesting avenue for further studies.

PROPHYLAXIS

Undoubtedly, laparoscopy can play a prophylactic role in the early detection of acute pelvic inflammatory disease and in the early diagnosis of unruptured tubal pregnancy. It is unlikely that hysteroscopy will be of much value under these circumstances. It is clear, however, that there is a compelling need for nonsurgical, reversible means of female sterilization.[60] Several hysteroscopic approaches are showing promise.

Satisfactory plug formation occurred in 71.5% of 239 women when hysteroscopically delivered formed-in-place silicone plugs were used.[61] Six of 35 patients who were excluded from this series because plug formation was deemed inadequate did become pregnant. Although somewhat cumbersome to insert, it is reasonable to think that the silicone formed-in-place plug may be more widely used in the future. A cervical plug was designed, which is anchored to the myometrium by four retractable spines.[62] Examination of the extirpated uteri of volunteers who had worn the device demonstrated some expansion of the tubal lumen and flattening of the endosalpingeal cells. The P-block plug[63] is retained in the isthmus because it absorbs fluid after insertion and swells. The device is in a developmental stage.

Preliminary studies were conducted with a nylon intratubal device that has an open loop at each extremity, which fixes it both in the tube and at the uterine ends.[22] Each loop has an elastic memory. The device can be fitted in the office using the MCH without anesthesia.

None of these devices is well enough developed to enter routine clinical practice. The woman who has been sterilized and now regrets the decision is no less in need of help than the involuntarily infertile patient. Perhaps the development of a truly reversible hysteroscopically delivered sterilization device will offer a fresh approach to this perennial problem.

SUMMARY

Hysteroscopy with either the panoramic or Hamou MCH is no longer a procedure looking for an indication. Once the appearances of the uterine cavity have been learned, it is a simple, low-risk technique. When combined with laparoscopy it offers the most thorough survey of the lower female genital tract.

It is becoming apparent that hysteroscopic detection of polyps and small submucous myomata in the infertile patient is of little prognostic significance. Hysteroscopy, however, has an emerging, definable role in the diagnosis and treatment of intrauterine adhesions and septa in patients who complain of infertility and recurrent pregnancy loss.

REFERENCES

1. Taylor PJ and Hamou J: Hysteroscopy, *J Reprod Med* 28:359-387, 1983.
2. Lindemann HJ: Historical aspects of hysteroscopy, *Fertil Steril* 24:230-242, 1973.
3. Barbot J, Parent B, and Dubuisson JB: Contact hysteroscopy: another method of endoscopic examination of the uterine cavity, *Am J Obstet Gynecol* 136:721-726, 1980.
4. Baggish MS: Contact hysteroscopy: a new technique to explore the uterine cavity, *Obstet Gynecol* 54:350-354, 1979.
5. Neuwirth RS: A new technique for and additional experience with hysteroscopic resection of submucous fibroids, *Am J Obstet Gynecol* 131:91-94, 1978.
6. Lindemann HJ and Mohr J: CO₂ hysteroscopy: diagnosis and treatment, *Am J Obstet Gynecol* 124:129-133, 1976.
7. Lindemann HJ: Symposium: advances in fiberoptic hysteroscopy, *Contemp Obstet Gynecol* 3(4):115-119, 1974.
8. Hulf JA et al: Blood carbon dioxide tension changes during hysteroscopy, *Fertil Steril* 32:193-196, 1979.
9. Obstetrician convicted in sterilization death is placed on probation, *Obstet Gynecol News* 9:4, 1979.
10. Menken FS: Eine neues verfahren mit vorrichtung zur hysteroskopie, *Endoscopy* 19:161-162, 1971.
11. Edstrom K and Fernstrom I: The diagnostic possibilities of a modified hysteroscopic technique, *Acta Obstet Gynecol Scand* 49:327-330, 1970.
12. Luengo J and Van Hall EV: Prevention of peritoneal adhesions by the combined use of Spongostan and 32% dextran 70: an experimental study in pigs, *Fertil Steril* 29:447-450, 1978.
13. Knudtson ML and Taylor PJ: Uberemplindichkeitsreaktion auf dextran 70 (Hyskon) wahrend einer hysteroskopie, *Geburtshilfe Frauenheilkd* 36:263-264, 1976.
14. Sciarra JJ and Valle RF: Hysteroscopy: a clinical experience with 320 patients, *Am J Obstet Gynecol* 127:340-348, 1977.
15. Siegler AM: A comparison of gas and liquid for hysteroscopy, *J Reprod Med* 15:73-75, 1975.
16. Siegler AM and Kemmann F: Hysteroscopy, *Obstet Gynecol Surv* 30:567-588, 1975.
17. Phillips JM: Hysteroscopy: an overview and history of intrauterine gas insufflation, *J Reprod Med* 16:329-333, 1976.
18. Salat-Baroux J et al: Microhysteroscopy complications. In Siegler AM and Lindemann HJ (eds): *Hysteroscopy, principles and practice,* Philadelphia, 1984, JB Lippincott.
19. Taylor PJ: Correlations in infertility: symptomatology, hysterosalpingography, laparoscopy and hysteroscopy, *J Reprod Med* 18:339-342, 1977.
20. Daniell JF and Miller W: Hysteroscopic correction of cornual occlusion with resultant term pregnancy, *Fertil Steril* 48:490-492, 1987.
21. Salat-Baroux J et al: *Notre experience sur 744 hysteroscopies, actualities gynecologiques,* Paris, 1981, Masson.
22. Hamou J and Taylor PJ: Panoramic, contact, and microcolpohysteroscopy in gynecologic practice. In Leventhal JM (ed): *Current problems in obstetrics and gynecology,* 6(2), Chicago, 1982, Year Book Medical Publishers.
23. Silber SJ and Cohen RS: Microsurgical reversal tubal sterilization: five-year follow-up (abstract), *Fertil Steril* 39:398, 1983.
24. Lindemann HJ: CO₂ hysteroscopes today, *Endoscopy* 11:94-100, 1979.
25. Siegler AM, Kemmann E, and Gentile GP: Hysteroscopic procedures in 257 patients, *Fertil Steril* 27:1267-1273, 1976.
26. Cohen MR and Dmowski WP: Modern hysterorscopy: diagnostic and therapeutic potential, *Fertil Steril* 24:905-911, 1973.
27. Taylor PJ and Graham G: Is diagnostic curettage harmful in women with unexplained infertility? *Br J Obstet Gynaecol* 89:296-298, 1982.
28. Fedorkow D, Taylor PJ, and Pattinson HA: Is diagnostic hysteroscopy adhesiogenic? *Int J Fertil,* 1990.
29. Taylor PJ and Cumming DC: Hysteroscopy in 100 patients, *Fertil Steril* 31:301-304, 1979.
30. Taylor PJ and Martin RH: Semen analysis in the investigation of infertility, *Can Fam Physician* 27:113-116, 1981.
31. Taylor PJ and Cumming DC: Laparoscopy in the infertile females. In Kistner RW (ed): *Current problems in obstetrics and gynecology,* vol 2, Chicago, 1979, Year Book Medical Publishers.
32. Templeton AA and Penny GC: The incidence, characteristics, and prognosis of patients whose infertility is unexplained, *Fertil Steril* 37:175-182, 1982.
33. Cumming DC and Taylor PJ: Historical predictability of abnormal laparoscopic findings in the infertile woman, *J Reprod Med* 23:295-298, 1979.

34. Taylor PJ and Gomel V: Endoscopy in the infertile patient. In Gomel V et al (eds): *Laparoscopy and hysteroscopy in gynecologic practice*, Chicago, 1986, Year Book Medical Publishers.

35. Siegler AM: Hysterography and hysteroscopy in the infertile patient, *J Reprod Med* 18:143-148, 1977.

36. Valle RF: Hysteroscopy in the evaluation of female infertility, *Am J Obstet Gynecol* 137:425-431, 1980.

37. Hamou J, Salat-Baroux J, and Siegler AM: Diagnosis and treatment of intrauterine adhesions by microhysteroscopy, *Fertil Steril* 39:321-326, 1983.

38. Mohr J and Lindemann HJ: Hysteroscopy in the infertile patient, *J Reprod Med* 19:161-162, 1977.

39. Rosenfeld DL: A study of hysteroscopy as an adjunct to laparoscopy in the evaluation of the infertile woman. In Phillips JM (ed): *Endoscopy in gynecology*, Downey, Calif, 1978, American Association of Gynecologic Laparoscopists.

40. Taylor PJ and Leader A: Laparoscopy combined with hysteroscopy in the management of the ovulatory infertile female, *Int J Fertil* 28:59-60, 1983.

41. Sugimoto O: Hysteroscopy. II. Normal endometrial findings, *Obstet Gynecol* 131:539-547, 1978.

42. Hamou J and Salat-Baroux J: Advanced hysteroscopy and microhysteroscopy: our experience with 1000 patients. In Siegler AM and Lindemann HJ (eds): *Hysteroscopy, principles and practice*, Philadelphia, 1984, JB Lippincott.

43. Sugimoto O: Diagnostic and therapeutic hysteroscopy for traumatic intrauterine adhesions, *Am J Obstet Gynecol* 131:539-547, 1978.

44. Taylor PJ, Cumming DC, and Hill PJ: Significance of intrauterine adhesions detected hysteroscopically in eumenorrheic infertile women and role of antecedent curettage in their formation, *Am J Obstet Gynecol* 139:239-242, 1981.

45. Foix A et al: The pathology of postcurettage intrauterine adhesions, *Am J Obstet Gynecol* 96:1027-1033, 1966.

46. Taylor PJ, Hamou J, and Mencaglia L: Hysteroscopic detection of heterotopic bone formation, *J Reprod Med* 33:337-339, 1988.

47. Malpas P: A study of abortion sequences, *J Obstet Gynaecol Br Emp* 45:932-949, 1938.

48. Poland BJ et al: Reproductive counseling in patients who have had a spontaneous abortion, *Am J Obstet Gynecol* 127:685-691, 1977.

49. Warburton D and Fraser FC: Genetic aspects of abortion, *Clin Obstet Gynecol* 2:22-35, 1959.

50. Glass RH and Golbus MS: Habitual abortion, *Fertil Steril* 29:257-265, 1978.

51. Stray-Pedersen B, Eng J, and Reikvam TM: Uterine T mycoplasma colonization in reproductive failure, *Am J Obstet Gynecol* 130:307-311, 1978.

52. Beer AE et al: Major histocompatibility complex antigens, maternal and paternal immune responses, and chronic habitual abortion in humans, *Am J Obstet Gynecol* 141:987-999, 1981.

53. Oelsner G et al: Outcome of pregnancy after treatment of intrauterine adhesions, *Obstet Gynecol* 44:341-344, 1974.

54. MacKay EV and Khoo SK: Reactions in the rabbit fallopian tube after plastic reconstruction. II. Histopathology, *Fertil Steril* 23:207-216, 1972.

55. Gomel V: Recent advances in surgical correction of tubal disease producing infertility. In Kistner RW (ed): *Current problems in obstetrics and gynecology*, vol. 1, Chicago, 1978, Year Book Medical Publishers.

56. Asch RH: Laparoscopic recovery of sperm from peritoneal fluid in patients with negative or poor Sims-Huhner test, *Fertil Steril* 27:1111-1114, 1976.

57. Hammerstein J, Koch U, and Zielske F: Investigation on sperm migration in the human female genital tract as a routine diagnostic method for sterility. Presented at the World Congress on Fertility and Sterility, Buenos Aires, 1974.

58. Gomel V: Microsurgical reversal of female sterilization: a reappraisal, *Fertil Steril* 33:587-597, 1980.

59. Taylor PJ and Leader A: Reversal of female sterilization: how reliable is the previous operative report? *J Reprod Med* 27:246-248, 1982.

60. Kessel E and Mumford SD: Potential demand for voluntary female sterilization in the 1980s: the compelling need for a nonsurgical method, *Fertil Steril* 37:725-733, 1982.

61. Reed TP, Erb RA, and DeMaeyer J: Tubal occlusion with silicone rubber-update 1980, *J Reprod Med* 26:534-537, 1981.

62. Hosseinian AH, Lucero S, and Kim MH: Hysteroscopic implantation of uterotubal junction blocking devices. In Sciarra JJ, Droegmueller W, and Speidel JJ (eds): *Advances in female sterilization techniques*, Hagerstown, Md, 1976, Harper & Row.

63. Sciarra JJ: Hysteroscopic approaches to tubal closure. In Zatuchini GI, Labbock MH, and Sciarra JJ (eds): *Research frontiers in fertility regulation*, Hagerstown, Md, 1980, Harper & Row.

14

Reconstructive Surgery versus Assisted Reproductive Technology: A Treatment Dilemma

··

DAVID G. DIAZ

ROBERT B. HUNT

Before the availability of assisted reproductive technology (ART), surgeons relied on reconstructive pelvic surgery to manage infertile women with significant pelvic disease. The incorporation of fine suture materials, the use of magnification, and the emphasis placed on gentle tissue handling led to excellent pregnancy rates in selected patients. Nevertheless, some pelvic conditions cannot be repaired surgically. A method was needed that could bypass diseased fallopian tubes and still permit fertilization.

In 1978 the pioneering efforts of Steptoe and Edwards culminated in the birth of the first human being known to have been conceived under laboratory conditions. The new technology of in vitro fertilization (IVF) had arrived. Many related procedures such as gamete intrafallopian transfer (GIFT) and zygote intrafallopian transfer (ZIFT) soon evolved. Pregnancy rates for IVF/embryo transfer (ET) have stabilized at 18% to 20% per attempt in the more successful clinics, but the live birth rate continues to remain at about 10% per attempt.[1,2]

As these revolutionary events were occurring, surgical treatment for infertility continued to evolve. Many reconstructive procedures performed by laparotomy were being accomplished by laparoscopy. These advances were aided by improved instrumentation and the availability of video and lasers.

Whether treatment is undertaken with microsurgery or ART, the diagnosis of tubal disease should not automatically be considered as the sole reason for infertility. A thorough investigation of the infertile couple must be performed to rule out other contributing factors.

GENERAL CONSIDERATIONS

Experienced IVF/ET centers and skilled reconstructive surgeons are not distributed uniformly, making access difficult at times. If a couple achieves a successful pregnancy after reconstructive surgery, they may try for another pregnancy, usually without further surgery. With the exception of cryopreservation, the couple undergoing IVF/ET will have to repeat the entire procedure for another attempt.

Whereas it may take months or years to determine if a couple will conceive after reconstructive pelvic surgery, they will know within 2 weeks after embryo transfer. Furthermore, ectopic pregnancies are more common in patients undergoing reconstructive pelvic surgery compared with those selecting IVF/ET.

With IVF/ET, additional information is gathered, such as whether fertilization actually has occurred. Oocytes that fertilize may be cryopreserved and transferred to the uterus or fallopian tube during subsequent cycles. With reconstructive pelvic surgery, we only know if an oocyte has fertilized when the serum human chorionic gonadotropin (hCG) level is positive.

As a group, patients over 40 years old treated with IVF/ET have had pregnancy rates between 5% and 8%. Many factors have been cited for these low figures, including poor response to ovulation-induction agents, decreased fertilization rates, and an overall decline in reproductive capacity. The donor egg program offers hope for some of these patients. Since many IVF centers refuse to accept these patients into their programs, reconstructive surgery may be their only option. Reasonable results have been attained in patients up to age 45 years who undergo tubal anastomosis for reversal of sterilization.[3]

Economic considerations are important to most infertile couples. Whereas many insurers cover most or all of the surgical charges, they extend coverage to include IVF/ET only in a few states. Hidden but important costs related to these procedures are associated with being taken out of the work environment. These patients must be available for treatment over a 2-week period. We recommend patients remain out of work for about 1 week after surgical laparoscopy and 4 to 6 weeks after laparotomy.

PROXIMAL AND MIDTUBAL OCCLUSION

Proximal tubal occlusion accounts for one third of tubal factor infertility. It may be caused by a disease process or by prior surgical intervention. Correction involves resecting the obstructed portion and establishing tubal patency by anastomosis or implantation. Midtubal obstruction is usually a result of previous sterilization procedure or conservative management of an ectopic pregnancy.

Two separate studies yielded a pooled pregnancy rate of 59% for pathologic cornual occlusion managed by anastomosis or implantation. The live birth rate was 50%, much higher than the 10% obtained by a single IVF/ET cycle.[4,5] We obtained a 70% (7/10) viable or continuing pregnancy rate in patients undergoing cornual anastomosis for pathologic occlusion. The results with reversal of tubal sterilization have been excellent, with a viable or continuing pregnancy rate as high as 65% (13/20) in patients undergoing anastomosis.

An intriguing procedure is transcervical cannulation of the oviduct (see Chapter 12). When more data are collected we will be able to place this technology in proper perspective.

DISTAL TUBAL DISEASE

The terminal portion of the fallopian tube is involved in several infertility-related disorders ranging from thin, filmy ("friendly") adhesions to complete occlusion of its distal pole with distortion of anatomic relationships. Possible causes of distal tubal disease include bacterial pathogens, endometriosis, and surgical trauma resulting in agglutination of the delicate fimbriae. Tissue edema followed by infiltration of leukocytes subsequently results in the characteristic acute and chronic salpingitis. The inflammatory response may be limited to the serosal surface of the fallopian tube or may account for extensive destruction of the mucosal folds and the microscopic cilia that line the ampullary portion. Consequently, the production of human tubal fluid, which is critical to the

normal transport of gametes, may be compromised secondary to tissue injury. Whatever the putative cause of tubal damage might be, the end result is a defective ovum pickup mechanism and suboptimal transport of gametes through the tubal lumen.

Several classifications correlate the degree of tubal disease to the likelihood of pregnancy. Variables include the extent of ovarian surface covered by adhesions, tubal wall thickness, diameter of the hydrosalpinx, and extent of mucosal damage. Rock et al,[6] in a retrospective study of 87 patients, developed such a classification, with mild disease defined as absent or small hydrosalpinx (15 mm diameter) easily recognized fimbriae when tubal patency was restored, no significant peritubal or periovarian adhesions, and hysterosalpingogram demonstrating normal rugal folds. Eighty percent of these patients achieved an intrauterine pregnancy. Moderate disease consisted of a hydrosalpinx 15 to 30 mm in diameter, portions of fimbriae not easily identified, the presence of perifimbrial or periovarian adhesions, few cul-de-sac adhesions, and absent rugal folds on preoperative hysterosalpingogram (HSG). The pregnancy rate in this group was 17%. Severe disease was characterized by a large hydrosalpinx (30 mm in diameter), total absence of fimbriae; dense pelvic or adnexal adhesions with a fixed ovary and tube, and obliteration of the cul-de-sac. A 5% pregnancy rate was achieved in this subgroup. It should be noted that these results reflect the use of laparotomy before the advent of advanced endoscopic equipment. Subsequent series have demonstrated superior results using the techniques of surgical laparoscopy.[7]

If an HSG has been performed, we review these films if we can obtain them. We look especially for evidence of proximal disease, ampullary mucosal folds, strictures, intratubal adhesions, and spillage and dispersion of the contrast medium. After we have completed the appropriate infertility evaluation, we schedule the patient for surgical laparoscopy. At that time we perform adhesiolysis and all other indicated reparative procedures that can be accomplished by laparoscopy, including salpingostomy.

When the status of the tubal epithelium cannot be ascertained by HSG or if extensive tubal damage is encountered at laparoscopy, direct inspection of the tubal lumen can be carried out by salpingoscopy (tuboscopy). This relatively new technology has evolved from the use of a modified, rigid hysteroscope to an ultrafine, flexible endoscope capable of visualizing the crucial distal one third of the tubal lumen. We use the Olympus 2.8mm, flexible endoscope and camera, which transmit a high-quality image of the tubal endothelium. The presence of intratubal adhesions or loss of normal landmarks can therefore be determined accurately. This information is useful in estimating the prognosis and planning future management. If tubal restoration and extensive adhesiolysis have been accomplished, tuboscopy should be performed at a later time after healing of the tube has occurred.

When bipolar block (proximal and distal obstruction) is encountered, many believe these patients should be considered only for IVF/ET based on surgical success rates of 5%. Some, however, disagree. If patients are selected by careful review of laparoscopic and tuboscopic findings and other fertility factors, an acceptable success rate should be obtainable. Of three such patients, two had viable pregnancies (RBH).

SUMMARY

Reconstructive pelvic surgery and IVF/ET are not mutually exclusive. The physician and infertile couple may be confronted with the dilemma of which to choose first. Often the decision rests ultimately on practical grounds such as availability, cost, insurance coverage, time lost from work, and age.

In the meantime, we should continue to evaluate our surgical and assisted reproductive technology results and report them honestly. Researchers must strive to improve what we are already doing and to look for new and better ways to accomplish our objectives. By continued and concerted efforts, we will improve our take-home infant rates with less emotional and physical stress on our patients.

REFERENCES

1. Navot D et al: The value of in vitro fertilization for the treatment of unexplained infertility, *Fertil Steril* 49:854, 1988.
2. Chetkowski RJ, Kruse LR, and Nass TE: Improved pregnancy outcome with the addition of leuprolide acetate to gonadotropins for in vitro fertilization, *Fertil Steril* 52:250, 1989.
3. Trimbos-Kemper TCM: Reversal of sterilization in women over 40 years of age: a multicenter survey in the Netherlands, *Fertil Steril* 53:575, 1990.
4. McComb P and Gomel V: Cornual occlusion and its microsurgical reconstruction, *Clin Obstet Gynecol* 23:1229, 1980.
5. Meldrum DR: Microsurgical tubal reanastomosis: the role of splints, *Obstet Gynecol* 57:613, 1981.
6. Rock JA et al: Factors influencing the success of salpingostomy techniques for distal fimbrial occlusion, *Obstet Gynecol* 52:591, 1978.
7. Gomel V: Laparoscopic tubal surgery in infertility, *Obstet Gynecol* 46:47, 1975.

15

Advanced Endoscopic Surgery: A Perspective

···

CARL J. LEVINSON

There has been a revolution in gynecologic surgery. It started in Europe in the early 1970s and reached the United States in the early 1980s and has since spread widely. Now it even involves general surgeons.

By definition, a revolution is the "complete and forcible overthrow of an established government" or "a radical and pervasive change in society and social structure, especially one made suddenly." In the circumstances to which I refer, the latter definition is more appropriate.

In 1984 DeCherney made a presentation comparing microsurgery with the American, French, and Russian Revolutions. He pointed out that there were four phases to a revolution. Phase one is marked by gross discontent. In phase two a violent reaction to the discontent results in the overthrow of the established regime. Law and order are finally established, and a new order rules. Shortly afterward, discontent with the new order grows, especially among the young, who frequently complain that it has not gone far enough.

With respect to laparoscopy, early pioneers such as Raul Palmer demonstrated the ease and effectiveness of the procedure, even with relatively crude instruments. From France and Germany (Bruhat and Semm) information progressed to Great Britain (Steptoe) and the United States (Cohen). In the 1960s culdoscopy was being performed in some centers, with great dissatisfaction because of the positioning and limitation of the endoscopic exploration. Even in the early stages of laparoscopy, the discontent spilled over, branding the procedure as a "gimmick."

In phase two the radical and pervasive change took place and, although not immediate, progression was rapid. At about the time the first formal organization dedicated to laparoscopy was being formed, centers in Kiel, Germany, and Clermont-Ferrand, France, were overthrowing the shackles that limited the practice of this technique. Whereas laparoscopy itself was a major transition from traditional laparotomy, a subset of the revolution developed in the late 1970s and early 1980s with the performance of advanced laparoscopic surgery. In phase three, a new order was established with codification of procedures and techniques, reports of results (particularly from abroad), and the emergence of pioneers in the new surgery. Standard equipment was soon to be supplemented by a new form of energy, the laser.

As might have been anticipated, there was much discontent with the new order, but surprisingly enough, it developed on both sides of the issue. Some indicated concern that these procedures were not for everyone, that they took too long, that laser is not only expensive, it is overkill, and that the operating room would not be able to handle the situation. A new subset of pioneers were expanding into unexplored areas: hysterectomy, node dissection, and, in 1990, cholecystectomy.

What effect did the revolution have? Although there are more important effects to be discussed, it became evident to me that there was less need to make rounds at the hospital. Procedures were performed in such a manner that patients could return home the same day. A survey of medical records at my own hospital indicated that approximately 50% of procedures performed by laparotomy in 1984 were performed by endoscopy in 1988 to 1989. Oophorectomy, salpingectomy, and ovarian cystectomy were performed by both laparoscopy and laparotomy. Patients who underwent laparoscopy spent only one third of the time in the hospital, required only 20% of the time for recovery, and were charged approximately 50%, compared with laparotomy.

Given all these circumstances, there was bound to be enthusiasm resulting in trial and experimentation and education and training resulting in more widespread use.

219

Other possible indications for laparoscopy were treatment of acute abscess, early treatment for acute pelvic inflammatory disease (PID), laparoscopic surgery for distal tubal disease, and methods to diagnose ovarian malignancies.

Advanced endoscopic surgery has several economies. Economy of time is achieved with experience. For example, it is not necessary to open and close the abdomen. Cosmetic economy is presented to the patient in the form of two, three, or four small (6 to 11 mm) incisions that generally heal with minimal (and often nonvisible) scarring. There is economy of discomfort in that most patients do not require excessive medication. The economy of function is evident in a recovery period of 1 to 5 days rather than 2 to 5 weeks. In this age of cost accounting, economy is realized in that the procedure is performed at lower cost than laparotomy.

Several special aspects are associated with advanced endoscopic surgery. Video recording is possible for education, and to facilitate assistance and interest. Exploration is complete in that the entire abdominal cavity from diaphragm to cul-de-sac can be examined easily. In the process, manipulation of all organs is greatly facilitated. The use of the laser adds a significant tool to cutting and coagulation. A variety of other energy sources are available to allow for electrosurgery and the use of mechanical devices. Although lavage and suction have been used regularly, they continue to have special value in endoscopic procedures and even greater significance in the therapy of acute PID and pelvic abscesses. Perhaps most significant is the fact that the procedure allows for diagnosis and therapy under the same anesthetic. (Preparation is necessary, however, involving full discussion with the patient preoperatively.)

FALLOPIAN TUBE

Laparoscopic surgery at the cornual end of the tube is, for the most part, inappropriate. A cornual pregnancy occasionally can be removed through the laparoscope, but this can be a formidable exercise and should be done only by experienced surgeons. Surgery at the isthmus is related to ectopic pregnancy or anastomosis. Anastomosis has been performed endoscopically but primarily as an experimental procedure using sutures at the 6 and 12 o'clock positions. In Europe this is augmented by the use of fibrin glue, which is applied to the serosa to hold the two sutured ends together. The success rate is relatively poor.

Most tubal surgery is performed at the distal end of the tube in situations where this portion may be partly or completely occluded. This can be performed with the laparoscope. Salpingolysis may be all that is necessary to free the distal tube. In so doing, a fimbrioplasty may

be accomplished. If the tube is completely occluded (hydrosalpinx), it is cleared of adhesions, and an incision can be made by laser, electrosurgery, or mechanical means. Once a passage is made into the tube salpingostomy, the incision can be extended by cutting or stretching. The extent and value of the mucosa are determined, and additional radial dissections are made as needed. The previously distended tube is checked once again for the free passage of dye. The serosa near the edge of the new stoma can then be contracted using bipolar current, endotherm, or a diffused laser beam. In this manner, the edges of the newly formed stoma are everted. Although some have attempted to suture the edges of the new stoma, this is generally not done, nor is it believed to be necessary. All of these procedures can be performed using the laparoscope.

ECTOPIC PREGNANCY

The ectopic (tubal) pregnancy is becoming more amenable to conservative and laparoscopic therapy. The diagnosis is made by a combination of appropriate suspicion, β-human chorionic gonadotropin levels, and ultrasound. In competent hands, virtually all such procedures can be managed with the laparoscope. Where such skill is not readily available, patients with great blood loss or shock should undergo laparotomy.

The endoscopic procedure is begun as a diagnostic laparoscopy, after which strategic decisions are made, assessing the amount of blood in the pelvis, evaluating the opposite tube, and noting the patient's desire for future pregnancy. Laparoscopic management may be conservative, removing just the products of conception, or radical, removing part or all of the tube. Dilute pitressin is injected into the mesosalpinx of the affected tube. An incision is made into the tube with laser, mechanical instruments, or electrosurgery. The products of conception are removed from the tube and from the abdomen. It is not necessary to suture the incision. It may be appropriate at this time to perform minor tubal repair on the opposite side, such as adhesiolysis. In my opinion it is not the appropriate time to perform major tuboplastic repair by fimbrioplasty or salpingostomy. All of the procedures described can be performed endoscopically.

Should it be necessary, partial or total salpingectomy can also be performed with the laparoscope. In the case of isthmic tubal pregnancy, both ends can be coagulated together with the attached mesosalpinx. The involved tube, with the products of conception, can then be removed. If the tube is damaged beyond repair, it can be removed, starting at the cornu and proceeding to the infundibular pelvic ligament. Major vessels are controlled by clips, electrosurgery, endotherm, or an Endoloop, and the tube is excised.

OVARIAN CYSTS

Ovarian cysts are particularly amenable to surgery by the laparoscope; however, this statement is not without its caveats. The spectre of malignancy must always be considered with every cyst. If malignancy is a consideration, washings should be done at entry into the peritoneal cavity, the other ovary should be inspected for papillary excrescences, and solid areas should be biopsied. It has never been established as to whether the spill of a malignant ovarian cyst into the peritoneum cavity has any effect on the prognosis for that patient.

Functional cysts should not be surgically treated. These should have been treated previously with observation or suppressive therapy.

Mucous or serous cystadenomas can generally be dissected free of the adjacent ovary using surgical instruments or the laser. Traction on the ovarian cyst with countertraction on the ovarian tissue is important. It is better to hold the cyst and to pull on the more solid ovary. Scissors are used for dissection. Once the cyst has been dissected free it can be emptied. This is best performed by inserting the trocar and sleeve directly into the cyst. The trocar is removed and replaced by the lavage-suction equipment. The interior of the cyst is washed and suctioned repeatedly. The collapsed cyst can then be grasped, dissected free of the ovary, and removed, cutting it into pieces if necessary. Should a portion of cyst remain within the ovary, this can be ablated. It is not necessary to close the ovary, although some surgeons prefer to do so. During the procedure, the ovary and pelvis are lavaged frequently and fluid is suctioned from the cul-de-sac. Hemostasis is obtained with the laser or with electrosurgery.

Dermoid cysts present a special problem, since rupture of their wall results in release of potentially noxious agents. The presence of fat, sebaceous material, and hair within the peritoneal cavity presents a hazard for immediate infection or long-term adhesion formation. Therefore the surgeon who chooses to remove a dermoid cyst by the laparoscope should have a clear-cut strategy.

A decision should be made early as to how the cyst will be removed: intact or ruptured, through the anterior abdominal wall, or through the cul-de-sac.

It should be dissected while intact. The dissection is easier, but traction on the cyst itself is obviously more difficult. The cyst is dissected free gently until it is almost free of the adjacent ovary. At this point, the surgeon has two options. First, the intact cyst can be removed and "parked" in the cul-de-sac. Subsequently, a culdotomy is performed and the cyst is removed. The cul-de-sac incision is then closed. The second choice is to open the cyst and remove its contents by means of alternating lavage and suction. It is then relatively easy to complete the dissection and remove the cyst through the abdominal wall. Under these circumstances it may be necessary to insert a larger 11-mm cannula into the suprapubic area. If necessary, scissors may be used to cut the cyst wall into segments that can be removed through the cannula.

Large ovarian cysts, potentially malignant ovarian cysts, dermoid cysts in young women in whom fertility is to be preserved, if the surgeon is not certain that the cyst can be removed cleanly, and any ovarian surgery that is beyond the surgeon's ability to remove endoscopically are treated by laparotomy.

Oophorectomy also can be accomplished by laparoscopy. The appropriate indications are as important as the technique. Blood vessels at the infundibular pelvic ligament and the utero-ovarian ligament can be controlled with bipolar current, clips, endotherm, or Endoloop. After excision, it may be difficult to remove the ovary, particularly if it is large. Biopsy, ovariolysis, and wedge resection also can be performed laparoscopically.

UTERUS

Until recently, several specific pathologic entities involving the uterus could not be treated by the laparoscope or hysteroscope. These have been slightly modified. The diffuse nature of adenomyosis makes it a condition to be treated by laparotomy. Extremely large myomata should be removed by laparotomy. Exceptions are lesions that can be shrunk adequately by the use of gonadotropin-releasing hormone.

Any surgery for malignancy (carcinoma, sarcoma) involving the uterus should be performed by laparotomy. Radical laparoscopic hysterectomy with node dissection has been described, but since no results have been reported after this procedure, appropriate surgery is still laparotomy.

Some myomata may be removed through the laparoscope, particularly small ones and those located subserosally. The word *remove* has two meanings here, however. The myomata may be removed from the uterus, and it is necessary also to remove them from the abdomen. The technique is much the same as by laparotomy: injection of vasopressin, incision, dissection of the myoma from the capsule, hemostasis at the base, and resuturing of the uterine wall (although in many cases suturing is not done). Large myomata involving the intramural area can also be removed with appropriate skill and equipment. They may be morcellated, cut into sections, or placed in the cul-de-sac to be removed by culdotomy. None of these procedures is especially easy. Myomas should not be removed "because they are there." If they are large and strategically placed, near the cornua, major vessels, or the cervix, laparotomy is probably a safer approach.

Submucosal myomata often can be removed with the hysteroscope. This endoscopic procedure should be reserved for those who are trained and for patients who have had recurrent abortions or abnormal bleeding.

Adhesions

Adhesions are the bête noire of pelvic surgery, whether they be primary (attributable to infection or endometriosis) or secondary (attributable to prior surgery). Laparoscopic adhesiolysis is possible for most adhesions, certainly those that are minimal and thin, as well as those that are moderate and mildly vascular. They can be managed with laser, electrosurgery, or mechanical techniques (scissors or knives). Laparotomy is appropriate for surgeons who have less experience with dense and vascular adhesions and for special circumstances of dense adhesions in particularly sensitive sites: the sidewall of the pelvic cavity (wherein reside the ureter and major vessels); the cul-de-sac, which may be bound down to the rectosigmoid; and the region of the tube and ovary where these two structures may be intimately bound by prior disease. Under these circumstances, vital organs are involved and there is increased chance for hemorrhage and organ damage. Often these adhesions are best treated by laparotomy.

Endometriosis

In the hands of experienced surgeons, virtually all conservative surgery for endometriosis can be performed by laparoscopy. This includes lysis of adhesions, coagulation of endometriosis, partial or complete resection of endometriomas, ablation of the base of an endometrioma where the cyst wall has not been completely removed, resection of endometriosis from peritoneal surfaces, and resection or ablation of endometriosis involving the serosa of the bowel.

Practical considerations dictate a more cautious approach to extensive disease. For those with less experience, laparotomy would be indicated for large endometriomas, particularly those bound down by dense adhesions; endometriomas or endometriosis intimately involved with the peritoneum overlying the ureter and iliac vessels; endometriosis involving the bowel where the depth of the lesion cannot be determined or appears to be extensive; and endometriosis involving a broad segment of sidewall, cul-de-sac, and rectosigmoid.

SUMMARY

Much experimentation has taken place in endoscopic surgery. As a result, appendectomy, hysterectomy, pelvic lymph node dissection, and cholecystectomy have been performed endoscopically. The evidence is clear: given the appropriate experience and instrumentation, these procedures can be performed. History has shown us that there is a progression of this experience. Initially, a procedure is performed by individuals or small groups. The technique is then duplicated in other centers, indicating feasibility. If the procedure is direct (e.g., salpingotomy to remove an ectopic tubal pregnancy), it becomes the standard of care. The response on the part of the medical profession is additional education, usually in the form of hands-on courses, further dissemination of information of the actual technique itself, increased awareness of the availability of the procedure, and, ultimately, widespread use of the procedure. Since these occur in hospitals that have teaching programs, it becomes a normal experience for the residents who ultimately adopt it as part of their routine training (e.g., use of the laser).

Given this format, it would not be unusual for these comments to be outdated by the time this book is published. By that time, I suspect that cholecystectomy will be performed by laparoscopy more frequently than by laparotomy, and even newer technical advances will have been made.

SELECTED READINGS

1. Baggish MS: *Endoscopic laser surgery*, New York, 1990, Elsevier.
2. Donnez J: *Laser operative laparoscopy and hysteroscopy*, Leuven, Belgium, 1989, Nauwelarts.
3. Dubuisson JB et al: Reproductive outcome after laparoscopic salpingectomy for tubal pregnancy, *Fertil Steril* 53:1004, 1990.
4. Keye W Jr.: The present and future application of laser to the treatment of endometriosis, *Fertil Steril* 47:208, 1990.
5. Mage G et al: Laparoscopic management of adnexal torsion, *J Reprod Med* 34:520-524, 1989.
6. Mage G et al: Use of CO_2 laser via laparoscopy. Presented at the third international congress for laser surgery, Graz, September 24-26, 1979.
7. Mage G et al: CO_2 laser microsurgery: five years' experience, *Microsurgery* 8:89-91, 1987.
8. Martin DC: CO_2 laser laparoscopy for endometriosis associated with infertility, *J Reprod Med* 31:1089-1094, 1986.
9. Nezhat C, Winer WK, and Nezhat F: Laparoscopic removal of dermoid cysts, *Obstet Gynecol* 72:2, 1989.
10. Nezhat C, Winer WK, and Nezhat F: Endoscopic infertility surgery, *J Reprod Med* 34:127, 1989.
11. Palmer R: La celioscopie gynecologique rapport du prof mocquot, *Acad Chir* 72:363-368, 1946.
12. Pouly JL et al: Conservative laparoscopic treatment 321 ectopic pregnancies, *Fertil Steril* 46:1093, 1986.
13. Reich H et al: Laparoscopic treatment of 109 consecutive tubal pregnancies, *J Reprod Med* 33:885-890, 1988.
14. Reich H and McGlynn F: Laparoscopic treatment of tubo-ovarian abscess, *Am J Obstet Gynecol* 151:1098, 1985.
15. Sanfilippo JS and Levine RL: *Operative gynecologic endoscopy*, New York, 1989, Springer-Verlag.
16. Semm K: *Operative manual for endoscopic abdominal surgery*, Chicago, 1987, Year Book Medical Publishers.

16

Open Laparoscopy

ROBERT B. HUNT

Although closed laparoscopy is generally a safe procedure, accidents do occur. To lessen the chance of injury I have converted entirely to open laparoscopy. If the steps described in this chapter are taken, the advantages are as follows:

1. Virtual elimination of aortic and iliac vessel injury.
2. Elimination of gas emboli.
3. Possible reduction in frequency of bowel injury.
4. Ability to release pneumoperitoneum rapidly in an emergency.
5. Marked reduction in frequency of failed laparoscopy and omental emphysema.
6. Elimination of postoperative fascial hernias at the site of laparoscopic entry.

Potential disadvantages of the technique are as follows:

1. Need to learn a new technique.
2. Increased surgery time.
3. Wound complications.
4. Possibly a larger surgical scar.

COMPLICATIONS
Blood vessel injury

The complication of large blood vessel injury is serious and potentially fatal. Of 99,204 laparoscopic procedures performed in France, there were 31 major internal vessel injuries: 20 with the Veress needle and 11 with the sharp trocar.[1] Another series reported 5 cases of major vessel injury.[2] One resulted in a laparotomy with repair of the right iliac artery; one in laparotomy and repair of the aorta, and the need to administer several units of blood; one in a second laparotomy, 22 U of blood, and a $500,000 lawsuit; one in permanent brain damage; and one in death. I strongly recommend changing to the open technique to prevent these injuries.

A survey in the United Kingdom by the Royal College of Obstetricians and Gynaecologists revealed 9 major vessel injuries per 10,000 procedures performed.[3] In 1975, 12 laparoscopists from United States, Great Britain, and Holland reported 19 such untoward events.[4]

The Centers for Disease Control monitored deaths from sterilization procedures from 1977 to 1981. Of the three associated with vascular injury, one each resulted from the Veress needle and sharp trocar, and one from inappropriate use of a scalpel to open the abdomen.[5]

One author collected over 100 injuries to the aorta or iliac vessels that were inflicted with either the Veress needle or sharp trocar.[6] Open laparoscopy performed as described in this chapter should eliminate major vessel injury.

Gas embolism

Although unusual, gas emboli do occur in closed laparoscopy. Three fatal cases were reported in 99,204 procedures.[1] Each patient had auscultatory findings of gas emboli, and one had the insufflation needle "stuck in the left common iliac vein."[1] Each accident was thought to have occurred during insufflation, and the author stressed the importance of performing the syringe security test in closed laparoscopies, as well as discontinuing the procedure if it is not going well. In addition, the author emphasized the need for the anesthesiologist and surgeon to monitor intraperitoneal pressure.

Six fatalities were caused by air embolism in 642 patients with laparoscopic complications.[7] The diagnosis is made by detection of a so-called mill wheel murmur and is treated by turning the patient on her left side and aspirating the ventricle by needle or cardiac catheterization.[8] Obviously, prevention is better. Open laparoscopy should avoid this complication.

Bowel injuries

Punctures of bowel do occur at laparoscopy. In a series of 1024 surgeons reporting on 125,560 sterilization procedures performed laparoscopically, the frequency of unrecognized and recognized bowel injuries was 0.11 and

0.31 per 1000 cases, respectively.[9] Surgeons who perform advanced surgical laparoscopy should expect a higher frequency, however, because of underlying disease and the complex techniques required to deal with the disease.

Of 99,204 laparoscopies in France, 31 resulted in gastrointestinal injury.[1] Five were trocar injuries after insufflation of bowel and 26 were pure trocar perforations. Two patients died of complications. Forty-seven instances were disclosed in a survey of 63,845 cases reported in the German literature.[10]

A collected series of 56,106 laparoscopies reported damage attributable to trocar or Veress needle in 20 cases: 9 stomach, 5 small bowel, and 6 large bowel.[8]

Open laparoscopy does not completely eliminate bowel injuries. Six were reported in 10,840 open laparoscopic procedures performed by 18 surgeons. Of these, 5 were known to be scalpel lacerations inflicted by sharply opening the peritoneum.[4] Another small bowel injury was caused by opening the peritoneum with a scalpel.[11] The technique described in this chapter avoids opening the peritoneum sharply.

In my experience, one colon and two small bowel injuries occurred with the trocar using the closed technique. Two of these would have been avoided had I used the open technique. I have produced two small bowel injuries at the site of entry using the open technique. In each of these two instances, the bowel was fused to the peritoneum at the umbilicus. That laparoscopic bowel injuries occur only in the hands of the inexperienced is not true. My first bowel injury occurred after 12 years of experience. In France, experienced laparoscopists performing closed procedures reported 58 insufflation injuries.[1]

Bowel injuries associated with open laparoscopy should be relatively infrequent. The one problem that may result in injury is bowel tightly fused to the parietal peritoneum at the site of entry.

Cardiac arrest

Cardiac arrest may occur with open or closed laparoscopy and has been estimated to occur in approximately 0.3 per 1000 cases.[8] Suggested causes are increased partial pressure of carbon dioxide (CO_2), vagal reflexes from abdominal distention, decreased venous return attributable to increased intraabdominal pressure, and gas emboli. Should cardiac arrest occur during the procedure, the intraabdominal gas can be released within seconds by the open technique with rapid restoration of normal intraperitoneal pressures and, it is hoped, correction of the dysrhythmia.[12]

Herniations

Herniations in closed laparoscopy at the site of primary trocar entry do occur and can be serious. They require repair by laparotomy.[13] A review of 56,106 laparoscopies disclosed 6 omental and 2 small bowel herniations at the site of trocar entry.[8]

Herniation through the fascia is avoided by the open technique since the fascial defect is closed. An extraperitoneal, subfascial herniation can occur with either open or closed technique, however. Therefore, regardless of the technique, the surgeon should always visualize the peritoneal cavity through the laparoscope as the instrument is withdrawn to prevent this complication.

Failed laparoscopy attempt

Inappropriate gas insufflation is a relatively common problem in closed laparoscopy. Two studies reported 4 per 1000 and 12 per 1000, respectively.[14,15] Of 276 patients, there were 12 (8%) failures to establish a pneumoperitoneum in another study.[16]

In a series of 56,106 patients, the laparoscopy could not be completed in 39 patients because of gas being placed either in the omentum or the preperitoneal space.[8]

Two national surveys by the American Association of Laparoscopists revealed failure rates of 11.3 per 1000 diagnostic procedures out of 36,411 procedures and 6.7 per 1000 for 76,842 sterilization procedures.[17] Other studies of over 1000 procedures reported a frequency of between 1 and 4 per 1000.[18,19] In three patients in whom the surgeon was unable to produce a satisfactory pneumoperitoneum, these laparoscopic procedures were completed successfully by converting to the open technique.[20]

It may be difficult to establish a pneumoperitoneum successfully in massively obese patients. Nine patients weighing more than 250 pounds had failed closed laparoscopy. The open technique allowed completion of the procedure in each patient.[21]

Wound complications

Patients generally do complain of slight incisional discomfort with the open technique, but this is not disabling. Wound cellulitis occurred in 3 of 175 patients undergoing open laparoscopy.[22] Only 3 of 150 patients experienced minor wound infections, with contamination from the navel being the probable cause in one case.[11] In a later series there were 2 minor wound infections in 630 open laparoscopies performed for tubal sterilization.[23] Of 10,840 open procedures, there were 18 wound infections, none of which required drainage.[4] The importance of cleansing the navel immediately before surgery and minimizing tissue trauma should be stressed. I have not experienced any wound infections requiring drainage out of 723 consecutive open laparoscopies over 3 years. I did explore the wound and remove the fascial suture in two of these patients to relieve pain, probably attributable to nerve entrapment. I have since changed to absorbable sutures.

Wound infections occur in closed as well as open laparoscopies. These infections were reported in 3 of 276 patients undergoing closed procedures.[16]

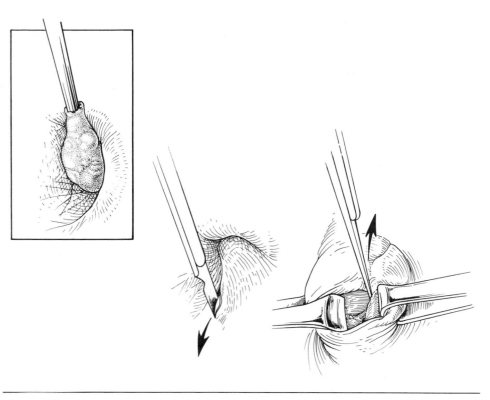

Figure 16-1
(Inset) The navel is cleansed with a cotton applicator in soaked antiseptic solution. The orientation shown is maintained throughout the figures. **A,** An incision is made in the inferior portion of the navel, taking care to incise only the skin. This vertical incision corresponds to Langer's lines. **B,** The incision is extended to the base of the navel.

In the technique shown in this chapter, the vertical incision is 1.5 cm in length, just large enough to accommodate a 1.0-cm laparoscope. Since the incision extends into the navel fossa and corresponds to Langer's lines, it is barely visible.

LEARNING OPEN LAPAROSCOPY

The surgeon can become proficient in open laparoscopy after approximately 20 procedures. In my experience surgery time is increased by about 3 minutes over the closed technique. A controlled study of four surgeons reported that minor surgical difficulties with the open technique dropped from 5.0% to 1.7% after the first 100 cases each surgeon performed.[24] Complications with the open technique were not, however, increased in these first 100 cases. Thus surgeons trained in closed laparoscopy can make the transition to the open technique safely.

Popularity

The open technique has not become popular. In 1982 only 4% of 124,560 procedures used this approach.[9] A 1988 survey by the same organization showed essentially no change in the percentage of cases being performed by the open technique.[25] I suspect the reason is that most surgeons performing laparoscopy have experienced few complications and therefore resist changing to an alternative procedure.

Currently the disposable trocar is championed by many. Although it offers some advantages over the standard trocar, it is expensive and does not prevent Veress needle and some trocar injuries.

One author described open laparoscopy using standard operating room instruments in 40 patients.[26] Another reported opening the peritoneum with finger dissection.[27] Other techniques have been described.[12,22,28]

By extending laparoscopic surgery to include rather complex procedures on patients with abnormal abdominal and pelvic anatomy, I hope the reader will consider using the open technique. In my view, if surgeons can prevent one major complication in their careers by using this technique, the extra 3 minutes required in each case is worthwhile.

Anesthesia

Although my experience with open laparoscopy has been with general anesthesia exclusively, local anesthesia is acceptable in the properly selected patient.

Text cont'd on p. 234.

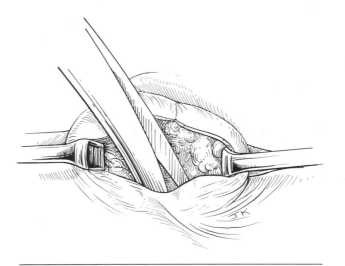

Figure 16-2
Fibrous tissue is divided with Metzenbaum scissors.

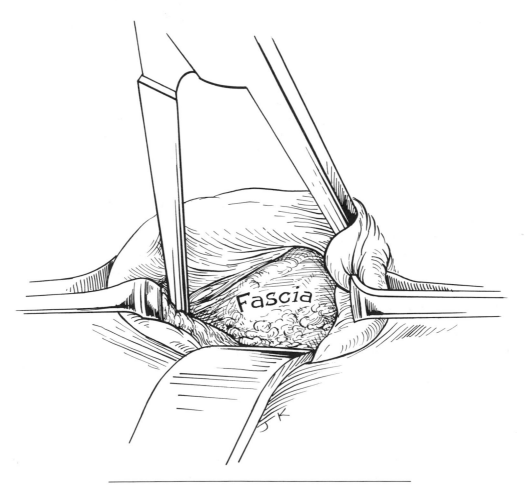

Figure 16-3
Subcutaneous tissue is cleared away with a fine hemostat.
The Alys clamps may be removed at this time if desirable.
The S retractor is an aid in the dissection.

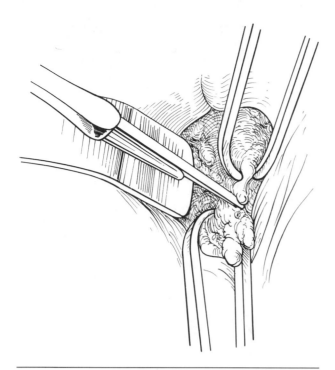

Figure 16-4
The S retractor is to the right of the navel, and Alys clamps grasp the fascia superiorly and inferiorly. The fascia is incised transversely with a scalpel. The skin is protected by the retractor.

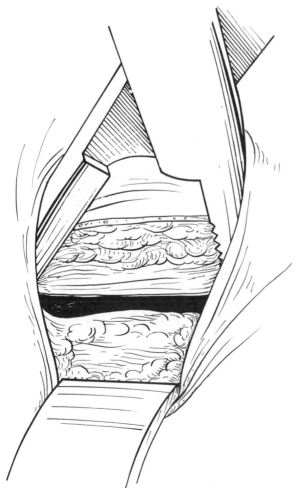

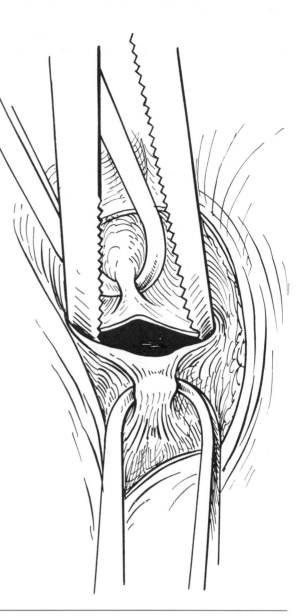

Figure 16-5
The tips of a hemostat are placed inside the fascial defect.

Figure 16-6
Alys clamps are removed and the hemostat opened slowly and widely. This enlarges the fascial defect. Significant bleeding is an unusual occurrence and usually ceases spontaneously. If achieving hemostasis is difficult, a suction tip should be used to expose the bleeding vessel.

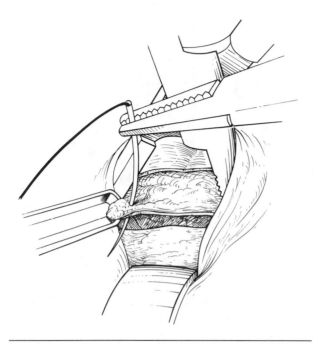

Figure 16-7
A figure-of-eight suture of 2-0 absorbable material is placed in the fascia. The hemostat and S retractor expose the surgical site.

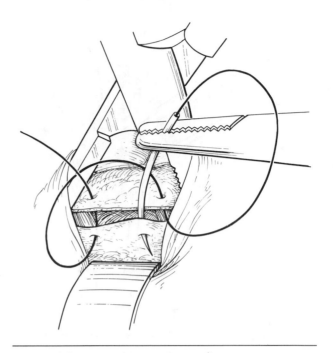

Figure 16-8
The fascial stitch is completed.

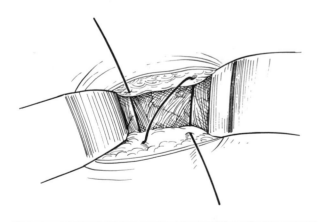

Figure 16-9
The S retractors are placed laterally through the fascial defect. The rectus muscles are visible beneath the fascia.

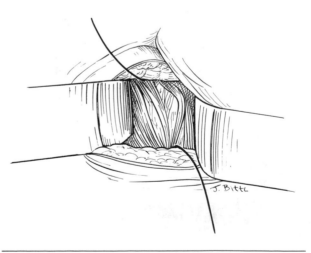

Figure 16-10
The S retractors are used to dissect posteriorly to the transversalis fascia.

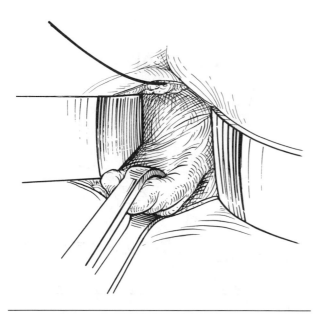

Figure 16-11
The transversalis fascia is grasped transversely with an Alys clamp.

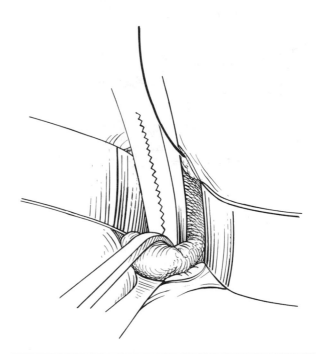

Figure 16-12
A Kelly clamp is pushed gently but firmly through the transversalis fascia and peritoneum. The jaws are directed inferiorly and anteriorly to relieve pressure on the Alys clamp and to direct the jaws away from the sacral promontory, major vessels, and bowel. Alternatively, the clamp may be advanced superiorly.

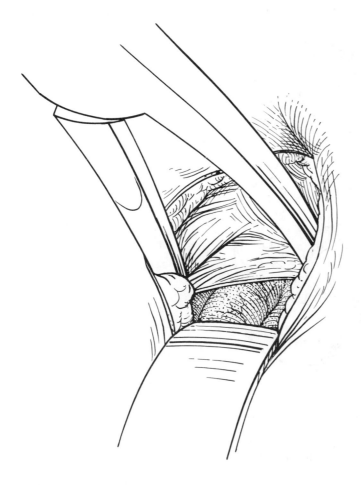

Figure 16-13
The jaws of the clamp are now opened slowly and widely, which enlarges the opening through the transversalis fascia and peritoneum.

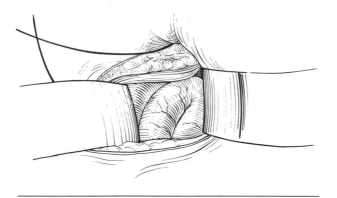

Figure 16-14
The S retractors are inserted inside the peritoneum and retracted laterally. This exposes the bowel.

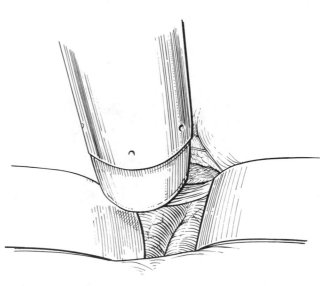

Figure 16-15
The Hasson cannula is inserted.

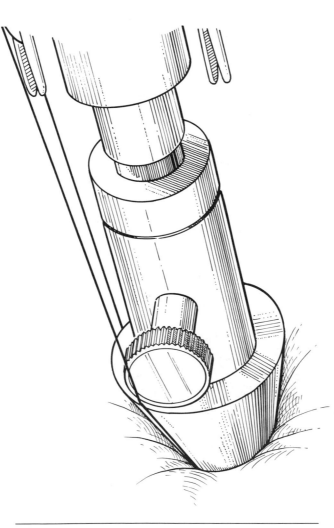

Figure 16-16
The cannula is now fully inserted. The two ends of the fascial suture are secured around one of the cannula cleats.

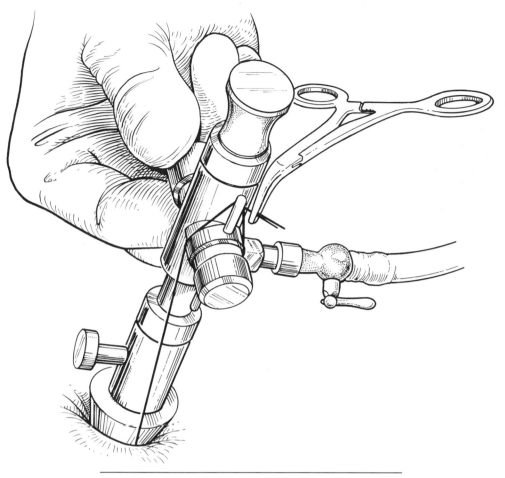

Figure 16-17
The cannula is in place and all connections completed.

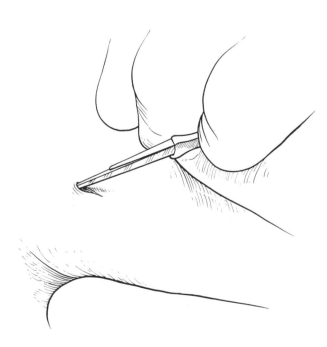

Figure 16-18
A small incision is made transversely in the right lower quadrant, just lateral to the deep epigastric vessels. The position of these vessels is determined by viewing them directly with the laparoscope from the peritoneal side.

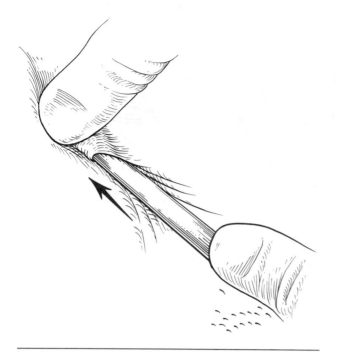

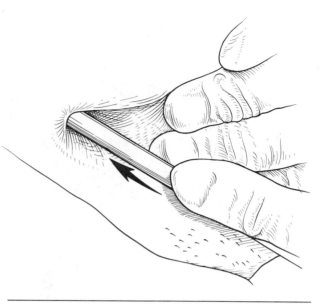

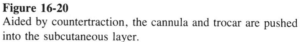

Figure 16-20
Aided by countertraction, the cannula and trocar are pushed into the subcutaneous layer.

Figure 16-19
The trocar is guided through the skin by the index finger of the opposite hand to prevent its slipping and lacerating the skin. Note the trocar is directed laterally and superiorly.

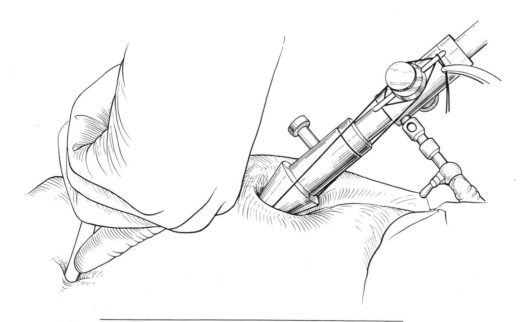

Figure 16-21
The trocar and cannula are redirected toward the pelvis in a position of function and inserted through the remaining layers of the abdominal wall just lateral to the deep epigastric vessels. The surgeon constantly observes progress by viewing directly through the laparoscope or off the video screen.

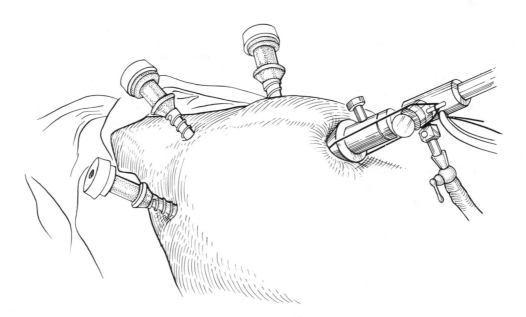

Figure 16-22
Three secondary cannulas have been positioned. The urinary bladder must be visualized laparoscopically before inserting the midline cannula to avoid bladder injury.

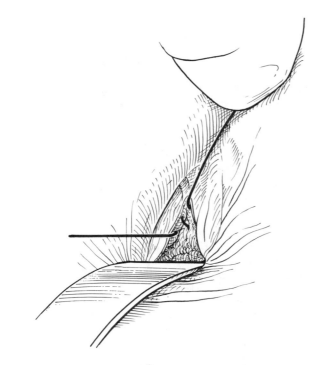

Figure 16-23
The laparoscopy has been completed and the laparoscope withdrawn from the abdomen as the surgeon views through it directly or off the videoscreen. The fascial stitch is being tied. Note the S retractor in the inferior side of the wound to prevent superficial layers becoming entangled in the suture. Any fascial defect greater than 7 mm should be sutured shut to prevent hernia. Interrupted subcuticular sutures of 4-0 absorbable material are placed to close the skin incisions.

Contraindications

Absolute and relative contraindications for open and closed laparoscopy are the same. Absolute contraindications are few, although many relative ones have been written about. Among these are excessive obesity, previous peritonitis, abdominal carcinomatosis or tuberculosis, hiatal hernia, cardiorespiratory disease, and previous pneumothorax. The surgeon will probably elect not to perform laparoscopy on the patient who is in shock from a significant hemoperitoneum, suffering from acute, generalized peritonitis, or experiencing intestinal obstruction. Great care must be taken in performing laparoscopy on patients with umbilical hernia, since 60% of these hernias have abdominal contents.[8]

Technique

Open laparoscopy is made easy because of the relatively thin abdominal wall at the navel, the so-called window to the peritoneum. Skin, anterior fascia, and linea alba, the two obliterated umbilical arteries, urachus, transversalis fascia, and peritoneum converge at the navel, and the subcutaneous fat is markedly reduced in thickness.[29,30,31,32] The procedure that is shown (Figures 16-1 through 16-23) is a modification of Hasson's method.[11,29,33,34]

SUMMARY

Open and closed laparoscopy both carry a low frequency of complications. The availability of disposable cannulas may give the surgeon a false sense of security. The Veress needle, with its associated dangers, is often used initially, and the sharp disposable trocar must still protrude into the abdomen for a short distance before being covered by a plastic material. Although not without problems, the open technique avoids many serious and potentially fatal complications. I urge every laparoscopist to become skilled in performing this technique.

REFERENCES

1. Mintz M: Risks and prophylaxis in laparoscopy: a survey of 100,000 cases, *J Reprod Med* 18:26, 1977.
2. Penfield AJ: Vascular injuries and their management. In Phillips JM (ed): *Endoscopy in gynecology*, Downey, Calif, 1978, American Association of Gynecologic Laparoscopists.
3. Chamberlain G and Brown JC (eds): *Gynaecological laparoscopy: the report of the confidential enquiry into gynaecological laparoscopy*, London, 1978, Royal College of Obstetricians and Gynaecologists.
4. Penfield AJ: How to prevent complications of open laparoscopy, *J Reprod Med* 30:660, 1985.
5. Peterson HB et al: Deaths attributable to tubal sterilization in the US 1977-1981, *Am J Obstet Gynecol* 146:131, 1983.
6. Penfield AJ: Open laparoscopy, surgical equipment and training in reproductive health. In Burkman RT, Magarick RH, and Waife RS, (eds): *Johns Hopkins program for international gynecology and obstetrics*, Baltimore, 1979, Johns Hopkins University Press.
7. Siegler AM: Trends in laparoscopy, *Am J Obstet Gynecol* 109:794, 1971.
8. Loffer FD and Pent D: Indications, contraindications and complications of laparoscopy, *Obstet Gynecol Surv* 30:407, 1975.
9. Phillips JM, Hulka JF, and Peterson HB: American Association of Gynecologic Laparoscopists' 1982 membership survey, *J Reprod Med* 29:592, 1984.
10. Bruhl W: Complications of laparoscopy and liver biopsy under vision: the results of a survey, *Ger Med Monoschr* 12:31, 1967.
11. Hasson HM: Open laparoscopy: a report of 150 cases, *J Reprod Med* 12:234, 1974.
12. Perone N: Conventional vs. open laparoscopy, *Am Fam Physician* 27:147, 1983.
13. Sauer M and Jarrett JC II: Small bowel obstruction following diagnostic laparoscopy, *Fertil Steril* 42:653, 1984.
14. Duignan NM: One thousand consecutive cases of diagnostic laparoscopy, *J Obstet Gynaecol Br Commonw* 79:1016-1024, 1972.
15. Kleppinger RK: One thousand laparoscopies at a community hospital, *J Reprod Med* 13:13, 1974.
16. Peterson EP and Behrman SJ: Laparoscopy of the infertile patient, *Obstet Gynecol* 36:363, 1970.
17. Phillips J et al: Gynecologic laparoscopy in 1975, *J Reprod Med* 16:105, 1976.
18. Hasson HM: Open laparoscopy vs. closed laparoscopy: a comparison of complication rates, *Adv Planned Parenthood* 13:41, 1978.
19. Uribe-Ramirez LC et al: Outpatient laparoscopic sterilization: a review of complications in 2,000 cases, *J Reprod Med* 18:103, 1977.
20. Dodson MG: The treatment of failed laparoscopy using open laparoscopy, *Int J Gynaecol Obstet* 22:331, 1984.
21. Holtz G: Laparoscopy in the massively obese female, *Obstet Gynecol* 69:423, 1987.
22. Sur S: Modified method of open laparoscopy, *J Reprod Med* 30:421, 1985.
23. Hasson HM: Open laparoscopy for tubal occlusion in the female, *Adv Contracept* 1:181, 1985.
24. Bhiwandiwala PP, Mumford SD, and Kennedy KI: Comparison of the safety of open and conventional laparoscopic sterilization, *Obstet Gynecol* 66:391, 1985.
25. Hulka JF, Peterson HB, and Phillips JM: American Association of Gynecologic Laproscopists' 1988 membership survey on laproscopic sterilization, *J Reprod Med* 35:584, 1990.
26. Grimes EM: Open laparoscopy with conventional instrumentation, *Obstet Gynecol* 57:375, 1981.
27. Grundsell H and Larsson G: A modified laparoscopic entry technique using a finger, *Obstet Gynecol* 59:509, 1982.
28. Treat M et al: A technique for open peritoneoscopy, *Surgery* 92:544, 1982.
29. Hasson HM: Window for open laparoscopy, *Am J Obstet Gynecol* 137:869, 1980.
30. McVay CB: *Anson & McVay surgical anatomy*, ed 6, vol 1, Philadelphia, 1984, WB Saunders.
31. Morton JH: Abdominal wall hernias. In Schwartz SI et al (eds): *Principles of surgery*, ed 2, New York, 1974, McGraw-Hill.
32. Warwick R and Williams PL: *Gray's anatomy*, ed 35, Philadelphia, 1973, WB Saunders.
33. A modified instrument and method for laparoscopy, *Am J Obstet Gynecol* 110:886, 1971.
34. Hasson HM: Open laparoscopy. In Sanfilippo JS, Levine RL (eds): *Operative gynecologic endoscopy*, New York, 1989, Springer-Verlag.

17

Advanced Laparoscopic Surgery

HARRY REICH

ROBERT B. HUNT

Diagnostic laparoscopy is the most common gynecologic procedure performed today. The technique enables the surgeon to confirm normal anatomy, to define and delineate existing disease, and to plan further surgical and medical therapy. Operative laparoscopy implies the performance of a surgical procedure often accomplished by laparotomy.

Laparoscopy is a method of access. Although the surgeon's hands are remote from pelvic structures, the magnified and well-illuminated view of these structures is excellent, similar to that obtained by use of the surgical microscope at laparotomy. Equipped with appropriate instrumentation, the well-trained laparoscopist can perform most intraabdominal gynecologic procedures endoscopically.

Patient advantages as compared with laparotomy include superior cosmetic result, shorter hospitalization, rapid recuperation, reduced hospital costs, and at least equivalent results. Advantages to the surgeon include intraoperative access to the rectum and vagina, a superb view of the pelvic structures, the opportunity to view tissue beneath fluid to achieve complete hemostasis and to evacuate blood clots, and a low complication rate. As with laparotomy, the surgeon must have a thorough understanding of pelvic anatomy, pathology, and physiologic effects of fluids and gases, and a working knowledge of the instruments.

A laparoscopic surgical procedure can be time consuming, often lasting more than 3 hours. Ample time must be alloted to perform the surgery and competent coverage of practice commitments made.

This is a chapter of techniques. Surgical results have been omitted to keep the chapter a reasonable length. Some procedures described are quite advanced, and the reader may prefer not to attempt them. Not all procedures currently done are discussed. We selected a broad range of procedures that we believe to be representative.

PREPARATION
Anesthesia

Close cooperation between the surgeon and anesthesiologist is mandatory. To select the optimal anesthetic agents that accomplish adequate relaxation yet rapid recovery with few sequelae from these procedures is a challenge. Special conditions associated with operative laparoscopy include a pneumoperitoneum coupled with 20 to 30 degrees of Trendelenburg and the use of large quantities of intraabdominal fluids. Proper padding must be placed to protect pressure points. The upper extremities are protected from brachial nerve injury by keeping the arms close to the sides and positioning padded shoulder braces to prevent patient slippage. The intravenous site and monitoring equipment must be applied to avoid interfering with the surgeon's work. In addition, the anesthetist must stay involved throughout the procedure, checking quantity of blood loss, amount of fluid absorbed, vital signs, expired carbon dioxide concentration, oximeter readings, body temperature, and the progress of the procedure. General endotracheal anesthesia is used in all cases of advanced laparoscopy in our institutions.

Surgeon

It is important that the surgeon who performs advanced laparoscopic procedures has extensive diagnostic laparoscopic experience, has attended courses dedicated to these techniques, and has worked with others who are adept at performing these procedures. Each time the surgeon implements any laparoscopic procedure, all retroperitoneal structures should be identified, including ureters; common, internal, and external iliac vessels; and rectum. In general the surgeon should undertake less difficult cases at first, such as an uncomplicated adhesiolysis or an unruptured ectopic pregnancy.

Hospital personnel

Optimally, one or two operating room nurses should visit a facility experienced in these procedures. Once the op-

235

erating room staff is convinced of the extraordinary value of laparoscopic surgery and can monitor the surgery by video, they will invariably become enthusiastic about it. Extensive in-service education is essential for them to be familiar with and troubleshoot equipment used. The recovery room and hospital nursing staff have to be aware of how these procedures vary from diagnostic laparoscopies, including surgical time, the instillation of large quantities of intraperitoneal fluid, and extensive dissection often required.

Patient preparation

The patient restricts food intake to a light diet during the day, clear liquids that evening, and is kept NPO after midnight the day of surgery. In addition, she is asked to ingest a bottle of magnesium citrate the afternoon before surgery, followed by a Fleet enema several hours later.

If extensive cul-de-sac disease is anticipated, a mechanical bowel preparation is recommended. The patient has the same dietary instructions but ingests 10 mg metochlopramide hydrochloride (Reglan), followed in 30 minutes by a polyethylene glycol-based isosmotic solution (GoLytely or Colyte) dissolved in 4 L water the afternoon before surgery. This results in rapid bowel cleansing by inducing diarrhea. Reglan promotes gastric emptying and reduces abdominal bloating and distention.

The patient arrives at the surgical unit 1 ½ hours before surgery. Interviews and a physical examination are conducted, consent forms (see Appendix A) and laboratory results are checked, and the patient changes into the appropriate attire and voids. The intravenous line is established. Last-minute questions are answered and the patient is ready for surgery.

Operating room

A suggested room set-up is diagrammed in Figure 17-1. When the operating room has been prepared, the patient is brought in. She is positioned on the operating table and her lower extremities placed in stirrups while she is still awake to reduce pressure points (Figure 17-2). Monitors are placed, medications are given, and the patient is anesthetized.

A suprapubic shave is not essential, although one author (RBH) prefers to do so. A Foley catheter fitted with a catheter plug is placed if desired, and the bladder intermittently emptied as necessary. Antibiotics are administered in procedures extending longer than 2 hours; one author (RBH) administers prophylactic antibiotics in all patients.

Initial surgical steps

A rectovaginal examination is performed. The patient is prepared and draped. An assessment hysteroscopy is done unless contraindicated, and appropriate intrauterine corrections are made. The hysteroscope is withdrawn and replaced with a cervical cannula and tenaculum for manipulation and lavage. Alternatively, a blunt curette may be used for manipulation. The Valtchev uterine mobilizer (Figure 17-3) is a superb instrument and is available from Conkin Surgical Instruments Ltd (Appendix B).

Initial laparoscopic assessment is performed. The upper abdomen is examined first. The patient is then placed in a 20- to 30-degree Trendelenburg position. A systematic assessment of each pelvic and lower abdominal structure is accomplished. A probe inserted through a secondary puncture site is often required. Pelvic abnormalities amenable to laparoscopic surgery are noted, and the necessary number of secondary incisions are made to correct them.

Ergonomics

The surgeon should be as comfortable as possible while performing these procedures. When using a videomonitor as the surgical guide, the operating table should be just above waist level. If the surgeon is viewing the surgical field directly through the laparoscope and is positioned to the patient's left, the table should be raised to the surgeon's shoulder level when surgery is being performed on the right side of the pelvis. The surgeon can then rest the right elbow on the patient's left shoulder brace. When performing surgery on the left side of the pelvis, the table will be lowered slightly, allowing the surgeon to obtain additional support by resting the right elbow on the patient's right shoulder brace. Alternatively, the surgeon may use a support positioned above the patient's neck and face (Figure 17-2). Additional comfort may be obtained by rotating the table slightly toward the surgeon and having the surgeon rest the left foot (forward) on a low stand. The surgeon will often find a back brace protects from overstressing the lower back.

INSTRUMENTATION AND TECHNIQUES
Aquadissection

A suction-irrigator-dissector (aquadissector) is one of the most valuable instruments used (Figure 17-4). It can be considered a substitute for the surgeon's fingers, since it is an excellent dissector. In addition, it is used to irrigate; evacuate smoke, blood, fluids, and debris; and suction-retract tissue, and is the primary instrument used for lysing acutely inflamed adhesions and evacuating abscess cavities.

Aquadissection is broadly defined as the use of hydraulic energy to perform surgical procedures.[1] The force vector is multidirectional, in contrast to the unidirectional mechanical energy applied by a rigid probe. Pressurized fluid displaces tissue, often creating cleavage planes in the least adhered spaces. Installation of pressurized fluid into closed spaces or behind enclosed areas produces distended tissue on tension, with resultant loss of elasticity. Thereafter, it is possible to divide this tissue safely.

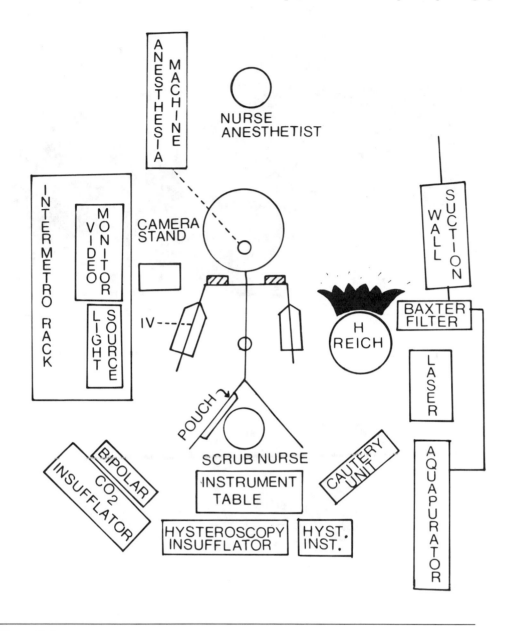

Figure 17-1
Operating room set-up used by one author.

The tip of the aquadissector is placed against the adhesed interface between the two structures to be separated. The pressurized fluid is released and used to develop a cleavage plane between these structures. The plane is extended either bluntly or with more fluid. Often, adhesions can be "weakened" with laser and the adhesiolysis completed with the aquadissector. Aquadissection is valuable in dissecting and distending the retroperitoneum for excision of peritoneal disease or in identifying and mobilizing retroperitoneal structures.

Suction-traction

This technique refers to the use of the suction capability of the aquadissector to retract pelvic structures and dis-

eased tissue. Examples are elevating the tube and ovary for inspection and retracting fibrotic cul-de-sac endometriosis for excision (Figure 17-5).

Scissors dissection

The principal technique for adhesiolysis is scissors dissection. The surgeon should have available both 3- and 5-mm, well-maintained scissors in straight, hooked, and microscissors designs (Figure 17-6).

Electrosurgery

High-frequency alternating electrical current in the unipolar mode can be used to cut, desiccate, or fulgurate tissue. To cut tissue, a nonmodulated, continuous,

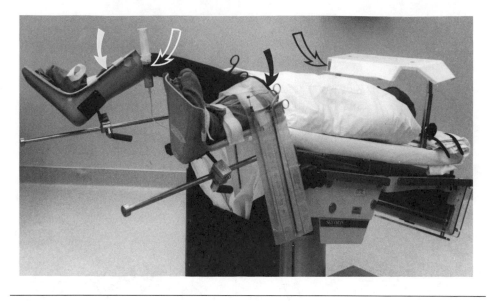

Figure 17-2
Mock operating room set-up showing Allen stirrups *(closed white arrow)*, indigo carmine *(open white arrow)*, Hunt instrument organizer *(closed black arrow,* available from Apple Medical), and chest support *(open black arrow).*

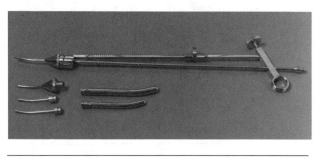

Figure 17-3
The Valtchev uterine mobilizer and accessories. (Available from Conkin Surgical Instruments Ltd.)

sinusoidal (cutting) current is selected. When passed through a laparoscopic knife or needle electrode, a high-power density results. The tissue effect on cells is one of exploding and vaporizing them.

In desiccation, tissue is heated to the boiling point using either a nonmodulated (cutting) current applied at low-power density or a modulated (coagulation) current in contact with tissue. Most electrosurgical generators have a blended mode whereby a combination of cutting and coagulating current may be applied, producing a cutting effect with some accompanying desiccation.

Fulguration refers to the use of the coagulation current applied in a noncontact mode; that is, a space exists between the active electrode and tissue. The current follows a path of least resistance, resulting in drying and shrinking of superficial cells with little penetration.

Whereas all three tissue effects can be accomplished with unipolar electrodes, only desiccation can be obtained with bipolar ones. Both cutting and coagulation waveforms can be passed through bipolar electrodes (Figures 17-7 and 17-8). Because desiccation is more uniform with the cutting current, it should be selected when using bipolar electrodes. The reader is referred to the excellent discussion of electrosurgery found in Chapter 6.

A 3-mm knife and a 1-mm needle electrode in the unipolar mode are excellent instruments for lysing adhesions and draining cysts (Figures 17-9 and 17-10). The power density of the knife electrode may be altered by applying the narrow or wide part of the instrument to the tissue treated. The surgeon must be aware that the newer electrosurgical generators, such as the Valleylab Force 2 and the Aspen Lab Excalibur, require a much lower power (wattage) setting than the older models.

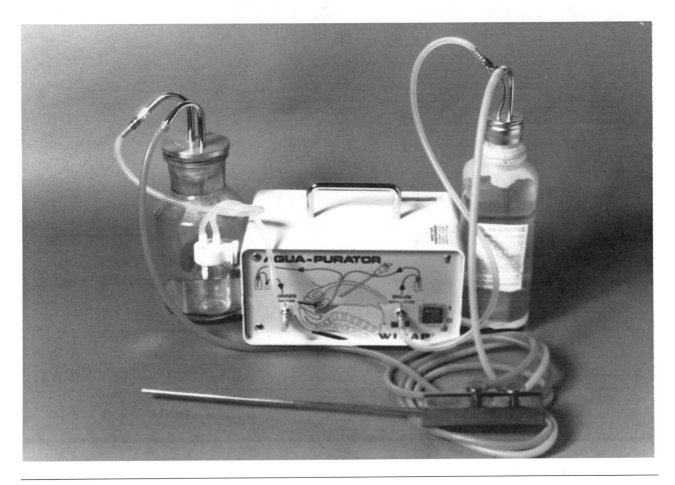

Figure 17-4
A suction-irrigation-dissection system. From Hunt RB: Operative laparoscopy. In Seibel MM (ed): *Infertility—a comprehensive text,* East Norwalk, Conn, 1990, Appleton & Lange.

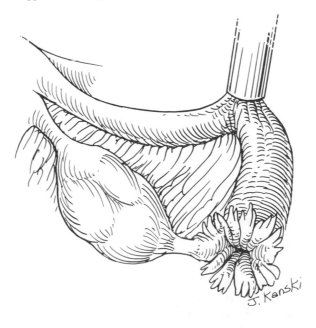

Figure 17-5
Suction-traction of the fallopian tube.

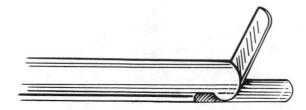

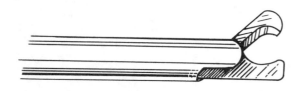

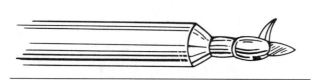

Figure 17-6
Straight scissors *(top)*, standard dissecting scissors *(middle)*, and microscissors *(bottom)*.

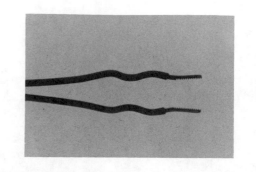

Figure 17-7
Modified Kleppinger bipolar forceps. The width of bipolar paddles is reduced by 50% and the insulation is extended to the paddles.

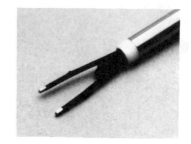

Figure 17-8
The Vancaillie microbipolar forceps. (Available from Storz Instrument Company.)

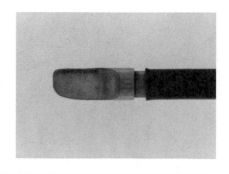

Figure 17-9
Unipolar knife electrode.

For lysing adhesions or draining cysts, pure cutting current (20-40 W) is selected to acquire a high degree of precision and to reduce thermal damage. A specific blood vessel may be occluded by pressing a knife, hook, or button electrode against it and momentarily applying a cutting or coagulation current for desiccation. Brief application of cutting current before pulling the electrode away from the vessel may prevent avulsing the char at the site of desiccation. Fulguration with noncontact coagulation current is used to control diffuse bleeding, such as that seen in the ovary after ovarian cystectomy.

Laser dissection

The carbon dioxide (CO_2) laser beam may be aimed through the surgical channel of a laser laparoscope. This converts the umbilical incision into a portal for performing surgery as well as observation. The perpendicular angle of the beam to the surgical field allows the surgeon to reach otherwise inaccessible sites and avoids the need to create yet another incision. The surgeon must ascertain that the laser beam is properly aligned. One way to do this is by placing transparent tape or stretching the surgeon's glove over the distal end of the laparoscope and observing the He-Ne beam as it exits the surgical chan-

Table 17-1 CO_2 Laser Power at Distal End of Scope

Power entering laparoscope	Power leaving laparoscope, i.e., at tissue	
Laser setting (W)	7.5-mm channel* (W)	5-mm channel** (W)
20	11	5
40	24	14
60	40	20
80	52	27
100	70	32

Sharplan 1100 laser (Tel Aviv, Israel)
*Sharplan or Storz laser laparoscope with 7.5-mm channel
**Wolf laser laparoscope with 5-mm Channel (Rosemont, Ill)

nel. The spot should be round, approximately 1 mm in diameter, and centered in the surgical channel. The surgeon must be aware that the beam will be adversely altered by tension on the laparoscope, irrigant on the laparoscope tip, and plume. The effectiveness of the CO_2 beam is reduced by the presence of moisture at the impact site. Also, the power delivered to tissue is reduced 30% to 50% with a 7.2-mm surgical channel and by 60% with a 5-mm one. In addition, an increase of power enlarges the spot size slightly and must be taken into account when calculating power density (Table 17-1).

A setting of 20 to 35 W superpulse through a 5-mm surgical channel and a spot size of 1.2 to 1.8 mm are adequate for most laser laparoscopic procedures. One author (HR) selects 80 to 100 W continuous mode for its diffuse hemostatic effect (3- to 4-mm spot size) during myomectomy and culdotomy. The limited thermal damage and shallow depth of penetration of the CO_2 laser make it ideal for vaporizing and excising lesions as well as for adhesiolysis.

There are many other choices of laser energy and delivery systems, such as the fiber lasers, including argon, postassium-titanyl-phosphate (KTP), and neodymium: yttrium-aluminum-garnet (YAG). Also available is the infraguide for the CO_2 laser. Research continues in developing new delivery systems and lasers of different and

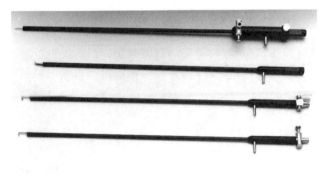

Figure 17-10
A variety of unipolar electrodes. (Available from Elmed.)

various wavelengths. We currently use the CO_2 laser for laparoscopic surgery.

HEMOSTASIS
Large vessels

Bipolar coagulation with high-frequency, low-voltage cutting current at 20 to 50 W power effectively desiccates large vessels such as the ovarian and uterine arteries.[2] The process seals these vessels adequate to withstand pulsating forces until healing permanently occludes them. Ideally, the bipolar forceps are positioned such

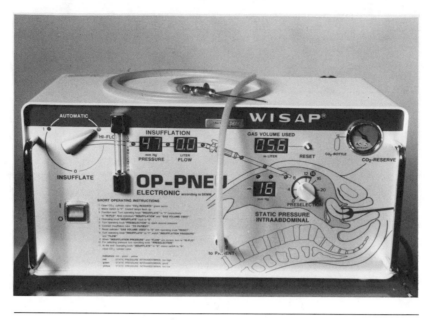

Figure 17-11
A rapid insufflator.

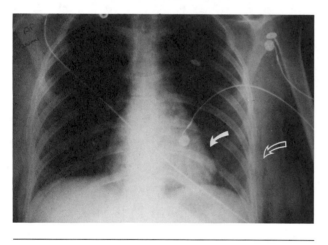

Figure 17-12
Pericardial *(closed arrow)* and subcutaneous *(open arrow)* gas is seen, resulting from too high intraperitoneal pressure at laparoscopy.

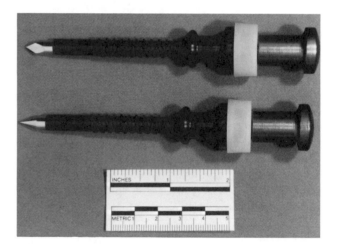

Figure 17-13
Hunt-Reich secondary cannulas of a screw design with simple, gas-tight seals. (Available with pyramidal or conical trocars from Apple Medical.)

that the vessel to be desiccated is completely occluded between its tips. The generator is then activated until desiccation is complete. Some generators contain meters that indicate when this end point has been reached.

The Kleppinger bipolar forcep has been modified by one author such that the tips are narrow and the insulation extended to lessen the possiblity of damaging nearby structures (Figure 17-7). Although superb for large vessel hemostasis, it works poorly beneath fluids. Other excellent bipolar forceps for small and large vessel hemostasis are available (Apple Medical and Karl Storz).

Small vessels

Bipolar desiccation of small vessels is an excellent technique. An instrument designed for this is the Vancaillie microbipolar forceps (Storz). It has a channel for irrigation and a fixed distance between electrodes (Figure 17-8). Irrigation is used to identify the bleeding vessel, which is contacted with one of the electrodes, after which current is applied. The vessel is effectively desiccated when the electrical current bridges the gap from one electrode to the other through Ringer's lactate solution.

Preventive hemostasis

Preventive hemostasis was popularized by Pouly et al[3] and consists of infiltrating tissue with a vasoconstrictor adjacent to areas where incisions are to be made. This in turn reduces the amount of energy needed to achieve hemostasis and thereby results in less tissue damage. An example of its use is in managing an ectopic pregnancy. Dilute vasopressin is constituted at a concentration of 20 U per 100 ml Ringer's lactate solution. A laparoscopic needle may be inserted through a secondary cannula and placed into the mesosalpinx. Alternatively, a 4.5-inch, 22-gauge spinal needle may be introduced through the skin at the pubic hairline, lateral to the inferior epigastric vessels, and inserted into the mesosalpinx. The needle should be positioned in the mesosalpinx 1 to 2 cm from the ectopic pregnancy as atraumatically as possible to avoid vascular injury. Dilute vasopressin is injected, inducing a visible swelling. The vasoconstrictive effect persists for approximately 2 hours, allowing natural hemostatic processes to occur. Vasopressin may be used similarly in other laparoscopic procedures.

Final hemostasis

To conclude the surgery, the abdomen is flooded with 2 to 5 L Ringer's lactate. To achieve adequate visualization, the tip of the laparoscope and aquadissector are manipulated together beneath the floating bowel and omentum. By alternatively irrigating and suctioning and with judicious use of the microbipolar coagulator, hemostasis is obtained. Once the fluid has been removed, including that accumulated in the upper abdomen, 2 L Ringer's lactate are placed in the abdomen and not removed. If hemostasis has been achieved, the fluid will remain clear. The Ringer's lactate floats pelvic and abdominal structures apart as the healing process begins; this should result in fewer postoperative adhesions.

Laparoscope

That the surgeon should have a variety of high-quality laparoscopes with an excellent light source (250 W or more) should not require emphasis. One author (HR) has five zero-degree laparoscopes: a 5-mm and a 10-mm viewing laparoscope; a 10-mm surgical laparoscope with a 5-mm surgical channel; a 10-mm laser laparoscope with a 5-mm laser channel; a 12-mm laser laparoscope with a 7.2-mm laser channel. The other uses 10-mm, 30-degree viewing laparoscope and a 10-mm laser laparoscope with a 5-mm laser channel.

Insufflation

A high-flow insufflator is imperative (Figure 17-11). For these 5- to 10-L per minute insufflators to be safe, they must be adjusted such that influx of the gas ceases when a preset intraperitoneal pressure is achieved, usually 10 to 15 mm Hg. A welcome feature is a single CO_2 supply tank, rendering unnecessary the continual refilling of an internal tank by the circulating nurse. High intraabdominal pressure may result in a pneumomediastinum (Figure 17-12).

Secondary cannulas

The surgeon will find short secondary cannulas, preferably of a screw design, easier to use than secondary cannulas of standard length[4] (Figure 17-13). Cannulas with trap doors should be avoided as these doors can damage delicate instruments. Short cannulas are currently available from Apple Medical and Wolf.

Suturing

The capability of pelvic suturing in surgical laparoscopy is an invaluable asset. Pioneered by Clarke[5] and Semm,[6] the technique greatly expands the number of procedures that can be done effectively. Among its applications are ovarian repair after cystectomy, eversion of mucosal flaps subsequent to salpingostomy, closure of salpingotomy after removal of an ectopic pregnancy, repair of the uterus succeeding myomectomy, covering a left pelvic sidewall defect with the rectosigmoid colon, and closure of peritoneal floor and rectosigmoid defects after resection of deeply invasive endometriosis. Sutures currently available are polydioxanone (Z-420, Ethicon), polyglactin (Ethicon special order), silk, and Gore-Tex. Others will soon be available.

The greatest difficulty is tying a secure knot once the suture has been placed. One option is to tie the knot intraperitoneally as an instrument tie (Figures 17-14 and 17-15). After the needle has been passed through the tissues to be approximated, the suture is pulled through until only a short segment remains. The longer segment is grasped with the contralateral needle carrier close to the needle. A double loop is then passed around the tip of the second needle carrier and the suture is tightened. Second, third, and fourth single loops are then placed alternately as with any instrument tie. The suture segment with the needle is then held with a needle carrier. A scissors is passed through the contralateral secondary cannula and the suture is cut. The surgeon must watch carefully as the needle is extracted through the cannula. The remaining suture segment is then cut and removed.

An alternative method of knot tying is illustrated. Once the suture has been placed, both ends of the suture, including the needle, are positioned outside the body and cannula. A single loop is made and the Clarke knot pusher (Marlow Surgical) is applied to one strand (Figure 17-16). The loop is then displaced inside the abdominal cavity through the open cannula with the knot pusher. Both ends of the suture are held on tension outside the

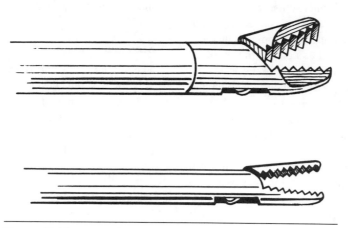

Figure 17-14
Needle carriers. Both the 5-mm (top) and 3-mm designs are shown.

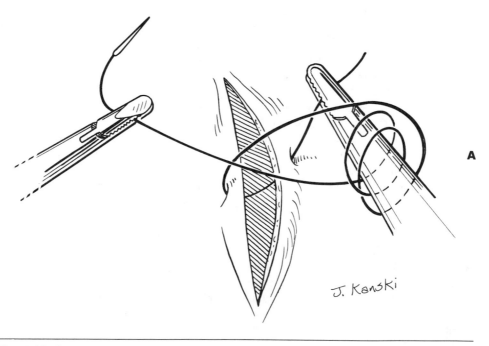

Figure 17-15
A, Knot tying. The 3-mm needle carrier is inserted through the left lower quadrant cannula and the 5-mm needle carrier through the right lower quadrant one. The suture is inserted into the abdomen with the 3-mm needle carrier. A surgeon's throw (double throw) is initially accomplished.

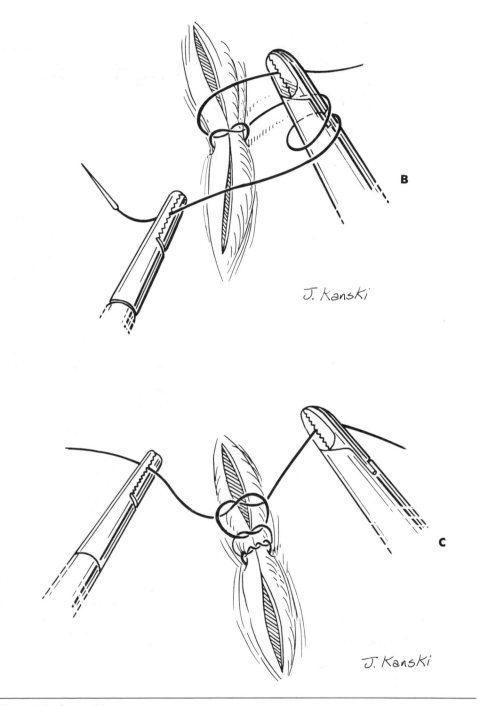

Figure 17-15, cont'd.
B, The second throw is a single one, placed to achieve a square knot. **C,** The third single throw completes the knot. A fourth single throw may be added.

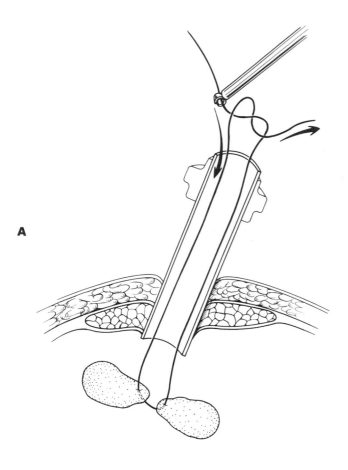

A

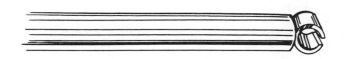

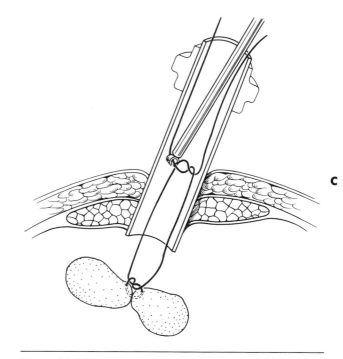

C

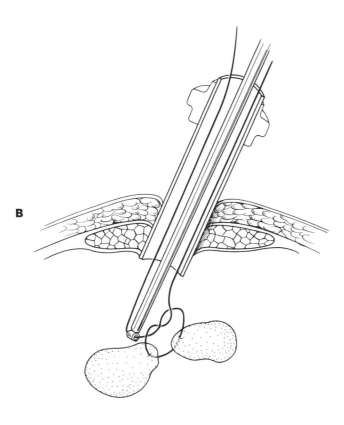

B

Figure 17-16
Knot tying. **A,** The suture has been passed through the tissues to be approximated. A single or double throw is achieved extraabdominally and one end seated in the Clarke knot pusher *(Inset)*. **B,** The suture is tightened with the Clarke knot pusher as necessary. **C,** The second throw is placed, completing a square knot. A third and a fourth throw may be placed.

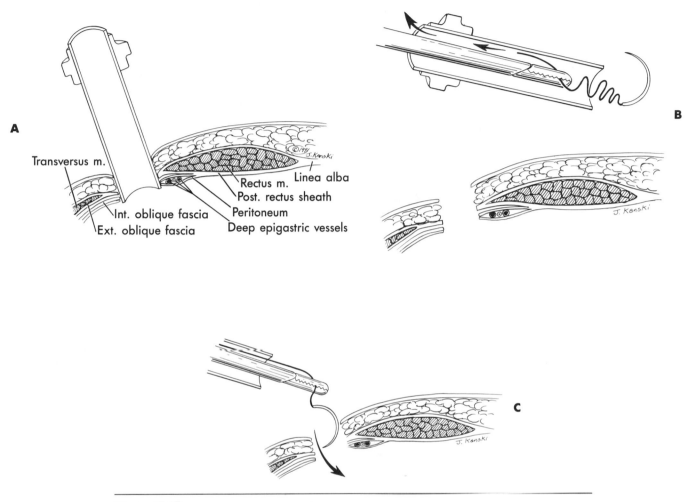

Figure 17-17
A, A 5.5-mm cannula is positioned just lateral to the deep epigastric vessels in the left lower quadrant. **B,** The cannula is removed, and the loose end of a suture, consisting of a curved needle too large to fit through the cannula, is drawn through the cannula with a needle carrier. **C,** The suture, needle carrier, and cannula are placed over the abdominal wall defect.

cannula as the knot pusher tightens the first loop, firmly approximating the tissue. The knot pusher is removed and, second and third loops are placed alternately in a similar manner to accomplish a secure surgical knot. With the knot complete, the suture ends are cut and removed. A third method of suturing (Figure 17-17), using a large curved needle in conjunction with the Topel needle holder (Cook Ob/Gyn), is advocated by one author (HR).

A loop ligature is also available (Endoloop from Ethicon). It consists of 0 chromic or plain catgut with a preformed slipknot. The device is inserted through a 5-mm secondary cannula and may be used to ligate large vascular pedicles, omentum, and appendix. It has no needle and is used only as a ligature.[7]

Disposable staples (U.S. Surgical Corporation) are used primarily for large vessel hemostasis. An automatic clip applicator contains 20 medium or 9 large titanium clips. This disposable unit is inserted through a 10-mm

Text cont'd on p. 251.

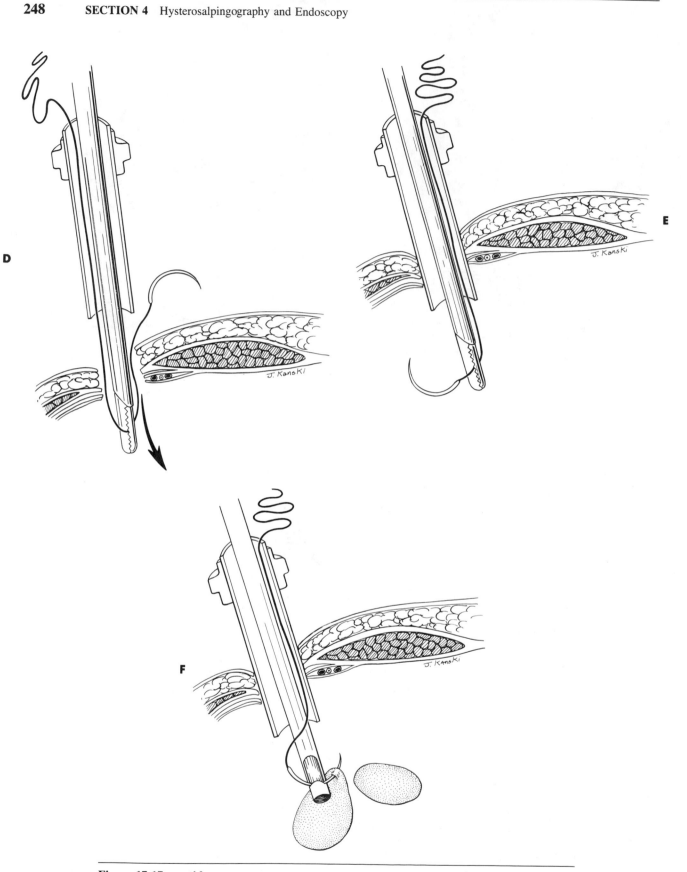

Figure 17-17, cont'd.
D, The needle carrier holding the suture is passed through the abdominal wall defect initially.
E, The needle and cannula have been advanced through the abdominal wall defect. **F,** The needle is grasped with a Topel needle carrier and the needle passed through the tissue to be sutured.

G

H

I

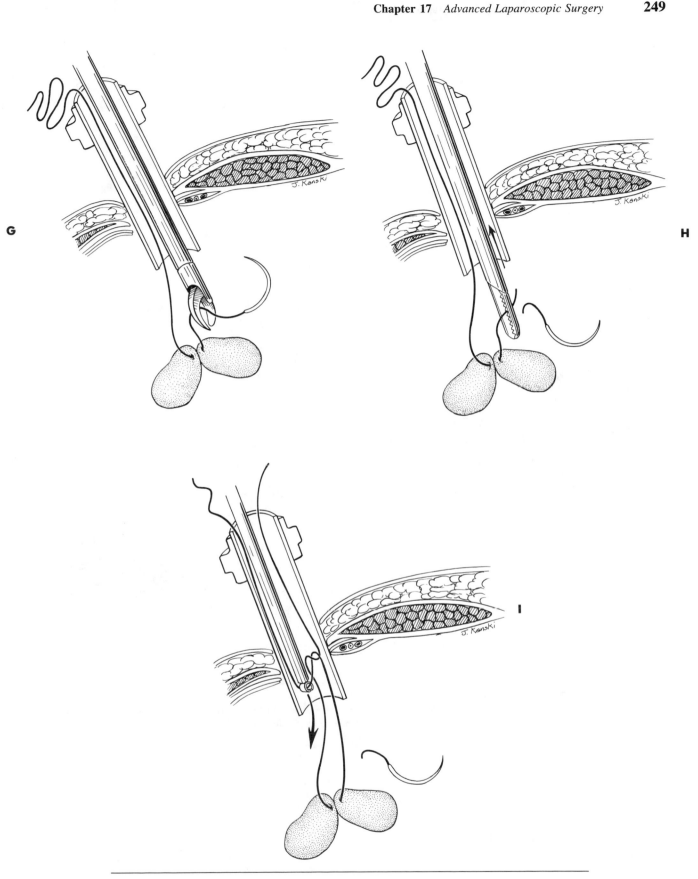

Figure 17-17, cont'd.
G, The needle is cut off and placed in a safe location. **H,** The second loose end is retracted through the cannula. **I,** The suture is tied as detailed in Figure 17-16.

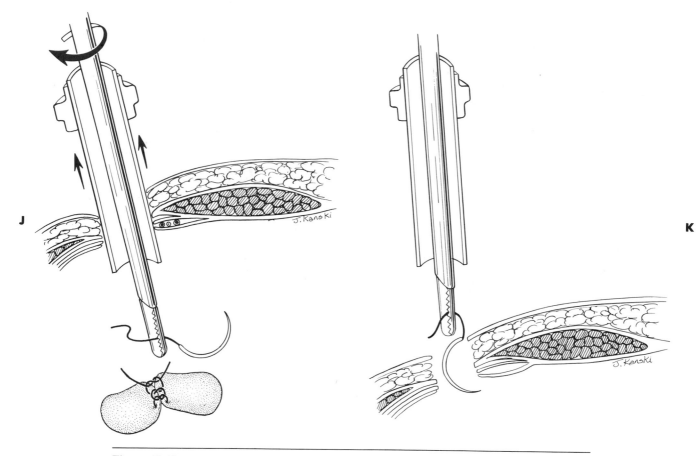

Figure 17-17, cont'd.
J, The suture attached to the needle is grasped with the standard needle carrier. **K,** The needle is extracted from the abdomen together with the needle carrier and secondary cannula.

cannula. To prevent slippage, the vessels must be dissected out before clips are applied. Much research is being done in clip development, and many new designs will undoubtedly be available soon.

Rectal, vaginal, and uterine probes

A rectal probe is available (Reznik Instruments, Inc.) and is useful when dissecting around the rectum (Figure 17-18). A moistened sponge on a sponge forceps is inserted into the posterior vaginal vault and aids the surgeon in identifying the vaginal apex correctly. If marked anteversion of the uterus is required, a no. 3 or 4 Sims blunt curet or Valtchev uterine mobilizer may be placed in the endometrial cavity and the task accomplished (Figure 17-19).

Additional instruments

Several types of instruments are useful in performing laparoscopic surgery. Some examples, including graspers and biopsy forceps, are shown in Figures 17-20 through 17-31.

Photography and videography

Documentation of the procedure by photography or videography makes good sense from medical, legal, and public relations standpoints. Also, many surgeons prefer performing surgery directly off the video screen, either with or without a beam splitter on the laparoscope. Whereas some depth perception and color differentiation are lost, this technique is much more comfortable for the surgeon. The authors use a beam splitter on the laparoscope and perform surgery off the video screen but use direct visualization when the clearest view is essential (see Chapter 30).

INCISIONS
Primary incisions

The thinnest area in the abdominal wall is the umbilicus, the so-called window of the peritoneum. This is the site for primary cannula placement.

When prepping, special care is taken to cleanse all debris from the umbilical fossa. With the surgeon standing on the anesthesized patient's left, the surgeon's left thumb is inserted into the umbilical fossa. The skin of the inferior portion of the umbilicus is grasped between the thumb and left forefinger. By externally rotating the wrist, the umbilical fossa is widened. With tension on the umbilicus maintained, the surgeon then incises the skin vertically with a no. 15 scalpel blade, beginning at the base of the navel and continuing inferiorly and in the midline. The vertical incision parallels Langer's lines and results in an almost undetectable scar. If the incision extends through the transversalis fascia, intraperitoneal injury is avoided, since the forefinger will control its

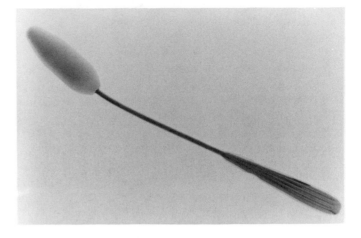

Figure 17-18
Rectal probe.

depth. Exercising the usual safety precautions, the Veress needle is inserted, the pneumoperitoneum established, and the primary trocar positioned.

If the surgeon is concerned over the possibility of abdominal adhesions, an open laparoscopy may be performed (see Chapter 16). If extreme periumbilical adhesions are suspected, the primary incision site may be placed at the left costal margin in the midclavicular line. After gastric emptying is accomplished by orogastric tube, the pneumoperitoneum is obtained with the Veress needle at the planned entry site, and the primary cannula introduced. If the umbilicus is observed to be free of adhesions or the adhesions are released, the primary cannula may be removed, the incision closed, and the primary site moved to the umbilical fossa as outline above. One problem with upper abdominal cannula placement is loosening of the parietal peritoneum, culminating in subcutaneous emphysema that can extend to the neck and face.

The wound is closed by placing interrupted 4-0 synthetic absorbable sutures in the fascia and approximating the edges. The skin is closed with the same material placed in an interrupted manner and with knots buried.

Secondary incisions

Two lower quadrant incisions are placed routinely. By visualizing the deep epigastric vessels from the peritoneal side, each incision is made just lateral to its respective epigastric vascular complex, usually at the superior margin of the pubic hairline (Figure 17-32). The trocar is inserted under direct laparoscopic vision to avoid unintended injury. One author prefers to position a 5-mm cannula in the left lower quadrant and a 3-mm one in the right lower quadrant. The other customarily places three 5-mm lower abdominal secondary cannulas, including one placed in the midline superior to the urinary bladder.

Text cont'd on p. 257.

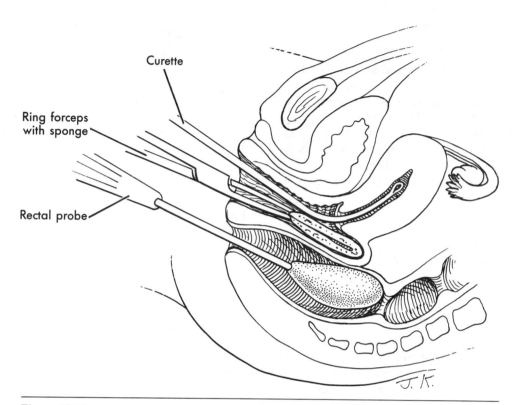

Curette

Ring forceps
with sponge

Rectal probe

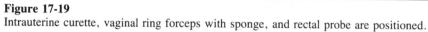

Figure 17-19
Intrauterine curette, vaginal ring forceps with sponge, and rectal probe are positioned.

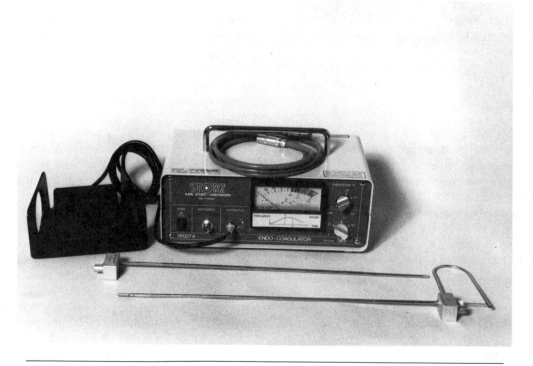

Figure 17-20
Endocoagulator and accessories.

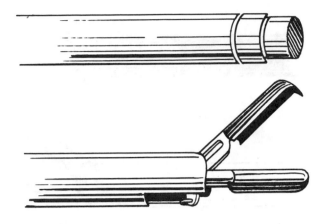

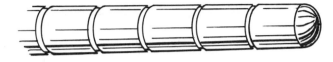

Figure 17-22
A standard calibrated probe. From Hunt RB: Operative laparoscopy. In Siebel MM (ed): *Infertility—a comprehensive text,* East Norwalk, Conn, 1990, Appleton & Lange.

Figure 17-21
Point coagulator *(top)* and crocodile forceps *(middle)* are designed for the endocoagulator. A standard Kleppinger bipolar forceps *(bottom)* is shown for comparison. From Hunt RB: Operative laparoscopy. In Siebel MM (ed): *Infertility—a comprehensive text,* East Norwalk, Conn, 1990, Appleton & Lange.

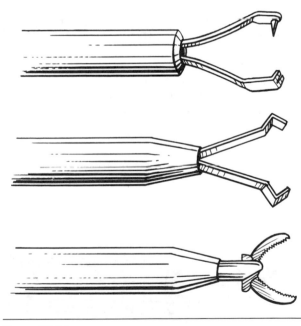

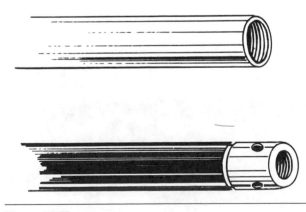

Figure 17-23
Suction cannulas. The top one is more suitable for aquadissection because of solid design without vents. (From Hunt RB: Operative laparoscopy. In Siebel MM (ed): *Infertility—a comprehensive text,* East Norwalk, Conn, 1990, Appleton & Lange.

Figure 17-24
An assortment of graspers. (From Hunt RB: Operative laparoscopy. In Siebel MM (ed): *Infertility—a comprehensive text,* East Norwalk, Conn, 1990, Appleton & Lange.

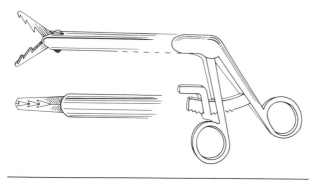

Figure 17-25
A ratcheted grasper, available in 3-mm and 5-mm sizes.

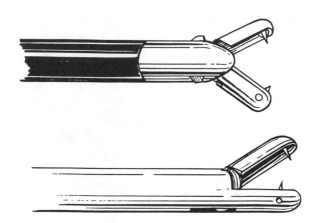

Figure 17-26
Double- (top) and single-action toothed forceps are illustrated. From Hunt RB: Operative laparoscopy. In Seibel MM (ed): *Infertility—a comprehensive text*, East Norwalk, Conn, 1990, Appleton & Lange.

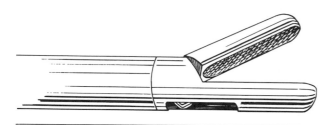

Figure 17-27
An 11-mm spoon forceps. From Hunt RB: Operative laparoscopy. In Siebel MM (ed): *Infertility—a comprehensive text*, East Norwalk, Conn, 1990, Appleton & Lange.

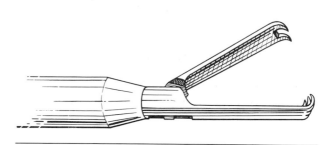

Figure 17-28
An 11-mm claw forceps. From Hunt RB: Operative laparoscopy. In Siebel MM (ed): *Infertility—a comprehensive text*, East Norwalk, Conn, 1990, Appleton & Lange.

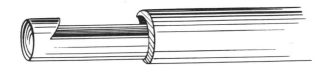

Figure 17-29
An 11-mm morcellator. From Hunt RB: Operative laparoscopy. In Siebel MM (ed): *Infertility—a comprehensive text*, East Norwalk, Conn, 1990, Appleton & Lange.

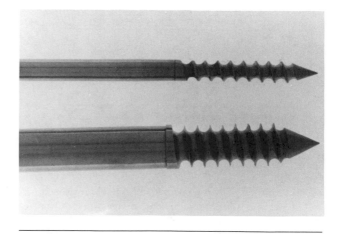

Figure 17-30
Small and large corkscrews for removing myomata. (Available from Reznik Instruments, Inc., Skokie, Ill.)

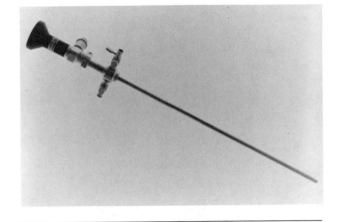

Figure 17-31
A 2.7-mm office hysteroscope used as a tuboscope.

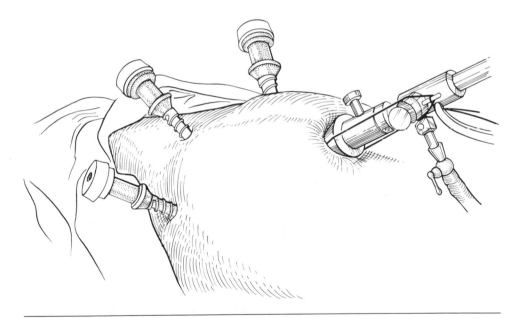

Figure 17-32
Placement of secondary cannulas by one author.

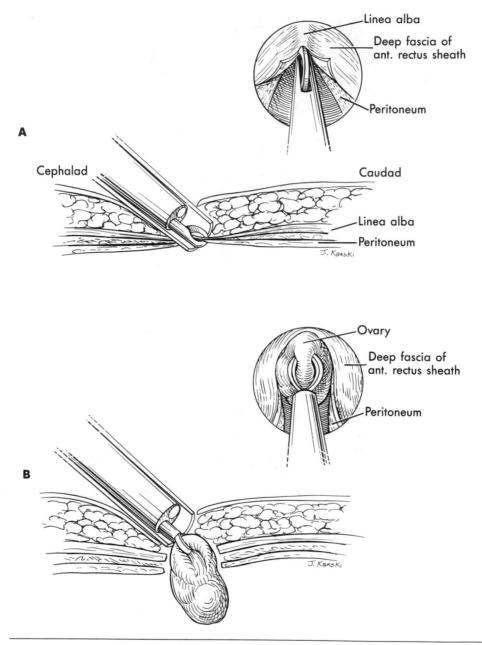

Figure 17-33

A, Removal of large tissue fragments. The peritoneum and deep fascia of the anterior rectus sheath are incised with laparoscopic scissors inserted through the operating channel of the surgical laparoscope. **B,** The tissue fragment is then removed through this enlarged umbilical incision by grasping it with a forceps and withdrawing the laparoscope.

We perform most laparoscopic procedures with the left hand, supporting the laparoscope with the right one.

Wound closure is accomplished with 2-0 material in the fascia if a 7-mm or larger instrument has been placed through it; otherwise only the skin is approximated. One author prefers to approximate the skin edges of these secondary incisions by applying Javid vascular clamps loosely to the wound edges for several minutes. The incisions are covered with collodion. Leakage of intraperitoneal fluid through the incision sites stops within 24 hours.

Incisions to remove large tissue fragments

Several options are available for removing large tissue fragments such as myomas and ovaries. One is to enlarge one of the secondary incision sites to accommodate a 11-mm cannula and remove the fragments by morcellation, or extraction with a Kocher clamp placed directly intraabdominally through the enlarged incision. The fascial defect must be approximated carefully to avoid a hernia.

If the tissue is not of a greater diameter than the surgical laparoscope, biopsy forceps can be inserted through the surgical channel and the tissue to be removed grasped. The forceps are withdrawn such that the tissue is partially contained in the surrounding 11-mm cannula. The cannula, laparoscope, biopsy forceps, and tissue are extracted through the primary incision with a single motion.

A third option is to extend the umbilical incision. A surgical laparoscope is required. The tip of the laparoscope is positioned in the trocar sleeve 1 cm from its peritoneal opening in the primary incision. The primary cannula is slowly withdrawn from the abdominal cavity. With scissors inserted through the surgical channel of the laparoscope, the peritoneum is visualized and incised inferiorly (Figure 17-33). The fascia is next viewed and cut with scissors inferiorly for approximately 1 cm. The skin incision is extended superiorly and in the midline to include the upper portion of the umbilical fossa. The tissue to be removed is now extracted through the enlarged incision as above.

A fourth option is laparoscopic culdotomy. This technique is particularly useful in dealing with cysts of uncertain cell type, including dermoids. To confirm the limits of the upper vagina, a blunt curette is placed in the uterus for anteflexion and a moistened sponge in the vagina for identification. The rectum is dissected off the posterior vaginal fornix if necessary with the aid of a rectal probe (Figure 17-18). With the vaginal apex and rectum clearly visualized and separated, a transverse incision is made in the vaginal apex with a knife electrode (30-40 W blended current) or CO_2 laser (3-mm spot size, 50-100 W continuous mode). Once the incision is deepened to the wet sponge, the tissue to be removed is placed over the vaginal incision. The mass may be pushed through the incision with a biopsy instrument inserted

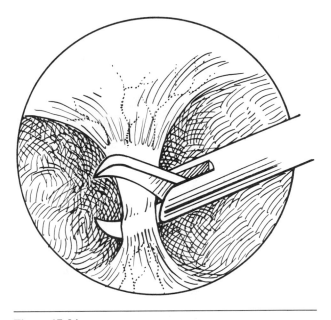

Figure 17-34
Adhesiolysis. Omental adhesions are dissected from the anterior abdominal wall after appropriate coagulation.

through a secondary cannula or pulled through the vaginal incision by inserting a laparoscopic biopsy instrument vaginally and extracting the mass. If the tissue contains cystic components, an 18-gauge needle may be inserted vaginally and the fluid removed. If the fluid is thick, as with a dermoid, the cyst may be opened vaginally and drained into the vagina. The mass is then extracted through the vaginal defect and removed. The culdotomy is closed vaginally with 0 absorbable sutures or laparoscopically with 4-0 absorbable material.

SURGERY
Adhesiolysis

Perhaps the most commonly performed advanced laparoscopic procedure is adhesiolysis. Pelvic and abdominal adhesions are associated with pain and infertility. Although no universal terminology exists, they are described as dense or filmy, broad or thin, opaque or translucent, and vascular or avascular.

Omental adhesions to parietal peritoneum are divided with scissors (Figure 17-34). Electrosurgery and laser should be avoided when the anatomy is unclear, since bowel may be contained within or behind the adhesions. If scissors are inserted through the surgical channel of a surgical laparoscope, the dissection is facilitated by rotating the laparoscope such that the scissors are flush with the parietal peritoneum. For dense adhesions, aquadissection is advantageous in developing planes necessary for safe scissor dissection. Finally, bleeding sites are located and sealed with bipolar desiccation.

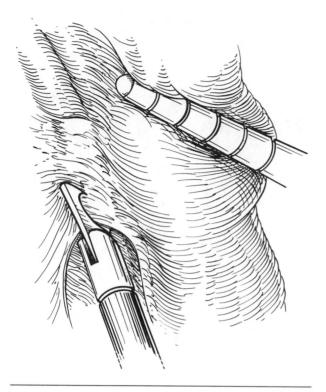

Figure 17-35
Mobilization of the rectosigmoid colon. Rectosigmoid adhesions are divided, releasing the colon from the lateral abdominal wall and pelvic sidewall. Great care must be taken not to cut the peritoneum.

The sigmoid colon is frequently adhered to the pelvic sidewall, obscuring visualization of the left adnexa. Mobilization of this structure begins superior to the pelvic brim. Lateral sigmoid attachments are divided with scissors, electrosurgery, or laser. Aquadissection develops the plane between the sigmoid and the common iliac vessels and their branches. With the rectosigmoid retracted medially, its attachments to the abdominal and pelvic sidewalls are released, dissecting superior to inferior (Figure 17-35). Care is taken to avoid injury to iliac and mesosigmoid vessels and the ureter.

Small bowel adhesions are divided by scissors. The bowel is retracted with atraumatic grasping forceps or by aquatraction. Often the planes can be located with aquadissection. The fluid delivered into adjacent tissue serves as a backstop should the CO_2 laser be used.

If the location of the ureter is unclear or if it is in the area to be dissected, it may be identified and mobilized as follows: the ureter is identified at the pelvic brim; the peritoneum is opened lateral to it (Figure 17-36); by a combination of scissors and aquadissection the peritoneal opening is extended inferiorly, maintaining a parallel lateral relation to the ureter; and with the medial peritoneal cut edge held by grasping forceps, the ureter is mobilized. Laser may also be used if desired. Identification and

mobilization can be continued to the level of the uterine vessels if necessary.

The ovary is often fused to the pelvic sidewall (Plates 5 and 6). The surgeon should preserve as much peritoneum as possible while liberating the ovary. Aquadissection is useful in developing space between the ovary and sidewall. Once planes are developed, adhesions can be divided with scissors. Dissection continues until the hilum of the ovary is reached. The ureter is almost always between the ovary and the sidewall in these cases, and great care must be taken to avoid harming it. Similarly, the surgeon should inflict as little ovarian damage as possible, particularly vascular compromise.

Second-look laparoscopy to release postoperative adhesions after a laparotomy are handled differently. Scheduled 1 to 3 weeks after the initial surgery, these newly formed adhesions separate much easier than at the time of the original surgery. Adhesion interfaces are identified laparoscopically and planes are developed by aquadissection. Usually the adhered structures can be separated with an excellent anatomic result.

Fimbrioplasty and salpingostomy

Laparoscopic adhesiolysis and salpingostomy can usually be accomplished with results equivalent to those obtained by laparotomy (see Chapter 21). The procedure is begun by performing a thorough adhesiolysis (Figure 17-37). Separating the distal tube from ovary is challenging. The surgeon must determine how far to dissect the tube to achieve mobility and preserve blood supply (Plates 7 and 8).

One author prefers to perform the procedure as follows (Figure 17-38). After mobilization, the tube is stabilized with a grasping instrument and the distal end opened. A 3-mm grasping forceps, followed by a 5-mm one, is inserted in the tubal ostium to dilate and stretch it. Avascular tissue is divided as necessary. The process is continued until ampullary mucosa protrudes and the tubal ostium is of adequate size. The technique can be varied by stabilizing the tube with grasping forceps introduced through either lower quadrant secondary cannula and incising the distal tube from the mesenteric to the antimesenteric side with scissors inserted through the midline secondary cannula (Figure 17-39).

Mucosal flaps are next everted. Several techniques can be used. The serosal side of the created flaps can be touched briefly with the point coagulator attached to the endocoagulator set at 100°C. Serosal contraction results in effective eversion of a thin-walled hydrosalpinx. A similar result can be obtained by suturing the mucosal flaps (Figure 17-39). A third option is to coagulate the serosal surface of the mucosal flaps superficially with the CO_2 laser at a setting of less than 5 W. One author everts the flaps with the point coagulator initially, then places one or two sutures at propitious points to complete the salpingostomy, if needed. Hemostasis is obtained by

Text cont'd on p. 262.

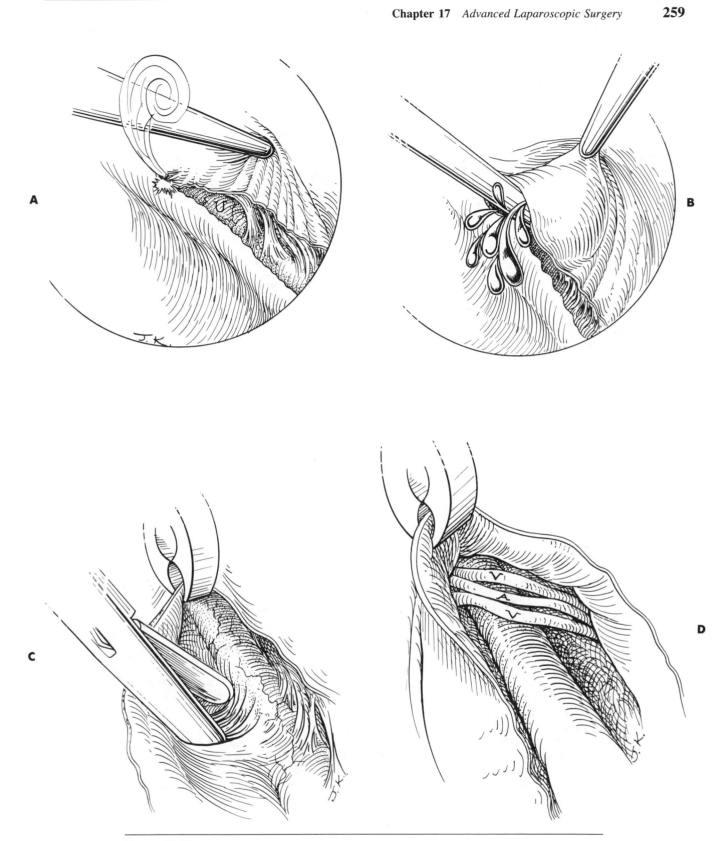

Figure 17-36
A, Ureteral dissection. The peritoneum overlying or medial to the ureter (U) is incised with the CO_2 laser. The peritoneum is retracted laterally to facilitate the dissection. **B,** Using grasping forceps and aquadissection judiciously, the ureter is released from the peritoneum. **C,** The ureter is released from surrounding tissue. **D,** The ureter is dissected down to the uterine veins (v) and artery (a).

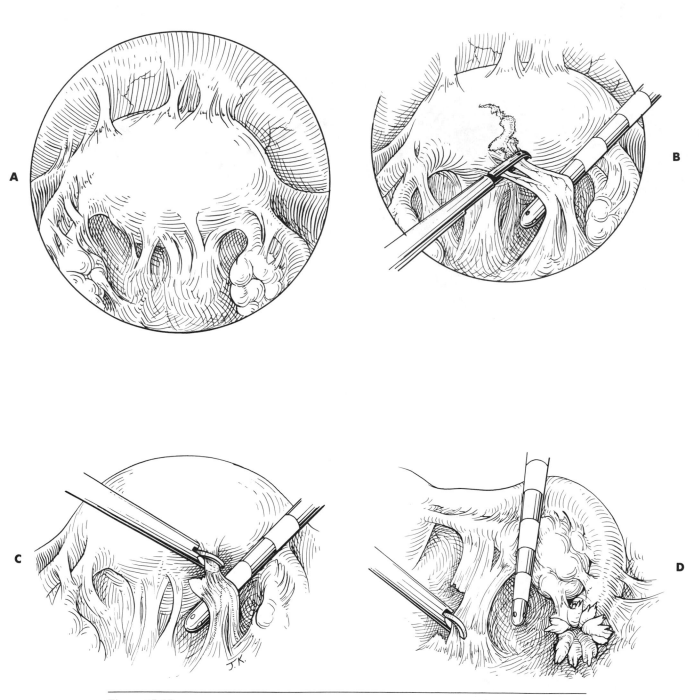

Figure 17-37
A, Salpingoovariolysis. Typical appearance of an adhesed pelvis. **B,** The cul-de-sac is first cleared of adhesions. Adhesions are coagulated with a crocodile forceps (endotherm). Bipolar forceps or laser may be used. A cul-de-sac free of adhesions provides a basin for collection and aspiration of fluids and gives wider access to the adnexal structures. **C,** Adhesions are next incised, then excised. **D,** The adnexal structures are next released from the pelvic sidewalls.

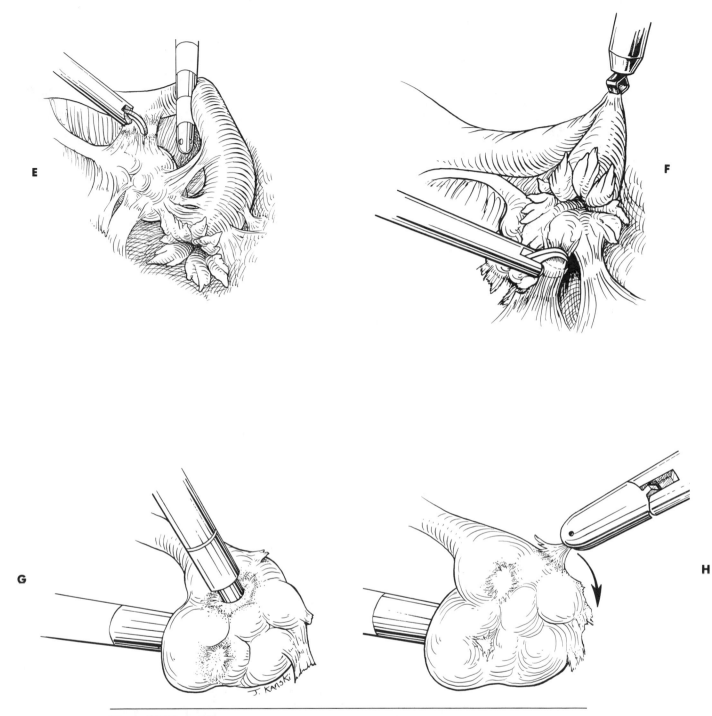

Figure 17-37, cont'd.
E, Adhesions binding the tube and ovary together are divided approximately 1 mm from tubal serosa. This provides a pedicle for coagulation should bleeding occur. **F,** Fimbriae are next released, cutting approximately 1 mm from the tube. **G,** The adhesions on the ovary are desiccated with a point coagulator (endotherm). A bipolar forceps with slightly separated paddles may be used. **H,** All adhesions are removed by stripping them away with biopsy forceps. Note the direction of biopsy forceps is parallel to the ovarian surface. (From Hunt RB: Operative laparoscopy. In Seibel MM, (ed) *Infertility—a comprehensive text*, East Norwalk, Conn, 1990, Appleton & Lange.)

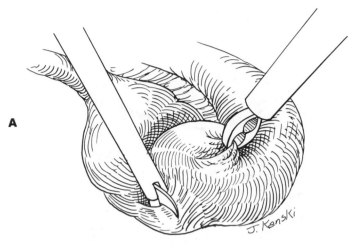

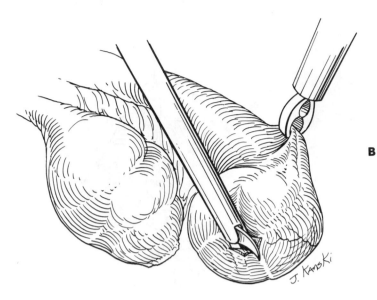

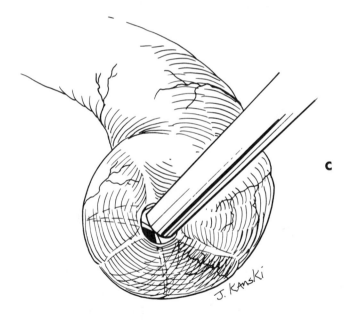

Figure 17-38
A, Salpingostomy. The distal tube is dissected sharply from
the ovary. The tube is lifted with a grasping forceps. **B,** The
distal tube is opened by scissors dissection. **C,** The opening
is enlarged by dilating with forceps.

identifying the arterial bleeders with irrigation and applying bipolar coagulation, taking care to impose minimal damage to nearby mucosa. Tuboscopy and tubal
lavage complete the procedure.

Ovarian cystectomy

Ovarian cystectomy, a frequently performed procedure,
can be accomplished laparoscopically in most cases

(Plates 9 through 12). Preoperative studies should include
an ultrasound and often measurement of CA 125 level.
The patient should be informed of the possibility of a
malignancy and possible modes of management. Other
unintended outcomes should be discussed, such as oophorectomy and ovarian failure.

The procedure begins with adhesiolysis. Peritoneal
washings for cell block are obtained if indicated. Once

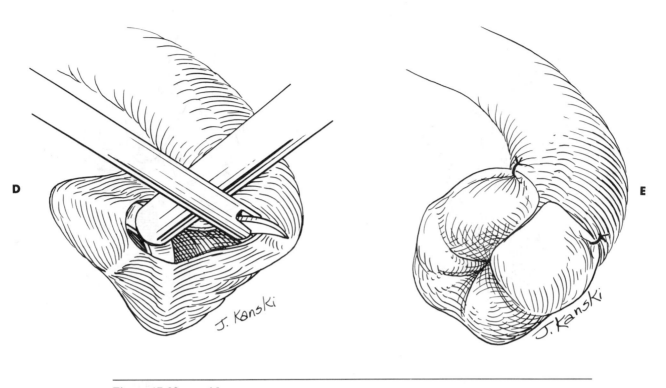

Figure 17-38, cont'd.
D, Incisions are made in thinned-out portions of the distal tube. **E,** The serosal flaps are everted by contraction of the serosa with endocoagulation or laser and sutured if needed.

the cyst is mobilized, the cortex is grasped with a biopsy instrument. The cortex is incised by laser or scissors, exposing the cyst wall. The incision is enlarged with scissors, and aquadissection is instituted to separate the cyst from the ovarian stroma. Once the cyst is dissected, it can be removed intact through a culdotomy incision. Alternatively, it may be opened, evacuated, thoroughly lavaged with the aquadissector, and removed (see "Incisions to remove large tissue fragments" on p. 257). If the cyst is opened intraperitoneally, the patient should be taken out of Trendelenburg position while the fluid is removed and the pelvis lavaged. Arterial bleeders are identified and desiccated. The ovary usually does not require suturing; however, if the edges gape widely, they can be loosely approximated with interrupted 4-0 synthetic absorbable sutures.

Ectopic pregnancy

Laparoscopic management of ectopic pregnancy is feasible in most cases. One group recommends laparotomy under the following conditions[3]:
1. Interstitial pregnancy.
2. Ectopic pregnancy larger than 6 cm.
3. HCG value greater than 15,000 mIU/ml.
4. Hemoperitoneum greater than 2000 ml.
5. Hemodynamic instability of the patient attributable to blood loss.

In selected women, alternatives to surgery include administration of methotrexate or expectant monitoring.[8]

Evacuation of hemoperitoneum

The 5-mm aquadissector is usually sufficient to evacuate the hemoperitoneum, including large clots. If the aquadissector is inadequate, a 11-mm cannula is inserted. A 1-cm air vent is cut into wall suction tubing 25 cm from the distal tip to prevent excessive suction pressure, and the tubing is inserted directly into the pelvis through the cannula. The clots are then aspirated. Rapid loss of pneumoperitoneum occurs with this technique.

Salpingectomy

Removal of the tube may be the procedure of choice when future fertility is not desired or in cases of tubal rupture or extensive damage. First, blood clots are removed and adhesions in the vicinity of the tube are divided. The tube is fixed with grasping forceps (Figure 17-40). Bipolar forceps and scissors are introduced successively to desiccate and sever the fallopian tube and its mesentery. Alternatively, an Endoloop ligature may be placed around the tube and tightened and the tube removed. Two additional loops should be placed around the pedicle to avoid delayed hemorrhage.

The tube containing the products of conception is removed by one of the methods described in "Incisions to

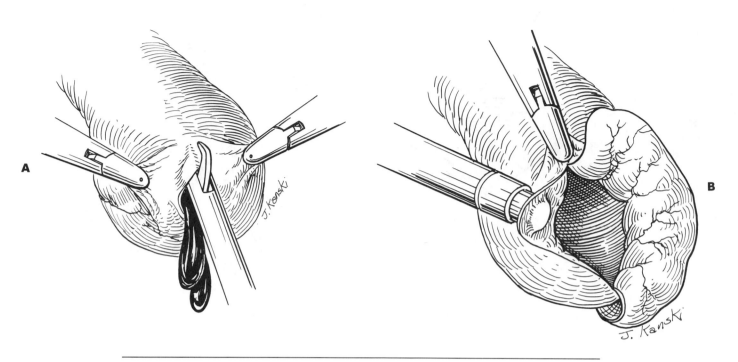

Figure 17-39

A, Salpingostomy. After the distal tube is mobilized and the adhesiolysis completed, a grasping forceps is placed on either side of the tube and gentle traction applied to each forceps. A single incision is made with scissors from the mesenteric to the antimesenteric side of the tube.

B, Each mucosal flap is everted with the endocoagulator at 100° C. To avoid damage to mucosa, contact with the serosa of each flap is brief but at several spots. Eversion occurs immediately. Occasionally, one or two sutures placed at propitious points will be necessary.

remove large tissue fragments" on p. 257. Care must be taken to retrieve products of conception that may extrude from the tube as it is extracted from the abdomen. These fragments should be collected and undergo pathologic evaluation.

Partial salpingectomy

With an isthmic ectopic pregnancy, a ruptured tube, or continued bleeding after salpingotomy, a partial salpingectomy may be performed. Bipolar forceps are inserted and the tube is desiccated on either side of the damaged site. These sites are divided. The underlying mesentery is desiccated and the tubal segment excised and removed (Figure 17-41). Alternatively, an Endoloop ligature may be placed around the segment and the tubal segment excised (Figure 17-42). Additional loops are placed around the pedicle to ensure hemostasis.

Salpingotomy

Tubal preservation is the usual objective in the patient with an unruptured ampullary ectopic pregnancy) Plates 13 through 16). The mesosalpinx is infiltrated with dilute vasopressin (see "Preventive hemostasis" on p. 243). With the tube stabilized, the serosa is incised on the antimesenteric side over the ectopic pregnancy for 1 to

2 cm (Figure 17-43). A knife or needle electrode connected to an electrosurgical generator set at 20 to 50 W is adequate for the incision. Alternatively, laser or a hooked scissors may be used. If the pregnancy is located inside the tube, the serosa-muscularis-mucosa is opened, and the products of conception are located and withdrawn with the aquadissector. Suction is used if the products of conception are viable and irrigation if they are nonviable and surrounded by blood clots. Occasionally, biopsy forceps are needed to dislodge pregnancy tissue, especially if the tissue is located in an extraluminal site between serosa and muscularis. Once the tissue has been removed, the tube is thoroughly irrigated distally and proximally with the aquadissector. The tube heals by secondary intention; however, if the edges gape widely, it is advisable to approximate them loosely with one or two sutures of 4-0 absorbable material.

Fimbrial evacuation of tubal pregnancy

Sometimes the ectopic pregnancy is located in or near the fimbriae. It can be removed by irrigation, suction, or grasping forceps.

Aquaexpression of tubal pregnancy

This technique consists of inserting the distal tip of the aquadissector into the tubal lumen through the fimbriated

Text cont'd on p. 268.

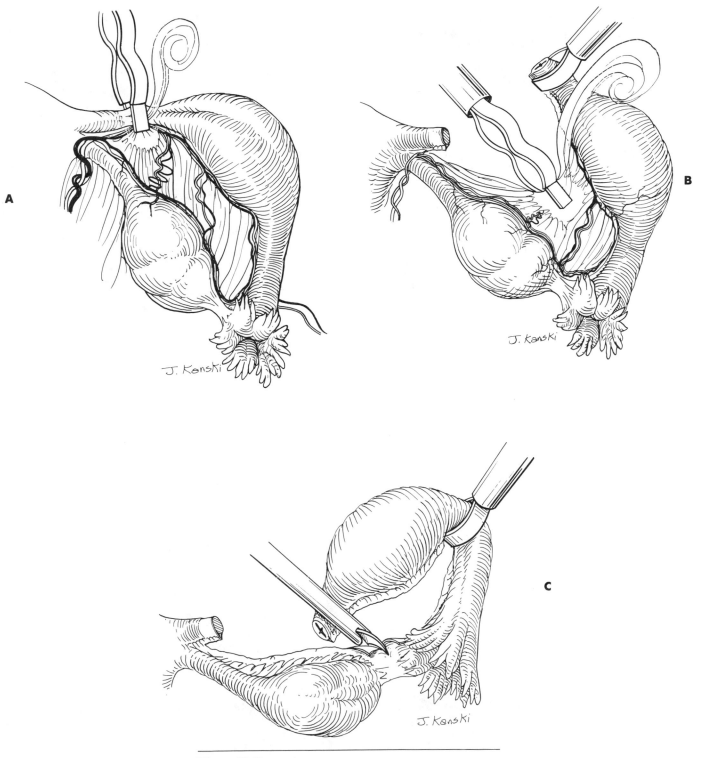

Figure 17-40
A, Complete salpingectomy for an ectopic pregnancy. The
proximal tube is desiccated. **B,** Desiccation and excision are
continued distally. Blood supply to the ovary is preserved.
C, The final steps of the excision process are completed.

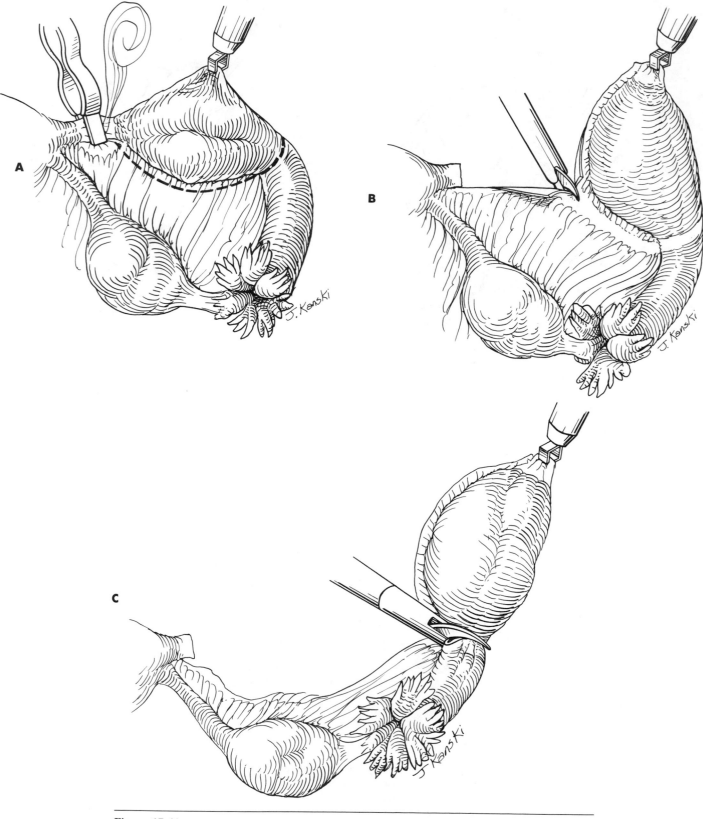

Figure 17-41
A, Partial salpingectomy for an ectopic pregnancy. The tube is desiccated just proximal to the ectopic gestation. **B,** The desiccation and excision process is continued. **C,** The distal tube is desiccated adjacent to the pregnancy and the tubal segment excised.

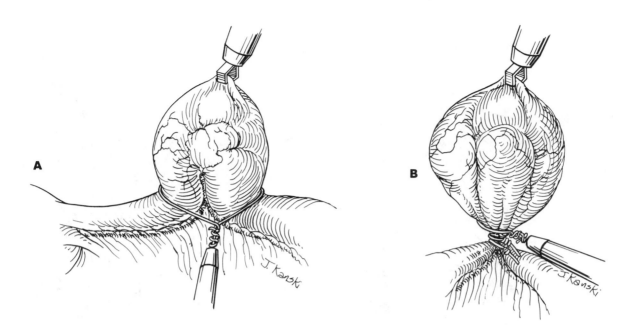

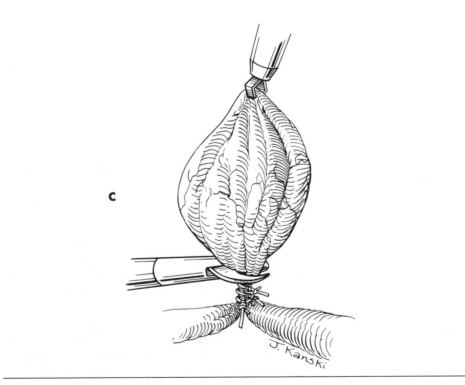

Figure 17-42
A, Partial salpingectomy for an ectopic pregnancy. The Endoloop is positioned around the ectopic pregnancy, and the involved tubal segment is lifted superiorly. **B,** The Endoloop has been
tightened securely, a second one placed similarly, and a third one is being tightened. **C,** The
tubal segment containing the ectopic pregnancy is excised.

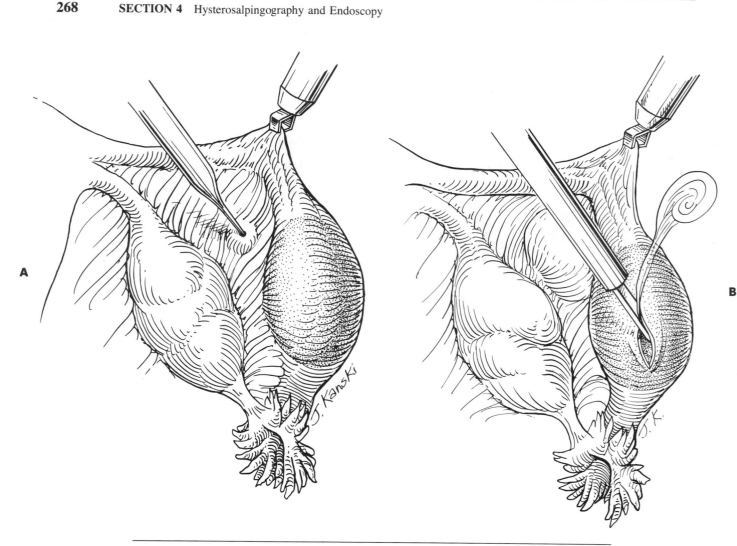

Figure 17-43
A, Salpingotomy for an ectopic pregnancy. One unit of dilute vasopressin is injected in the mesosalpinx. **B,** The tube is opened.

end to extract a nonviable ampullary pregnancy with surrounding blood clot. The pregnancy is dislodged and irrigated out of the tube with the pressurized fluid from the aquadissector (Figure 17-44). Theoretically, this technique would not be successful for extraluminal ectopic pregnancy.

Interstitial ectopic pregnancy

An interstitial ectopic pregnancy is evacuated with loss of the proximal tube. Judicious use of dilute vasopressin in the uterine wall may be helpful, and suturing may be necessary. Tubal patency can be established by microsurgery after 3 months if desired.

Endometriosis

This enigmatic disease is among the most difficult to treat. Surgical management of advanced disease often results in pain relief for varying lengths of time, and may result in a successful pregnancy.

Peritoneal implants

Islands of disease may be treated by electrosurgery, endocoagulation, laser ablation, or excision. One author uses the CO_2 laser (30-40 W superpulse), a knife electrode (20-60 W unipolar cutting current), or scissors to encompass the lesion by an elliptical incision (Figure 17-45). The cut edge is lifted superiorly and the lesion undermined by aquadissection. This displaces underlying structures, allowing for safe resection of the lesion.

The process of identifying endometriosis continues until the entire pelvis and lower abdomen have been evaluated and the lesions removed. Small lesions can be vaporized with the CO_2 laser, desiccated with bipolar forceps, or drained with a needle electrode using unipolar cutting current followed by vaporization of the base with laser.

Ovarian endometrioma

The removal of this lesion usually requires some modification to the technique described in "Ovarian cystec-

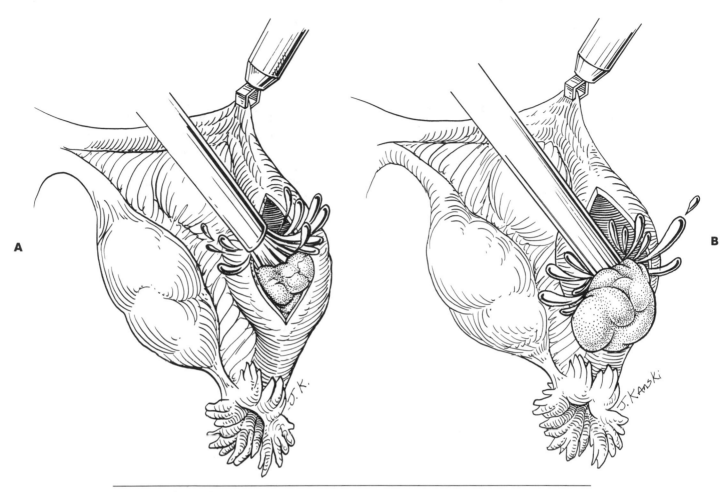

Figure 17-43, cont'd.
C, The ectopic gestation is dissected free by a combination of aquadissection and aquatraction.
D, The ectopic pregnancy is removed.

tomy" on p. 262 mobilization of the ovary often results in rupture of the cyst. When this occurs, the following steps may be taken (Figure 17-46): all endometrioma fluid is aspirated from the pelvis and adhesiolysis completed; two grasping forceps placed through either lower quadrant secondary cannulas stabilize the superior edge of the ovarian defect and the ovarian cortex lateral to it; a scissors is introduced through a low midline secondary cannula, and an incision is made in the ovarian cortex between the two grasping forceps; the incision is deepened until the endometrial cyst wall is reached; the grasping forceps are repositioned and a plane is developed between the cyst wall and ovary; and with a combination of scissors and aquadissection and by continually relocating the forceps, the entire cyst wall can be dissected out of the ovary with relative facility. It is removed from the abdomen by one of the techniques described in Incisions to Remove Large Tissue Fragments on p. 257.

Partial and complete cul-de-sac obliteration

This finding is associated with the presence of retrocervical fibrotic endometriosis located in the following sites: upper vagina, rectum, rectovaginal space, space between the upper vagina and the cervix, and one or both uterosacral ligaments.

To determine if cul-de-sac obliteration is partial or complete, a sponge stick is inserted vaginally and pressed against the posterior vaginal fornix. Partial obliteration is present when superior rectal tenting is present but the vagina protrudes between the rectum and the inverted U of the uterosacral ligaments. When the rectum and fibrotic nodules cover this area, cul-de-sac obliteration is complete (Figure 17-47). Excision of disease in this area is potentially hazardous and should be attempted only by one experienced in advanced laparoscopy. The dissection is as follows.

The rectal probe, vaginal sponge stick, and uterine curette are positioned. If the ureter is not identified, it is

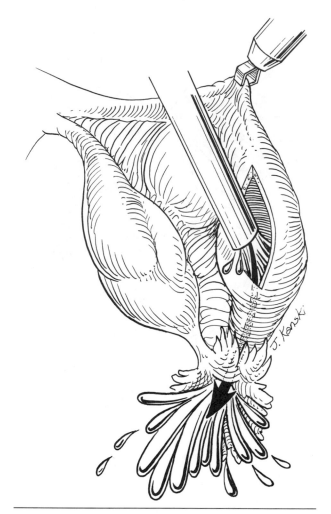

Figure 17-43, cont'd.
E, The tubal lumen is thoroughly lavaged.

located at the pelvic brim and traced into the pelvis (see "Adhesiolysis" on p. 257). The rectal serosa is opened at its junction with the cul-de-sac lesions by laser or scissors (Figure 17-47). The rectum is then carefully dissected away from the posterior uterus, cervix, and vagina using a combination of laser, electrosurgery, scissors, and aquadissection. The dissection continues until the loose areolar tissue of the rectovaginal space is reached. Great care must be exercised when dissecting near the uterine vessels, since opening them can produce life-endangering hemorrhage.

Attention is directed to the posterior vagina, identified by the vaginal sponge stick. Endometriosis is excised from it by the same technique as the rectal dissection (Figure 17-47). If the disease goes full thickness through the vaginal wall, it must be excised en bloc, taking a full-thickness section from the vaginal wall. This opening can be closed by vaginal or laparoscopic suturing. The excision, coagulating, and vaporizing process continues

superiorly along the posterior cervix and uterus until all visible or palpable disease is removed or destroyed.

Attention is next focused on the rectum (Figure 17-47). Endometriotic nodules infiltrating the rectal muscularis are excised with laser, usually with the surgeon's or assistant's finger located rectally just beneath the lesion. After the dissection is completed, the rectum may be reperitonealized by plicating the uterosacral ligaments and lateral rectal peritoneum across the midline with 4-0 or 5-0 absorbable sutures. A rectal perforation can be identified by injecting betadine solution with an Asepto syringe inserted through the anus and observing the rectum laparoscopically. Enterotomy may be closed by laparoscopy or laparotomy in these bowel-prepped patients.

Oophorectomy

Occasionally it is necessary to remove an ovary, such as one severely damaged by endometriosis or pelvic inflammatory disease. The procedure begins by adhesiolysis. Next the common iliac vessels and its branches and the ureter are identified (see "Adhesiolysis" on p. 257). The ovary is grasped, and the mesovarium and utero-ovarian ligament are desiccated and divided (Figure 17-48). The ovary is then removed as described in "Incisions to remove large tissue fragments" on p. 257.

If a salpingo-oophorectomy is to be performed, the same techniques are used. The infundibulopelvic ligament, mesovarium, mesosalpinx, utero-ovarian ligament, and proximal tube are desiccated and divided (Figure 17-49).[2] Salpingectomy is described in the section, "Ectopic pregnancy" on p. 263. Alternatively, an Endoloop may be placed around the tube and/or ovary and the structure(s) excised. Two additional loops are placed around the pedicle to ensure hemostasis.

Myomectomy

Intramural and subserosal myomas less than 5 cm in diameter are frequently amenable to laparoscopic resection (Plates 17 and 18). Gonadotropin-releasing hormone analogs have expanded the number of patients falling into this category. When given over 3 to 6 months before surgery, the myomas often decrease to as much as half their original size, rendering an otherwise inoperable lesion operable.[9] Either a preoperative hysterosalpingogram or hysteroscopy is advisable. If significant blood loss is expected, the patient is asked to donate blood for autologous transfusion, and/or a cell saver is requested.

The serosa and myometrium overlying the myoma are incised with scissors or a knife electrode at 30 W cutting current (Figure 17-50). A corkscrew is then fixed into the substance of the myoma and tension placed on the tissue. The pseudocapsule surrounding the myoma is incised and the myoma dissected out of its bed by aquadissection. Fibrous adhesions and blood vessels are di-

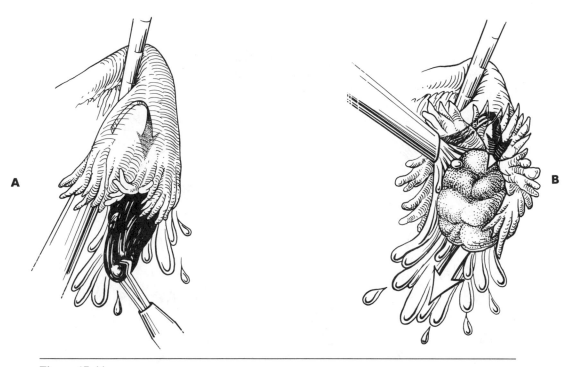

Figure 17-44
A, Fimbrial evacuation of an ectopic pregnancy implanted in the distal tube. **B,** Aquaexpression of an ectopic pregnancy implanted in the distal tube.

vided and desiccated as they are encountered using endotherm, unipolar blended, or bipolar current. Alternatively, the CO_2 laser at 50 to 100 W continuous wave may be used.

Once released, the myoma can be removed by one of the techniques described in "Incisions to remove large tissue fragments" on p. 257. Persistent bleeders are identified with the aquadissector and desiccated with bipolar coagulation. If there is diffuse oozing, vasopressin and/or fulguration may be used. The uterine defect is closed with 4-0 or 5-0 synthetic absorbable sutures.

Surgical management of polycystic ovaries

Wedge resection by laparotomy is associated with significant postoperative adhesion formation. Laparoscopic treatment of polycystic ovaries is advocated by some and is usually reserved for patients who fail to conceive by medical means.

The ovary is stabilized and manipulated with a grasping forceps (Figure 17-51). Numerous symmetrically placed openings are drilled through the ovarian capsule and into the ovarian stroma, draining follicles as they are encountered (Plates 19 and 20). These openings can be made with various energy sources, including laser and electrosurgery. If the latter is selected, the generator is set at 20 to 60 W cutting current. Approximately 30 small openings are made in each ovary.

Pelvic and tubo-ovarian abscess

This enormously destructive process must be managed aggressively if damage to pelvic organs is to be limited. Laparoscopic diagnosis and treatment have been ideal (Plates 20 and 21).[10,11] In the process developed by one author, intravenous antibiotics are administered beginning 2 to 24 hours before surgery. Laparoscopic assessment begins by examining the upper abdomen. The patient is placed in 20-degree Trendelenburg position, and the pelvis is examined laparoscopically. A grasping forceps or blunt probe is inserted through the right lower quadrant cannula and is used for traction and retraction. The aquadissector is inserted through the left lower quadrant cannula. With these two instruments, the omentum, small and large bowel, tubes, ovaries, and uterus are gently separated. As purulent fluid is encountered, the patient is placed in 10-degree Trendelenburg position to prevent upper abdominal soilage. The abscess cavity is thoroughly debrided with the biopsy and grasping forceps and aquadissector. Culture material is obtained from inflammatory debris and removed with biopsy forceps, and from exudate in the vicinity of the tubal ostia, collected with a bronchoscope cytology brush. Grasping forceps are inserted into the fimbrial ostia and the opening is gently dilated. Retrograde irrigation is performed with the aquadissector. The quality of ampullary mucosa is noted. Tubal lavage is performed through a cervical

Text cont'd on p. 276.

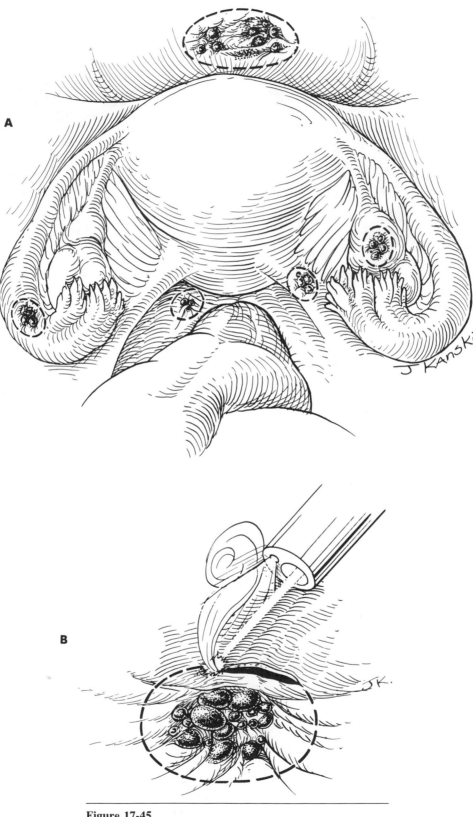

Figure 17-45
A, Resection of endometrial implants. Peritoneal implants
are noted. **B,** An implant is circumscribed by the CO_2 laser.

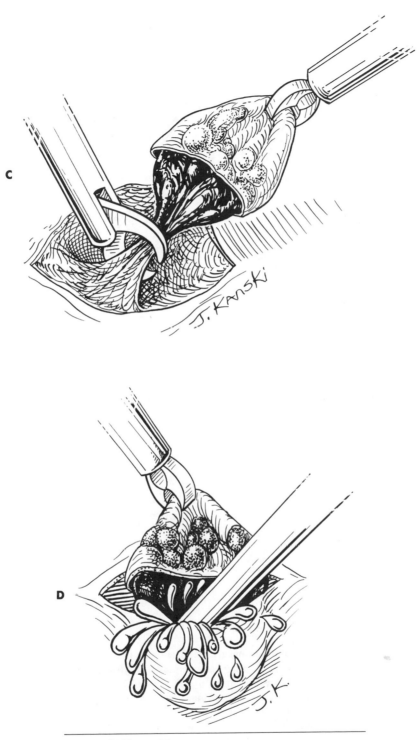

Figure 17-45, cont'd.
C, The diseased peritoneum is lifted superiorly and dissected by aquadissection. **D,** The implant is excised and the defect left open.

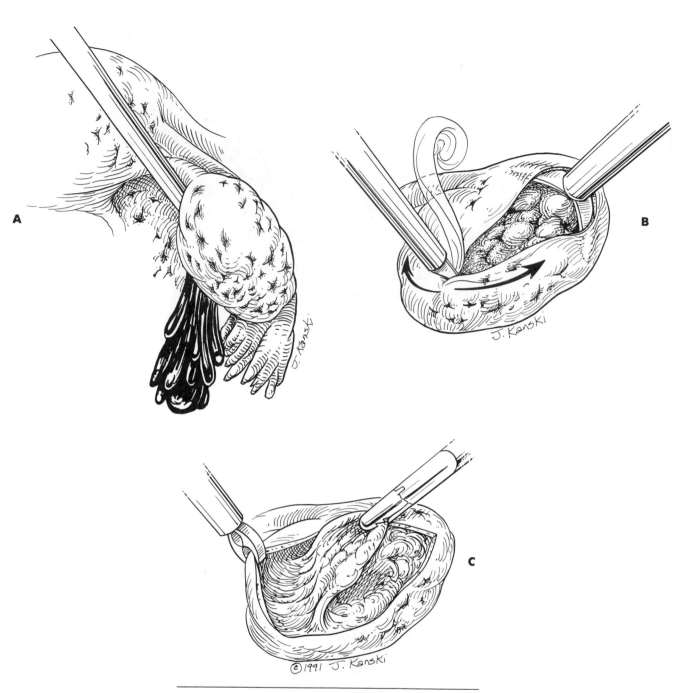

Figure 17-46

A, Resection of an endometrioma. The ovary is mobilized by aquadissection. **B,** The ovarian cortex overlying the endometrioma is incised with a knife electrode. The edges of the ovarian defect are kept separated by an open grasping instrument. **C,** The endometrioma is removed carefully by traction and countertraction. The surgeon must constantly observe tissue tension to avoid lacerating the ovary.

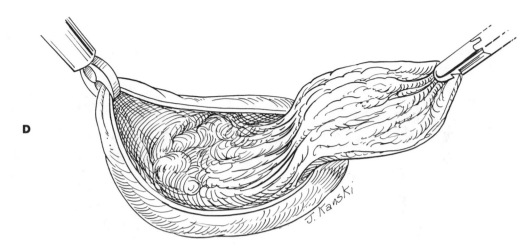

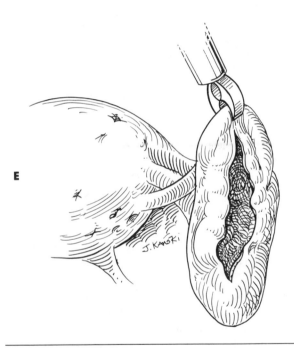

Figure 17-46, cont'd.
D, The process continues until the endometrioma is completely removed from the ovary. **E,** The appearance of the ovary after the endometrioma has been excised. Suturing is not required usually.

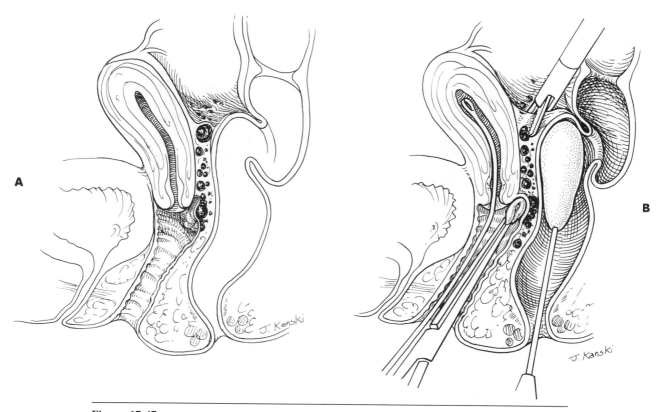

Figure 17-47
A, Cul-de-sac obliteration. Complete cul-de-sac obliteration is illustrated. **B,** With the uterus anteverted and the vaginal sponge stick and rectal probe in place, the rectum is dissected away from the endometriosis. Frequent rectal examinations may be required to assist in this part of the dissection.

cannula. Often the tube will appear to have proximal obstruction. This may be due to edema associated with acute inflammation.

The final step is copious lavage with the aquadissector, beginning with 2 L Ringer's lactate placed in the upper abdomen and 1 L on either side of the falciform ligament. Reverse Trendelenburg will cause purulent material to flow from the upper abdomen to the pelvic cavity, where it is aspirated. The patient is then placed in the Trendelenburg position again and the irrigation and aspiration process continued. As many as 15 L Ringer's lactate may be used to cleanse the abdomen and pelvis thoroughly. After an "underwater examination" to obtain final hemostasis, 2 L of Ringer's lactate are placed in the abdomen and the skin incisions closed.

The reader should note that all dissection in the acutely inflamed pelvis and abdomen is performed gently and with blunt instruments. Sharp dissection has a limited role in these procedures. The more acute the infection, the easier the dissection; however, chronic abscesses also can be treated by this method.

After surgery the patient continues to take antibiotics. Recovery generally is rapid. The patient's temperature is usually normal after the first postoperative day, and the diet is progressed as tolerated. She is discharged as soon as vital signs are normal and she is comfortable. She is examined 1 week after surgery, and all restrictions are lifted.

COMPLICATIONS

As we continue to extend laparoscopic surgery to include patients with advanced disease, we expect to have more complications. The reader is also referred to Chapters 16 and 29.

Hernia

Failure to close fascial defects greater than 7 mm may result in a postoperative hernia. If possible, these incisions should be closed.

Infection

Infection is an unusual postoperative complication after advanced laparoscopic surgery. Occasionally, a skin incision becomes infected. Its diagnosis and treatment are outlined in Chapter 16.

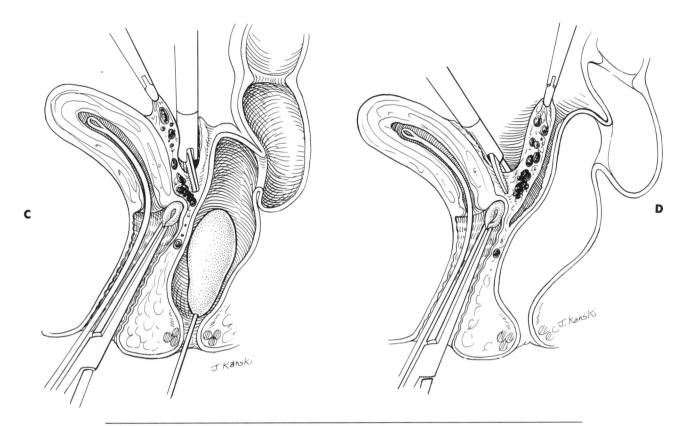

Figure 17-47, cont'd.
C, The dissection continues into the rectovaginal septum. Note traction on the endometriotic tissue to facilitate the process. **D,** The endometriosis is excised from the posterior uterus, cervix, and vagina, and the specimen is removed.

Dissemination of cancer

Although cancer cells may theoretically implant in other areas when a malignant cyst is aspirated, the risk seems to be minimal provided the malignant process is treated appropriately.

Fluid overload

Theoretically, overexpansion of the vascular system can occur during lengthy laparoscopic procedures. Although as many as 30 L Ringer's lactate solution have been placed in and aspirated from the abdomen during some procedures, and 2 L are left in the abdomen at the conclusion of the procedure, fluid overload is an unusual event. When encountered, diuretics should correct the condition promptly.

Subcutaneous and subfascial emphysema and edema

Manipulation of instruments loosens the parietal peritoneum and provides access to the subcutaneous and subfascial spaces by fluid and gas. Marked vulvar swelling can develop, requiring a Foley catheter. Similarly,

mediastinal, neck, and facial emphysema may develop. These complications usually clear spontaneously within 24 to 48 hours.

Large vessel injury

The increased intraabdominal pressure caused by insufflation, decreased venous pressure resulting from Trendelenburg, and retroperitoneal hematoma may obscure injury to a major vessel. To avoid a potentially disastrous complication, the surgeon should examine the distal aorta and the iliac vessels at the start and finish of every laparoscopic procedure. If a retroperitoneal hematoma is noted, the overlying peritoneum should be incised, the clot evacuated with the aquadissector, and, if bleeding persists, proper consultation obtained and the vessel repaired.

Epigastric vessels

By direct laparoscopic visualization from the peritoneal side at the time of introduction of the secondary trocars and cannulas, these injuries should be rare. Should one

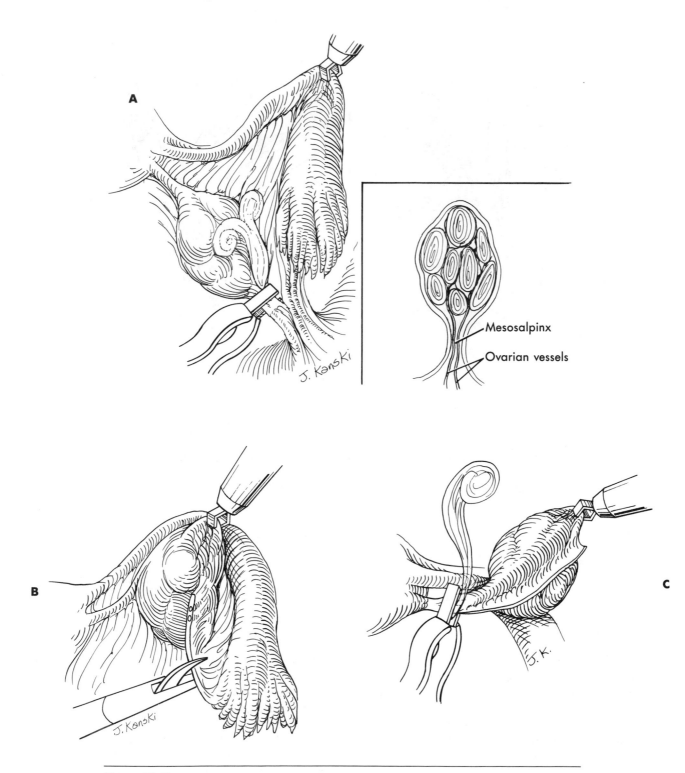

Figure 17-48
A, Oophorectomy. The mesovarium is illustrated (inset). The blood supply to the ovary is desiccated. Note the tube is lifted superiorly. **B,** The desiccation-excision process is continued. Note the ovary is lifted superiorly. **C,** The utero-ovarian ligament is desiccated and divided, and the ovary removed.

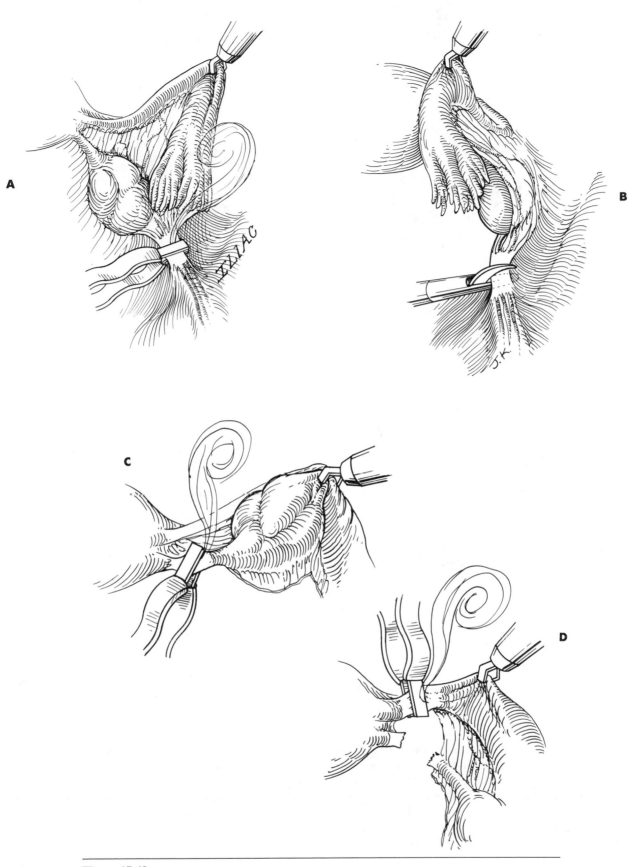

Figure 17-49

A, Salpingo-oophorectomy. The tube is lifted superiorly and desiccation of the infundibulopelvic ligament accomplished. Note the iliac vessels. **B,** The infundibulopelvic ligament is divided. The cut is made slowly to detect any vessels that may not have been occluded by desiccation. **C,** The utero-ovarian ligament is desiccated. **D,** The utero-ovarian ligament has been divided and the proximal fallopian tube is desiccated. The tube is next divided and the specimen removed.

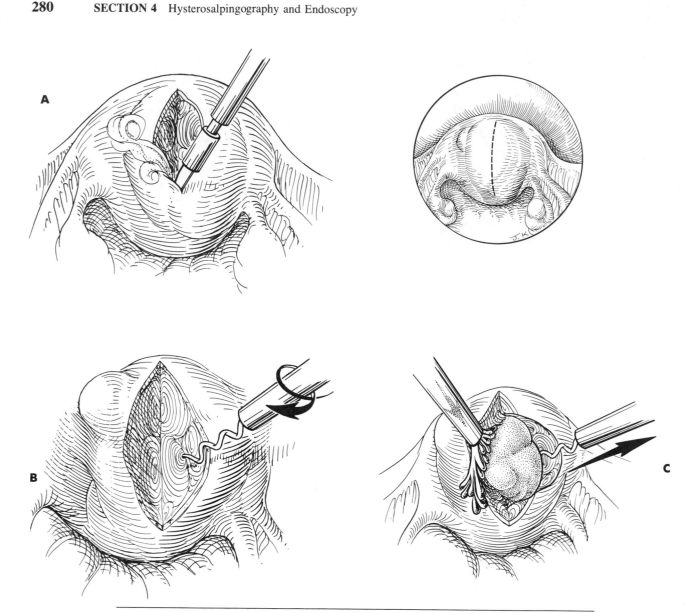

Figure 17-50
A, Myomectomy. The seromuscular incision is deepened to include a portion of the myoma *(inset)* The line of incision. **B,** A corkscrew is embedded in the myoma. **C,** The myoma is dissected from the pseudocapsule by traction and aquadissection.

of these vessels be damaged, pressure can be placed on it with the cannula by depressing the portion of the cannula outside the patient until occlusion occurs and holding it for 5 to 10 minutes. Pressure can also be applied to the vessel laceration site by inserting a Foley catheter through the cannula, inflating its balloon after the cannula is removed, and securing the catheter tightly above the skin with a hemostat.

If this does not correct the problem, the bleeding site can sometimes be desiccated from the peritoneal side with bipolar forceps superior and inferior to the injury site. The inferior portion of this vessel can be rapidly

identified where the ipsilateral round ligament curves around the vessel and enters the internal ring. A third approach is to place a large needle and suture through the abdominal wall full thickness, encompassing these vessels, and tying the suture. If needed, a second suture may be placed such that the vessels are ligated superior and inferior to the injury. This is done under laparoscopic visualization to avoid viscus injury. If these approaches do not solve the difficulty, the abdominal incision is enlarged and the bleeding vessel(s) sutured under direct vision.

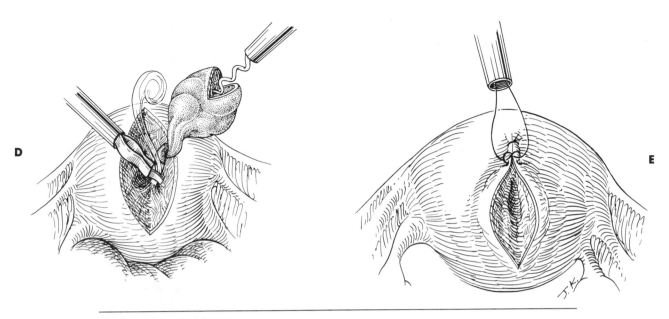

Figure 17-50, cont'd.
D, The vascular pedicle of the myoma is desiccated and the myoma removed. **E,** The uterine defect is closed with sutures.

Gastrointestinal

Although gastrointestinal complications are discussed in Chapter 16, a few additional comments are in order. The routine use of an orogastric tube should lessen the possibility of a trocar injury to the stomach. Should such injury occur, the defect may be closed with a purse-string suture of 4-0 absorbable suture placed laparoscopically.

Injury to the small or large bowel at the insertion of the insufflation needle or primary trocar may go unrecognized. In addition to inspecting the bowel at the beginning and end of the procedure, the primary cannula should be withdrawn slowly from the abdomen, with the distal end of the laparoscope still within the abdomen. By viewing through the laparoscope as it is slowly removed from the abdomen, the surgeon will detect bowel impaled on the laparoscope or a juxtaposed injured bowel segment. These injuries require immediate repair.

Intraoperative small and large bowel injury may occur. Serosal lesions can be repaired laparoscopically. Full-thickness damage usually requires laparotomy, although laparoscopic repair may be accomplished in selected instances. Appropriate consultation in the operating room should be sought in these situations.

Thermal damage is particularly worrisome, since the extent of injury is often unknown. If the area appears small and was caused by the bipolar forceps or the endocoagulator, the surgeon may elect to reinforce the site with a purse-string suture of 4-0 or 5-0 material. A unipolar electrical injury is potentially more serious and may require immediate bowel resection and repair. If in doubt,

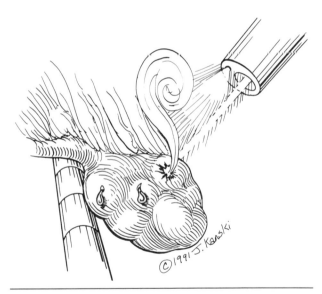

Figure 17-51
The ovary is supported and multiple follicles drained.

consultation should be sought and the appropriate steps taken.

Ureter

Intraoperatively, 5 ml indigo carmine may be injected intravenously to determine if the ureter is intact. The dye should appear in the urinary tract within 10 minutes of injection.

Should the patient develop flank pain or unusual pelvic pain after surgery, a kidney ultrasound or intravenous pyelogram should be performed. Thermal injury produces ureteral narrowing and resultant hydronephrosis. Prompt diagnosis sometimes allows successful placement of a ureteral stent for 1 to 3 months and may result in a cure without further surgery.

Urinary bladder

The secondary trocar can perforate the bladder, particularly if previous lower abdominal surgery has distorted the anatomy. The diagnosis is confirmed if gas appears in the Foley catheter, provided one is in place. If the urinary bladder is not seen at laparoscopy, it may be filled transurethrally with dilute indigo carmine for identification. A similar technique will identify a bladder perforation.

When injury to the bladder has occurred, it may be closed with a purse-string 4-0 or 5-0 synthetic absorbable suture placed laparoscopically, provided it is not adjacent to the ureter. Distending the urinary bladder with dilute indigo carmine will ascertain whether a water-tight seal exists. If the defect is small, continuous catheter drainage for 7 to 10 days should be adequate for healing to occur. The patient is treated with an appropriate urinary tract antimicrobial after surgery.

SUMMARY

Advanced laparoscopic surgery is a rapidly changing field, with new instruments and techniques being developed all the time. We urge those interested in either learning or furthering their expertise in advanced laparoscopic surgery to attend the meetings available, to keep abreast of the literature, and to observe colleagues skilled in this exciting surgical modality. Only then can we offer our patients the best care we know how to give.

REFERENCES

1. Reich H: Laparoscopic treatment of extensive pelvic adhesions, including hydrosalpinx, *J Reprod Med* 32:736, 1987.
2. Reich H: Laparoscopic oophorectomy and salpingo-oophorectomy in the treatment of benign tuboovarian disease, *Int J Fertil* 32:233, 1987.
3. Pouly JL et al: Conservative laparoscopic treatment of 321 ectopic pregnancies, *Fertil Steril* 46:1093, 1986.
4. Reich H and McGlynn F: Short self-retaining trocar sleeves for laparoscopic surgery, *Am J Obstet Gynecol* 162:453, 1990.
5. Clarke HC: Laparoscopy—new instruments for suturing and ligation, *Fertil Steril* 23:274, 1972.
6. Semm K: Tissue-puncher and loop-ligation—new ideas for surgical therapeutic pelviscopy (laparoscopy) endoscopic intraabdominal surgery, *Endoscopy* 10:119, 1978.
7. Hay DL et al: Chromic gut pelviscopic loop ligature: Effect of the number of pulls on the tensile strength, *J Reprod Med* 35:260, 1990.
8. Leach RE and Ory SJ: Modern management of ectopic pregnancy, *J Reprod Med* 34:324, 1989.
9. Schlaff WD et al: A placebo-controlled trial of a depot gonadotropin-releasing hormone analogue (leuprolide) in the treatment of uterine leiomyomata, *Obstet Gynecol* 74:856, 1989.
10. Henry-Suchet J, Soler A, and Loffredo V: Laparoscopic treatment of tubo-ovarian abscesses, *J Reprod Med* 29:579, 1984.
11. Reich H and McGlynn F: Laparoscopic treatment of tubo-ovarian and pelvic abscess, *J Reprod Med* 32:747, 1987.

UTERINE SURGERY

18

Uterine Reconstructive Surgery

MARIAN D. DAMEWOOD

JOHN A. ROCK

Uterine reconstructive surgery requires a thorough understanding of the anatomy and physiology of the uterus, as well as the principles of healing of the smooth muscle of the uterine wall. With current diagnostic techniques, an accurate diagnosis of the extent of uterine disease is often possible. Using the principles of microsurgery, the uterus usually can be restored to near normal configuration. Often when considering a uterine reconstructive procedure, a decision as to the length and depth of the incision(s) is necessary. Moreover, the surgeon in some instances must determine if a less than complete resection (i.e., partial myomectomy) is in order; if an extensive procedure were performed, infertility or perhaps hysterectomy might result. The ability to make this judgment can be acquired only through study and experience.

Uterine surgery has traditionally taken an abdominal approach, and contemporary techniques have been expanded to include the hysteroscope for procedures previously reserved for laparotomy. Surgical hysteroscopy now includes surgery on the septate uterus, uterine synechiae, and submucous myomas. In addition, medical therapy with gonadotropin-releasing hormone (GnRH) analogs has been used successfully in the treatment of myomata uteri, which formerly were thought to be amenable only to surgical therapy.

Basic principles of uterine and reconstructive surgery should help the surgeon formulate an approach to the evaluation and selection of patients for the procedures. The surgical techniques described have been developed and found useful at Johns Hopkins.

UTERINE ANATOMY AND SMOOTH MUSCLE HEALING PROCESSES

The uterus is a muscular organ in the true pelvis. It lies between the rectum and bladder and measures 7 to 7.5 cm in length, 4.5 to 5 cm in width, and 2.5 to 3 cm in thickness. The uterine cavity has an average depth of 6 to 7 cm and a capacity of 3 to 8 ml.

The uterus comprises three layers: the perimetrium (serosa), the myometrium, and the endometrium. The perimetrium is continuous with the broad ligament laterally and the bladder and rectal reflection anteriorly and posteriorly, respectively. The myometrium is composed of three layers of smooth muscle fibers. the outer layer (stratum supravasculare), which is chiefly longitudinal; the middle layer (stratum vasculare), in which fibers are in circular arrangement and contain many blood vessels; and the inner layer (exaggerated muscularis mucosae) where thin muscle strands are arranged obliquely and longitudinally. The endometrium is a mucous membrane composed of tubular glands, stroma, fine connective tissue, and a fine, delicate vasculature (Figure 18-1).

The uterus has a dual blood supply, receiving branches from both the uterine and ovarian arteries. As the uterine artery courses through the uterine body, a series of radial arteries branches from it. Each radial artery branches into straight arteries that extend only to the basal layer of the endometrium and into spiral arteries that are usually coiled and extended through the endometrium. In the superficial layer of the endometrium, "lakes" are formed by capillaries. Venous return is primarily through small veins that drain these capillary plexuses. The vascular picture is quite dynamic, with proliferation and regression associated with cyclic menstruation.

Few publications are available concerning the healing of the nonpregnant uterus. This is due in part to the lack of surgical specimens for histologic study immediately after uterine reconstruction. In particular, one study noted that studies of sections from healing uterine incisions revealed a mass of connective tissue with scattered areas of muscle bundles.[1] Hartwell[2] summarized the healing process as follows:

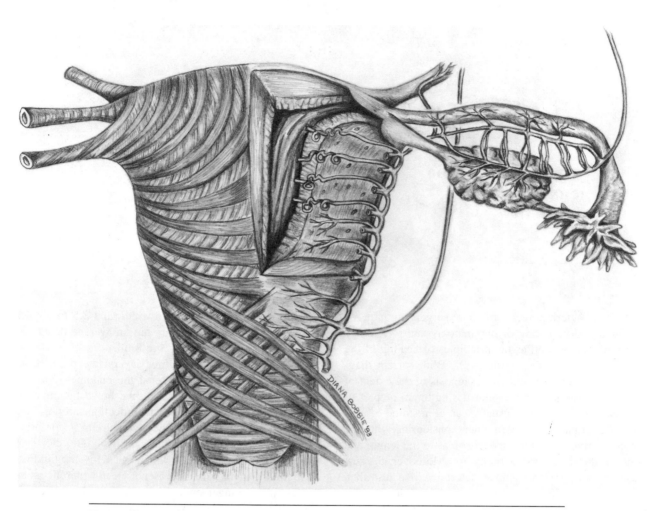

Figure 18-1
Diagrammatic representation of the uterine anatomy. The wall of the uterine body is composed of three layers: serosal, muscular, and mucosal. The muscular layer is made up of involuntary muscle fibers arranged in an interlacing fashion. Radial arteries branch in the inner third of the myometrium into straight and coiled (spiral) arteries. The straight arteries pass as far as the basal endometrium, and the spiral arteries follow a coiled course through the endometrium.

1. Healing by outgrowth of fibroblasts from preexisting structures does not occur.
2. A healing cicatrix is formed by exudate cells or macrophages.
3. Fat is of great importance in healing.
4. Determination of healing fibrosis is directly related to physical forces. That is, the healing of the uterus may be disturbed by hematoma formation, infection, improper suturing, and constitutional disease.

Siegel[3] emphasized the importance of carefully approximating the layers of the uterus to avoid incorporating the decidua or endometrium. Inaccurate approximation may result in adenomyosis, which may subsequently interfere with healing of the uterine musculature. In addition, studies have revealed that connective tissue formation after incision into the pregnant uterus is abundant and greater in amount than in the nonpregnant uterus.

No prospective studies have carefully delineated the importance of the depth and length of uterine incisions during myomectomy; nor have correlations been made between the integrity of the uterine scar and subsequent pregnancy success.

Uterine rupture after myomectomy is a rare event. Postoperative infection[4] or an extensive myomectomy[5] with entry into the uterine cavity is considered indication for cesarean section.

We believe that cesarean section is not necessarily required for delivery after myomectomy. Our clinical experience and that of others supports the view that vaginal delivery may be anticipated unless uterine scars are known to have been weakened by postoperative infection. Invasion of the endometrial cavity and the extent of myomectomy appear to be of secondary importance in determining the necessity for cesarean section. Nevertheless, care and consideration must be given to the potential risks of vaginal delivery. In our own series of 28 term pregnancies, cesarean section was performed in 12, with 16 patients having vaginal delivery without a major obstetric problem. The principal indication for cesarean section was a previous extensive myomectomy or a history of postoperative endometritis.

GENERAL DIAGNOSTIC TECHNIQUES

Major improvements in diagnostic techniques have afforded greater accuracy in identifying uterine factors that contribute to infertility. Hysterosalpingography (HSG) remains an important diagnostic procedure for the investigation of the infertile couple,[6] enabling physicians to establish tubal patency as well as to locate intrauterine abnormalities. Image intensification with fluoroscopy enhances the ability to visualize the uterine cavity in areas suspicious for synechiae, submucous myomata, or points of tubal obstruction. Congenital anomalies are usually detected initially on the HSG.

Hysteroscopy has become a major diagnostic procedure to evaluate and treat uterine abnormalities. The development of new media for uterine distention and the application of fiberoptics allow high-intensity light to be delivered salely through the hysteroscope and have broadened the indications for hysteroscopy.[7,8] Present diagnostic applications include the evaluation of women with abnormal uterine bleeding or a uterine irregularity to delineate the presence of organic pathology such as endometrial polyps, submucous myomata, and suspected uterine synechiae. The procedure also may be used to evaluate the patient with repeated abortion and in particular, to determine the extent of congenital uterine anomalies.[9] Surgical hysteroscopy has expanded the scope of uterine reproductive surgery. This technique requires additional skill in the manipulation of instrumentation such as uterine biopsy forceps, scissors, and coagulation instruments. Repeated hysteroscopic observation may be performed after lysis of uterine synechiae to determine if uterine scarring has resolved. At the same time, further lysis may be performed if necessary.

Although the findings of HSG may not always be confirmed by hysteroscopy, it is considered the definitive screening procedure. A hysteroscopic attempt to localize the lesion should be undertaken when a uterine defect is noted or suspected on HSG.[6,10] When numerous lesions are present, as with uterine synechiae or endometrial polyps, the relationship among particular ones can be studied more readily with a combination of HSG and diagnostic or operative hysteroscopy.

INSTRUMENTATION

The basic instrument set for exploratory laparotomy is that used for uterine surgery. In general, when performing a myomectomy, atraumatic forceps are necessary to grasp the uterine musculature while promoting hemostasis (Figure 18-2). A microsurgical instrument set should be available for more delicate reconstructive procedures, such as careful approximation of the uterine serosa and resection of associated endometriosis. Although chromic sutures may be used to approximate the uterine muscle, rather fine, nonreactive, absorbable sutures should be used to approximate the serosa.

ABDOMINAL RECONSTRUCTION OF THE UTERUS
Congenital uterine anomalies

Congenital uterine anomalies are usually a result of failure of lateral fusion or lack of absorption of a vertical uterine septum. Nonobstructive congenital uterine anomalies are most often noted during a diagnostic evaluation for repeated pregnancy loss (Figure 18-3). Obstructive uterine defects will still destroy any residual reproductive potential. When uterine anomaly is suspected, a thorough preoperative evaluation is indicated. An intravenous pyelogram may detect associated renal anomaly. When the vagina is patent, HSG is useful to determine the uterine configuration. Ultrasound examination may provide measurements of the uterus and vagina when an obstructive membrane is present.[11,12] Patients with uterine anomalies often require several procedures, especially if they have an associated vaginal anomaly. Since this discussion addresses only the repair of uterine anomalies, the reader is referred to a contemporary review of surgical management of associated vaginal anomalies.[13]

OBSTRUCTIVE FAILURE OF LATERAL FUSION
Noncommunicating rudimentary uterine horn

If obstruction occurs in the region of the cervix, the reservoirlike action of the vagina to accommodate cyclic menstrual blood is lost, and symptoms are often acute from retention. If the cervix is well formed on the unobstructed side, consideration may be given to anastomosing the obstructed to the unobstructed side (Figure 18-4). In anomalies of this type, it is sometimes technically impossible to repair the obstructed side and leave a functioning uterus. Therefore in some instances it may be necessary to remove the horn (Plates 23 and 24).

At times, the obstructed and isolated horn of the uterus will have a small connection to the unobstructed uterus. When this occurs, early removal is desirable so that retrograde menstruation will not cause endometriosis and compromise subsequent reproduction.

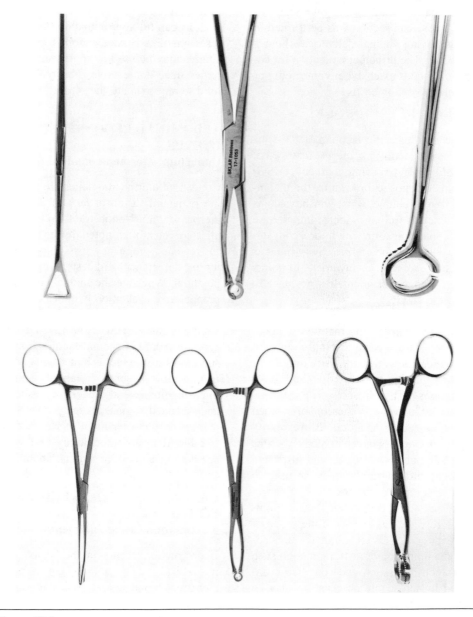

Figure 18-2
Atraumatic clamps from left to right: Pennington clamp (J. Sklar Manufacturing Co., order no. 17-2957), Pratt T forceps (J. Sklar Manufacturing Co. order no. 17-1055), and atraumatic ring clamp (special order).

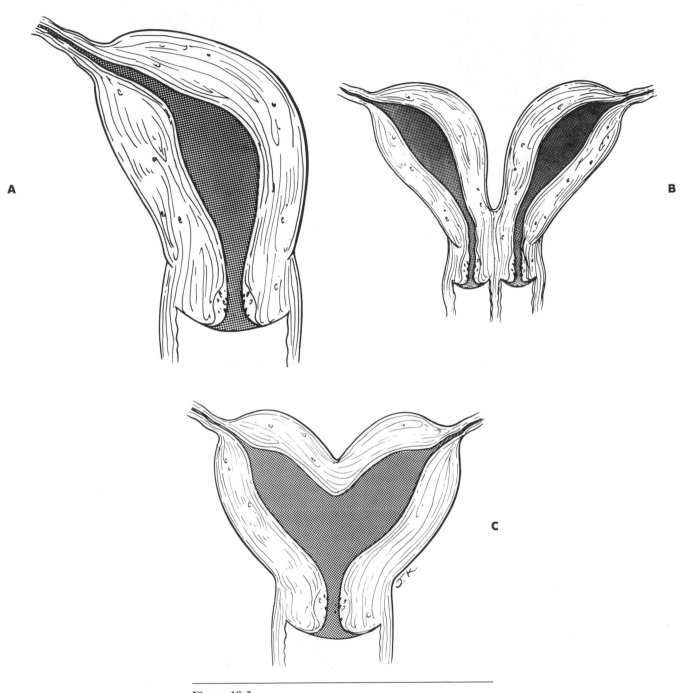

Figure 18-3
A, Unicornuate uterus. **B,** Uterus didelphys. **C,** Bicornuate uterus.

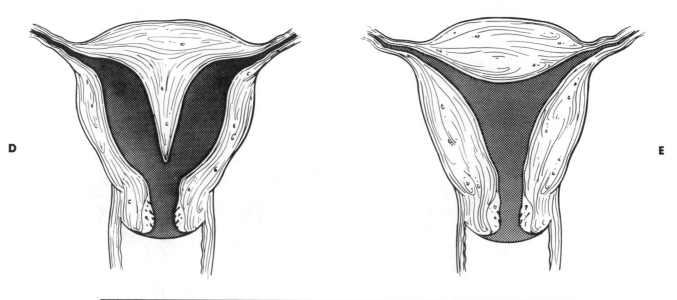

D **E**

Figure 18-3 cont'd.
D, Septate uterus. **E,** Arcuate uterus. (From Hunt RB and Seigler AM: *Hysterosalpingography: techniques and interpretation,* Chicago, 1990, Mosby–Year Book.

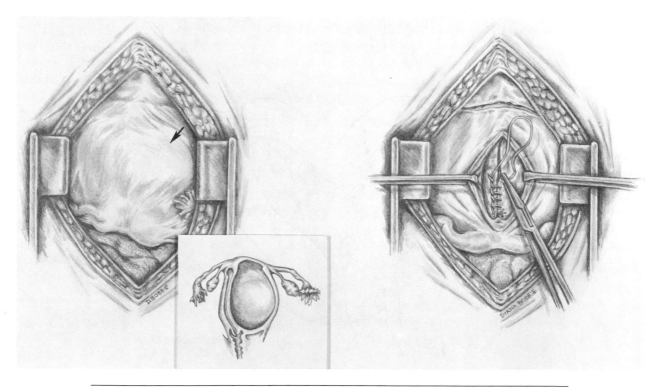

Figure 18-4
Unification of an obstructed noncommunicating uterine horn. Note the asymmetric uterine bulge *(arrow).* The uterine septum may be excised and the cavities united. Alternatively, hemihysterectomy may be performed.

Fortunately, in some instances of rudimentary horns with obstruction the cavity of the uterus fails to communicate with the fallopian tube so that menstrual blood has no opportunity to spill. Excision of these horns gives complete relief of symptoms.

A few pregnancies have been observed in an obstructed rudimentary horn. Essentially, all were in young women who were exposed to pregnancy before the monthly accumulation of trapped menstrual blood had destroyed the function of the obstructed horn. In these instances, by necessity, sperm ascended through the unobstructed side. All such patients had symptoms of an ectopic pregnancy. In more instances the rudimentary horn was surgically excised, but in others this was difficult because of the attachment of the horn to the functioning side.

When there is failure of lateral fusion of the mullerian ducts with unilateral obstruction, absence of the ipsilateral kidney is the rule. Thus an intravenous pyelogram is a useful diagnostic tool and may clarify the diagnosis in obscure circumstances.

NONOBSTRUCTIVE FAILURE OF LATERAL FUSION
Didelphic and unicornuate uteri

Women with nonobstructed failure of lateral fusion involving both the uterus and vagina (uterus didelphys) have no symptoms related to menstruation (see Figure 18-3, *B*). However, dyspareunia may be a problem because of the vagina's narrowness. If so, it may be necessary to remove the septum. This is not particularly difficult, although sometimes the septum is very thick and contains a large number of blood vessels that must be secured. At times the two vaginal cavities are asymmetric, so that vaginal function is normal and satisfactory on one side but most difficult on the other.

Overall reproduction seems to be modestly compromised in patients with didelphic uteri. Information is anecdotal and consists of case reports or small series recording examples of primary infertility, pregnancy wastage, and premature labor. Examples of simultaneous pregnancies in each uterus have been reported; some patients enjoyed a satisfactory outcome for both pregnancies. The older literature contains examples of vaginal deliveries with sequential labor, with significant intervals between onset of labor and birth. An interval of 24 hours is not unusual, and intervals of several days have been reported. Cesarean section would be performed almost routinely at the present time. There is no indication for surgical intervention in a didelphic condition except to remove a longitudinal vaginal septum, which might cause dyspareunia.

The reproductive history of a patient with a unicornuate uterus is not different from that of one with a di-

delphic uterus (Figure 18-3, *A*). This is not surprising, since a didelphic uterus is just a symmetrically inversed duplication of a unicornuate uterus.

Reproduction may be compromised by infertility, pregnancy wastage, and premature labor; however, most pregnancies seem to result in a healthy child.[14,15] Cerclage has been reported favorably in cases of repeated miscarriage and premature labor.

A comprehensive study of reported material on both the unicornuate and didelphic uterus should be undertaken. Existing data are probably biased because of the report of only abnormalities.

Bicornuate and septate uteri

A symmetric nonobstructed double uterus (i.e., septate or bicornuate) may cause a problem in reproduction (Figure 18-3, *C* and *D*). Generally, the difficulty is not in becoming pregnant but arises from abortion, which is often repeated, or from premature labor. In the event pregnancies are carried to term, obstetric malpresentation and difficulties in delivery are not unusual. Primary infertility in a patient with a symmetric double uterus is sometimes observed, but the etiologic relationship between infertility and the anomaly is unknown.

Identifying the type of symmetric double uterus without obstruction is of great importance. It is necessary to distinguish between the bicornuate and the septate uterus, since the former is usually associated with minimal reproductive problems, whereas the latter is almost always the type that is involved with reproductive failure. Two distinct horns may be felt when palpating a bicornuate uterus. The exterior configuration of the septate uterus may be essentially normal, and many of these uteri cannot be recognized at laparotomy. In some patients there may be the slightest midfundal indentation. On pelvic examination, one can suspect a septate uterus because of its broadness.

Ultrasonography may be helpful, but cannot be expected to make the critical distinction between a bicornuate and a septate uterus, nor can they be distinguished by HSG. As may be inferred from these comments, it is seldom that a bicornuate uterus requires surgical reconstruction.

A special situation pertains to the anomalies associated with and probably caused by exposure in utero to diethylstilbestrol (DES) (Figure 18-5). Kaufman and associates[16] called attention to a uterus shaped like a T with some variations in many DES-exposed patients. Haney and coauthors[17] described the lesion in detail. Although the reproductive performance of these uteri has not been specifically determined, pregnancy in DES-exposed women usually has an unfavorable outcome.[18] Nevertheless, repeated pregnancy wastage does not appear to occur and thus there is no indication for surgical intervention.[19]

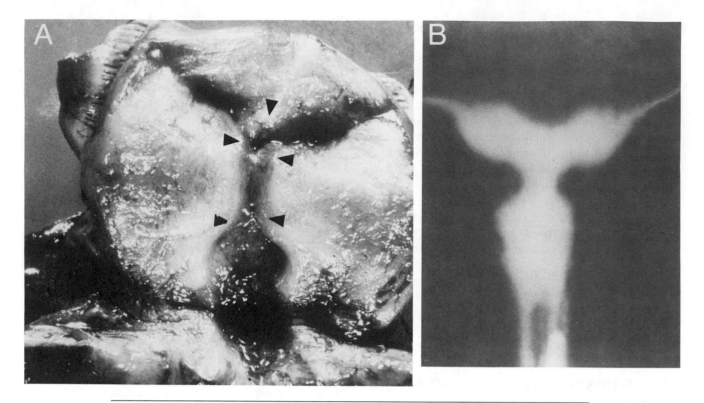

Figure 18-5
A, Gross specimen of a DES-exposed uterus. The characteristic lateral protuberances *(arrowheads)* can cause the lateral shadows seen on the HSGs in these women. From Winfield AC and Wentz AC (eds): *Diagnostic imaging of infertility,* Baltimore, 1987, Williams & Wilkins.
B, The HSG of this DES-exposed uterus closely corresponds with the extirpated specimen in **A.**

The diagnosis of reproductive wastage attributable to a double uterus is made by exclusion. In view of the fact that reproduction in a double uterus, particularly of the bicornuate type, may be essentially normal, it is necessary to determine whether one particular uterus is responsible for the reproductive problem. It is important in making the diagnosis that all other causes of repeated miscarriage be excluded. Thus investigation should include male factors and such female factors as cervical incompetence, chronic illness, luteal defects, and other endocrine disorders of the adrenal and thyroid that sometimes result in pregnancy wastage. In addition, the evaluation should require the exclusion of fetal factors, particularly karyotypic anomalies in one or other potential parents that may result in a genetically defective zygote.[20]

The characteristic history is an early-midtrimester loss associated with mini-labor starting with cramps and followed by bleeding. In a primigravid woman, labor may last up to 6 hours or even more, resulting in the delivery of a well-formed but not viable fetus. When miscarriages occur in the first trimester or when there is a history of lack of recognition of an embryo, it is necessary to suspect a genetic etiology. On the other hand, histories that differ from the typical one described above are sometimes encountered. In the absence of other causes of miscarriage, such patients may deserve uterine unification.

ABDOMINAL METROPLASTY

At present, surgical hysteroscopy is used primarily to resect a uterine septum. Thus abdominal metroplasty is no longer routinely performed except in cases of a very broad septum or during the Strassmann procedure for a bicornuate uterus. However, the three principal types of metroplasty (Figure 18-6) are reviewed as part of a complete discussion of reproductive uterine surgery.

The original Strassmann procedure is unsuitable for correcting the defect in a septate uterus. Strassmann[21] performed surgery only on a bicornuate uterus, since he worked in an era before HSG, and the diagnosis usually was made on the basis of bimanual examination and exploration of the endometrial cavity by curet. Tompkins[22] and others recommended a metroplasty beginning with a midline fundal incision in the uterus (i.e., median bivalve incision). The septum is then incised.

The exterior configuration of the uterus may be quite normal in a septate uterus. In the Tompkins procedure, however, the incision may be made precisely in the groove that can be palpated on the anterior fundal portion

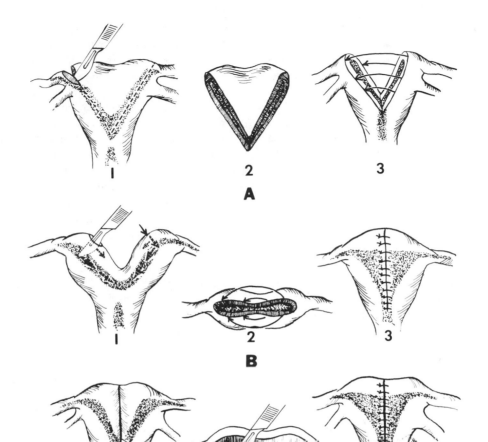

Figure 18-6
Unification of a double uterus. **A,** Jones wedge metroplasty. **B,** Strassmann unification procedure. **C,** Tompkins' fundal bivalve metroplasty. From Rock JA and Zacur HA: The clinical management of repeated early pregnancy wastage, *Fertil Steril* 39:123, 1983.

of the uterus. The anterior fundal incision is then carried downward approximately 5 cm, at which point the knife enters the endometrial cavity (Plates 25 through 29). The horns of the uterus may separate spontaneously or by gentle pressure on the incision itself, beginning at the point at which the endometrial cavity was first entered. At the point where the horns separate, the uterus will evert itself and each horn will appear to be converted into a semicylinder.[22] The uterus is then in a position to be sutured into a complete, single uterine body. The incisional closure is begun with two anterior sutures placed at the base of the incision at which the horn separation has occurred. Two posterior sutures are also placed in the corresponding posterior surface of the uterus. The uterine corpus is sutured together with a horseshoe-type incision closed by interrupted sutures of

catgut (2-0) on an atraumatic tapered needle. The uterine cavity should approximate a normal configuration at the completion of the procedure. During a Tompkins metroplasty it is important to avoid both traumatizing the myometrium and including the endometrium with the myometrial suture whenever possible.[23] After the suture line is completed, the uterine serosa is closed with running 3-0 polyglactin suture that covers the previous suture. In addition, when the initial incision is made the surgeon should not carry it to the point of the oviduct ostia, since the uterus may have oviducts entering a short distance from each other, and a very thin myometrium may exist in this location.

After the metroplasty is completed, several authors include a modified uterine suspension or plication of the round ligaments to provide uterine support and avoid adhesions.[23] A solution of 20 mg of dexamethasone and 200 ml of high-molecular-weight dextran also has been added to the peritoneal cavity to decrease adhesion formation.[23] Alternatively, one may cover the suture line with oxidized cellulose.*

Excision of the septum by wedge, or the Jones technique, has been quite satisfactory in our hands (Figure 18-7). The exterior configuration of the uterus may be quite normal, or a median raphe may be noted. Duplication of the uterus can often be confirmed by palpation.

For the procedure of the Jones metroplasty it is convenient to outline the incision with a suitable dye such as brilliant green (Figure 18-7, A). The markings help ensure that the incision is in the right place, since after the original incision is made, the uterine fundus often becomes distorted. The position of the brilliant green and the lines of incision depend on the radiographic appearance of the configuration of the cavity (Figure 18-7, C). Before making the incision, three temporary sutures can be placed, one on each side at the insertion of the round ligaments and one directly in the midline in the area that will be subsequently removed.

To control bleeding, dilute vasopressin, 5 U per 100 ml saline, may be injected into the anterior and posterior uterine walls before making the uterine incision (Figure 18-7, B). This produces blanching and diminishes blood loss during the procedure.

The uterine septum should be surgically excised as a wedge (Figure 18-7, D). The incisions begin at the fundus of the uterus. In approaching the endometrial cavity, care must be taken that the cavity is not transected (Figure 18-7, E). The original incisions at the top of the fundus are usually within 1 cm, and sometimes even less, of the insertion of the fallopian tubes. If the incision is directed toward the apex of the wedge, however, there seems to be little danger of transecting the tube across its interstitial transit in the myometrium.

After the wedge has been removed, the uterus may be closed in three layers with interrupted stitches: chromic catgut (2-0) on an atraumatic tapered needle is convenient, although synthetic absorbable materials are satisfactory. Two sizes of needles are used: a half-inch needle for the inner and intermediate layers, and a large needle, three-quarters half-round, for the outer muscular layers. The inner layer of stitches must include about one third of the thickness of the myometrium, since the endometrium itself is too delicate to hold a suture and it will cut through. The suture is placed through the endometrium-myometrium in such a way that the knot is tied within the endometrial cavity (Figure 18-7, F through H). While the suture is being tied, an assistant presses to-gether the two lateral halves of the uterus manually and with the guy sutures to relieve tension on the suture line and reduce the possibility of cutting through. The stitches are placed alternately anteriorly and posteriorly. After the first few are placed and before the first layer is completed, the second layer can be started so as to reduce tension. As surgery proceeds, the third layer can be inserted in the serosa both anteriorly and posteriorly (Figure 18-7, I through K). Finer, nonreactive suture material may be used to approximate the serosal edges of the uterus more precisely and prevent adhesion formation to the suture line (Figure 18-7, K and L).

At the conclusion, the uterus appears near normal in its configuration. The striking feature is usually the proximity of the insertions of the fallopian tubes. Special care must be taken not to obstruct the interstitial portions of the tubes while placing the fundal myometrial and serosal sutures. In the Tompkins procedure the same steps may be used to avoid adhesions.

The final size of the reconstructed uterine cavity seems to be unimportant; many times it is quite small compared with a normal uterus. Of more importance seems to be the symmetry; that is, a very small symmetric cavity seems to function quite normally. Postoperative films often show small "dogears," which are leftover tags from the original bifid condition. They do not seem to interfere with function. Although an endometrial cavity that looks normal on x-ray examination after such a procedure cannot be considered normal, it seems to function quite normally.

Duplication may only rarely involve the cervix. No attempt should be made to unify the cervix, since an incompetent cervical os will result. Surgical reconstruction must be applied only to the corpus, leaving the septum intact at the lower uterine segment.

Healing in the nonpregnant uterus is not to be compared with healing after a cesarean section, since myometrial healing after a term delivery takes place in a uterus that is undergoing involution. Thus it might be expected that cesarean section wounds are less firmly healed than incisions in the nonpregnant uterus. Nevertheless, most patients who have had surgical reconstruction of a double uterus are delivered by cesarean section as a matter of precaution. Patients with repeated abortion have had a long disappointing obstetric experience. They are often in their thirties, and to minimize the risk of an obstetric catastrophe, an elective cesarean section before onset of labor seems the most conservative course to avoid the possibility of a uterine rupture.[24]

To allow the uterine incision the best possible opportunity to heal, a delay of 9 months in becoming pregnant after surgical reconstruction is recommended. During this interval, it has been thought inadvisable to prescribe oral contraceptives because of their progestational effect on the myometrium and the possibility that healing under

---

*Interceed, Johnson and Johnson.

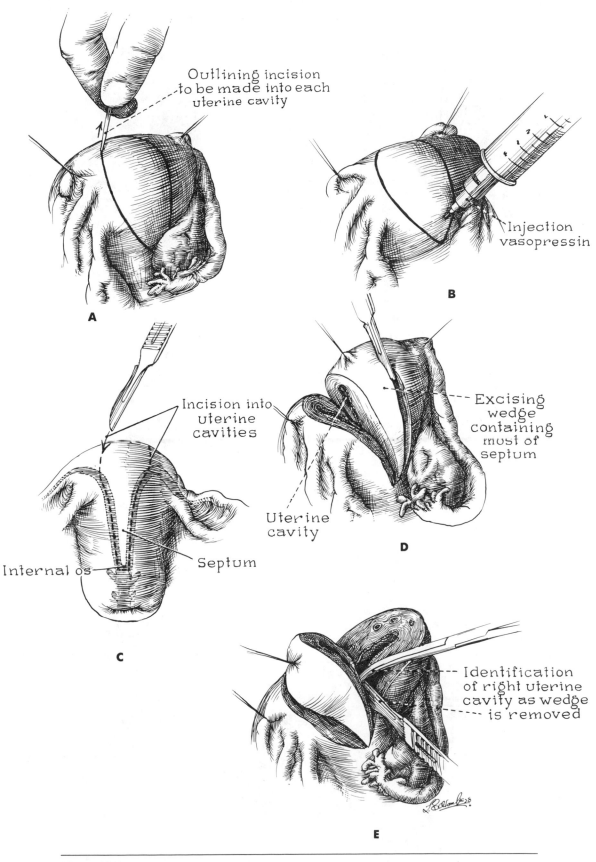

Outlining incision to be made into each uterine cavity

A

Injection vasopressin

B

Incision into uterine cavities

Internal os

Septum

C

Excising wedge containing most of septum

Uterine cavity

D

Identification of right uterine cavity as wedge is removed

E

Figure 18-7

Various steps in the operative pair of septate uterus by excision of a wedge. From Jones HW Jr and Rock JA: *Reparative and contructive surgery of the female generative tract,* Baltimore, 1983, Williams & Wilkins.

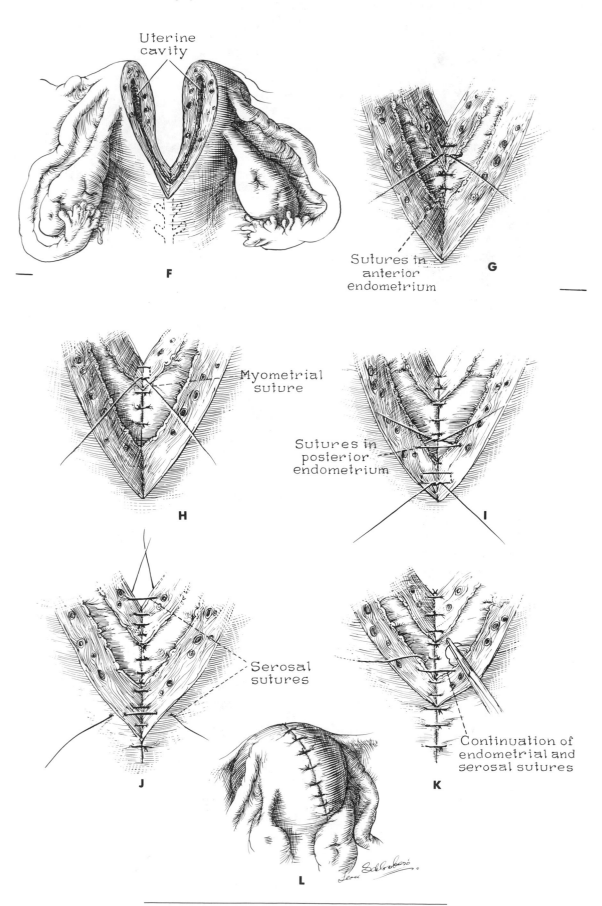

Uterine
cavity

F

Sutures in
anterior
endometrium   **G**

Myometrial
suture

H

Sutures in
posterior
endometrium   **I**

Serosal
sutures

J

Continuation of
endometrial and
serosal sutures   **K**

L

Figure 18-7 cont'd.

this circumstance would be similar to postpartum healing. Therefore mechanical contraception with diaphragm or condom is recommended.

Term delivery was reported in 77% of patients after this procedure,[25] with 73% of all pregnancies carried to term. More recent results further support the efficacy of the wedge metroplasty (Table 18-1). Similar results are established with the Tompkins procedure, with 66.7% of patients conceiving. Postoperative salvage rate in these patients was 77.8%. Pregnancy salvage rates may not rise from a particular technique of metroplasty, however, but may be related to careful patient selection.

FIBROMYOMATA UTERI

Leiomyomata alone are an infrequent cause of infertility.[26] Many women with fibroids have no difficulty with reproductive function; however, approximately 40% of women with multiple myomata have a history of infertility, repeated miscarriage, or premature labor.[27]

The major indications for myomectomy include infertility, repeated abortion, hypermenorrhea, ureteral compression, pelvic pain or pressure, frequency, and preservation of reproductive capacity. Of 1022 patients with myomata, 5% required myomectomy.[28] Alternatively, roughly 5% of infertile patients have fibroids that may be in part responsible for infertility.[29] Nine (18%) of 51 patients with infertility thought to be due to myomata underwent abdominal myomectomy to enhance their fertility. Thus fibroids are an infrequent indication for the procedure to enhance or preserve fertility. Studies are lacking that document the number of patients with significant fibromyomata who have had a term delivery.

The mechanisms by which myomata uteri interfere with reproductive function are unknown. Leiomyomata are uncommonly single tumors. They are most often multiple and generally originate from the myometrium. Their location in the uterus may be more important with respect to reproductive function than their presence. Intramural or submucous myomata may cause elongation or distortion of the endometrial cavity, subsequently increasing the distance of absolute sperm transport. Mechanical obstruction of the uterotubal junction may occur in the cornual region, with possible interference with uterotubal transport by disturbance of delicate neuromuscular mechanisms.[26] Myometrial irritation may occur from degeneration of intramural or submucous myomata or torsion of pedunculated fibroids.[30] Vascular compromise of the straight and radial arteries necessary for endometrial nutrition may result from submucous myomata. Pressure exerted by the lesions may cause chemical alterations in uterine fluid, impairing nidation and blastocyst implantation. Endometrial changes ranging from atrophy to hyperplasia were reported in up to 80% of patients with myomata.[31-33] It is suggested that a combination of these factors may be responsible for infertility. The observation

Table 18-1 Reproductive performance with double uterus before and after wedge metroplasty

Patients	Number (%) before	Number (%) after
With adequate follow-up	62	58
Pregnant	62 (100)	56 (96)
With living children	4 (6)	47 (82)
Total pregnancies	165	77
Term	0	59 (77)
Premature	9 (5)	4 (5)
Abortion	156 (95)	14 (18)
Living children	4 (2)	58 (75)

Data from the Johns Hopkins Hospital (1936-1983).

that 40% to 50% of patients conceive after myomectomy supports the fact that the neoplasms do interfere with conception.

The presence of myomata uteri in the setting of infertility does not always suggest an etiologic association. Other causative factors should be ruled out before abdominal or hysteroscopic myomectomy. Evaluation of semen count and motility, documentation of ovulation, evaluation of the luteal phase, and observation of the cervical mucus, as well as documentation of tubal patency, should be performed before surgical intervention. In patients with habitual abortion, a karyotype and an appropriately timed endometrial biopsy should also be performed.[20]

A hysterogram is particularly useful to evaluate the relationship of the tumors to the endometrial cavity and to document patency or distortion of the fallopian tubes. Hysteroscopy is an important adjunctive procedure to establish the presence of submucous myomata. Preoperative HSG is of limited value in predicting the feasibility of a myomectomy or the probability of pregnancy success after surgery.[34]

An intravenous pyelogram may be useful to determine displacement or distortion of the uterus, especially when the myomata are large and fill the pelvic cavity.

GnRH analogs as presurgical adjuncts to myomectomy

Again, traditional therapy for symptomatic myomata uteri has been surgical. Success of myomectomy, however, appears to be inversely related to tumor size, and up to 15% of patients may experience recurrent tumors.[26] Encouraging results have been achieved with the administration of a GnRH agonist as a potential alternative to hysterectomy or myomectomy in symptomatic premenopausal women or as a presurgical adjunct to myomectomy.[35] Suppression of the hypothalamic-pituitary-ovarian axis with GnRH analogs has been undertaken increasingly as treatment for estrogen-dependent conditions such as fibroids and endometriosis. Continuous administration of these agents results in down-regulation of the hypothalamic-pituitary-ovarian axis subsequent to decreased release of the gonadotropins follicle-stimulating hormone (FSH) and luteinizing hormone (LH). Efficacy of GnRH analog therapy, particularly with respect to myomata uteri, is associated with the decreased concentrations of bioactive FSH and LH, resulting in reduced concentrations of circulating estradiol and estrone. Since leiomyomata are clinically estrogen dependent, GnRH agonists administered continuously produce a medical "oophorectomy" and reduce tumor growth and volume.[36]

Administration of analogs such as buserelin has achieved significant reduction of fibroid volume as determined by pelvic ultrasound, with reductions of up to 91.2% of fibroid volume.[37] The hypoestrogenic state induced by leuprolide was effective in reducing total uterine volume, total fibroid volume, and nonmyomatous uterine volume after 6 months of therapy.[38] An average decrease of 40% in fibroid volume was achieved by several groups after 6 months of analog therapy.[39-42] The reduction achieved in any one individual fibroid may be variable and range from 0% to 100% as a result of heterogeneous leiomyomata composition.[35] The majority of size reduction appears to be achieved within 3 months of therapy and is correlated with the degree of a hypoestrogenic state achieved during therapy.[40]

Several advantages of medical therapy of fibroids with GnRH are apparent. Anemia may be improved because of the hypoestrogenic state and absence of uterine bleeding. Autologous blood donation may then be possible. The shrinkage of the fibroid and vascular compromise of the tumor may be associated with a more straightforward surgical technique with respect to location of the capsule and resection of the myoma from the uterine body. Additional randomized clinical trials are necessary to address this consideration, although preliminary data suggest enhanced surgical technique.

The GnRH analogs are administered by the subcutaneous, intramuscular or intranasal route. Treatment usually is initiated on cycle days 1 through 5. Clinical monitoring of therapy includes a pelvic examination, assessment of symptoms, and ultrasonography for myomata uteri every 1 to 3 months. Baseline bone density may be measured initially and possibly at 6- to 12-month intervals in patients at high risk for osteoporosis. Major side effects include hot flushes, headaches, and vaginal dryness. The suppression achieved by GnRH analogs is reversible, with menstruation occurring in a mean of 33 days after discontinuation of the agents.[42]

Several studies have addressed potential alterations in bone mineral density with the use of selected GnRH analogs. One group reported that bone mass did not change significantly after 6 months of intranasal or subcutaneous therapy.[43] In patients who received a 6-month course of the agents for myomata uteri and endometriosis, bone mineral density measured by dual-photon absorptiometry was not significantly altered.[44] The detectable change in bone mineral density after 6 months was approximately 0.5% in each of the four locations measured.[44] Implications of GnRH therapy for myomata uteri include the following[45]:

1. Reduced blood loss at surgery.
2. Facilitation of surgical technique.
3. Reduced risk of blood transfusion.
4. Increased preoperative hemoglobulin concentrations in iron-deficient women.
5. Increased probability of a hysteroscopic approach.

Abdominal myomectomy

The surgical technique of abdominal myomectomy is based on the observation that myomata do not invade the uterine myometrium but rather exert pressure on the surrounding tissues as they enlarge. This results in distortion and displacement of the myometrium rather than infiltration. The thinned-out myometrium that encapsulates the myoma, or pseudocapsule, provides a well-defined plane of cleavage between the fibroid and the capsule (Plates 30 and 31).

Hemostasis

Hemostasis is a major consideration at the time of uterine surgery. Myomectomy can often result in considerable blood loss. Various methods to control the uterine vascular supply have been employed. The use of a rubber tourniquet around the uterus at the lower uterine segment, placed through a small incision beneath the round ligaments, was first introduced by Rubin.[46] Alternatively, a Bonney clamp may be used to compress the ascending branches of the uterine artery and stabilize the uterus.[47] Lock[48] suggested the use of a rubber-shod sponge forceps to occlude the uterine and ovarian vessels. With these methods of compression, the release of pressure-producing clamps was recommended by the authors every 20 minutes to prevent possible ischemic necrosis of the uterine wall and to avoid the release of free histaminelike substances that may accumulate within the uterus during myomectomy.

Vasopressin may lessen blood loss because of arteriolar vasoconstriction. Dillon[49] suggested vasopressin injection at the junction of the uterus with the myoma or its pedicle. With a dose of 2 U per 10 ml solution, the effect lasted approximately 30 minutes, at which time additional injections were needed. Arterial bleeding was not masked. With the administration of vasopressin, 72% of patients requiring myomectomy did not require blood replacement, as compared with 43% of controls. Ingersoll and Malone[50] also found vasopressin injection satisfactory for minimizing blood loss, and our experience has been quite similar. Nevertheless, careful dissection and prompt suturing with application of direct pressure to bleeding vessels by the surgical assistant are necessary to aid in minimizing blood loss. Additional approaches include the use of an autologous transfusion service. A cell saver available allows the blood drained during surgery to be collected for return to the patient intraoperatively.

Allis-Adair or large T clamps may be used on the incised myometrial walls to minimize bleeding. Gentle traction between the fibroid and its pseudocapsule allows careful dissection in the plane of cleavage. In this manner, under direct vision, fibers between the fibroid and its pseudocapsule may be carefully lysed. Twisting, pulling, and blunt finger dissection to shell out the tumor should be avoided, since they usually result in excessive bleeding and perhaps the unnecessary invasions of the endometrial cavity. Furthermore, if the dissection is taken laterally, uncontrolled bleeding may occur in the broad ligaments, occasionally resulting in damage to the ureters. Particular care must be taken if myomata are adjacent to the interstitial portion of the oviducts, since inadvertent occlusion may occur if sutures are placed carelessly so as to encircle the intramural portion of the fallopian tube.

Myometrial incision

The uterine incision should be placed so that as many fibroids as possible may be removed through it. Traction sutures may be placed at the junction of the round ligaments to elevate the uterus. A single vertical incision is useful in exposing the maximum number of tumors. The location of the incision will necessarily vary, but consideration should be given to the fact that vessels supply the uterus by horizontal concentric loops (Figure 18-1). As the incision is extended, the myometrium usually retracts over the surface of the tumor. Often a tenaculum may be applied to the fibroid to elevate it.

The myometrial incision may be determined by the size and location of the fibroid. Fundal fibroids may have a broad or thin base. An elliptical incision easily exposes the pseudocapsule (Figure 18-8, *A* through *C*). Multiple subserous fibroids may pose a problem. Generally, four to five may be removed through a single incision. With the best technique, two to three incisions may be required for complete removal of multiple myomata.

Developing a cleavage plane

Vessels along the incised myometrial edge should be suture-ligated. Small bleeders along the incision may be controlled with the placement of Allis-Adair or T clamps. Proper placement of the T clamp may be useful for traction also, allowing easy dissection with Metzenbaum scissors along the pseudocapsule (Figure 18-8, *D*). If additional visualization is needed, the T clamp may be advanced and readjusted. The fibroid may be held under traction with a tenaculum to expose the attachments at its base. A Kelly clamp applied to the base will free the tumor and allow suture ligation of the pedicle (Figure

18-8, *E*). This technique is particularly useful to avoid the risk of tissue retraction where hemostasis could be achieved only with the blind placement of deep sutures. The remaining accessible fibroids are removed.

Repairing the myometrial defect

Meticulous ligation of bleeders results in minimal bood loss; however, a warm moist pad may be useful in limiting blood loss from small unidentified vessels while the uterine musculature is being repaired. If the uterine cavity is entered, the endometrium should be approximated carefully with interrupted sutures of 3-0 chromic catgut placed so that the knots are positioned within the uterine cavity. The uterine defect may be closed in two layers. The endometrium must be approximated carefully to prevent the development of adenomyosis, which may ultimately weaken the uterine scar. A purse-string suture is sometimes useful to obliterate the dead space at the base of the defect (Figure 18-8, *F*). The first layer of interrupted 2-0 chromic catgut sutures is placed so as to close the defect in the uterine wall and establish hemostasis (Figure 18-8, *G*). Care should be taken to ensure that each suture extends down to the base of the uterine defect, thus preventing hematoma formation. Depending on the size of the defect, an additional layer of suture may be necessary to approximate the myometrium. Redundant myometrium should be excised to achieve a better approximation of the serosa. The serosa may be approximated with subcuticular sutures.

Preventing adhesions

A single vertical incision is less likely to result in adhesions than are several incisions. Although all myomata cannot always be removed through one incision, often other fibroids can be removed, mobilizing them toward the primary incision.[26] With posterior uterine incisions, uterine suspension may be preferable to prevent retrofixation. Mobilizing the round ligaments to bring the broad ligament over the incision, placing omental or peritoneal grafts, or using oxidized cellulose over a posterior incision, may prevent adherence of the small bowel or sigmoid colon to the uterus. Minimizing postoperative adnexal adhesions should be a primary concern when selecting the incision site. It may be necessary to leave some myomata with the realization that tubo-ovarian adhesions would surely result if removal was attempted. Attention to surgical principles of limiting blood loss and avoiding adhesion formation will result in minimal surgical morbidity and an excellent anatomic result.

1. To limit blood loss
   a. Use vasopressin myometrial injection.
   b. Place atraumatic hemostasis clamps on the incised myometrial wall.
   c. Use moist pads to compress small bleeders.
   d. Avoid digital blunt dissection of fibroids.
   e. Use autologous transfusions.

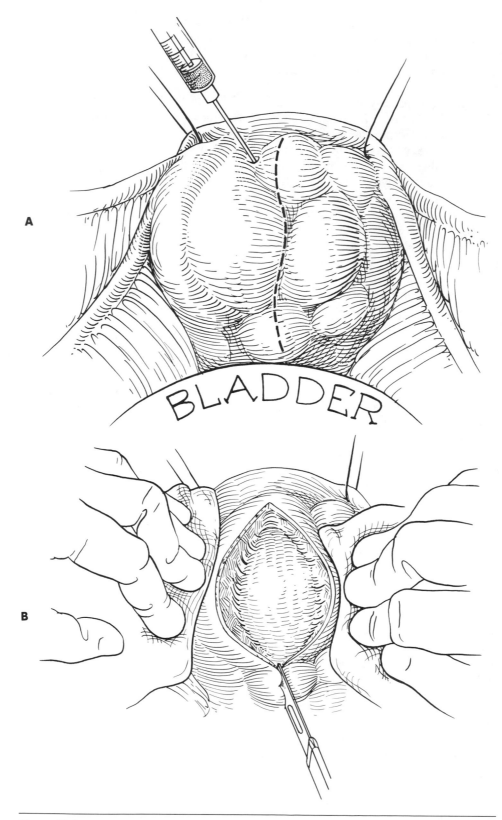

BLADDER

Figure 18-8
Technique of myomectomy. **A,** The myometrium is injected with a dilute solution of vasopressin
(1:20 dilution). **B,** A single longitudinal incision provides access to many myomata. As the
outer layer of the myometrium and pseudocapsule are incised, a well-defined cleavage plane can
be identified between the fibroid and the capsule.

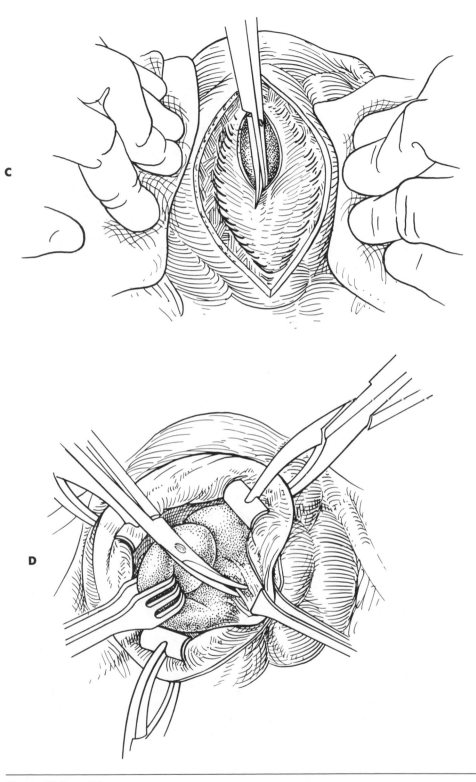

Figure 18-8 cont'd.
C, The cleavage plane is developed with Metzenbaum scissors. **D,** T clamps are applied and may be advanced for proper visualization. A tenaculum applied to the myoma aids dissection.

E

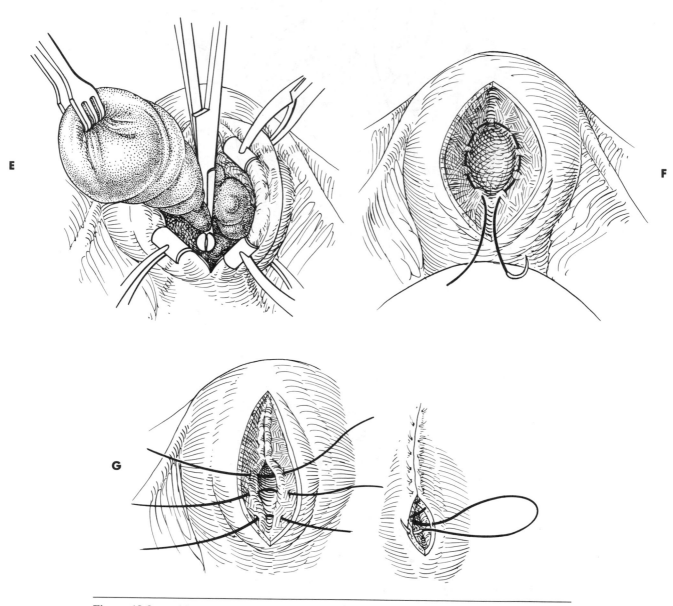

F

G

Figure 18-8 cont'd.
E, A Kelly clamp is applied to the base of the pedicle and the myoma is excised. Other accessible myomata are excised similarly. **F,** A purse-string suture obliterates the dead space at the base of the uterine defect. **G,** The myometrial defect is closed in one or two layers with interrupted sutures of 2-0 chromic catgut. The serosa is then approximated with nonreactive 3-0 absorbable sutures.

f. Use hematologic cell saver and recirculation during surgery.
2. To avoid adhesion formation
   a. Use atraumatic technique and nonreactive suture to close the serosa.
   b. Select fibroids that may be removed without increasing the risk of adnexal adhesions.
   c. Perform a uterine suspension and/or omental-peritoneal graft or use oxidized cellulose when appropriate.

Laparoscopic myomectomy

The evolution of surgical techniques applied to laparoscopy has allowed a variety of procedures to be performed through the laparoscope. Occasionally during a diagnostic laparoscopy for pelvic pain or infertility, a small myoma may be found emanating from the uterine body. With the availability of sophisticated equipment, particularly instruments providing hemostasis such as bipolar coagulators, endocoagulators, and the carbon dioxide or neodymium:yttrium-aluminum-garnet (Nd:YAG) laser, small subserosal or intramural myomas may be removed with minimal blood loss.

Laparoscopic myomectomy involves injecting saline or dilute vasopressin into the base and capsule of the myoma. The capsule is then incised and capsular tissue is reflected back with grasping forceps. The capsule is carefully stripped off the myoma and the myoma is grasped with large forceps or secured with a corkscrew. The myoma is removed by gentle twisting and traction after thorough hemostasis at the level of the pedicle has been achieved. The pedicle is then incised with laparoscopic scissors. Usually, point coagulation or laser application at the myoma base controls bleeding at this location. In some situations, endosutures may be used to close a large defect in the uterine serosa (see Chapter 17).

Results

A term pregnancy rate in the range of approximately 40% to 50% may be expected after myomectomy in patients with primary infertility.[50-53] Of 75 patients with a uterus greater than twice normal size, 49% conceived after myomectomy and 40% delivered term infants.[54] Roughly two thirds of these patients had primary infertility of an average duration of 4 years. The majority of pregnancies occurred within the first 2 years after myomectomy.

We recorded a similar experience in 67 patients treated with myomectomy between 1930 and 1975.[52] Thirty-six (54%) of 67 patients conceived; 28 (42%) had a term delivery that resulted in a living child. Eight-two percent of the patients who conceived did so within the first 2 years after myomectomy. Of the 46 patients in the study, 42 had a preoperative hysterogram, which showed a distorted endometrial cavity in 9. Of these, five had secondary infertility and three had primary infertility. The remaining 33 had endometrial cavities that were normal by HSG. Correlation between the distortion of the endometrial cavity and pregnancy success could not be demonstrated. An update of our patient series between 1951 and 1983 revealed an acceptable pregnancy success rate after myomectomy (Table 18-2).

Recurrence of fibromyomata after myomectomy may occur in an appreciable number of patients. Clinical reports indicate that it is between 14% and 45%.* Among 49 women who underwent myomectomy, 22 (44.9%) required hysterectomy within 1 to 18 years.[28] Fourteen (63.6%) of these 22 patients required hysterectomy for recurrence of myomata that were responsible for symptoms. In the Johns Hopkins study, 28% of patients required additional surgery for the recurrence of fibromyomata.[52] Less than one half of these patients, however, required hysterectomy. In general, recurrence is a measure of the thoroughness of the surgeon's search for all myomata, including seedlings, at the time of the original procedure. Every attempt should be made to remove each fibroid carefully. Occasionally, an exploratory incision may help to identify a suspected fibroid that can be palpated within the uterine musculature.

As a rule, an incision in the nonpregnant uterus heals far better than one in the gravid uterus. Although some surgeons feel that myomectomy is an absolute indication for delivery by cesarean section, we have been less stringent. Vaginal delivery may be anticipated unless the uterine scars are known to have been weakened by postoperative infection or if several incisions were required for a rather extensive myomectomy. Of the 28 term pregnancies in our series, 16 patients delivered vaginally without complications and 12 were delivered by cesarean section.[52]

SURGICAL HYSTEROSCOPY FOR UTERINE REPAIR

The hysteroscope has become an important diagnostic as well as therapeutic tool in the study of uterine function and fertility. In a series of 210 patients with infertility, intrauterine abnormalities were demonstrated in 34.3%.[57] The types of intrauterine problems subsequently diagnosed on hysteroscopy are noted in Table 18-3. Furthermore, the majority of findings in these cases may be treated with the hysteroscope. Resection of submucous myomata, uterine adhesions, and polyps, and correction of the subseptate uterus may be accomplished through the hysteroscope or resectoscope.

Uterine synechiae

The phenomenon of intrauterine synechiae was identified by Heindrich Fritsch in 1894 when he published the first observation of total atresia of the uterine cavity resulting from curettage for postpartum bleeding. Full recognition

*References 28,30,52,55,56.

Table 18-2 Rate of conception and total number of term pregnancies and abortions after myomectomy

Type of infertility	Number of patients	Number (%) of pregnancies	Number (%) of term deliveries	Number of abortions
Primary	45	19 (42)	16 (36)	3
Secondary	21	16 (76)	12 (57)	4
Totals	66	35 (53)	28 (42)	7

Data from Johns Hopkins Hospital (1936-1983).

Table 18-3 Hysteroscopic findings in 58 patients with abnormal uterine bleeding

Hysteroscopic findings	Number (%) of patients
Submucous leiomyomas	9 (15.5)
Intramural leiomyomas*	5 (8.6)
Endometrial polyp†	5 (8.6)
Thick and irregular endometrium‡	3 (5.3)
Intrauterine adhesions	3 (5.3)
Uterine septum	3 (5.3)
Arcurate uterus	2 (3.4)
Adenomyosis	2 (3.4)
Endocervical polyp	1 (1.7)
Placental remnants	1 (1.7)
Isthmic adhesions	1 (1.7)
Normal uterine cavity	23 (39.5)
Totals	58 (100)

*One case associated with adenomyosis, and another associated with intrauterine adhesions.

†One case associated with uterine septum.

‡In one patient the histopathologic diagnosis was endometrial polyp. From Tozzini RI and Pineda RI: Selection of patients for hysteroscopy: experience with 300 operations. In Siegler AM and Lindemann HJ (eds): *Hysteroscopy, principles, and practice,* Philadelphia, 1984, JB Lippincott.

of this syndrome resulted from several publications by Asherman[58-60] describing its clinical features. Although this syndrome has several eponyms, including Asherman's syndrome, the term *intrauterine synechiae* has gained wide use and acceptance.[61]

The definition of intrauterine synechiae requires the presence of an adherence to the anterior and posterior uterine wall that results in complete or partial obliteration of the cavity. Depending on the extent of the synechiae, specific clinical symptoms may result. Numerous articles have described etiology, symptoms, and therapy.[61-65]

The frequency of intrauterine synechiae is not known, although it is possible to determine the rate of occurrence in certain patient groups. For example, 20% to 25% frequency was observed in all patients treated with dilatation and curettage within 2 months postpartum.[66] Frequency has been estimated as 1.5% of all patients who have had

hysterograms[67] and 68% of women with infertility after two or more curettages.[59] Roughly 5% of all hysterograms done for repeated abortion revealed intrauterine adhesions.[68]

Surgeons in certain countries have reported a high prevalence of uterine synechiae thought to be due to an increased rate of postabortal infection.[69,70] This may be related to tuberculosis of the genital organs, which is not uncommon in some areas.

Intrauterine synechiae were observed at hysteroscopy in 192 of 7000 patients evaluated for abnormal bleeding, infertility, and/or uterine pathology.[63] All those with synechiae had a history of uterine manipulation, and 63 reported a history of postcurettage infection. It is not possible to determine the overall incidence of women with reproductive difficulty attributable to uterine synechiae until a reference population is established of these patients who have delivered uneventfully.

The etiology of uterine synechiae may be considered from three viewpoints. Although a congenital abnormality has been considered as an etiologic factor, it has not been documented in the literature.[71] Trauma is the most frequent antecedent event: puerperal dilatation and curettage results in the highest prevalence.[72] Less frequently, synechiae may result from diagnostic curettage, myomectomy, cesarean section, caustic abortifacients, uterine packing, metroplasty, and hysterotomy. Dilatation and curettage between the second and fourth weeks postpartum was reported to result in the greatest frequency of uterine synechiae.[66] This appeared to be the vulnerable phase, since curettage during the first week resulted in low frequency. Thus a hypoestrogenic state after delivery or abortion may result in poor endometrial proliferation and may predispose to the formation of intrauterine adhesions.

Although Asherman[58] originally reported that adhesions resulted from mechanical forces, others considered infection to be the primary etiologic factor.[68] The authors noted that cornual adhesions were located where the curet was unable to reach but perhaps where infection could easily spread. An endometrium refractory to estrogen was viewed as a possible explanation for this observation.

Pelvic angiography in patients with significant intrauterine synechiae revealed widespread vascular occlusion of myometrial arteries in 7 of 12 patients.[73] These authors suggested that such findings could explain the poor obstetric history in some patients, as well as their greatly reduced menstrual flow. Furthermore, they theorized that hypomenorrhea could be a reflection of atrophy or fibrosis of the uterine cavity attributable to infection or extensive vascular damage.

Asherman[58,59] hypothesized that sustained myometrial contractions could cause narrowing of the isthmus, resulting in adhesions between opposing endometrial surfaces. A more reasonable explanation states that trauma to the basal layer of the uterine mucosa and myometrium results in granulation tissue that persists for several days. If granulation tissue from opposing walls is joined, forming a bridge of tissue, this may become infiltrated by myometrium and covered by endometrium.[66] The resulting synechiae or scarring may involve a large portion of the uterine cavity or may be scattered throughout the fundus. When the endometrial cavity is significantly reduced in size, hypomenorrhea may result.

Traumatic damage to and infection of the endometrium may cause corporal or cervical synechiae or both, which may result in hypomenorrhea-amenorrhea, a symptom of Asherman's syndrome. Originally, menstrual insufficiency was thought to be a frequent sign of uterine synechiae.[74,75] Contemporary reports reveal that menstrual irregularity may occur in only 20% of affected women.[22,64,76] A close correlation was demonstrated between the severity of menstrual insufficiency and the extent of corporal adhesions.[62]

Secondary amenorrhea may be due to complete obliteration of the uterine cavity or stenosis or atresia of the internal os; under these circumstances, the ovarian cycle may continue, but the endometrium becomes refractory to hormonal stimuli. Seldom does hematometra occur. Simple cervical dilation may restore menstruation in 4 to 5 weeks. This menstrual insufficiency may be explained by two pathophysiologic mechanisms: reduction of endometrial bleeding area and possible atrophic changes and unresponsiveness of the endometrium, possibly related to a visceral reflex originating in the area of the internal os.[62] Furthermore, the occurrence of severe dysmenorrhea with hypomenorrhea when adhesions are located in the isthmic area may be related to the mechanical obstacle to free flow of menstrual blood. Adenomyosis may account for pain in approximately 25% of patients with intrauterine synechiae.[77]

Additional symptoms that are commonly recognized are infertility and abortion. Over 80% of patients in our series whose symptoms were diagnosed as uterine synechiae complained of repeated pregnancy loss.[64] Various theories for this association with infertility have been set forth. Adhesions may impede sperm migration or create an unsuitable endometrial environment for the blastocyst. In some instances the synechiae may actually obliterate the internal os. It has also been hypothesized that adhesions may cause occult or missed abortion or, on occasion, intrauterine fetal demise. In one group of patients, disastrous pregnancy outcomes were abortion, 33%, premature labor, 33%, and ectopic pregnancies, placenta accreta, and placenta previa, 33%.[78] Of 18 pregnancies in 17 patients treated for Asherman's syndrome, only 6 resulted in an uncomplicated term delivery.[79] Four patients had premature delivery and neonatal death, three had placenta accreta and postpartum hemorrhage, and one had a cervical pregnancy. Two had incomplete or missed abortion. These studies, together with those by others,[80-82] indicate a high prevalence of fetal wastage in patients who have been treated for intrauterine synechiae.

The diagnosis may be visually confirmed by hysteroscopy, however, HSG remains an important adjunct. Synechiae are recognizable by their lacunar pattern with sharply angulated edges (Figure 18-9). When performing HSG, it is important to inject only 2 ml of dye so as not to obscure the view.[72]

Other methods, such as sounding the uterine cavity, progesterone withdrawal, and a careful history, may aid in establishing the diagnosis. Sounding with a uterine probe may allow exploration of the uterine cavity with detection of synechiae as irregularities. Failure to bleed with progesterone after proper estrogen priming is suggestive of endometrial sclerosis; however, the differential diagnosis must also include other disease entities, such as hypogonadotropic hypogonadism and premature ovarian failure, which must be excluded. The biphasic basal body temperature chart in the presence of amenorrhea is highly suggestive of an unresponsive uterus attributable to endometrial sclerosis.[58]

Occasionally it is possible to disrupt synechiae with the endometrial curet when exploring the cavity. Grossly, synechiae are bands identified between the anterior and posterior uterine walls. Histologic examination of the band or scar reveals a core of endometrial tissue with fibrosis of a variable degree surrounded by superficial epithelial cells. Synechiae may contain inflammatory cells. Examination of areas of endometrium away from the synechiae may reveal inactive endometrial glands with fibrosis; however, some areas may have glands that retain their cyclic activity.

Hysteroscopic lysis

Therapy for uterine synechiae has as its goals the restoration of normal menstrual function and the restoration of fertility. Although almost all authors agree that lysis of synechiae is beneficial, little agreement exists as to the choice of adjunctive treatment, such as the use of prostheses and hormonal therapy. Because of the lack of trials with carefully controlled, randomized treatment groups, it has not been possible to determine the efficacy of any particular regimen; however, it is important to establish a uniform approach.

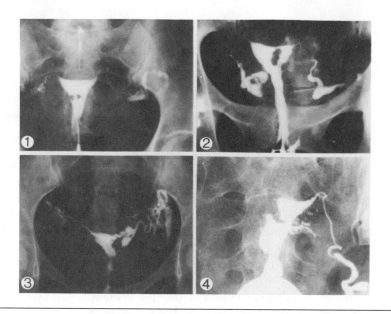

Figure 18-9
Intrauterine synechiae classified by hysterography according to Toaff and Ballas.[62] (1) Grade I—small defect well inside the uterus. (2) Grade II—medium sized defect occupying one fifth of the uterine cavity. (3) Grade III—several defects involving one third of the cavity, which is asymmetric because of marginal adhesions. (4) Grade IV—large filling defect occupies most of the uterine cavity and has resulted in tubal obstruction.

The extent of intrauterine adhesions can be delineated and the amount of uterine cavity obstruction demonstrated by hysteroscopy, and almost all of them can be incised under visual control. When the hysteroscope is introduced into the endocervix, the adhesions may be identified. The instrumentation includes the hysteroscope, with the lens and tips at an angle of 25 to 30 degrees to allow viewing of the ostia.[83] The diagnostic hysteroscope is usually 5 mm in diameter and the surgical hysteroscope at least 7 mm in diameter, often requiring cervical dilatation. A surgical channel for flexible or semirigid instruments is present with the surgical hysteroscope. An Nd:YAG or argon laser will fit through the hysteroscope for incision of uterine adhesions. The resectoscope features a 90-degree wire loop attached to an electrical generator set at 40-W cutting current. The resectoscope is inserted into a insulated hysteroscope sheath, allowing approximately 4 cm range of movement of the wire loop within the field.[83]

The surgical hysteroscope is used with Hyskon (32% dextran 70, 10% dextrose USP) to obtain a clear image of the adhesions when the uterine cavity is moderately dilated by the solution. High-molecular-weight dextran provides excellent visualization, although carbon dioxide may be used safely for diagnostic hysteroscopy. Although uterine bleeding may not be present, the use of dextran may osmotically draw fluid into the intravascular space. Abrupt volume expansion has resulted in pulmonary edema, with subsequent disseminated intravascular coagulation in a number of cases.[84-86] For this reason we do not recommend more than 300 ml of distention medium to be used during a procedure.

Transhysteroscopic lysis of synechiae under direct visualization is the preferred therapeutic modality. Curettage is useful in removing the fragments of tissue that remain after lysis. After the hysteroscope is introduced into the endocervix, the adhesions, once identified, should be separated at their midpoint (Figures 18-10 and 18-11). The central adhesions should be approached first, regardless of density. The outline of the uterine cavity can be delineated and marginal and sidewall adhesions may be approached. When the synechiae are lysed with the conventional hysteroscope, blood may obscure vision with loss of orientation within the cavity. Bleeding may be reduced with the resectoscope and a flushing system.

After surgery, agglutination of the anterior and posterior walls of the uterine cavity should be prevented. In our experience a 3-ml Foley catheter placed for 10 days in the uterine cavity with broad-spectrum antibiotic coverage has provided a satisfactory solution of this problem. In addition, a conjugated estrogen regimen for 25 days (days 1-25) with medroxprogesterone acetate for 10 days

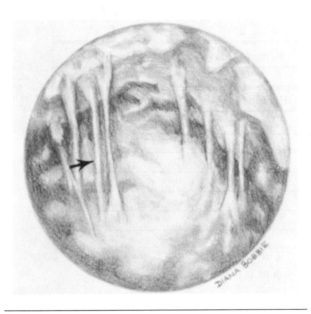

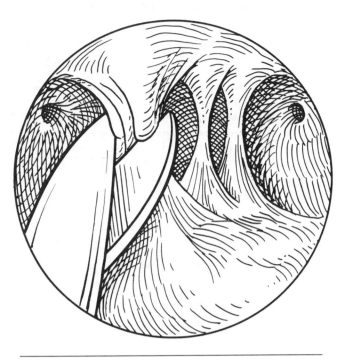

Figure 18-10
Intrauterine synechiae as visualized through the hysteroscope. Arrow shows the point of lysis with the hysteroscopic scissors.

Figure 18-11
Intrauterine adhesions divided with hysteroscopic scissors.

(days 16-25) starting after surgery will promote endometrial proliferation and healing. A repeat hysterogram, hysteroscopy, or both in 3 months is recommended to determine if synechiae have reformed.

Results. It is difficult to compare pregnancy rates in different patient series because of the large number of treatment regimens and the use of different adjunctive therapies. Furthermore, strict definition of criteria used for diagnosis are lacking. Various types of adjunctive therapy have been administered and several kinds of intrauterine devices used.

Observations based on reports during the 1980s reflect pregnancy success rates in the range of 30% to 50%.[7,87] The Johns Hopkins experience with hysteroscopic lysis of adhesions has been comparable (Table 18-4). Although several authors[63] recommended a classification system based on correlation of defects revealed by hysterogram, other investigators have not been able to demonstrate a direct correlation between extent of adhesions and pregnancy success.[88] The hysteroscope has provided not only an excellent means of diagnosis but a method to classify the extent of disease under direct visualization. A useful system for categorization based on the amount, character, and site of adhesions is shown in Figure 18-12.[89]

Although correlation between the hysterogram and hysteroscopic findings has been poor, direct correlation between menstrual patterns and the degree of endometrial

Table 18-4 Reproductive performance of women with intrauterine adhesions before and after therapy

Reproductive performance	Number (%) before therapy	Number (%) after therapy
Patients with adequate follow-up	31	31
Patients pregnant	31 (100)	26 (84)
Patients with living children	9 (29)	20 (65)
Total pregnancies	79	29
Term	9	21
Premature	6	2
Abortion	64	6
Spontaneous	56	5
Induced	8	1

Data from the Johns Hopkins Hospital (1936-1983).

scarring has been demonstrated. Perhaps with a standard classification, variables comparisons among regimens may be possible.

THE SEPTATE UTERUS

As previously discussed, mullerian fusion defects have been associated with repeated pregnancy wastage in the first and second trimesters. The septate or subseptate

THE AMERICAN FERTILITY SOCIETY CLASSIFICATION OF INTRAUTERINE ADHESIONS

Extent of Cavity Involved	<1/3	1/3 - 2/3	>2/3
	1	2	4
Type of Adhesions	Filmy	Filmy & Dense	Dense
	1	2	4
Menstrual Pattern	Normal	Hypomenorrhea	Amenorrhea
	0	2	4

Prognostic Classification   HSG· Score   Hysteroscopy Score   Additional Findings: _____

Stage I   (Mild)   1-4   _____ _____   _____

Stage II   (Moderate) 5-8   _____ _____   _____

Stage III (Severe)   9-12   _____ _____   _____

Figure 18-12
American Fertility Society classification of intrauterine adhesions.

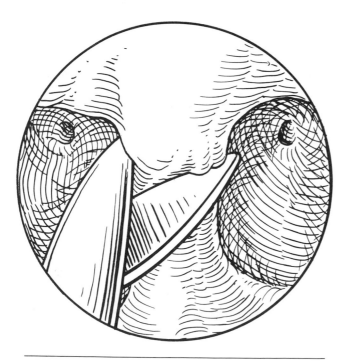

Figure 18-13
The uterine septum is divided with hysteroscopic scissors.

uterus, once managed by abdominal metroplasty, now can be successfully corrected with the surgical hysteroscope with the transcervical resection technique. Concomitant laparoscopy may also be performed to denote the external contour of the uterus.

The surgical approach includes incision of the septum with scissors under direct visualization (Figure 18-13) or with electrosurgery using the resectoscope (Figure 18-14). The Nd:YAG laser also has been used successfully. As the walls of the septum separate and retract, the contour of the uterine cavity becomes evident. Although minimal bleeding usually occurs from the avascular septum, a 3-ml balloon may be inserted for hemostasis if excessive bleeding is encountered. Several series have reported satisfactory degrees of septal resection as revealed by postoperative hysterogram.[90,91] The hysteroscopic procedure offers the patient a shorter hospitalization, ultimately avoiding the necessity for a cesarean section in a subsequent pregnancy. A delay of 2 to 3 months before attempting pregnancy is suggested to allow complete resorption of septum remnants.[7]

SUBMUCOUS MYOMATA

Hysteroscopy is often performed in the management of submucous fibromyomata uteri. This procedure is useful not only in preoperative assessment but in the resection of submucous myomata (Figures 18-15 and 18-16). The development of the panoramic surgical hysteroscope has allowed resection of these lesions with an electrosurgical wire loop, scissors, and Nd:YAG laser with excellent anatomic results.[92] The resecting hysteroscope is essentially a modification of the urologic resectoscope.[93] Hyskon is often used as a distending medium. Cutting or blended current best suited for resection of submucous

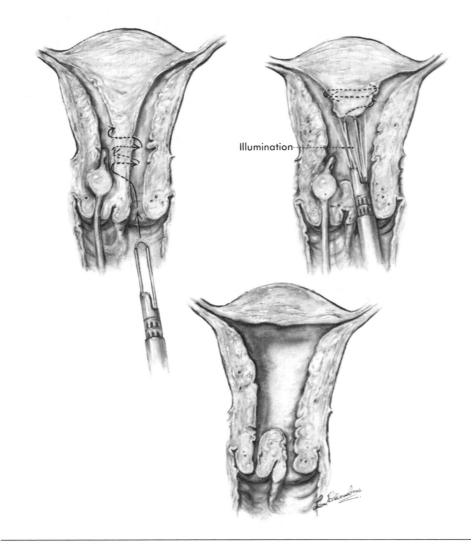

Illumination

Figure 18-14
Lysis of complete septum leaving the cervical septum intact. Modified from Siegler AM: Hysteroscopic metroplasty. In Siegler AM (ed): *Therapeutic hysteroscopy: indications and techniques,* St. Louis, 1990, Mosby–Year Book.

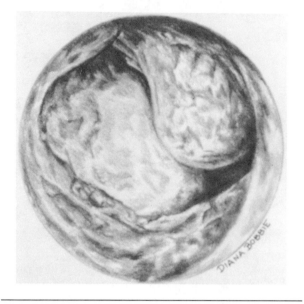

Figure 18-15
Hysteroscopic view of submucous fibroids. If quite large, the uterotubal os may not be visualized. The fibroid may be shaved down in several layers with the resectoscope.

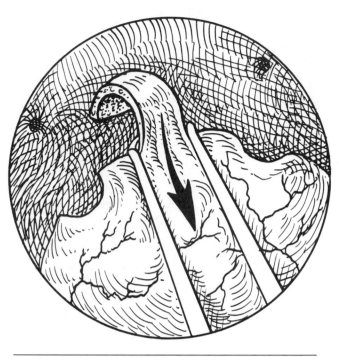

Figure 18-16
The submucous fibroid is resected with a resectoscope.

myomata is 60 to 120 W, which results in a 2-mm depth of injury. These instruments provide visual control for a transcervical excision of the predunculated myoma and a resection of the sessile one. Indications for myomectomy by hysteroscopic resection include the presence of a submucous myoma that is symptomatic, with menorrhagia unresponsive to therapy. In addition, as previously discussed, submucous myomata may be associated with repeated pregnancy wastage. Therapy with GnRH analogs is particularly useful to reduce the size of lesions before the surgical procedure. The majority of reduction in fibroid size appears to occur after 3 months of analog therapy.

The technique described by Neuwirth[93] uses dextran 70 or Hyskon, which is injected from a 15-ml syringe or a controlled foot-pedal injection system into the hysteroscopic cannula. A standard oblique telescope and the urologic resectoscope sheath with electrosurgical current of 60 W for the cutting loop are used. The tumor is shaved down as close as possible to the level of endometrial cavity in several layers, with fragments removed as they are shaved off. As noted, the cutting current itself results in a 2-mm depth of injury. Laparoscopy is used for visual control and to avoid perforation of the uterus, as well as to displace the bowel from the posterior uterine surface.

The size of a pedunculated tumor can be reduced with the cutting current until the tumor itself can pass easily through the cervix and the base coagulated at the level of the pedicle. The balloon of an inflated Foley catheter of large diameter may be inserted temporarily into the uterine cavity to control bleeding from the myoma or pedicle base. Transabdominal myomectomy may now be reserved for submucous myomata in the cornual region or for tumors of such magnitude as to not be approachable through the hysteroscope.[94] The major risks of surgical hysteroscopy include uterine perforation, infection, and electrosurgical injury; however, morbidity is reduced compared with that of abdominal myomectomy. In one series,[93] over 80% of patients retained their uterus and did not undergo a subsequent hysterectomy.

OTHER APPLICATIONS OF SURGICAL HYSTEROSCOPY

The majority of hysteroscopic procedures are performed for intrauterine synechiae, septate uterus, or submucous myomata. The hysteroscope also has been employed to retrieve lost intrauterine devices and remove polyps. In the future, microhysteroscopy may be used to analyze endometrial tissue from a pathologic perspective.

REFERENCES

1. Kerr JMM: Wounds of the gravid and non-gravid uterus: a study of uterine scars, *Proc R Soc Med* 17:123-131, 1924.
2. Hartwell SW: Surgical wounds in human beings. A histologic study of healing with practical applications. II. Fibrous healing, *Arch Surg* 21:76-96, 1930.
3. Siegel I: Scars of the pregnant and nonpregnant uterus. I. Histologic comparison of scars two weeks postoperatively, *Am J Obstet Gynecol* 64:301-308, 1952.

4. Munnell WW and Martin FW: Abdominal myomectomy, advantages and disadvantages, *Am J Obstet Gynecol* 62:109-120, 1951.

5. Finn WF and Muller PF: Abdominal myomectomy: special reference to subsequent pregnancy and to the reappearance of fibromyomas of the uterus, *Am J Obstet Gynecol* 60:109-116, 1950.

6. Siegler AM: Hysterosalpingography. In Wallach EE and Kempers RD (eds): *Modern trends in infertility and conception control*, Chicago, 1985, Year Book.

7. Siegler AM and Valle RF: Therapeutic hysteroscopic procedures, *Fertil Steril* 50:685, 1988.

8. Mencaglia L, Perino A, and Hamou J: Hysteroscopy in perimenopausal and postmenopausal women with abnormal uterine bleeding, *J Reprod Med* 32:577, 1987.

9. Valle RF: Hysteroscopy in the evaluation of female infertility, *Am J Obstet Gynecol* 137:425, 1980.

10. Hunt RB and Siegler AM: *Hysterosalpingography: techniques and interpretation,* Chicago, 1990, Year Book.

11. Pennes DR, Bowerman RA, and Silver TM: Congenital uterine anomalies and associated pregnancies: findings and pitfalls of sonographic diagnosis, *J Ultrasound Med* 4:521, 1985.

12. Worthen NJ and Gonzalez F: Septate uterus: sonographic diagnosis and obstetric complications, *Obstet Gynecol* 64(Suppl 3):34, 1984.

13. Rock JA: Mullerian anomalies. In Rock JA and Thompson JD (eds): *Telinde's operative gynecology*, ed 7, Philadelphia, 1991, JB Lippincott.

14. Jones HW Jr: Reproductive impairment and the malformed uterus, *Fertil Steril* 36:137, 1981.

15. Rock JA and Schlaff WD: The obstetric consequences of uterovaginal anomalies, *Fertil Steril* 43:681, 1985.

16. Kaufman RH et al: Upper genital tract changes associated with exposure in utero to diethylstilbestrol, *Am J Obstet Gynecol* 128:51, 1977.

17. Haney AF et al: Diethylstilbestrol-induced upper genital tract abnormalities, *Fertil Steril* 31:142, 1979.

18. Barnes AB et al: Fertility and outcome of pregnancy in women exposed in utero to diethylstilbestrol, *N Engl J Med* 302:609, 1980.

19. Stillman RJ and Miller LC: Diethylstilbestrol exposure in utero and endometriosis in infertile females, *Fertil Steril* 41:369, 1984.

20. Rock JA and Zacur HA: The clinical management of repeated early pregnancy wastage, *Fertil Steril* 39:123, 1983.

21. Strassmann EO: Operations for double uterus and endometrial atresia, *Clin Obstet Gynecol* 4:240, 1961.

22. Tompkins PT: Traumatic intrauterine synechiae, *Am J Obstet Gynecol* 83:1599, 1962.

23. Gray SE, Roberts DK, and Franklin RR: Fertility after metroplasty of the septate uterus, *J Reprod Med* 29:185, 1984.

24. Rasmussen PE and Pedersen OD: Metroplasty and fetal survival, Acta Obstet Gynecol Scand 11:117, 1987.

25. Rock JA and Jones HW Jr: The clinical management of the double uterus, *Fertil Steril* 28:798, 1977.

26. Buttram VC and Reiter RC: Uterine leiomyomata: etiology, symptomatology, and management, *Fertil Steril* 36:433, 1981.

27. Rubin IC: Uterine fibromyomas and sterility, *Clin Obstet Gynecol* 1:50, 1958.

28. Ranney B and Frederick I: The occasional need for myomectomy, *Obstet Gynecol* 53:437, 1979.

29. Barter RH and Parks J: Myoma uteri associated with pregnancy, *Clin Obstet Gynecol* 1:519, 1958.

30. Malone LJ and Ingersoll FM: Myomectomy in infertility. In Behrman SJ and Kistner RW (eds): *Progress in infertility*, ed 2, Boston, 1975, Little, Brown & Co.

31. Jacobson FJ and Norbert E: Uterine myomata and the endometrium, *Obstet Gynecol* 7:206, 1956.

32. Bolck F: Die pathologie der uterusmyome, *Arch Gynaekol* 195:166, 1961.

33. Deligdish L and Loewenthal M: Endometrial changes associated with myomata of the uterus, *J Clin Pathol* 23:676, 1970.

34. Weinstein D, Aviad Y, and Polishuk WZ: Hysterography before and after myomectomy, *Am J Roentgenol* 129:899, 1977.

35. Maheux R et al: LH-RH agonist and uterine leiomyoma: a pilot study, *Am J Obstet Gynecol* 152:1034, 1985.

36. Maheux R et al: Regression of leiomyomata uteri following hypoestrogenism induced by repetitive luteinizing hormone-releasing hormone agonist treatment: preliminary report, *Fertil Steril* 42:644, 1984.

37. Maheux R: LH-RH agonists—how useful against uterine leiomyomas? *Contemp Obstet Gynecol* 28:66, 1986.

38. Schlaff WD et al: A placebo controlled trial of a depot GnRH analog (leuprolide) in the treatment of uterine leiomyomata, *Obstet Gynecol* 74:857, 1989.

39. Coddington CC, Collins RL, Shawker TH, et al: Long-acting gonadotropin hormone-releasing hormone analog used to treat leiomyomata uteri. *Fertil Steril* 45:624, 1986.

40. Friedman AJ, Barbieri RL, Benacerraf BR, et al: Treatment of leiomyomata with intranasal or subcutaneous leuprolide, a gonadotropin-releasing hormone agonist, *Fertil Steril* 48:560, 1987.

41. Friedman AJ, Barbieri RL, Doublilet PM, et al: A randomized, double-blind trial of gonadotropin-releasing hormone agonist (leuprolide) with or without medroxyprogesterone acetate in the treatment of leiomyomata uteri, *Fertil Steril* 49:404, 1988.

42. Friedman AJ, Harrison-Atlas D, Barbieri RL, et al: A randomized, placebo-controlled, double-blind study evaluating the efficacy of leuprolide acetate depot in the treatment of uterine leiomyomata ,*Fertil Steril* 51:251, 1989.

43. Comite F, Jensen P, Lewis A, et al: GnRH analog therapy in endometriosis: Impact on bone mass. Presented at the 34th annual meeting of the Society for Gynecologic Investigation, Atlanta, March 18-21, 1987.

44. Damewood MD et al: Interval bone mineral density with long-term gonadotropin-releasing hormone agonist suppression, *Fertil Steril* 52:596, 1989.

45. Damewood MD and Rock JA: Reproductive uterine surgery, *Obstet Gynecol Clin North Am* 14;4:1049, 1987.

46. Rubin IC: Progress in myomectomy: surgical measures and diagnostic aids favoring lower morbidity and mortality, *Am J Obstet Gynecol* 44:196, 1942.

47. Bonney V: Abdominal myomectomy. In Hawkins J and Stallworthy J (eds): *Bonney's gynecologic surgery,* ed 8, Baltimore, 1974, Williams & Wilkins.

48. Lock FR: Multiple myomectomy, *Am J Obstet Gynecol* 104:642, 1969.

49. Dillon TF: Control of blood loss during gynecologic surgery, *Obstet Gynecol* 19:428, 1962.

50. Ingersoll FM and Malone LJ: Myomectomy: an alternative to hysterectomy, *Arch Surg* 100:557, 1970.

51. Malone LJ: Myomectomy: recurrence after removal of solitary and multiple myomata, *Obstet Gynecol* 34:200, 1969.

52. Babaknia A, Rock JA, and Jones HW Jr: Pregnancy success following abdominal myomectomy for infertility, *Fertil Steril* 30:644, 1978.

53. Berkley A, DeCherney A, and Polan M: Abdominal myomectomy and subsequent fertility, *Surg Gynecol Obstet* 152:319, 1983.

54. Malone LJ and Ingersoll FM: Myomectomy. In Behrman SJ and Kistner RW (eds): *Progress in infertility,* ed 1, Boston, 1968, Little, Brown & Co.

55. Brown AB, Chamberlain R, and TeLinde RW: Myomectomy, *Am J Obstet Gynecol* 71:759, 1956.

56. Israel SL and Mutch JC: Myomectomy, *Clin Obstet Gynecol* 1:455, 1958.

57. Gallinat A: Carbon dioxide hysteroscopy: principles and physiology. In Siegler AM and Lindemann HJ (eds): *Hysteroscopy principles and practice,* Philadelphia, 1984, JB Lippincott.

58. Asherman J: Amenorrhea traumatica (atretica), *J Obstet Gynaecol Br Emp* 55:23, 1948.

59. Asherman J: Traumatic intrauterine adhesions, *J Obstet Gynaecol Br Emp* 57:892, 1950.

60. Asherman J: Traumatic intrauterine adhesions and their effects on fertility, *Int J Fertil* 1:49, 1957.

61. Klein SM and Garcia CR: Asherman's syndrome: a critique and current review, *Fertil Steril* 24:722, 1973.

62. Toaff R and Ballas S: Traumatic hypomenorrhea-amenorrhea (Asherman's syndrome), *Fertil Steril* 30:379, 1978.

63. Sugimoto O: Diagnostic and therapeutic hysteroscopy for traumatic intrauterine adhesions, *Am J Obstet Gynecol* 131:539, 1978.

64. Berquist CA, Rock JA, and Jones HW Jr: Pregnancy outcome following treatment of intrauterine adhesions, *Int J Fertil* 26:107, 1981.

65. Schenker JG and Margalioth EJ: Intrauterine adhesions: an updated appraisal, *Fertil Steril* 37:593, 1982.

66. Eriksen J and Koestet C: The incidence of uterine atresia after postpartum curettage, *Dan Med Bull* 7:50, 1960.

67. Dmowski WP and Greenblatt R: Asherman's syndrome and risk of placenta accreta, *Obstet Gynecol* 34:288, 1969.

68. Rabau E and David A: Intrauterine adhesions: etiology, prevention and treatment, *Obstet Gynecol* 22:626, 1963.

69. Comninos A and Zourlas P: Treatment of uterine adhesions (Asherman's syndrome), *Am J Obstet Gynecol* 105:862, 1969.

70. Oelsner G et al: Outcome of pregnancy after treatment of intrauterine adhesions, *Obstet Gynecol* 44:341, 1974.

71. Gibbs E: Endometrial sclerosis, *JAMA* 188:390, 1964.

72. Bergman P: Traumatic intrauterine lesions, *Acta Obstet Gynecol Scand* 40(Suppl 4):1, 1961.

73. Polishuk WZ et al: Vascular changes in traumatic amenorrhea and hypomenorrhea, *Int J Fertil* 22:189, 1977.

74. Musset R and Solomon Y: Traumatic menstrual disturbances after curettage, *Rev Fr Gynecol Obstet* 48:311, 1953.

75. Netter A et al: Traumatic uterine synechiae. A common cause of menstrual insufficiency, sterility, and abortion, *Am J Obstet Gynecol* 71:368, 1956.

76. Sweeny WF: Intrauterine synechiae, *Obstet Gynecol* 27:284, 1966.

77. Carmichael DE: Asherman's syndrome, *Obstet Gynecol* 36:922, 1970.

78. Forssman L: Posttraumatic intrauterine synechiae and pregnancy, *Obstet Gynecol* 26:710, 1965.

79. Jewelewicz R et al: Obstetric complications after treatment of intrauterine synechiae (Asherman's syndrome), *Obstet Gynecol* 47:701, 1976.

80. Bergman P: Treatment of sterility of intrauterine origin, *Clin Obstet Gynecol* 2:852, 1959.

81. Wood J and Pena G: Treatment of uterine adhesions (Asherman's syndrome), *Am J Obstet Gynecol* 105:862, 1969.

82. Georgakopoulos P: Placental accreta following lysis of uterine synechiae (Asherman's syndrome), *J Obstet Gynaecol Br Commonw* 81:730, 1974.

83. Carson SA: Operative hysteroscopy, *Contemp Obstet Gynecol* 34:35, 1989.

84. Zbella EA, Moise J, and Carson SA: Noncardiogenic pulmonary edema secondary to intrauterine instillation of 32% dextran 70, *Fertil Steril* 43:479, 1985.

85. Leake JF, Murphy AA, and Zacur HA: Noncardiogenic pulmonary edema: a complication of operative hysteroscopy, *Fertil Steril* 48:497, 1987.

86. Carson SA et al: Hyperglycemia and hyponatremia during operative hysteroscopy with 5% dextrose in water distension, *Fertil Steril* 51:341, 1989.

87. Valle RF and Sciarra JJ: Intrauterine adhesions: hysteroscopic diagnosis classification, treatment, and reproductive outcome, *Am J Obstet Gynecol* 158:1459, 1988.

88. Buttram VC and Turati G: Uterine synechiae: variations in severity and some conditions which may be conducive to severe adhesions, *Int J Fertil* 22:98, 1977.

89. March CM, Israel R, and March AD: Hysteroscopic management of intrauterine adhesions, *Am J Obstet Gynecol* 130:653, 1978.

90. Chervenak FA and Neuwirth RS: Hysteroscopic resection of the uterine septum, *Am J Obstet Gynecol* 141:351, 1981.

91. Daly DC et al: Hysteroscopic resection of uterine septum in the presence of a septate cervix, *Fertil Steril* 39:569, 1983.

92. Neuwirth RS and Amin HK: Excision of submucous fibrids with hysteroscopic control, *Am J Obstet Gynecol* 126:95, 1976.

93. Neuwirth RS: A new way to manage submucous fibroids, *Contemp Obstet Gynecol* 12:101, 1978.

94. Neuwirth RS: Hysteroscopic management of symptomatic submucous fibroids, *Obstet Gynecol* 62:509, 1983.

TUBAL SURGERY

19

Tubal Implantation

CARL J. LEVINSON

FUNG LAM

Indications for the implantation procedure persist. These few paragraphs will provide an update, although the basic techniques remain the same.

Before 1975, implantation was performed at the cornual site. Although still occasionally performed at this location, the posterior uterine wall has proved to be more suitable. Original reports proposed an incision into the posterior wall, but the use of a borer (reamer) to provide two small 1-cm openings into the uterine cavity has made the procedure simpler, results in fewer complications, and leaves the patient less likely to require a cesarean section.

Indications remain the same. That is, proximal tube disease results in obstruction of the cornual area but does not lend itself to anastomosis of the cornual region to the distal isthmus or ampulla. In the 1970s, monopolar laparoscopic tubal cautery resulted in similar occlusion, but this problem no longer exists clinically. Before any repair, at least one hysterosalpingogram (HSG) and a laparoscopy are necessary to establish the diagnosis of occlusion with reasonable certainty.

Recent approaches to cornual occlusion have opened other possibilities. The basic premise is that the occlusion can be alleviated by the passage of a splint, usually plastic, by way of the uterus through and past the blocked area. This is accomplished radiographically, passing the splint through the cervix into the corpus, aiming at the tubal ostium, and passing it into the tube under fluoroscopic control. Others have used hysteroscopy, passing the splint under direct vision and carefully placing it into the tubal ostium. The results have been variable, the numbers are small, and no pathologic specimens are obtained. The techniques and surgeons are variable.

Recent personal experience has been limited by the number of appropriate cases. Unipolar sterilizations requiring reversal are rare; most other cases can be performed by microsurgical anastomosis. Canalization is successful in some cases that might otherwise have come to surgery. I have performed 7 seven cases in the past 5 years (1985-1989), involving 11 tubes, 4 bilateral, and 3 unilateral. Seven of the 11 tubes were patent at subsequent HSG. Two patients (28.5%) became pregnant; one delivered vaginally, and the other by cesarean section. There was no evidence of obstetric rupture in the patient who underwent cesarean section. No ectopic pregnancies occurred.

Repair of cornual tubal obstruction is the most difficult and challenging of all fertility surgery. Microsurgical techniques are necessary if a cornual-isthmic or cornual-ampullary anastomosis is performed and are of great value for an implantation procedure. Cornual anastomosis is successful if the remaining portion of the tube is patent and reasonably free of disease, with up to a 60% success rate.[1] Implantation should be reserved for those patients in whom an anastomosis is not possible.

Although approximately 20% of all fertility procedures to 1975 were for implantation, most modern microsurgeons perform this procedure in a smaller percentage of cases.[2] In a personal series of 950 major infertility surgeries, only 68 (7%) have been implantations, many of these referred specifically for the procedure.

Reassessment of implantation resulted from several developments of the past decade, which follow:

1. Microsurgery has added a new dimension to fertility tubal surgery.
2. The ability to reverse sterilization has given us the opportunity to perform surgery on patients in whom the cornu of the tube has been destroyed by unipolar electrosurgery.
3. New experimental work has revealed more basic information regarding the anatomy, physiology, and pathology of the uterotubal junction (UTJ).

These aspects have greatly improved results that were previously poor. It is necessary to point out a lack of success from combined implantation procedure and distal repair on the same tube.

ANATOMY AND PHYSIOLOGY

The intramural or "interstitial" portion of the tube runs through the myometrium of the cornu of the uterus and connects the isthmic tube to the endometrial cavity. The complexity of the area can be imagined by considering the number of forces in play over a 1- to 2-cm area: cilial action, secretions, hormonal (estrogen, progesterone, medications), prostaglandins, and nerves.

The endosalpinx of the intramural tube is partially ciliated. Its length is generally 1 to 2.5 cm, its diameter may vary from 200 to 600 μm. Its course is sinuous, with an occasional right angle. This combination of small diameter and convolution makes probing difficult, if not impossible. Excess probing may result in the creation of false passages, with more destruction than reconstruction.

The musculature is complex, representing a transition from three uterine muscle layers to a much thinner isthmic musculature. At the junction with the isthmus there is the occasional appearance of a sphincter-like anatomic structure (discussed below).

The cornu is noted for its vascularity, deriving its blood supply from both the ascending uterine artery and the confluence of vessels derived from the ovarian artery. Therefore careful hemostasis is required.

Does the UTJ contain a sphincter? Anatomically, this is an inconstant finding, and the answer is probably no. A temporary block at this point is often seen on hysterosalpingogram, however; therefore the functional answer may be yes. There is an increase of adrenergic nerve fibers to this area. The issue remains unresolved.

It is not necessary for the UTJ to be present for sperm to pass, for conception to occur, or for the embryo to pass back into the uterus and implant. Numerous factors are involved in transportation of sperm, including contractility of the uterus and tube, uterine and tubal fluids, and cilial action. The UTJ may be a barrier to sperm in some animals but appears to act in a more selective fashion in humans, perhaps choosing to transport the more motile sperm. There is conflicting evidence as to whether resection of the UTJ enhances polyspermic fertilization by allowing more sperm to come in contact with the ovum. Passage of the ovum is delayed at the ampullary-isthmic junction (AIJ) but not at the UTJ. It is difficult to explain the reasons for delayed passage (questionably attributable to sphincteric activity); enhanced passage, which is due to an absent UTJ; and direction of the ovum to the implantation site, as well as many other phenomena.

EXPERIMENTAL DATA

Much experimental work has been done, most of it recently, in an attempt to determine the function of the UTJ and adjoining tubal areas. Whereas broad conclusions may be reached, many of the specifics still elude us. Mroueh[3] transected the UTJs of rabbits and implanted the tubes into the uterine wall. Fifty percent of the tubes were blocked and 50% remained patent. There were no pregnancies. Ova were found within the tubes. David, Brackett, and Garcia[4] resected 1.5 cm of rabbit isthmus. The tube was then anastomosed with nylon to the uterine horn (0.25 to 0.5 cm of uterus and 1.25 cm of tube were involved). The nidation index was 0.96 on the control side, compared with 0.41 on the surgery side. Using pigs, Hunter and Leglise[5] resected the isthmus and then performed an anastomosis. Eleven of the 21 animals showed patency to sperm. Although fertilization did occur, there was also an increase in polyspermia. These authors did the same procedure on rabbits. Ovulation occurred in 14 of 18 animals. The conclusion was that there was some inhibition of sperm entry into the tube.

Perez and Eddy[6] resected 50% to 100% of the isthmus and then did an anastomosis. The nidation of index for the control group was 0.68 implantations. If 50% of the isthmus were removed, this dropped to 0.44. If 100% were removed, it dropped to 0.27. Perez, Rajkumar, and Eddy[7] resected 5 mm of isthmus, which included the UTJ. There was a nidation index of 82%. Winston[8] resected 50% to 100% of rabbit isthmus. The nidation index was less in both groups, with no difference between them. McComb, Newman, and Halbert[9] removed the proximal 1 to 2 cm of the tube and implanted the distal isthmus in rabbits. Fifty percent of the animals achieved a pregnancy; however, the nidation index for the control group was 0.81 whereas it was only 0.28 for the surgery group. These same authors removed the isthmus in some of the animals, removed the isthmus and AIJ in another group, and removed the isthmus, AIJ, and a segment of ampulla in the third group. As a control, they transected the opposite side and did an anastomosis. Conclusions reached as a result of this study were that if only the isthmus was removed, fertilization was decreased by approximately 60%. Also, if more than 53% of the total tube was removed, no pregnancy occurred. Therefore one could conclude that the decrease in fertility is related to the length of the tube (isthmus), but that even if the entire isthmus were removed, some fertility persisted.

Paterson and co-workers[10] resected only the isthmus in one group of pigs and the isthmus and AIJ in another. The nidation index was the same for both groups (0.64) but was less than the control group (0.92).

Theory holds that the UTJ is basically an entry point from the tube into the uterus and does not, either by endocrine or anatomic function, delay passage of the fertilized egg. Should the fertilized egg pass into the uterine cavity too soon, the number of implantations will decrease.[11] Experimental work shows that the nidation index in animals is decreased if the UTJ and/or surrounding areas are removed, but the extenuating circumstances of the experimental design make it difficult to determine whether the UTJ is the prime reason for sustaining the egg within the tube. Indeed, the entire isthmus may be removed without completely inhibiting fertilization and implantation. Finally, cornual-ampullary anastomoses as well as ampullary implantations have resulted in pregnancies. Therefore there is evidence that the UTJ, the isthmus, and the AIJ are not entirely necessary for a pregnancy to occur. Halbert, McComb, and Bourdage[12] showed that pregnancy rates in rabbits were decreased simply by transecting the isthmus and reanastomosing it without removal of any portion of the tube.

Considering the complexity of the forces acting on the UTJ, it is not surprising that any interference of a surgical nature with it and the isthmus results in a diminution of pregnancy rates. It would be significant (and clinically important) to be able to specify what happens to the pregnancy rate if a certain amount of tube is removed. This information is not forthcoming, nor is it likely to be in the near future. Although pregnancies could possibly occur with less than 50% of the distal tube remaining, the percentage is very low. The more tube that remains, the better the prognosis.

DIAGNOSTIC TECHNIQUES

The diagnosis of cornual occlusion can be made by one of several techniques. The hysterosalpingogram is a relatively safe and simple procedure that can be done on an outpatient basis. It has been reported to have a possible therapeutic as well as diagnostic value.[13] For these reasons, it should be done as the first approach to determine whether there is a cornual occlusion. Aqueous or oily medium may be applied under gentle pressure. Regardless of whether a true sphincter exists, false evidence of occlusion at the cornua is often seen, which may be due to adrenergic nerve stimulation. Antispasmodic drugs (glucagon, amyl nitrite) have been used with varying degrees of success. In addition to true occlusion and spasm, other reasons for cornual occlusion include the following:

1. Technical problems such as poor cervical occlusion.
2. Obstruction of the tubal ostium by polyps.
3. Occlusion by an air bubble.
4. An excessively large uterus with poor filling pressure.

If hysterosalpingogram demonstrates cornual occlusion, chronic infection is the most likely etiology. Laparoscopy is then indicated, which requires general anesthesia and entry into the abdominal cavity. Although more accurate, it should be the second procedure for determining tubal patency unless there is a direct primary need for observation (e.g., suspected endometriosis). The procedure also will indicate whether there is distal tubal disease and assist in determining whether surgical repair is indicated.

With the patient anesthetized, tubal spasm usually can be ruled out. Before the procedure a well-fitted cannula (Kahn, Jarcho, or HUI) is placed and methelyne blue or indigo carmine is injected. Under direct observation, the tube is observed with respect to fill and spill. Again, the pressure should be steady and applied with the uterus in various positions.

Hysteroscopy may also be performed. With this technique the tubal ostium can be observed and occasionally cannulated. Polyps can be observed, as can any other abnormal architecture that might occlude the ostium. Dye can then be injected if a concurrent laparoscopy is performed. Although hysteroscopy has proved to be of some value, hysterosalpingogram and laparoscopy remain the standard approach to evaluating cornual occlusion. (The Rubin procedure using carbon dioxide insufflation has received a modest resurgence of interest and is a reasonable screening test, but has severe limitations in determining whether one or two tubes are occluded and the exact site of such obstruction.)

Hysterosalpingography provides many false positive results, for example, evidence of cornual occlusion that subsequently proves to be false. This may occur in as many as 30% to 40% of examinations showing occlusion.[14] Therefore confirmation by laparoscopy is indicated.

At laparotomy, a needle can be passed through the fundus into the uterine cavity, the cervix being occluded with a Buxton or Bonney clamp; dye is then injected into the cavity. This approach will occasionally indicate a patent tube previously considered to be occluded; however, there are technical problems. Finding the cavity with the needle is occasionally difficult for the inexperienced; dye is often injected into the myometrium.

CORNUAL OCCLUSION

Cornual occlusion is not a common finding. Etiologic factors include:

1. Infection (postabortion, postpartum, cases of unexplained occlusion, possible relationship to intrauterine device use).
2. Salpingitis isthmica nodosa, presumed by many to be infectious in origin.
3. Trauma (previous tubal ligation, myomectomy, uterine suspension or other surgery).
4. Endometriosis.
5. Spasm.

Pathologic evaluation of the resected UTJ indicates inflammation in 40% to 67% of patients. The figure is even higher if salpingitis isthmica nodosa is considered to be of infectious origin.[15,16] The underlying factor has prognostic importance. If chronic pelvic inflammatory disease is the basic case, primary surgical repair is indicated. If endometriosis is suspected, one report shows that resolution of the occlusive problem may occur with the therapeutic use of danazol, obviating the need for surgery.[17]

PROCEDURES

Numerous variations of the theme of restoring tubal patency have been developed in the past 88 years since the first reported case done in 1893 by Watkins and reported by Ries.[18] In principle, the approach has been sustained for almost 100 years; the diseased cornu is excised and the patent remaining tube is developed and implanted.

Today there are two basic procedures to restore patency at the UTJ,[14] outlined as follows:

I. Implantation (macrosurgical and microsurgical)
  A. Cornual
   1. Closed
   2. Open
  B. Posterior wall
   1. Closed
   2. Open
II. Anastomoses (microsurgical)

If intramural tube remains, it is possible to anastomose the patent isthmic or ampullary tube as described by Gomel[1] (Figure 19-1, *A*). The option is to insert a portion of the patent tube (isthmus or ampulla) into a site in the uterus (Figure 19-1, *B*). This site can be prepared by sharp excision/incision or by the use of a reamer or borer. The sites in the uterus used thus far have been the cornu (with the obstruction excised) or the posterior wall. This can be done blindly (closed) or visually (open) by incising the uterus and viewing the insertion and implantation. In the closed technique, the approximation of the endosalpinx and endometrium is assumed rather than visualized.

Closed cornual implantation

Closed techniques include use of a reamer, sharp dissection and excision, and blunt dissection. Holden and Sovak[19] described the use of a reamer (similar to a cork-borer) to remove the diseased cornu and provide a passage into the uterine cavity (Figure 19-2). Two of the first three patients had patent tubes postoperatively, one of whom delivered vaginally without complication. Green-Armytage[20] added the concept of splinting the tubes throughout their length and into the uterus after using the reamer.

In contrast, the original sharp dissection of Watkins was the procedure employed by Bonney[21] and Palmer[22] but without splinting (Figure 19-3). Modifications were made by Moore-White,[23] who used a probe to place the tube, and by Mulligan, Rock, and Easterday,[24] who wedged the cornu (rather than core it out); they also used the splint.

Blunt dissection techniques were described. Rommer[25] did not excise the occluded tube but merely pushed a Kocher clamp through the cornu, creating a passage for the tube. Wirtz[26] reversed this approach, pushing a cannula through the cervix into the uterine cavity and then through the cornu by blunt dissection. This was done on each side. A single splint was then placed through one tube into the uterine cavity and out through the opposite tube.

Open cornual implantation

The theoretic advantage to opening the uterus is to allow visual approximation of the endosalpinx to endometrium. Halban[27] used posterior wall incision, through which he guided the reamer into the uterine cavity at the cornu and implanted the tube. The posterior wall was then closed. Polowe[28] followed a similar procedure using an anterior vertical incision into the uterus. The open technique was used by Shirodkar[29] and Stallworthy.[30] They made an incision across the fundus from cornu to cornu (Figure 19-4). Johnstone[31] actually bivalved the uterus with an anterior-posterior incision, reamed out the cornual area, and brought the tube into direct view for implantation.

Open posterior-wall implantation

Peterson, Musich, and Behrman[32] were the first to develop a noncornual site for implantation of the tube. Thus far, only the posterior uterine wall has been used. There was a need (mid 1970s) to reconstruct tubes destroyed during sterilization by laparoscopic unipolar cautery, many of which were occluded at the cornual site. This group conceived of using the posterior wall by making the transverse incision at the level of the utero-ovarian ligaments and implanting the tubes at the angles of the incision (Figure 19-5). In this procedure the endometrial mucosa could be visualized. The distance from the tube to the uterine cavity was as short as or shorter than that to the cornu so that tension was less. The concept was a novel approach to an old problem. The original description pointed out the frequent need for grafts over the incision and the absolute need for cesarean section because of the risk of dehiscence at the implantation site.

Closed posterior-wall implantation

In modification of the posterior wall approach, the incision is replaced by two apertures made by the borer at the level of the utero-ovarian ligaments. Bleeding is diminished and the risk of pregnancy and dehiscence can be lessened, but the visual approximation of endometrium and endosalpinx must be forgone. This technique is described in detail later (Plates 32 and 33).

Microsurgical anastomosis

Winston[8] and Gomel[1] have been strong proponents of cornual anastomosis (cornual-isthmic, cornual-ampullary) for reconstruction of the tube if the intramural area

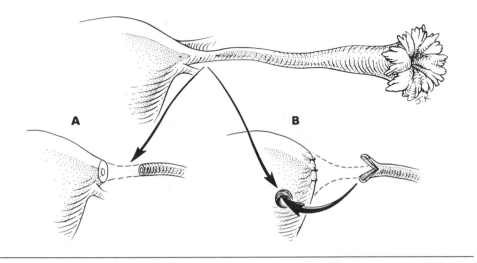

Figure 19-1
The two principal procedures for correcting cornual block are **A,** anastomosis and **B,** implantation.

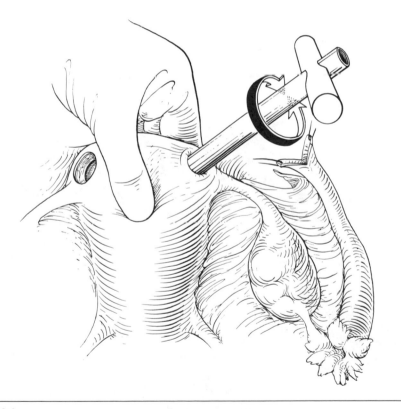

Figure 19-2
Traditional site for implantation (at the cornua) using a borer. (Modified from Musich and Behrman 1983. Reprinted with permission of the publisher, the American Fertility Society.)

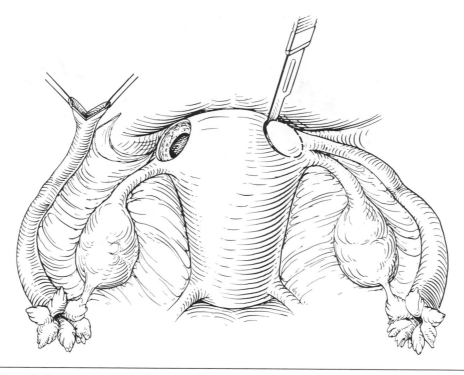

Figure 19-3
Traditional site for implantation (at the cornua) using a scalpel. (From Musich and Behrman, 1983. The American Fertility Society.)

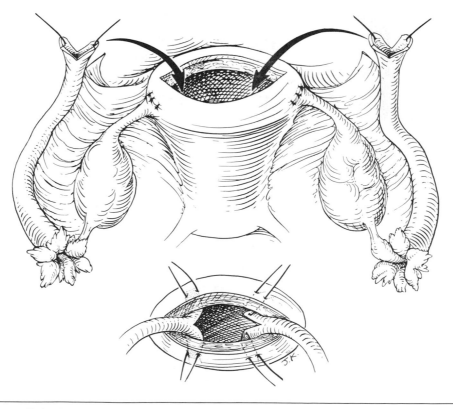

Figure 19-4
Implantation site (at the fundus) reached by a transverse fundal incision. (From Musich and Behrman, 1983. The American Fertility Society.)

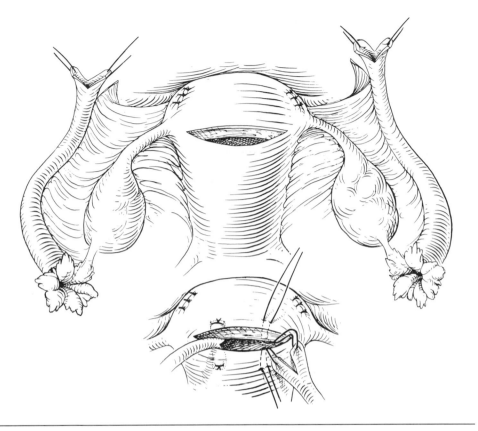

Figure 19-5
Posterior uterine wall site for implantation through a transverse incision. (From Musich and Behrman, 1983. The American Fertility Society.)

is occluded. Gomel especially advocated shaving the cornu, even down to the endometrial cavity, with subsequent anastomosis. He has developed a special scalpel and techniques to facilitate this. The results are excellent in his hands, taking into consideration that this (especially cornual-ampullary anastomosis) is the most difficult of all microsurgical procedures. Winston summarized the advantages of an anastomosis: patency can be obtained; the blood supply to the area is preserved; maximal tubal length is used; and there is no need for cesarean section with subsequent pregnancy. Furthermore, if there is function in the UTJ, it will be preserved.

IMPLANTATION USING A BORER
General preparation

The patient is placed under general anesthesia. The legs are temporarily put into stirrups so that the bladder may be catheterized with a Foley catheter and a Harris uterine injector (HUI) can be placed within the uterine cavity. The balloon of the HUI is then distended and the distal end is attached to a syringe filled with indigo carmine. The patient's legs are put down and she is prepared and draped as for any abdominal procedure.

A Pfannenstiel incision in made unless a previous vertical incision exists. The peritoneal cavity is entered, the

bowel is packed off with wet laparotomy pads, and a self-retaining Kirschner retractor is put in place. Any adhesions are lysed using a microelectrode. Once the tubes and ovaries are freed, the cul-de-sac is packed with Kerlex gauze to provide a platform for the tubes and ovaries.

Dye is injected slowly to note whether any passes into the isthmus. The surgical microscope is put in place. An incision in made into the isthmus approximately 0.5 to 1 cm from the cornu. Another attempt is made to inject dye. Should the dye not appear, progressive incisions are made toward the endometrial cavity (Gomel has designed a curved blade specifically for this purpose) (Figure 19-6). After each incision, an attempt is made to pass dye. If the incision has been made well into the cornual wall and there is no passage of dye (Figure 19-7), an implantation procedure is planned. Any remnant of the scarred proximal portion of the tube is excised.

Preparation of the proximal portion of the distal segment

Under the surgical microscope, a probe is passed through the fimbriated end of the tube and passed proximally. Patency must be determined. If the tube is not open to a probe or the flushing of fluid, incisions are made until

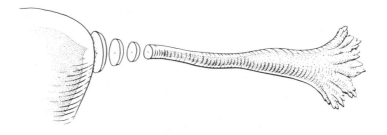

Figure 19-6
Progressive incisions are made toward the uterus to determine patency proximally.

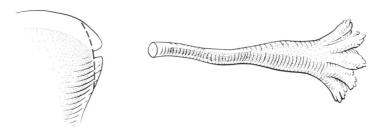

Figure 19-7
Occlusion persists well into the cornual wall.

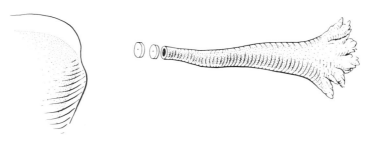

Figure 19-8
If a probe cannot be passed or if the tube cannot be flushed,
incisions are made proximally until a patent segment is
reached.

a patent segment of tube is reached (Figures 19-8 and
19-9).

Lateral tubal incisions, approximately 1 cm long, are
made through the tube at the 9 and 3 o'clock positions,
dividing the tube into a mesenteric and antimesenteric
half. In this matter, a fishmouth is fashioned (Figure 19-
10). The mesosalpinx is dissected back for at least 1 cm
(Figure 19-11). Hemostasis is obtained by electrocautery
except for bleeders on the endosalpinx. A 2-0 absorbable
suture is placed through each half of the fishmouth, serosa
through endosalpinx, encompassing a substantial amount
of tissue (Figure 19-12). (It will be necessary to put this
area under some tension as it is being brought into the
uterine cavity and tied.) This newly fashioned portion of

the tube is placed on the Kerlex gauze, temporarily set
aside, and irrigated frequently.

Preparation of the uterine wall

Any defect at the cornu is now closed. The surgical
microscope is removed; at this juncture, a head loupe is
often of value. The HUI is removed to avoid having a
foreign body within the uterine cavity. If the uterus is
not sufficiently elevated, a Buxton clamp can be placed
around the cervix to facilitate such elevation.

A solution is prepared by diluting 1 ml of vasopressin
(Pitressin) with 5 ml of normal saline. At the level of the
utero-ovarian ligament on the posterior uterine wall, approximately 2 to 3 ml is injected on either side using a

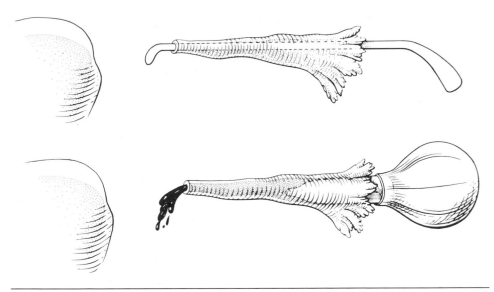

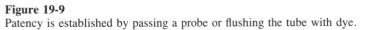

Figure 19-9
Patency is established by passing a probe or flushing the tube with dye.

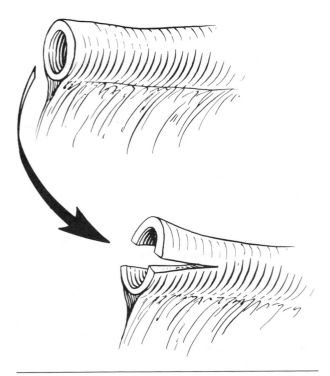

Figure 19-10
By dividing the tube into mesenteric and timesenteric halves,
a fishmouth is formed.

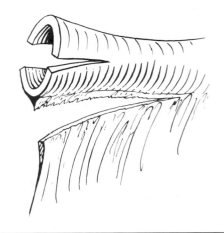

Figure 19-11
The mesosalpinx is incised and dissected back for 1 cm.

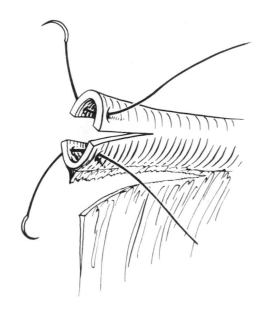

Figure 19-12
An absorbable suture is placed through each half of the fish-mouth.

25- or 30-gauge needle (Figure 19-13). This results in a blanching of the uterine wall. Maximum effectiveness occurs in 2 minutes.

The uterus is elevated either with a hand or the Buxton clamp. A Holden borer (reamer) with a diameter of 1 cm or, occasionally, a 0.7-cm borer is inserted into the serosa at the level of the ovarian ligament with slight angulation toward the midline (Figure 19-14, *A*). The borer is rotated inward; a sharp edge will facilitate entry. Entry is signaled when there is a feeling of a slight "pop" and a sudden diminution of resistance. The borer can be removed and usually contains a complete core of myo-metrium (Figure 19-14, *B*). Bleeding is minimal and remains so during the procedure. If the uterine segment does not come out with the borer, it can be removed with forceps. Occasionally, a small attached edge requires sharp cutting. Implantation on the opposite side is per-formed in the same manner at the same time.

Implantation

The fishmouth end of the tube is positioned so that the one suture through the mesenteric half faces downward and the one through the antimesenteric half faces upward (Figure 19-15). The lower suture is more difficult and should be placed first. The original needle should be removed and the suture placed on a no. 4 Mayo needle with a fairly heavy needle holder. The needle is placed in reverse fashion so the needle holder grasps the needle near the tip. The threaded needle is placed (blunt end first) through the new opening into the uterine downward, through the endometrium and myometrium, and exiting

at the serosa (Figure 19-16, *A*). The opposite thread of the same suture is placed on the Mayo needle and the procedure repeated but with the exit point approximately 3 to 5 mm from the previous one. Both ends are clamped.

A similar procedure is performed with the suture on the antimesenteric half, but the needle is directed upward. Thus the individual sutures will exit at 180 degrees from each other. The needle eye is used as the leading edge because it much less likely to make a false passage; however, it is more difficult to grasp the needle near its rounded tip (Figure 19-16, *B*).

Gentle traction is required to bring the proximal por-tion of the distal tube close to, and then into, the new opening in the uterus. As this is done, the sutures are gently pulled, easing the fishmouth into the uterine cav-ity. The procedure can be facilitated with microforceps (Figure 19-16, *C*). Sutures of 2-0 material are used to minimize the possibility of cutting through the tube or breaking the suture in the process of tying. When the sutures are *snug,* they are tied, thereby splaying the tube within the endometrial cavity (Figure 19-17). This po-sitioning has been confirmed experimentally and by hys-teroscopic evaluation. Occasionally, the aperture at the level of the serosa is too large. It can be partially closed with a 4-0 suture; 6-0 absorbable sutures are then used to appose the serosa of the tube to the serosa of the uterus. If careful peritonealization is accomplished, grafts are unnecessary (Figure 19-18).

Ancillary procedures

Both the surgical loupes and surgical microscope are of value. The loupes are used when the tubes and ovaries are mobilized. The microscope is used to determine tubal patency, to prepare the fishmouth, and to place the sutures through the tubes. Loupes are once again used while boring into the uterus, implanting the tubes, and ap-proximating the serosal edges.

Lavage is performed throughout the procedure, em-ploying a 1:1:5 solution consisting of 1000 ml of Ring-er's lactate, 1000 mg of hydrocortisone acetate, and 5000 IU of heparin. This solution prevents the formation of small clots and keeps the field clean. Patients receive one dose of doxycycline, 100 mg intravenously, preop-eratively and two doses postoperatively. The Horne reg-imen of pharmacologic doses of dexamethasone and pro-methazine is not used.

Splints are not used. Concomitant surgery is avoided. A retroverted uterus is anteverted by simple ventral sus-pension or by triplication of the round ligaments (using Tevdek 2-0 suture).

Complications

Complications are relatively few with all implantation procedures except for the failure to achieve a pregnancy. Of the rarely reported intraoperative complications, bleeding is noted most frequently.

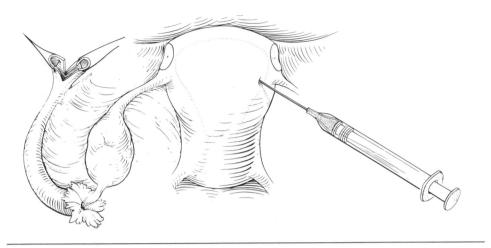

Figure 19-13
Vasopressin solution is injected on both sides of the posterior uterine wall at the level of the utero-ovarian ligament.

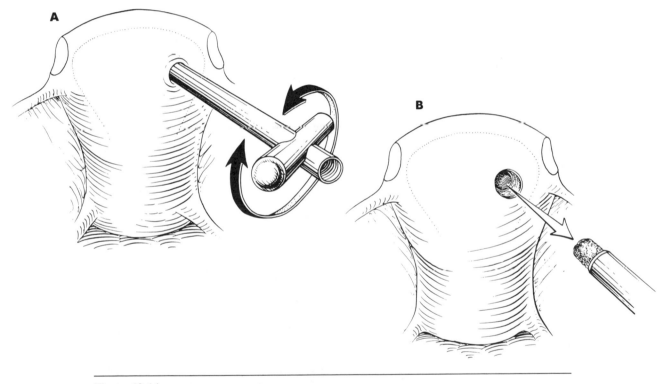

Figure 19-14
A, The borer is inserted into the serosa. **B,** When it is removed, the borer usually contains a complete core myometrium.

Bleeding from the mesosalpinx may occur if the incision across the tube is too extensive. This can be controlled by electrosurgery or with small clamp and suture. Bleeding from the uterine incision site may be extensive if a vasoconstrictive agent is not used. (It is surprising that postoperative bleeding is not more frequent than reported, anticipating that it would occur when the vasoconstrictive agent was no longer effective.) Postoperative hemorrhage and infection are also unusual, al-

though we have occasionally seen patients 7 to 14 days postoperatively with complaints of lower abdominal pain and a tender periuterine area, but no fever and no leukocytosis. These patients are generally treated with a course of antibiotics for 5 to 7 days prophylactically. If splints are used, occasionally a second surgical procedure is required to remove them.

Delayed postoperative bleeding is reported rarely. It appears to have been more common when prostheses

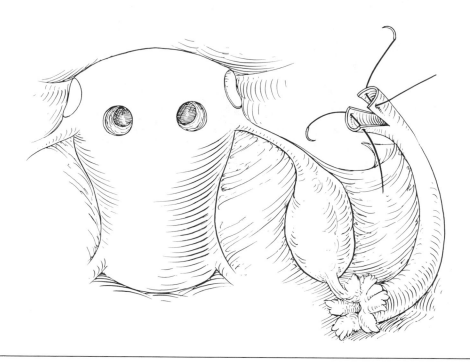

Figure 19-15
Positioning of the fishmouth end of the tube: the mesenteric half faces downward and the anti-mesenteric half faces upward.

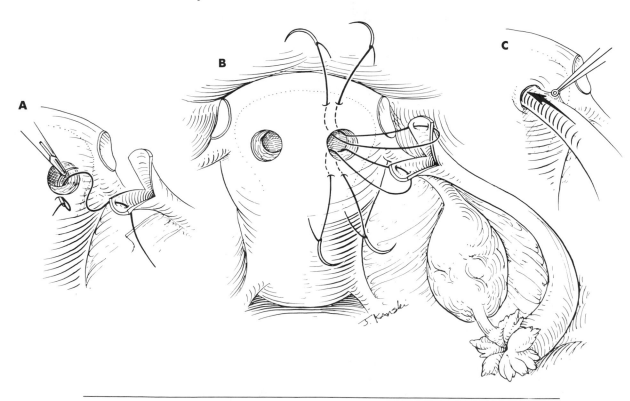

Figure 19-16
A, Placement of the threaded needle through the newly bored opening of the uterus. **B,** The sutures of the two valves of the fishmouth are drawn through the new opening and then through the uterine wall. **C,** The fishmouth is eased into the uterine cavity, aided by the use of microforceps.

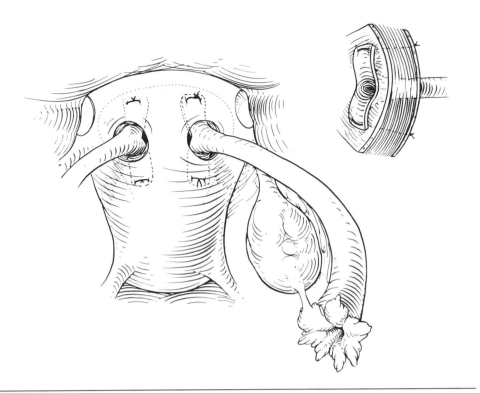

Figure 19-17
Final position of the tubes in the uterine cavity. (*Inset*) Inside view.

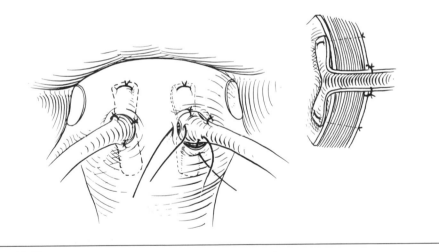

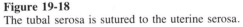

Figure 19-18
The tubal serosa is sutured to the uterine serosa.

were used. In our series, within 3 months all but one patient had returned to a presurgical menstrual pattern. Endometriosis at the implantation site was previously reported but has not been noted in any recent series. Ectopic pregnancies are minimally increased over the usually quoted 1 per 100 pregnancies; longer-term follow-up indicated approximately 2% to 4% ectopic pregnancies. Many series report none at all. The rate is expected to be higher in patients in whom the implantation procedure is performed for chronic pelvic inflammatory diseases than in those with prior tubal sterilization.

Uterine rupture after implantation has been reported. Exact figures are not available, but it must be recalled that several techniques are being compared. Green-Armytage[33] noted one such episode in 25 years of experience. Grant[34] noted only 1 in 73 cases.

Until the use of the posterior wall incision, it was recommended that delivery be performed by the vaginal

Table 19-1 Outcome of tubal implantations based on etiology of infertility

Etiology of infertility	Number of patients	Viable pregnancy (no./%)	Spontaneous abortion (no./%)	Ectopic pregnancy (no./%)
Sterilization	38	26/68.4	2/5.3	2/5.3
Inflammation	27	10/37	4/14.8	2/7.4
Myoma	1	1/100	—	—
Endometriosis	2	—	—	—
Totals	68	36/52.9	6/8.8	4/5.9

route, reserving cesarean section for obstetric indications only. Peterson, Musich, and Behrman[32] however, reported several instances of dehiscence at cesarean section and, as a result, advised surgical delivery for all of their patients. Although we avoid the posterior incision by using the borer, for a time most of our patients were delivered by cesarean section based on the experience of the Peterson group. Only two bulges were noted, however. Therefore although special care is indicated, we recommend vaginal delivery if the reamer technique has been used, much as did Green-Armytage.[33]

Failure

The purpose of implantation is to provide a viable child to the patient, not to provide patency from cervix to ovary. Failure primarily results from several possible causes, which include the following:

1. Closure of the site of implantation because of fibrosis.
2. Postoperative infection with subsequent closure.
3. Chronic pelvic inflammatory disease within the tubes, from preexisting disease.
4. Other fertility problems.
5. An excessively shortened tube.
6. Disturbance of the relationship between the tube and the ovary.
7. The use of a prosthesis with destruction of the endosalpinx and cilia.

Certain technical errors may also occur, including the following:

1. Dislocation of the tube from the endometrial cavity due to tension.
2. Poor implantation technique so that endosalpinx and endometrium do not fuse.
3. Hemorrhage as a result of inadequate hemostasis.

Since the UTJ cannot be visualized easily, it is difficult to determine the exact cause of most failures.

Results

The disease process is probably the most important etiologic factor in determining the prognosis for an implantation procedure. Trying to see the forest (later to observe the trees), the following seems evident:

1. Implantation procedures performed for reversal of sterilization have an excellent prognosis.
2. Implantation procedures performed for infectious disease and/or salpingitis isthmica nodosa manifested purely at the cornua have a reasonably good prognosis.
3. If the implantation procedure is performed for chronic infection that may involve other areas of the tube, particularly the fimbriated end, or associated with other pelvic disease such as endometriosis, a very poor prognosis can be anticipated.

Shirodkar[29] attempted to relate success to the degree of pathologic change. His findings indicated that 40% of patients with involved cornual-isthmic tube would become pregnant, compared to less than 10% if the adnexa were also fixed by adhesions or the fimbriae were affected.

The exact type of surgery, if properly performed, may not be a significant feature.

The above having been stated, the trees should be examined. Even close scrutiny of many series results in confusing data. The reasons, which are readily apparent, follow:

1. General surgical techniques and conditions have changed considerably over the past 80 years.
2. Large numbers of surgeons have used a wide variety of techniques.
3. Very few series are "pure" since they mix surgical techniques, types of cases, concurrent disease, and ancillary measures.
4. Numerous causes of infertility may exist. How does one compare the results of the surgical technique if the reamer is used in one patient whose husband's sperm count is 28 million per ml, and a sharp excision is used in another where the count in 89 million per ml.
5. The site of the block may be juxtamural, intramural, or juxtacavity. This fact is not usually stated.

6. The very decision as to which patient will have an implantation procedure as compared with an anastomosis reflects possible prejudicial judgment and may even reflect variations in skill and training on the part of the physician.
7. Ancillary measures vary widely, including methods to prevent adhesions, use of antibiotics, macrosurgical versus microsurgical techniques, and the use of stents or no stents.

If more than one procedure is performed or if different procedures are performed on the same patient, it is difficult to evaluate the results and relate them to any particular phase of the procedure. Furthermore, these are not recorded uniformly. Patency rates are given, but we are not told the technique by which they are determined or when they were determined. Fertility rates are often given, but no statement is made regarding the use of other fertility therapy. Rarely is the use of donor insemination or ovulation induction ever mentioned. Tubal length is often ignored, so no determination can be made as to the value of preserving the isthmus; where this has been done, there are conflicting results. Other factors not considered include the following:

1. The relationship of the tube to the ovary.
2. The histology of the excised cornu, which does not always support the diagnosis.
3. Age, race, and parity.
4. The duration of the disease and the infertility.

Even a computer may not be able to sort out these many issues. Some of the comparative issues involved in implantation procedure are best discussed according to the general technique used.

The reamer and sharp dissection have both been used extensively, with or without splints and other modification, for implantation into the cornual area. Results are similar, although there appears to be some advantage to the reamer. It makes little difference whether splints are used or whether the uterus is opened. Patency rates are well over 50%, often over 90%. Pregnancy rates varied from 14% to 100% (in a small series) but averaged 30% to 40% term deliveries overall. Williams[35] reported a pregnancy rate of 22% after isthmic implantation for reversal of sterilization, as compared with 11% for patients having the procedure for disease processes. In a summary of 355 surgeons doing 681 implantation procedures, the pregnancy rate was only 15%.[12] This probably represents the prognosis when the procedure is performed by a large number of general gynecologists.

Few address the issue of whether the isthmus or the ampulla is inserted. Rock[36] suggested a marked advantage to inserting the ampulla, while Cohen and coworkers[37] found a slight advantage to using the isthmus, and Palmer[22] found a 10% increase in pregnancy rate if the isthmus was used.

Results of 68 tubal implantations

Since 1976, I have performed 73 tubal implantations using the posterior wall and borer technique. Sixty-eight of these patients have been followed for 1 year. In 60 patients, implantation was bilateral; it was unilateral in 8. The etiologic factors leading to obstruction have changed considerably between 1976 and 1983. Initially, most of the procedures were performed for patients who requested reversal of unipolar sterilization. Subsequently, most have been performed for occlusion secondary to inflammation.

Outcomes of the procedures with respect to etiology of infertility are shown in Table 19-1.

SUMMARY

The implantation procedure for restoring tubal patency where cornual occlusion exists has been alternately extolled and decried. Until 1975, all such implantations were performed at the cornual site. At that time an innovation was introduced by Peterson, Musich, and Behrman, who used an incision into the posterior wall of the uterus and implanted the tubes into the angle of the incision. Based on this concept, but using a circular incision made with a borer, the new procedure yields superior results if performed after sterilization and good results if performed for chronic obstruction attributable to inflammation. Thus in the face of cornual obstruction, two options are available to the fertility surgeon and the patient: anastomosis at the cornu, particularly if isthmic tube remains patent, and posterior wall implantation, most suitable for the distal isthmus and ampulla.

REFERENCES

1. Gomel V: *Microsurgery in female infertility*, Boston, 1983, Little, Brown & Co.
2. Kistner RW and Patton GW: *Atlas of infertility surgery*, Boston, 1975, Little, Brown & Co.
3. Mroueh A: Effect of tubal implantation on rabbit fertility, *Fertil Steril* 20:928-932, 1969.
4. David A, Brackett BG, and Garcia CR: Effects of microsurgical removal of the rabbit uterotubal junction, *Fertil Steril* 20:250-257, 1969.
5. Hunter RHF and Leglise PC: Tubal surgery in the rabbit: fertilization and polyspermy after resection of the isthmus, *Am J Anat* 132:45-52, 1971.
6. Perez LE and Eddy CA: Ovum transport and fertility following microsurgical removal of the isthmus and utero-tubal junction (UTJ) in rabbits (abstract), *Biol Reprod* 22:72A, 1980.
7. Perez LE, Rajkumar K, and Eddy CA: Fertility and ovum transport after microsurgical removal of the uterotubal junction in rabbits, *Fertil Steril* 36:803-807, 1981.
8. Winston RML. Tubal anastomosis for reversal of sterilization in 45 women. In Brosens and Winston RML (eds): *Reversibility of female sterilization*, ed I. New York: Grune & Stratton, 1978, pp. 55-67.
9. McComb PF, Newman H, and Halbert SA: Reproduction in rabbits after excision of the oviductal isthmus, ampullary-isthmic junction, and uteroisthmic junction, *Fertil Steril* 36:669-677, 1981.

10. Paterson PJ et al: Fertility and tubal morphology after microsurgical removal of segments of the porcine fallopian tube, *Fertil Steril* 35:209-213, 1981.

11. Chang MC: Effects of delayed fertilization on segmenting ova, blastocysts and fetuses in rabbits (abstract), *Fed Proc* 11:24, 1952.

12. Halbert SA, McComb PF, and Bourdage RJ: The structural and functional impact of microsurgical anastomosis on the rabbit oviductal isthmus, *Fertil Steril* 36:653-658, 1981.

13. Wabby O, Sobrero AJ, and Epstein JA: Hysterosalpingography in relation to pregnancy, *Fertil Steril* 17:520, 1966.

14. Musich JR and Behrman SJ: Surgical management of tubal obstruction at the uterotubal junction, *Fertil Steril* 40:423-441, 1983.

15. Hellman LM: Tubal plastic operations, *J Obstet Gynaecol Br Emp* 63:852-860, 1956.

16. Crane M and Woodruff JD: Factors influencing the success of tuboplastic procedures, *Fertil Steril* 19:810-820, 1968.

17. Ayers JWT: Hormonal therapy for tubal occlusion: danazol and tubal endometriosis, *Fertil Steril* 38:748-750, 1982.

18. Ries E: Nodular forms of tubal disease, *J Exp Med* 2:347-389, 1987.

19. Holden FC and Sovak FW: Reconstruction of the oviducts: an improved technic with report of cases, *Am J Obstet Gynecol* 24:684-695, 1932.

20. Green-Armytage VB: Tubo-uterine implantation, *J Obstet Gynaecol Br Emp* 64:47-49, 1957.

21. Bonney V: The fruits of conservatism, *J Obstet Gynaecol Br Emp* 44:1-12, 1937.

22. Palmer R: Etude analytique de 44 cas d'implantation tubouterine, *Mem Acad Chir* 77:216-220, 1951.

23. Moore-White M: Four cases of re-implantation of the fallopian tubes, *J Obstet Gynaecol Br Emp* 58:381-384, 1951.

24. Mulligan WJ, Rock J, and Easterday CL: Use of polyethylene in tuboplasty, *Fertil Steril* 4:428-435, 1953.

25. Rommer JJ: Surgery in the treatment of sterility, *Urol Cutan Rev* 52:586-590, 1948.

26. Wirtz JW: Experience with a method for implantation of the fallopian tubes into the uterus, *Aust NZ J Obstet Gynaecol* 5:7-11, 1965.

27. Halban J: *Gynakologische Operationslehre*, Berlin, 1932, Urban & Schwarzenberg.

28. Polowe D: A new technique for reconstruction of the oviducts, Am J Surg 68:208-211, 1945.

29. Shirodkar VN: Further experiences in tuboplasty, *Aust NZ J Obstet Gynaecol* 5:1-6, 1965.

30. Stallworthy J: Fertility, infertility, and sterility. In Bourne A and Claye A (eds): *British gynaecological practice*, London, Heinemann, 1963.

31. Johnstone JW: Implantation of the fallopian tubes for sterility, *J Obstet Gynaecol Br Emp* 62:410-416, 1955.

32. Peterson EP, Musich JR, and Behrman SJ: Uterotubal implantation and obstetric outcome after previous sterilization, *Int J Fertil* 23:254, 1978.

33. Green-Armytage VB: Discussion on modern methods of salpingostomy, *Proc R Soc Med* 53:1009, 1960.

34. Grant A: Infertility surgery of the oviduct, *Fertil Steril* 22:496-503, 1971.

35. Williams GFJ: Tubo-uterine implantation with special references to reversal of sterilization, *Lancet* 1:825-827, 1969.

36. Rock JA: Uterotubal implantation. In Reyniak JV and Lauersen NH (eds): *Principles of microsurgical techniques in infertility*, New York, 1982, Plenum.

37. Cohen J et al: Results of a prospective study on surgical therapy of tubal infertility (abstract), *Fertil Steril* 28:284, 1977.

20

Tubal Anastomosis

· ·

ROBERT B. HUNT

DAVID G. DIAZ

Anastomosis of the fallopian tube is applicable to repair certain localized or segmental obstructions, such as those caused by salpingitis isthmica nodosa, endometriosis, or previous tubal sterilization. The basic principle of repair is the same for all disease states: excision of abnormal tissue; adequate hemostasis with preservation of the vascular tree; and a precise, tension-free anastomosis.

PREOPERATIVE STUDIES AND COUNSELING

When the couple considering anastomosis is seen for consultation, we review their evaluation up to that point. A physical examination is performed on the woman, obtaining necessary cultures and a Papanicolaou (Pap) smear if appropriate. We next outline any additional testing and discuss with the couple the proposed procedure. It is essential that the surgeon allow ample time to answer all the couple's questions. After the consultation is completed, a comprehensive letter is dictated to the couple, with a copy to the referring physician, covering the following points:

1. Additional testing needed and, if applicable, outside records requested.
2. The proposed procedure in understandable terms, including removal of organs if applicable.
3. The length of hospitalization and the time required to recover completely.
4. Plans for follow-up, such as advisability of a postoperative tubal patency study.
5. The possibility of an ectopic pregnancy or spontaneous abortion after surgery.

This letter is extremely important for a number of reasons. First, it gives us an opportunity to review the couple's case history again to ascertain that we have not omitted an important step in the evaluation, such as a postcoital test or semen analysis, ovulation assessment, or the need for genetic counseling. Second, the couple has an opportunity to read this summary in the privacy of their home. This prompts them to discuss the proposed procedure, to work with us to complete their evaluation, and to have a realistic expectation of a successful outcome. Third, this policy instills confidence in the couple, may result in a better outcome, is greatly appreciated by the referring physician, and documents the preoperative process for legal purposes.

When the couple schedules the surgery, they are mailed the appropriate informed consent form(s) (see Appendix A). Before surgery this document must be signed by the couple and returned to us to be incorporated into the woman's office record.

INSTRUMENTS AND MATERIALS
Magnification

Some have advocated tubal anastomosis without the use of magnification in selected cases for tubal reversal.[1] Rock et al[2] found that loupes and the surgical microscope yielded similar pregnancy results when the procedure was performed by experienced tubal surgeons and was limited to anastomosis of isthmic or ampullary segments. Gomel[3] was a strong proponent of using the surgical microscope for this procedure, finding an increase in pregnancy rates from 31% to 64.4%. Winston[4,5] also supported this practice. Diamond[6] reported a 4.7 times improvement in pregnancy rates in patients undergoing correction of cornual occlusion by anastomosis with the aid of the surgical microscope, as compared with tubal implantation. Pauerstein[7] also supported the use of the surgical microscope.

Sutures

Tissue reactions to synthetic absorbable and nonabsorbable sutures have been studied extensively. Whereas minor differences in these have been noted, all the materials tested seem to render satisfactory results.[8-12] One author (RBH) prefers nylon (Sharpoint) and polybutester (Davis & Geck) for the following reasons: excellent color contrast, monofilament material, strength, memory, and the availability of superb tapered needles with cutting tips.

PATHOLOGIC CORNUAL OCCLUSION

The rationale of cornual anastomosis for correction of pathologic cornual occlusion was established by Ehrler.[13] He noted that the intramural portion of the fallopian tube was usually preserved in proximal tubal disease. On the basis of this observation, he recommended cornual anastomosis as an alternative to tubal implantation (Plates 34 and 35). Although Ehrler's results after anastomosis were poor, his concept led to the refinement of the technique.

If either cornual anastomosis or tubal implantation seems to be indicated, we favor anastomosis for several reasons. First, there is less disturbance of the vascular tree. Also, tubal length is preserved. Finally, the patient may often deliver vaginally.

The four most frequently diagnosed disease states encountered in pathologic cornual occlusion are obliterative fibrosis (38.1%), salpingitis isthmica nodosa (23.8%), chronic tubal inflammation (21.4%), and endometriosis (14.3%).[14] To achieve continued postoperative tubal patency, all diseased tissue must be resected. This usually means a portion of the intramural segment and most or all of the isthmus. We find tissue quality often improves at the junction of the isthmus and ampulla. By transecting the tube at this site before it widens into the ampulla, we usually have healthy tubal segments remaining with little luminal disparity. A precise, tension-free anastomosis is then performed.

If the tube is diseased along its entire length, careful judgment must be exercised in deciding how much to excise to allow for a technically satisfactory anastomosis and for pregnancy to occur. We leave at least 2 cm of the ampulla with its attached fimbriae in these cases.

Transcervical selective cannulation of the fallopian tubes to relieve proximal tubal obstruction has become available.[15] When appropriate, we offer this procedure to patients before anastomosis. The technique is described in Chapter 12.

Some have supported the use of danazol to correct pathologic cornual occlusion. In one series, 5 of 12 patients achieved patency and 1 of 12 conceived after treatment.[16]

TUBOTUBAL ANASTOMOSIS FOR REVERSAL OF STERILIZATION

Patients who request sterilization reversal do so for a number of reasons. One study found these reasons, in decreasing frequency, to be change of marital status, crib death, desire for more children in the same marriage, a family tragedy, and psychologic factors.[3] Two studies found 90% of women requesting reversal of sterilization did so to have children in a new marriage or to have more children in the same marriage.[17,18]

In addition to the standard infertility studies, the patient considering reversal of sterilization should be considered for diagnostic laparoscopy, particularly if the sterilization included use of coagulation or consisted of a partial salpingectomy or fimbriectomy. The surgeon should obtain a copy of the sterilization and pathology reports if possible. Frequently, however, these reports are at variance with the findings at laparoscopy, including nonabsorbable sutures placed distal to the site of the ligation, an additional segment of tube included in the ligation, fimbrial occlusion, and extensive adhesions.[3] We usually perform the diagnostic laparoscopy at the time of the reversal.

Whether a hysterosalpingogram (HSG) should be obtained before the reversal procedure is controversial. Although some believe it is not warranted, we believe it is.[19] Examples of its value are discovery of a uterine septum or intrauterine synechiae, proximal tubal disease, such as polyps or salpingitis isthmica nodosa, and an ampullary segment ligation.

The woman's age is often an issue in counseling. Our cutoff age for surgery is 45 years. This policy is supported by a study of 78 patients undergoing reversal of sterilization between ages 40 and 45.[20] Of these, 34 (44%) patients had live births. Before performing the surgery, the surgeon should counsel these couples concerning genetic disorders. In women 40 years or older and in those who have recently developed long cycles, it is prudent to measure follicle-stimulating hormone levels to rule out impending ovarian failure.

At the time of anastomosis, the surgeon should remember that patients commonly have disease in the proximal tubal segment adjacent to the ligation site.[21-24] These abnormalities include polyps, chronic inflammatory changes, and endometriosis. If possible, we excise 0.5 to 1.0 cm of proximal tube adjacent to the site of ligation and inspect the cut section under the highest power of the microscope. One must not excise a segment of distal tube distal to the ligation site, since it is not diseased in this area and an enormous luminal disparity would result.

One author obtained a 61.1% pregnancy rate after reversal of sterilization when the only or longer oviduct was 4 cm or less. The mean time for conception to occur was 19.1 months in these short oviducts.[3] Another study was not so encouraging. If the longer tube was greater than 7 cm, the delivery rate was 75%.[25] If the longer tube was shorter than 7 cm, it fell to 16%. Yet another report found a significant improvement in patients undergoing reversal of sterilization when the longer oviduct was greater than 4 cm.[21] Although the minimal tubal

Table 20-1 Results of cornual anastomosis

Diagnosis	Number of patients	Number (%) IUP (viable or ongoing)	Number (%) EP	Number (%) Ab	Number (%) no preg
Path cor occ	10	7(70)	1(10)*	1(10)	2(20)
Bipolar bl	3	2(67)	0	0	0
Reversal	20	13(65)	1(5)	2(10)	4(20)

*This patient had a viable intrauterine pregnancy subsequently.

IUP = intrauterine pregnancy; EP = ectopic pregnancy; Ab = abortion; path cor occ = pathologic cornual occlusion; bipolar bl = bipolar blockage.

length, particularly ampullary length, required for humans to conceive after reversal of sterilization has not been determined, we prefer at least a 2.0-cm ampulla with healthy fimbriae on the longer tube.

FOLLOW-UP OF ANASTOMOSIS

We continue to monitor these patients carefully after surgery. At 1 month we see them for their surgical checkup. At 4 months we perform an HSG unless contraindicated. We usually see the patients every 2 months afterward, performing indicated studies and observations to maximize their chances of conceiving. We recommend a follow-up laparoscopy at 18 months if adhesions are suspected. In one study, approximately one half of patients who conceived did so in the first 10.2 months after surgery for reversal of sterilization.[3] Others found the mean interval for pregnancy to occur to be 8.4 months.[18] The length of time required to conceive appeared to be inversely related to the total length of the reconstructed oviducts.

CAUSES OF FAILURE

Many factors contribute to lack of a successful pregnancy after tubal anastomosis. If adhesions are present at the time of surgery, particularly thick, vascular ones, they do have a tendency to recur after surgery and can prevent pregnancy. Another cause is failure to excise microscopic disease in the proximal tubal segment, including salpingitis isthmica nodosa, endometriosis, fibrosis, and chronic salpingitis.[26] Among the causes of failure of cornual anastomosis procedures, as well as those in other parts of the tube, are reocclusion due to preexisting disease, faulty technique, postoperative infection or adhesions, inadequate tubal length, and disturbance of tubo-ovarian relationships.[21,27]

One study revealed that of 32 reversal procedures that failed to result in pregnancy, 6 patients had bilaterally occluded tubes and 3 had severe ovulatory dysfunction.[28] In 11 women the failure to conceive was unexplained, and in 12 the husband had not previously fathered a child. The authors thus concluded that an undefined male factor is responsible for many failures. The reproductive system is a dynamic one and many aspects of it may change significantly from time to time.

RESULTS

The viable pregnancy rates after cornual anastomosis for correction of pathologic cornual occlusion have been excellent. Fifteen (57.7%) of 26 patients achieved pregnancies that reached the viable stage.[29] In a second series, 27 (56.2%) of 48 patients had term pregnancies after surgery.[30] A third series reported 36 (44%) of 82 patients were delivered of a term pregnancy.[31] The ectopic pregnancy rates were 15.4%, 6.2%, and 7%, respectively. A collected series of 506 patients undergoing cornual anastomosis for proximal occlusion revealed 274 (54%) achieved intrauterine pregnancies and 18 (3.6%) ectopic pregnancies.[32] One author's (RBH) most recent results for cornual obstruction are shown in Table 20-1.

Reversal of sterilization has produced many reports of superb results. Of 118 patients undergoing tubotubal anastomosis, 93 (78.8%) achieved a term pregnancy and 2 (1.7%) experienced an ectopic pregnancy.[30] A collected series of 1803 patients revealed 1149 (63.7%) intrauterine pregnancies and 68 (3.8%) ectopic gestations.[32]

RESEARCH

Continuing research in reproductive surgery has been conducted using a tissue adhesive material for tubal anastomosis in selected cases. Preliminary studies using the rabbit model reported tubal patency and pregnancies after isthmic-isthmic anastomosis with this technique.[33]

One group followed 28 women in whom tubotubal anastomosis was achieved with fibrin glue combined with a single tubal stitch.[34] Thirteen intrauterine and three ectopic pregnancies resulted. A study compared uterine horn anastomosis in rabbits using fibrin sealant, 9-0 polyglycolic acid sutures, and a combination of the two.[35] Pregnancy rates were identical for the sealant and microsutures (95%), and that with the combination was slightly lower (85%).

Pregnancy rates in rabbits with anastomosis of uterine horns by a single continuous suture were compared with those using a two-layer anastomosis with interrupted su-

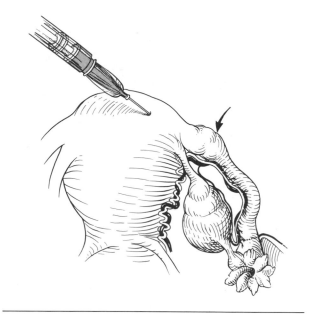

Figure 20-1
Typical cornual thickening *(arrow)* seen in salpingitis isthmica nodosa. The myometrium is injected with 1 to 2 U of vasopressin.

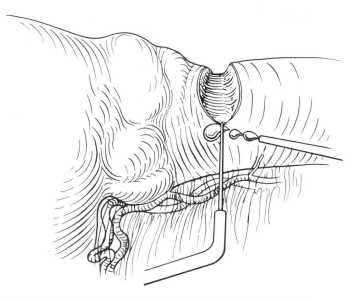

Figure 20-2
With microelectrode, scissors, or laser, the serosa is incised.

tures.[36] The advantage of the single-layer closure was shortened surgery time. Anecdotal reports of tubotubal anastomosis by laparoscopy exist.

The carbon dioxide (CO_2) laser was advocated as an alternative to incising the tube in preparation for anastomosis.[37] However, the same authors found the CO_2 laser inappropriate for anastomosing fallopian tubes by welding the tissues. Similarly, the argon laser yielded poor surgical results when rat uterine horn segments were approximated by photocoagulation.[38]

Whether the use of tissue adhesives, fibrin glue, or laser welding will compare favorably to the already excellent results achieved by microsurgical anastomosis remains to be seen.

TECHNIQUE OF CORNUAL ANASTOMOSIS

The example of cornual obstruction depicted is that of salpingitis isthmica nodosa, manifested by thickening at the cornu (Figure 20-1). After the pelvis is prepared as outlined in Chapter 9, approximately 1 U dilute vasopressin (20 U in 100 ml lactated Ringer's) is injected into the uterine fundus near the cornu. This reduces small vessel bleeding and consequently allows better visualization of the surgical site. Because vasopressin sometimes produces significant hypertension, the anesthesiologist should be alerted each time it is to be injected.

The tube is transected at mid-isthmus. The surgeon begins the transection by developing a peritoneal tract over the tube with a microscissors, microelectrode, or

laser (Figure 20-2). The dissection is carried out under continuous irrigation with heparinized lactated Ringer's solution (5000 U/L lactated Ringer's). Bipolar coagulation is used as needed.

The dissection is continued until the serosa covering the tube has been completely incised (Figure 20-3). The incision is continued to include serosa overlying the mesosalpinx for approximately 5 mm beneath the tube. The dissecting rod and forceps are an enormous help in rotating the tube to facilitate development of the peritoneal tract.

Next the tube is cut transversely with a straight iris scissors or laser (Figure 20-4). Great care is taken to avoid damaging the nutrient vessels coursing just beneath the tube and parallel to it. These vessels are important in providing tubal perfusion.

To lessen tissue damage, significantly bleeding vessels are coagulated with the bipolar unit (Figure 20-5). Irrigation defines the vessel and allows the surgeon to coagulate it. The identification and coagulation process begins superiorly to prevent blood from obscuring open vessels positioned inferiorly. Tiny vessels and those located adjacent to mucosa should not be coagulated. Bleeding will cease spontaneously once the anastomosis is completed.

If bleeding is brisk and the cut end of the vessel is not seen, gentle pressure on the tube between the thumb and forefinger will stop the bleeding and allow the surgeon, with the aid of irrigation, to identify and coagulate the vessel.

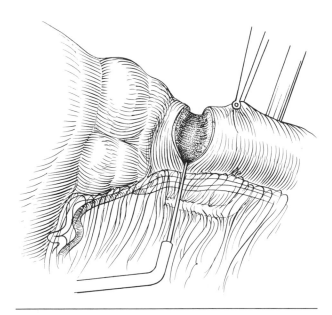

Figure 20-3
The peritoneal incision continues.

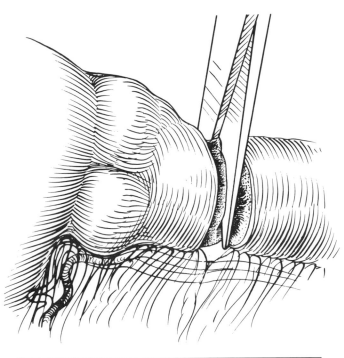

The proximal portion of the tube is grasped with a heavy toothed forceps and lifted superiorly (Figure 20-6). The tube is dissected from its underlying mesosalpinx by incising the peritoneum on either side of the meso-salpinx and the connective tissue underlying the tube. It is essential to preserve the nutrient vessels beneath the tube. The only ones that require bipolar coagulation and division are branches that penetrate directly into the tube. Using microscissors, microelectrode, or laser, the tube is cut transversely with a straight iris scissors or laser (Figure 20-4).

To lessen tubal damage, significantly bleeding vessels are coagulated with the bipolar unit (Figure 20-5). Irrigation defines the vessel and allows the surgeon to coagulate it. The identification and coagulation process begins superiorly to prevent blood from obscuring open vessels postioned inferiorly. Tiny vessels and those located adjacent to mucosa should not be coagulated. Bleeding will cease spontaneously once the anastomosis is completed.

If bleeding is brisk and the cut end of the vessel is not seen, gentle pressure on the tube between the thumb and forefinger will stop the bleeding and allow the surgeon, with the aid of irrigation, to identify and coagulate the vessel.

The proximal portion of the tube is grasped with a heavy toothed forceps and lifted superiorly (Figure 20-6). The tube is dissected from its underlying mesosalpinx by incising the peritoneum on either side of the meso-

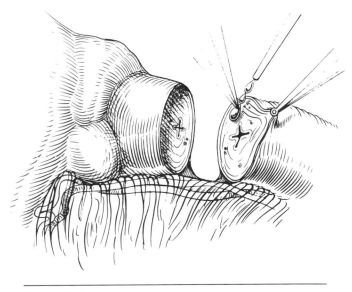

Figure 20-5
Bipolar coagulation of vessels is accomplished. Because it is nonconductive, glycine may be used for irrigation (Richard M. Soderstrom).

salpinx and the connective tissue underlying the tube. It is essential to preserve the nutrient vessels beneath the tube. The only ones that require bipolar coagulation and division are branches that penetrate directly into the

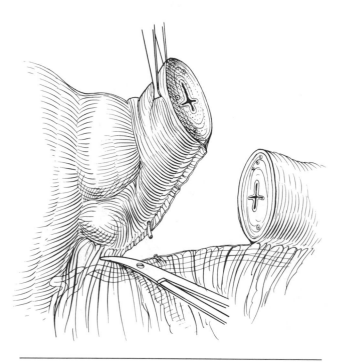

Figure 20-6
The proximal tube is lifted superiorly and dissected from the mesosalpinx, taking care to spare the nutrient vessels.

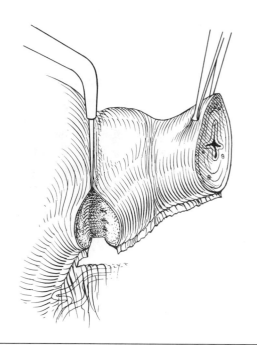

Figure 20-7
A peritoneal incision is made over the cornu.

tube. Using microscissors, microelectrode, or laser, the dissection is continued to the cornu. A dissecting rod is helpful in manipulating the tube throughout the dissection.

The proximal stump is pulled away from the uterus and a peritoneal tract developed over the cornu (Figure 20-7). Note that the nutrient vessels curve inferiorly to become a part of the uterine artery and vein complex. The blades of the iris scissors are placed in the peritoneal tract at an angle to avoid damage to the underlying vessels, and the tube is transected in a single cut (Figure 20-8). Bleeding is controlled by bipolar coagulation. Occasionally, a large venous sinus is encountered. Coagulation of it will result in excessive tissue damage, yet lack of hemostasis. It is best to close the sinus with a 8-0 suture.

Although tubal lavage may determine patency, normal tissue is seldom found at the site of transection in pathologic cornual occlusion. To dissect further into the cornu, a 6-0 suture is placed through the lumen of the tube with a tapered needle (Figure 20-9). Gentle traction is placed on the suture, and the dissection is continued just outside the circular muscle of the tube. Each time the surgeon has dissected 2 mm of tube, the section is transected and the tube inspected under the highest magnification (Figure 20-10). The steps are repeated until healthy tissue and a normally patent tube are observed. If the surgeon's view of the surgical site is hampered by bleeding, ad-

ditional vasopressin is injected. If visibility is poor due to working in a "hole," crescents of myometrium overlying the intramural tube are excised to provide a wider field of view.

Ideally, characteristics that the intramural tube prepared for anastomosis should exhibit include the following:

1. When the tube is lavaged, the stream of indigo carmine should be cylindric with uninterrupted egress. If not, a no. 0 or 1 monofilament suture or similar stent is inserted into the intramural tube and threaded gently into the uterine cavity. Often the stream will become normal when the stent is withdrawn (Figure 20-11).

2. The tubal mucosa should appear velvety and lightly stained with indigo carmine.

3. The tubal musculature should be well perfused.

4. The myometrium surrounding the tube should be devoid of fibrosis or other pathologic conditions.

When retrograde lavage with a cannula inserted through the fimbriae does not exhibit satisfactory flow through the transected end, additional tube must be excised. The medial portion of this lateral segment is grasped with the heavy toothed forceps, the peritoneum is incised on either side of the mesosalpinx, and the tube is dissected away from the underlying vessels (Figure 20-12). Bipolar coagulation is performed as necessary.

When the tube seems normal by appearance and palpation, a peritoneal tract is developed with the aid of ring forceps and a dissecting rod (Figure 20-13). The tube is

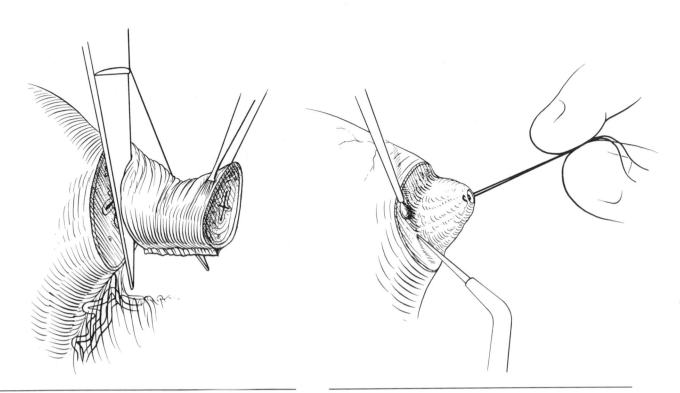

Figure 20-8
The proximal tube is excised with iris scissors.

Figure 20-9
A 6-0 suture is placed through the intramural tube and dissection continued.

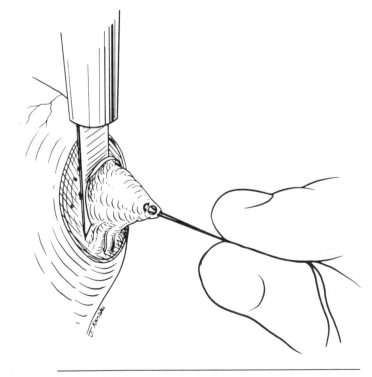

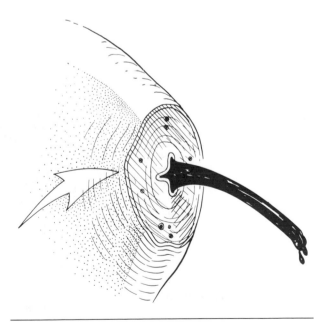

Figure 20-10
A segment of intramural tube is excised with a disposable ophthalmic scalpel.

Figure 20-11
A steady stream of indigo carmine exits the cut tubal lumen.

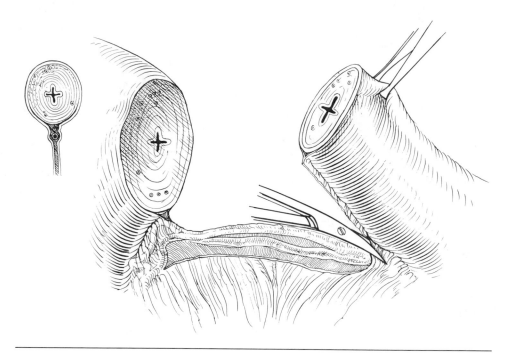

Figure 20-12
Distal tube is dissected from its underlying mesosalpinx and nutrient vessels.

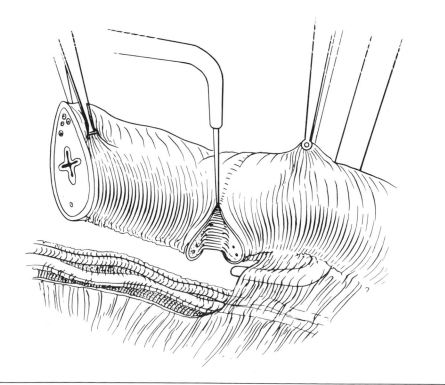

Figure 20-13
A peritoneal incision is made over the isthmus.

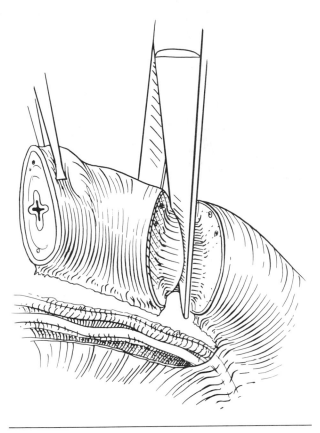

Figure 20-14
The dissected tubal segment is excised with iris scissors.

next transected with iris scissors, taking care not to cut the underlying vessels (Figure 20-14). Hemostasis is achieved, and patency is determined by retrograde lavage. The mucosa should appear healthy and the muscularis devoid of scar. If the cut end of the tube does not meet these criteria, additional tissue should be removed. Often an otherwise unhealthy appearing tube becomes normal in appearance at the ampullary-isthmic junction. This is fortunate, since it avoids excessive luminal disparity. Figure 20-15 illustrates a patent distal segment after dissection and transection of the proximal end.

At this point in the procedure, proximal and distal segments are prepared for anastomosis. Stay sutures of 6-0 material on a tapered needle are placed (Figure 20-16). It is essential to ascertain that the sutures are planned to align the lumina. To do otherwise will result in misalignment and possible failure of the anastomosis. The stay sutures are held with fine hemostats.

If the site of anastomosis is under tension, this must be released or the tubal lumen may become stenosed and eventually occlude. To bring the cut ends of the tube closer together to facilitate tying fine microsurgical sutures, the surgeon may perform several maneuvers. First, the peritoneum on either side of the mesosalpinx may be incised widely. Second, a sponge may be placed lateral

to the uterus on the contralateral side and lateral to the adnexa on the ipsilateral side. Third, if the proximal tubal segment is positioned superior to the distal segment, vaginal packing may be removed to bring the two segments into the same horizontal axis.

With the microscope properly centered and focused, the actual anastomosis begins. An 8-0 or 9-0 suture is placed in the 6 o'clock position extramucosally on the proximal segment and similarly in the distal segment, with the knot outside the tubal lumen (Figure 20-17). If the distal segment consists of ampulla at the site of anastomosis, a tiny bit of mucosa may be incorporated. The knot is tied and cut. Stay sutures may be tied at this time or later (Figure 20-18).

The first of two lateral sutures is placed but not tied, followed by placement of the second one (Figures 20-19 and 20-20). One or both lateral sutures are tied, and the 12 o'clock suture is placed. All sutures are now tied, including stay sutures (Figures 20-21 through 20-23). Patency is tested by transcervical or transuterine lavage. If the myometrial defect is large, it is partially closed and the serosal layer is then approximated (Figure 20-24). If additional sutures are required to close the mesosalpinx, they are placed at this time. Only the anterior mesosalpinx is closed. The overall tubal length is determined and recorded for statistical purposes. The completed anastomosis is shown in Figure 20-25.

TECHNIQUE OF TUBOTUBAL ANASTOMOSIS

Figure 20-26 depicts the typical appearance of the fallopian tube after ligation with a Falope ring. The anastomosis technique varies little whether coagulation, partial salpingectomy, a clip, or a ring was used for the sterilization (Plates 36 through 41).

The procedure begins with removal of the Falope ring. It is grasped with heavy toothed forceps, the peritoneum surrounding the ring is opened, and the ring is excised (Figure 20-26). A fibrous band of tissue joins the proximal and distal segments of fallopian tube. The band is grasped and lifted superiorly. It is then dissected away from the mesosalpinx until the proximal segment is reached (Figure 20-27). The surgeon prepares the proximal segment for anastomosis (see Figures 20-6 through 20-8). It is necessary to excise 0.5 to 1.0 cm of tube at the site of sterilization, since this section is usually diseased. Because this is an isthmic-ampullary anastomosis, the tube is transected at approximately a 30-degree angle. Again, care is taken to avoid damaging the underlying vascular tree.

Attention is now turned to the lateral segment. The fibrous band attached to it is lifted and dissected to the medial portion of the lateral segment (Figure 20-28). Using the fibrous band as traction, a cap of serosa is excised from the proximal ampulla (Figure 20-29). Note that none of the muscularis is excised and the tubal

Text cont'd. on p. 344.

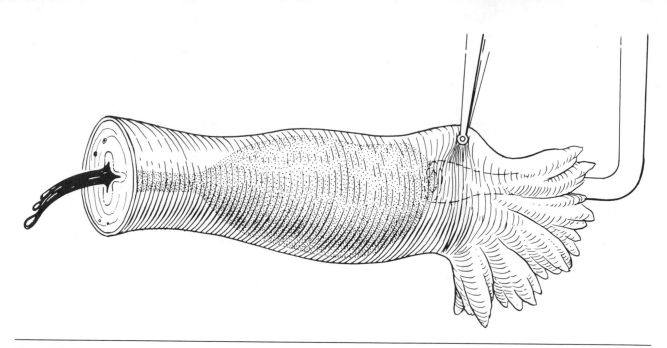

Figure 20-15
Retrograde lavage confirms patency.

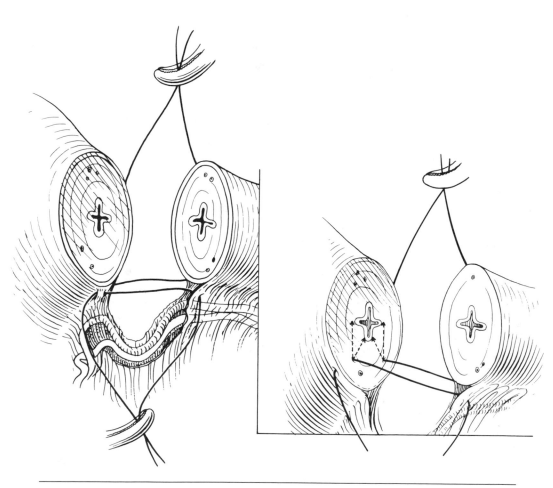

Figure 20-16
Segments of fallopian tube satisfactory for anastomosis remain. Stay sutures are placed and secured with fine hemostats. *(Inset)* They must be placed to accurately align the tubal lumina.

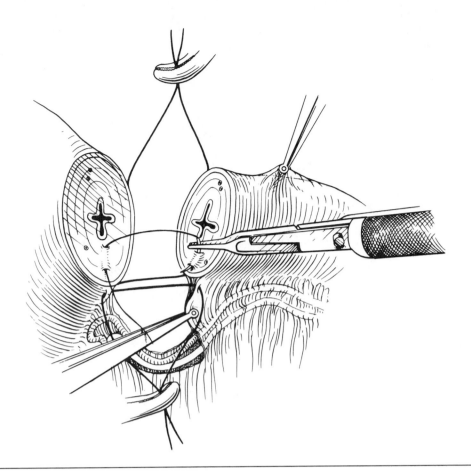

Figure 20-17
The 6 o'clock suture is positioned using a tapered needle with a cutting tip.

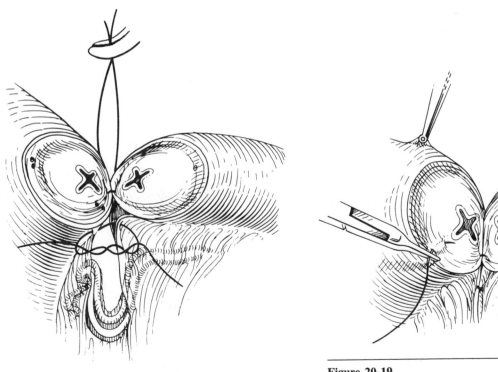

Figure 20-18
The 6 o'clock suture is tied. The stay sutures may be tied at this time or later.

Figure 20-19
The first lateral suture is placed.

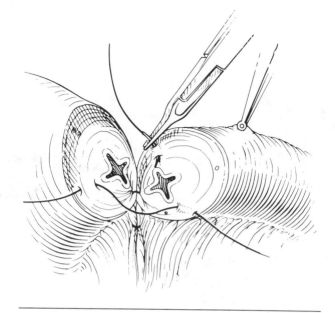

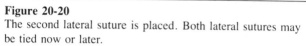

Figure 20-20
The second lateral suture is placed. Both lateral sutures may
be tied now or later.

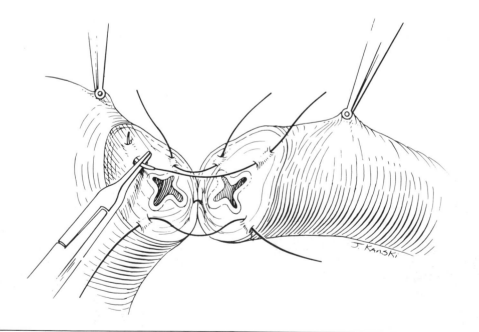

Figure 20-21
The 12 o'clock suture is placed.

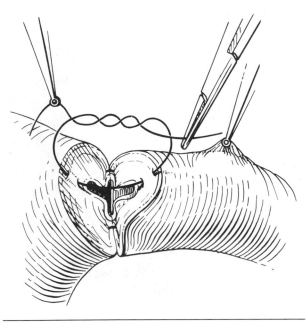

Figure 20-22
The lateral and 12 o'clock sutures are tied. Note the so-called surgeon's knot.

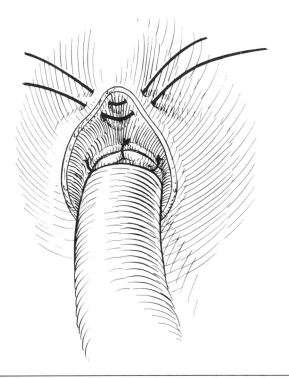
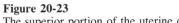
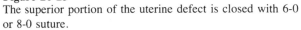

Figure 20-23
The superior portion of the uterine defect is closed with 6-0 or 8-0 suture.

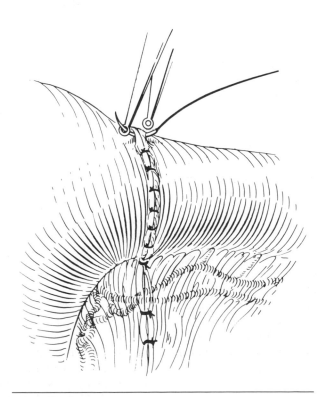

Figure 20-24
Serosal sutures are placed. A technique to facilitate grasping the needle tip is illustrated.

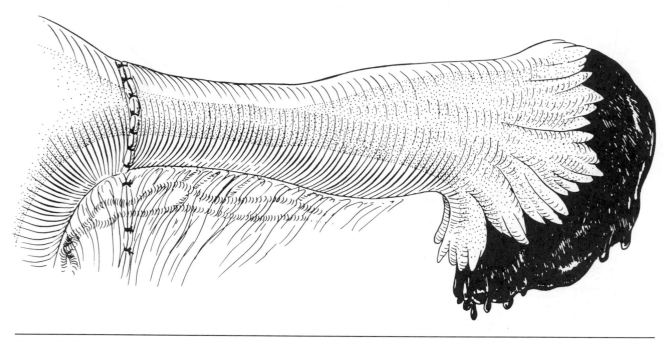

Figure 20-25
Indigo carmine flows through the fimbriae. Optimally, this is done before serosal closure.

mucosa is not exposed. When dissecting the ampulla, the microelectrode is not used to avoid thermal damage to the mucosa through this very thin muscle layer.

The most medial portion of the ampulla is grasped with a ring forceps and this tiny portion of ampulla excised (Figure 20-30). If the mucosa is not yet exposed, this step is repeated. Retrograde lavage often helps identify the most medial portion of the ampullary lumen. Also the cannula may be advanced the length of the ampulla to determine the most medial portion. After the ampullary mucosa is exposed, patency is documented by retrograde lavage.

Stay sutures of 6-0 material are placed to align the tubal lumina and to relieve tension on the anastomosis (Figure 20-31). Four sutures of 9-0 material are placed, avoiding the isthmic mucosa but incorporating a tiny bit of ampullary mucosa with the ampullary muscularis. All sutures are tied (Figure 20-32). After patency is confirmed, serosal sutures of 8-0 material are placed and tied and additional sutures are placed in the serosa of the mesosalpinx as required.

When placing the inner layer of sutures, progress may be hampered by ampullary mucosa draping over the surgical site. The excessive mucosa may be brushed back into the ampullary lumen as each suture is placed. Another suggestion is to lift the 3 and 9 o'clock sutures superiorly and return the mucosa to the ampullary lumen by irrigation or ring forceps.

Luminal disparity

Occasionally, a large luminal disparity exists between the tubal segments. To correct this disparity, we perform

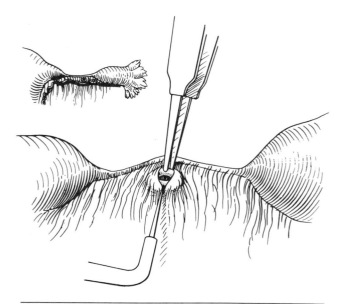

Figure 20-26
The fallopian tube after Falope ring ligation. The ring is being removed.

several steps. First, the proximal stump is cut approximately a 30-degree angle. Second, two or three sutures of 9-0 material are placed transversely in the distal segment and tied (Figure 20-33). This should narrow the ampullary lumen so that much less disparity exists, perhaps 3:1. The standard anastomosis is then performed (Figures 20-34 and 20-35). These techniques for correcting tubal luminal disparity are simple to perform and

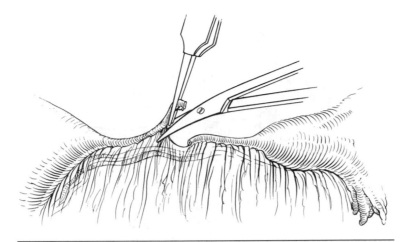

Figure 20-27
The fibrous band joining the tubal segments is divided and
dissected toward the proximal tube.

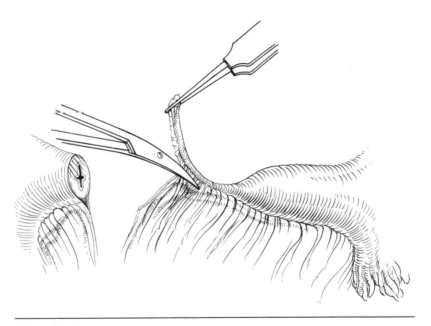

Figure 20-28
The fibrous band is dissected toward the distal tubal segment.

require minimal dissection, with little damage to the fallopian tube.

Ampullary obstruction

Causes of ampullary stenosis or obstruction include tubal ligation, partial salpingectomy, and salpingotomy for ectopic pregnancy (Figure 20-36). To correct this problem, the fibrous band or narrowed tube connecting the ampullary segments is divided and dissected away from the longitudinal vessels beneath it (Figure 20-37). A peritoneal tract is made over the proximal segment with microscissors and the tube is transected. Again, care is taken to avoid damaging the underlying vessels (Figure 20-38). Because there is no luminal disparity, the cut is perpendicular to the long axis of the tube. A similar procedure is performed on the distal segment (Figure 20-39). A standard anastomosis is carried out (Figures 20-40 and 20-41), usually requiring approximately six sutures on the inner layer. Patency is documented.

If at least 2 cm of distal ampulla with healthy fimbriae remains, and if the proximal tube is deciliated or otherwise damaged, the surgeon should consider resecting the proximal ampulla and performing an isthmic-ampullary anastomosis.

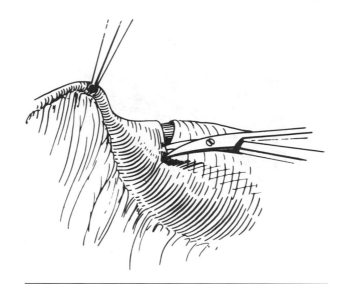

Figure 20-29
A serosal cap is excised.

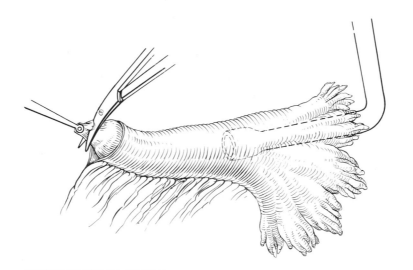

Figure 20-30
The medial portion of the ampulla is grasped with ring forceps and a tiny portion is excised.

CHECKING TUBAL PATENCY

Leakage at the anastomosis site occurs often and is acceptable, provided adequate flow of indigo carmine out of the distal end of the tube is observed and there is no tension at the anastomosis site. What is not acceptable is leakage with no spillage of dye at the distal end of the tube. If it appears that dye fails to flow into the proximal tube, and the uterus is not expanding as dye is injected, the lavage apparatus should be checked, perhaps removing the intrauterine catheter and converting to transuterine lavage with a Hunt lavage needle (Apple Medical). If the uterus is expanding with the injection of indigo car-

mine and the proximal tubal segment still does not fill, the surgeon may gently massage the myometrium in the vicinity of the cornu, which sometimes results in release of the obstruction. If these maneuvers are not successful in establishing flow into the proximal segment, the surgeon may elect not to undo the anastomosis and resect additional proximal tube under the following circumstances: the proximal tubal segment was determined to be patent earlier in the procedure; the surgeon is confident the anastomosis is technically satisfactory; and the preoperative HSG revealed a normal proximal segment.

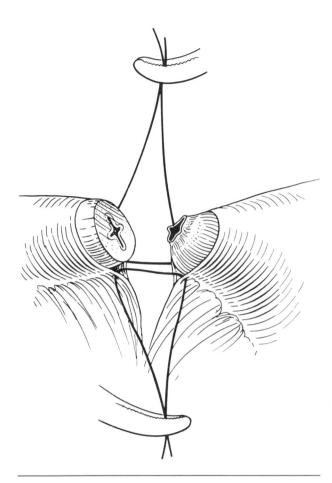

Figure 20-31
The proximal tube has been cut at a 30-degree angle. The luminal disparity is acceptable.

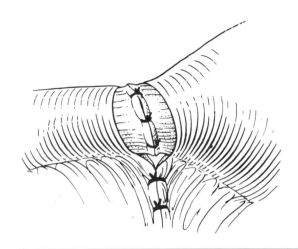

Figure 20-32
The inner layer of sutures of 9-0 material has been placed and tied. Serosal and additional mesosalpinx sutures complete the anastomosis.

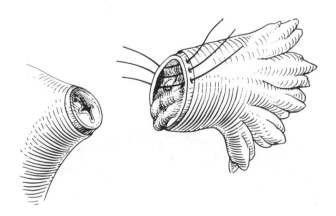

Figure 20-33
Transverse sutures are placed to correct a luminal disparity unacceptable for anastomosis.

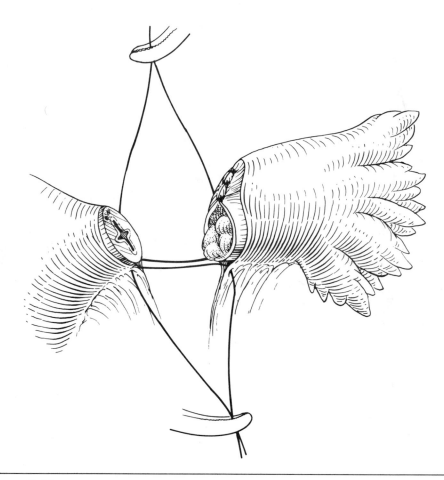

Figure 20-34
The anastomosis is begun with placement of stay sutures.

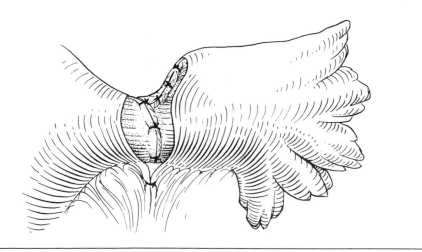

Figure 20-35
The inner layer of the anastomosis is complete and stay sutures are tied. The serosal sutures are placed next.

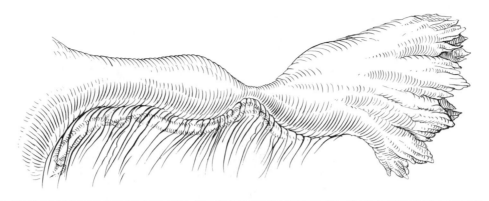

Figure 20-36
Ampullary obstruction is illustrated.

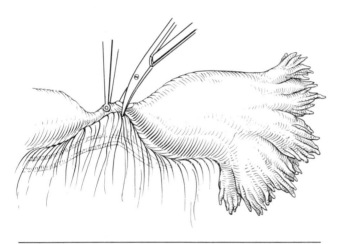

Figure 20-37
The fibrous band is divided.

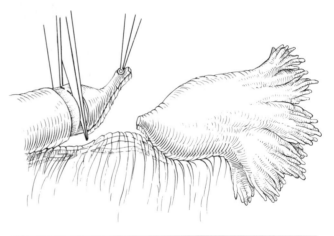

Figure 20-38
The tube is cut vertically with iris scissors.

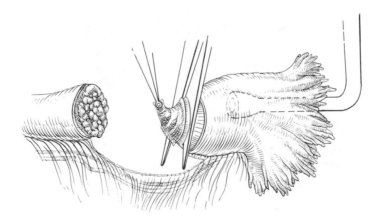

Figure 20-39
The distal segment is prepared similarly.

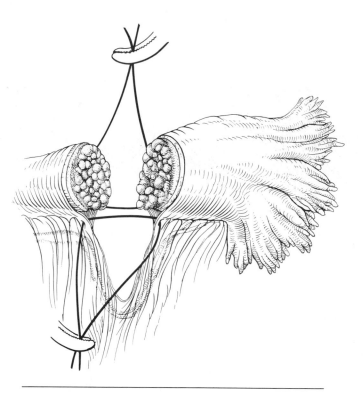

Figure 20-40
Stay sutures are placed and secured with small hemostats.

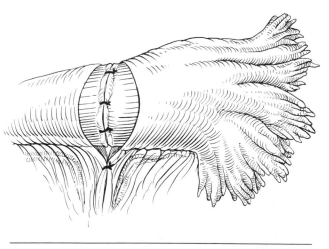

Figure 20-41
The inner layer of 9-0 sutures are placed and tied. Serosal approximation with 8-0 sutures completes the anastomosis.

SUMMARY

The techniques illustrated in this chapter represent a condensation of the ideas of many of our colleagues as well as our own refinements. The steps are standardized and apply to most conditions requiring tubal anastomosis. They are reproducible and have served our patients well over several years.

REFERENCES

1. McCormick WG, and Torres J: A method of Pomeroy tubal ligation reanastomosis, *Obstet Gynecol* 47:623, 1976.
2. Rock JA et al: Comparison of the operating microscope and loupe for microsurgical tubal anastomosis: a randomized clinical trial, *Fertil Steril* 41:229, 1984.
3. Gomel V: Microsurgical reversal of female sterilization: a reappraisal, *Fertil Steril* 33:587, 1980.
4. Winston RML: The future of microsurgery in infertility, *Clin Obstet Gynaecol* 5:607, 1978.
5. Hedon B, Wineman M, and Winston RML: Loupes or microscope for tubal anastomosis? An experimental study, *Fertil Steril* 34:264, 1980.
6. Diamond E: A comparison of gross and microsurgical techniques for repair of cornual occlusion in infertility: a retrospective study, 1968-1978, *Fertil Steril* 32:370, 1979.
7. Pauerstein CJ: Why has not man a microscopic eye? *Fertil Steril* 34:289, 1980.
8. Neff MR, Holtz GL, and Betsill WL Jr: Adhesion formation and histologic reaction with polydioxanone and polyglactin suture, *Am J Obstet Gynecol* 151:20, 1985.
9. Gomel V, McComb P, and Boer-Meisel M: Histologic reactions to polyglactin-910, polyethylene, and nylon microsuture, *J Reprod Med* 25:56, 1980.
10. Laufer N et al: Macroscopic and histologic tissue reaction to polydioxanone, a new, synthetic, monofilament microsuture, *J Reprod Med* 29:307, 1984.
11. Leader A et al: Histologic reaction to a new microsurgical suture in rabbit reproductive tissue, *Fertil Steril* 40:815, 1983.
12. Sojo D, Pardo JD, and Nistal M: Histology and fertility after microsurgical anastomosis of the rabbit fallopian tube with nylon and polyglactin sutures, *Fertil Steril* 39:707, 1983.
13. Ehrler P: Anastomose intramurale de la trompe, *Bull Fed Soc Gynecol Obstet* 17:866, 1965.
14. Fortier KJ, and Haney AF: Pathologic spectrum of uterotubal junction obstruction, *Obstet Gynecol* 65:93, 1985.
15. Rosch J et al: Selective transcervical fallopian tube catheterization: technique update, *Radiology* 168:1, 1988.
16. Claman P et al: Danazol therapy for proximal obstruction of the oviduct, *J Reprod Med* 31:687, 1986.
17. Leader A et al: A comparison of definable traits in women requesting reversal of sterilization and women satisfied with sterilization, *Am J Obstet Gynecol* 145, 1983.
18. Grunert GM, Drake TS, and Takaki NK: Microsurgical reanastomosis of the fallopian tubes for reversal of sterilization, *Obstet Gynecol Surv* 58:148, 1981.
19. Groff TR, Edelstein JA, and Schenken RS: Hysterosalpingography in the preoperative evaluation of tubal anastomosis candidates, *Fertil Steril* 53:417, 1990.
20. Trimbos-Kemper TCM: Reversal of sterilization in women over 40 years of age: a multicenter study in the Netherlands, *Fertil Steril* 53:575, 1990.
21. Rock JA et al: Tubal anastomosis following unipolar cautery, *Fertil Steril* 37:613, 1982.
22. Stock RJ: Postsalpingectomy endometriosis: a reassessment, *Obstet Gynecol* 60:560, 1982.
23. Vasquez G et al: Tubal lesions subsequent to sterilization and their relation to fertility after attempts at reversal, *Am J Obstet Gynecol* 138:86, 1980.
24. Donnez J et al: Tubal polyps, epithelial inclusions, and endometriosis after tubal sterilization, *Fertil Steril* 41:564, 1984.
25. Hulka JF, and Halme J: Sterilization reversal: results of 101 attempts, *Am J Obstet Gynecol* 159:769, 1988.
26. Gomel V: Causes of failed reconstructive tubal microsurgery, *J Reprod Med* 24:239, 1980.
27. Musich JR, and Behrman SJ: Surgical management of tubal obstruction at the uterotubal junction, *Fertil Steril* 40:423, 1983.
28. DeCherney AH, Mezer HC, and Naftolin F: Analysis of failure of microsurgical anastomosis after midsegment, non-coagulation tubal ligation, *Fertil Steril* 39:618, 1983.
29. McComb P: Microsurgical tubocornual anastomosis for occlusive cornual disease: reproducible results without the need for tubo-uterine implantation, *Fertil Steril* 46:571, 1986.
30. Gomel V: *Microsurgery in female infertility*, Boston, 1983, Little, Brown & Co.
31. Donnez J, and Casanas-Roux F: Prognostic factors influencing the pregnancy rate after microsurgical cornual anastomosis, *Fertil Steril* 46:1089, 1986.
32. Sotrel G: *Tubal reconstructuve surgery*, Philadelphia, 1990, Lea & Febiger.
33. Gauwerky JFH et al: Morphology and fertility after reanastomosis of the rabbit fallopian tube with fibrin glue, *Hum Reprod* 3:327, 1988.
34. Rucker K et al: Tubal anastomosis using a tissue adhesive, *Hum Reprod* 3:185, 1988.
35. Schroeder E et al: Fibrin sealant in experimental tubal microsurgery, *Int J Fertil* 32:250, 1987.
36. Hurwitz A et al: A single continuous suture as a possible alternative to the interrupted suture for tubal anastomosis, *Int J Fertil* 35:125, 1990.
37. Choe JK et al: Clinical and histologic evaluation of laser reanastomosis of the uterine tube, *Fertil Steril* 41:754, 1984.
38. Lyon DR et al: A comparison between argon laser and microsuture anastomosis of the rat uterine horn, *Fertil Steril* 47:329, 1987.

21

Adhesiolysis, Fimbrioplasty, and Salpingostomy

ROBERT B. HUNT

HUGO C. VERHOEVEN

HANS W. SCHLOSSER

In contrast to the excellent results achieved after microsurgical anastomosis for reversal of sterilization, the pregnancy outcome after repair of postinfectious tubal disease is not encouraging. Although anatomic reconstruction results in tubal patency in most instances, alteration of tubal function remains the stumbling block to a successful pregnancy.

Because infertile patients are strongly motivated, successful pregnancy rates in the range of 20% to 25% after salpingostomy often do not discourage them from selecting surgical repair. Since in vitro fertilization (IVF) has a successful pregnancy rate of approximately the same in the more successful clinics, we encourage patients to consult with our IVF colleagues before electing surgery. Surgery and advanced reproductive technologies (ART) are not mutually exclusive; therefore patients frequently choose both routes.

PREOPERATIVE EVALUATION

Before performing surgery for distal tubal disease, the surgeon must carefully evaluate each couple. Included should be a test of sperm status (postcoital test and/or semen analysis), ovulation documentation (progesterone level, basal body temperature record, and/or properly timed endometrial biopsy), and assessment of the uterus and fallopian tubes (laparoscopy, hysterosalpingogram, and/or hysteroscopy). The surgeon should devote ample time for discussion with the couple, emphasizing expectations of achieving a successful pregnancy, the problem of ectopic pregnancy, and other options, including IVF and adoption. They should be provided with an informed consent sheet similar to that in Appendix A.

It is particularly important in patients with postinflammatory conditions to detect harmful bacteria before corrective surgery. One group cultured pelvic tissues and fluids at the time of pelvic surgery on asymptomatic infertile patients.[1] The patients were divided into three groups. In group 1, 7 (23.3%) of 30 patients with findings of chronically inflamed pelvic structures, adhesions, and/or tubal obstructions cultured positive for *Chlamydia trachomatis* (CT). In group 2, 6 (15.4%) of 39 patients without signs of inflammation but with pelvic adhesions and/or tubal obstruction were found to have CT. Of 49 patients without signs of inflammation and without adhesions or tubal obstruction, only 1 (2%) cultured positive for CT. Of great concern was the absence of correlation between positive intraabdominal and lower genital tract cultures. Based on the findings of this superb study, one can make a strong case for recommending antibiotic treatment of every infertile couple falling in groups 1 and 2, unless medically contraindicated.

A few absolute contraindications to reconstructive tubal surgery exist. These include known genital tuberculosis, absence of both ampullary segments, ovarian failure, malignancy, and active pelvic inflammatory disease (PID).

To avoid excessive intraoperative bleeding and harming unsuspected pregnancy, the surgery is scheduled to be performed, when possible, before ovulation but after menses have ceased.

Hysterosalpingography

Hysterosalpingography (HSG) provides valuable information. It detects intrauterine abnormalities, leads one to suspect proximal and distal tubal disease, and allows the surgeon to estimate tubal health by the presence or absence of mucosal folds. In fact, in one study the most significant preoperative indicator for a successful pregnancy was the presence or absence of mucosal patterns on HSG.[2] The pregnancy rates after surgery was 60.7% among patients with mucosal patterns on HSG, compared with 7.3% for those without patterns. A review of 300 infertile patients revealed that only women with normal mucosal patterns on HSG and tubes that were normal size or only slightly dilated conceived after surgery.[3] In addition, the HSG may detect proximal tubal disease such as salpingitis isthmica nodosa.

Hysteroscopy

Hysteroscopy is a complementary procedure. It allows the surgeon to diagnose precisely such intrauterine conditions as submucous myomata, intrauterine synechiae, intrauterine polyps, and certain congenital anomalies. Either HSG or hysteroscopy should be included in the evaluation.

Diagnostic laparoscopy

Laparoscopy provides extremely valuable information to determine the status of pelvic structures and prognosis before reconstructive surgery. Most sequelae of distal tubal disease can be corrected at laparoscopy by a surgeon skilled in advanced laparoscopic techniques.

Tuboscopy

Tuboscopy should be performed at laparoscopy or laparotomy in the patient with distal tubal obstruction (Plates 42 and 43). This small endoscope is inserted through an incision in the distal end of the tube, and the tube is distended with fluid or a gaseous medium. The ampulla is examined for the presence of mucosa, strictures, and intratubal adhesions. One study divided patients with hydrosalpinges into two groups.[4] Of 79 patients with normal or subnormal mucosa diagnosed by tuboscopy, 26 (33%) had subsequent normal pregnancies. Of 57 with abnormal mucosa at tuboscopy, none had successful intrauterine pregnancies. The authors suggest the HSG provides important information of the status of the intramural and isthmic sections of the tube, whereas tuboscopy allows the surgeon to assess the ampulla most accurately. Since tuboscopy can be performed at laparoscopy, the surgeon can better counsel the patient if subsequent repair is contemplated. If salpingostomy is performed at the time of tuboscopy, the surgeon can better estimate the chances of a successful pregnancy outcome.

Microbiopsy

Efforts have been made to determine tubal health by performing microbiopsy of the ampullary mucosa at the time of surgery.[5] Because ampullary mucosa is not damaged uniformly, a random microbiopsy does not necessarily allow the surgeon to infer to what degree the tube has been damaged.[4]

SURGICAL LAPAROSCOPY

The credit for this innovative technique is due largely to the persistent development and dissemination of information by Semm. Although large series are not yet available, term pregnancy rates seem to be comparable with those for microsurgical procedures by laparotomy for distal tubal disease. There continues to be a diversity of opinion, however. For example, one author advocated surgical laparoscopy for salpingo-ovariolysis and selected cases of fimbrioplasty but microsurgery by laparotomy for salpingostomy.[6] Others took a contrary view, expressing the belief that surgical laparoscopy offers significant advantages over laparotomy in treating postinflammatory conditions.[7,8] The trend seems to be shifting rapidly to surgical laparoscopy based on economic considerations and patient preference.[9,10]

LAPAROTOMY
Microsurgery versus conventional surgery

Winston[11] presented an elegant paper on the superiority of microsurgery as compared with conventional surgery. After reviewing the literature, he concluded that term pregnancy rates were doubled and patency rates definitely improved with microsurgery. Another group used their own patients who had undergone conventional surgery for distal tubal disease for controls and compared them with patients undergoing the same procedures using at least 10 X magnification.[12] In all categories microsurgery yielded superior results. A third group demonstrated the superiority of microsurgical over macrosurgical technique, achieving a pregnancy rate of 18.2% with macrosurgery and 55.6% with microsurgery.[13]

The necessity of the surgical microscope to perform superior tubal surgery was challenged in an excellent review by Pauerstein.[14] Winston[15] countered in a follow-up article, but acquiesced that use of the surgical microscope is valuable in tubal anastomosis but not routinely required in correcting distal tubal disease sequelae.

General considerations

Tubal lavage is performed either by inserting an intrauterine catheter or by transuterine lavage using a 20-gauge needle. Vaginal packing is sometimes helpful, and an indwelling Foley catheter is a must. A desirable irrigant is warm, heparinized lactated Ringer's solution (5000 U/L) for intraperitoneal irrigation.

During the procedure, the surgeon may prefer to be on the side opposite to the adnexa being worked on. This involves changing sides during the procedure, which is a minor inconvenience. The initial adhesiolysis is performed with approximately 2 to 3 X loupe magnification and a headlight. If increased magnification is necessary, the surgical microscope is brought into the operating field.

Because surgical research has demonstrated that peritoneal defects heal from the base up and ischemia is a potent stimulus for postoperative adhesions, the surgeon should peritonealize with restraint and without tension.[16] When satisfactory hemostasis has been achieved, that anatomic site should be placed at rest to avoid precipitating additional bleeding.

Tissue to be excised should be held by heavy, toothed forceps to avoid damaging the more delicate instruments. Adhesions attached to the fallopian tube and other pelvic structures should be divided 1 to 2 mm from the involved structure to allow for retraction and to lessen the chance of injury to that structure if additional coagulation is required. When adhesiolysis has been completed under magnification, the surgeon should examine the site without magnification to locate additional adhesions. Irrigation is helpful in locating small, actively bleeding vessels.

If an ovary or tube is to be removed, it should be done last, after the other pelvic structures have been repaired. This allows the surgeon to make a more informed judgment as to whether the organ in question should be removed.

Peritoneal platforms should be developed as one of the last steps in the procedure. This avoids unnecessary stress to tissues making up the platforms.

To assess pregnancy rates, a standardized system of classification should be used, such as one offered by the American Fertility Society.

Adhesiolysis

Figure 21-1 shows a typical view of pelvic structures damaged by PID. The omentum is adherent to the uterus as well as to adnexal structures. Both fallopian tubes are blocked distally, and many adhesions bind the pelvic structures together.

Using loupe magnification augmented by a headlight, the surgeon begins the procedure by separating adhesed structures in the cul-de-sac (Figures 21-2 and 21-3). Adhesions involving omentum, bowel, and uterus may be divided by electrosurgery, laser, scissors, or scalpel dissection. Bleeding is best controlled by bipolar coagulation (Figure 21-2 [inset]). Dissection is greatly facilitated by keeping the uterus in sharp anteflexion and retracting the bowel cephalad, thus placing the structures to be separated under tension. When performing electrosurgery in the vicinity of bowel and ureter, great care must be taken to avoid electrical injury to these structures. Frequent irrigation at the surgical site facilitates the dissection and allows the surgeon to obtain precise hemostasis. Adhesions should be excised when appropriate.

The omentum is sometimes thick and chronically inflamed. A partial omentectomy should be considered. It is performed by isolating, ligating, and dividing omental vessels (Figure 21-3 [inset]). Synthetic absorbable ligatures (2-0 or 3-0) are used. Extreme care must be taken to ligate each vessel securely, since postoperative bleeding could be disastrous.

An alternative method of dealing with omentum adhered to the pelvic structures, but not thickened or inflamed, is to fold it back on itself (omentopexy) after it has been dissected. This folded portion is sutured to the underlying proximal omentum with interrupted 3-0 synthetic absorbable sutures, taking care to avoid omental vessels. This technique minimizes the risk of postoperative bleeding and avoids ischemic tissue pedicles.

Once the rectosigmoid and omentum have been dissected, they are positioned cephalad with abdominal packs. If a vertical abominal incision is used, it should not extend superior to the navel, since this makes displacing the bowel more difficult.

The adnexa are next released from the lateral pelvic sidewall. A Teflon rod is placed beneath these adhesions to facilitate the dissection, and to protect the ureter and major blood vessels (Figure 21-4).

Each adnexa is dissected free, a sump drain positioned in the pelvis, and Kerlex gauze soaked in heparinized lactated Ringer's solution carefully placed in the posterior cul-de-sac overlying the drain (Figure 21-5). A silicone mat, inserted beneath each adnexa, provides an unencumbered background on which to work.

Next, a laparotomy pad saturated in heparinized lactated Ringer's solution is placed anterior to the uterus, beneath the adnexa to be worked on, and overlying the contralateral adnexa (Figure 21-6). This centers the adnexa of immediate interest in the surgical field and keeps the contralateral adnexa moist and out of danger.

With the aid of magnification, adhesions are divided by microscissors, microelectrode, or the appropriate laser. Atraumatic forceps, such as ring forceps, are used to secure the tube, and toothed forceps are used to place adhesions under tension (Figure 21-7). The dissecting rod is of inestimable help during this part of the dissection. The surgeon must avoid striking the Teflon-coated rod directly with the carbon dioxide laser, however, since it will damage the rod and release noxious fumes.

Adhesions that remain attached to the ovary are then folded over a dissecting rod and excised (Figure 21-8, *A*). Adhesions adherent to the ovary are coagulated with bipolar coagulation and stripped away with forceps (Figure 21-8, *B*).

Fimbrioplasty

Often the fimbriated end of the tube is altered after infection or pelvic surgery. One such alteration is a ring of scar tissue that has compressed the fimbriae, which are folded inward by the process. If the condition is severe, the tube may resemble a hydrosalpinx; however, during tubal lavage, dye drips from the end of the tube, in contrast to the complete obstruction of a hydrosalpinx.

The surgeon continues removing adhesions between the tube and ovary (Figure 21-9). Scar tissue is next excised from the distal end of the tube by microelectrode

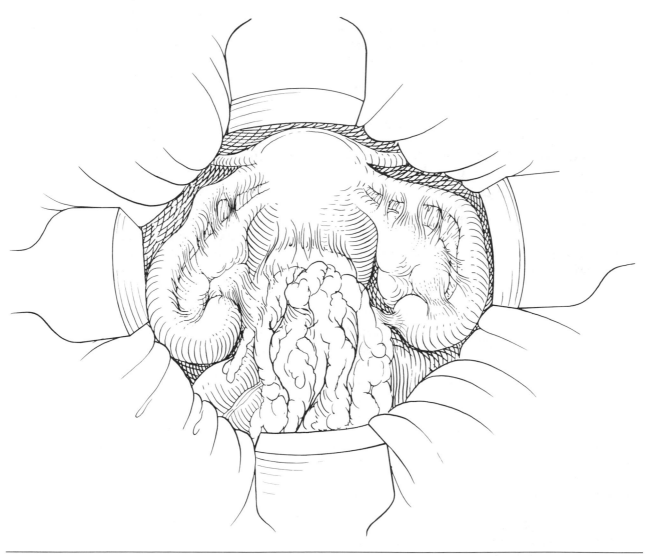

Figure 21-1
Pelvic structures after pelvic inflammatory disease.

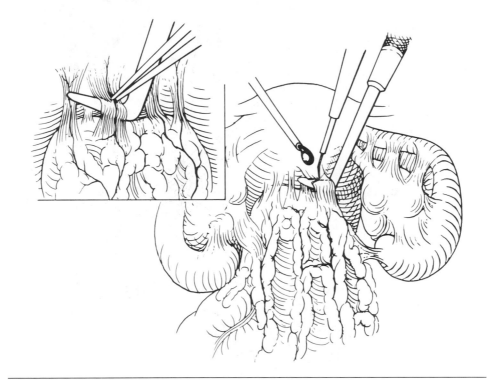

Figure 21-2
Adhesions between the omentum and uterus are divided. *(Inset)* Blood vessels are coagulated with long bipolar forceps.

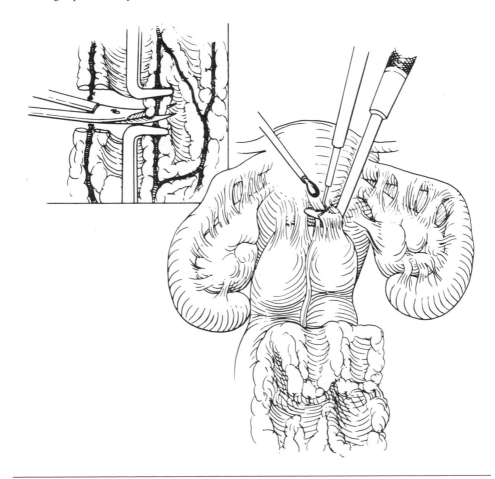

Figure 21-3
The omentum is folded back on itself and the rectosigmoid is released from the uterus. *(Inset)* A partial omentectomy is performed.

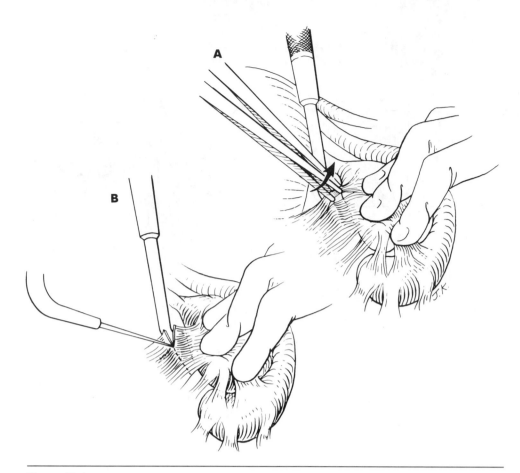

Figure 21-4
A, The adnexa is released from the lateral pelvic sidewall with bipolar forceps. **B,** Adhesions are lifted with a Teflon rod and divided with a needle electrode.

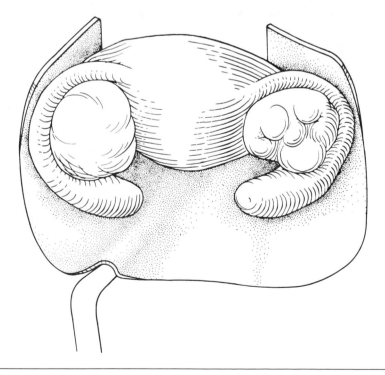

Figure 21-5
An unencumbered background is established with the silicone mat. Note the sump drain.

or microscissors (Figure 21-10). The fimbriated end is calibrated with Bakes dilators, beginning with a no. 3 and advancing to a no. 4 or 5. A careful search for mucosal bridges is made, and these are either teased apart or coagulated with bipolar forceps and sharply divided (Figure 21-11).

When tubal phimosis is encountered, the antimesenteric border is incised with the microelectrode, microscissors, or the appropriate laser (Figure 21-12). Care is taken to prevent damage to the mucosa. The length and direction of the incision is planned to provide an ample ostium, yet maintain excellent perfusion and proper geometry and produce minimal mucosal damage. Once the incision is made, the mucosal edges are everted to a slightly exaggerated degree and fixed with fine sutures (Figure 21-13).

Salpingostomy

One author (RBH) prefers the technique of salpingostomy developed by Kosasa and Hale,[17] who have achieved superb term pregnancy results with it. After the adhesiolysis is accomplished, the surgeon focuses on the distal end of the tube. This is frequently tightly adherent to the ovary and should be released with microelectrode, microscissors, or the appropriate laser (Figures 21-14 and 21-15). The distal end of the tube is stabilized with a Babcock forceps and distended with indigo carmine. The distal tube is incised with a microelectrode and the opening enlarged with a fine hemostat (Figures 21-16 and 21-17). Microscissors or laser may also be used. The edges created by the incision are grasped with fine hemostats and rotated outward, providing a marked mucosal eversion (Figure 21-18). If mucosal bridges are encountered, they should be divided. The mucosa is fixed to the serosa with 6-0 sutures (Figure 21-19). The eversion and suturing process is repeated until all mucosa has been everted (Figures 21-20 through 21-22). Figure 21-23 shows repair of tubal and ovarian defects. After completing the salpingostomy, it is desirable to inspect the interior of the tube with a tuboscope. This provides the surgeon with valuable prognostic information. A conventional technique of salpingostomy is shown in Plates 44 through 49.

In spite of laparoscopic screening, the surgeon sometimes encounters a thick-walled hydrosalpinx, requiring modification of the technique. The serosa and tubal muscularis are incised but not through the mucosa (Figure 21-24). The fibrotic and thickened ampullary serosa and musculature are excised distally (Figure 21-25). Approximately four incisions are made in the mucosa, and the flaps are sutured to the corresponding serosal sites (Figures 21-26 and 21-27).

An alternative technique is to excise the very distal end of this thickened tube (Figure 21-28). Approximately four incisions are made full thickness, and the edges are everted and fixed with fine sutures (Figure 21-29).

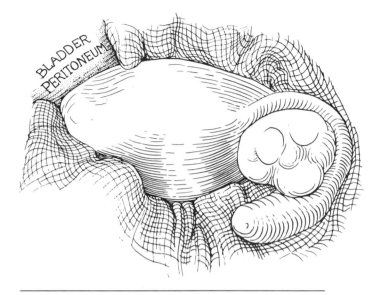

Figure 21-6
The right adnexa is elevated and the left adnexa covered.

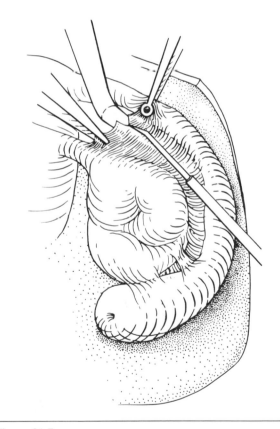

Figure 21-7
Ring and toothed forceps lift the adhesions, which are divided one layer at a time over a Teflon rod. This step and many of the succeeding ones can be performed with microscissors or the appropriate laser.

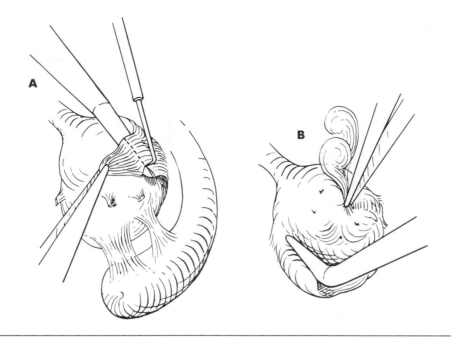

Figure 21-8
Ovarian adhesions are removed. **A,** They are folded over the Teflon rod and excised. **B,** The adhesions are coagulated with bipolar forceps and stripped away with ring forceps.

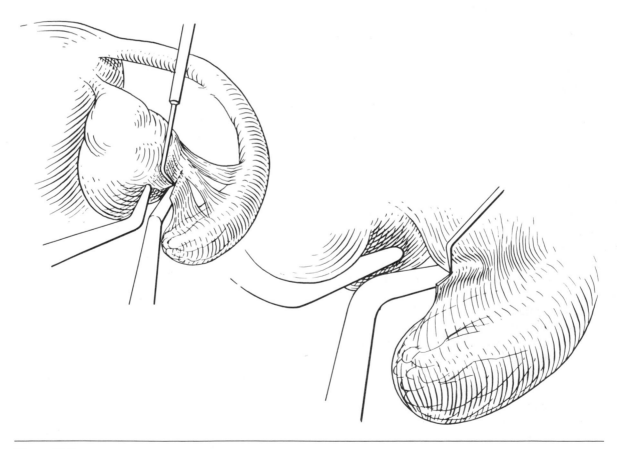

Figure 21-9
Adhesions between the fallopian tube and ovary are excised.

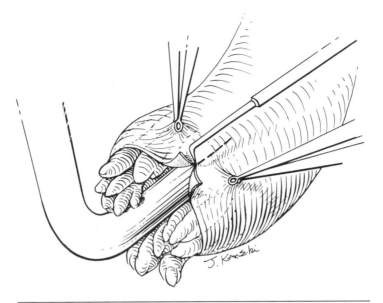

Figure 21-10
Fibrous tissue from the distal tube is excised.

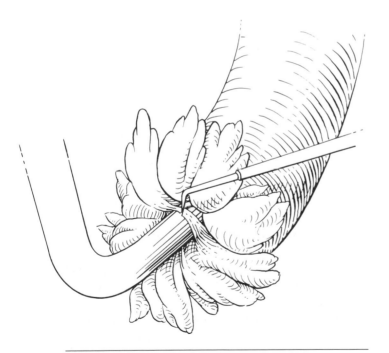

Figure 21-11
Mucosal bridges are coagulated and divided.

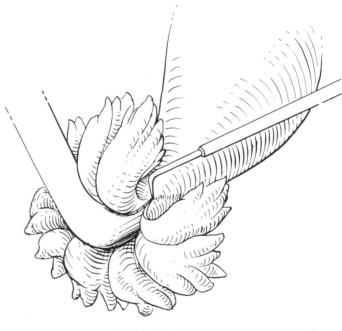

Figure 21-12
Tubal phimosis is corrected by incising the distal tube on the antimesenteric side.

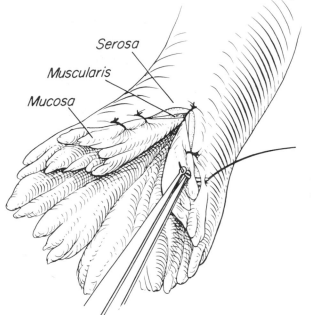

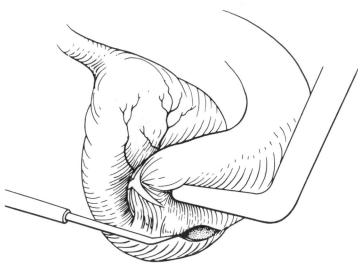

Figure 21-14
The distal tube is mobilized from the ovary by microscissors, microelectrode, or laser.

Figure 21-13
Approximation of mucosa to serosa with fine sutures completes the repair. Note the exaggerated eversion of the ampullary mucosa to prevent recurrent phimosis.

Peritoneal platforms

Once the adnexal surgery has been completed, the surgeon should consider ways to prevent the ovary from adhering to the pelvic sidewall and posterior broad ligament. One technique is to develop peritoneal platforms (Figure 21-30) using 2-0 or 3-0 synthetic absorbable sutures. The suture is begun approximately 5 mm below the inferior surface of and beneath the lateral one third of the ovary. It is placed through the peritoneum, piercing it with several shallow bites parallel to the inferior surface of the ovary. The suture is then placed in the uterine musculature approximately 1 cm inferior to the uterine insertion of the uterovarian ligament and tied. The resulting peritoneal platform rotates the ovary away from the pelvic sidewall and posterior broad ligament. The surgeon must locate the ureter and place the suture lateral to it. It is necessary to avoid piercing major blood vessels when placing the suture. This is accomplished by piercing the peritoneum superficially. If a uterine suspension is to be performed, the surgeon should factor this in when placing the peritoneal platform suture, thus avoiding undesirable tissue tension.

Uterine suspension

A uterus fixed in retroversion by adhesions may cause dyspareunia and possibly hamper ovum pick-up. In this situation the surgeon should consider suspending the uterus after adhesiolysis (Plates 50 through 52). The con-

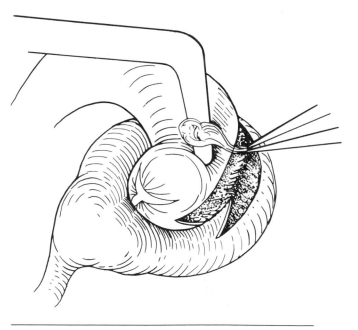

Figure 21-15
Hemostasis is achieved with bipolar coagulation.

cept of round ligament triplication is shown in Figure 21-31. The round ligament is considered to consist of three equal segments. The middle section is reversed and fixed at the respective uterine and internal ring insertions of the round ligament with permanent suture of 0 size. Care must be taken to avoid occluding the proximal tube

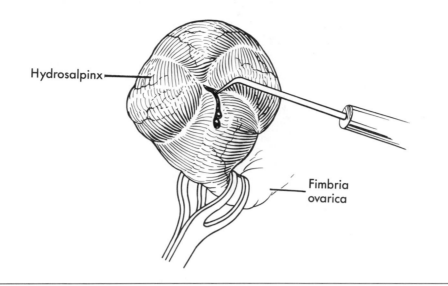

Figure 21-16
The fimbria ovarica is stabilized with a Babcock forceps, and the distal tube is opened with a microelectrode.

or piercing a major blood vessel in the vicinity of the internal ring. An additional suture of the same material is placed at the midpoint of the triplicated ligament to prevent the three round ligament bundles from separating. All sutures must be tied to approximate but not to overpower tissues and thus avoid postoperative adhesion formation at the ischemic sites. The surgeon may elect to plicate the uterosacral ligaments to antevert the uterus further. A completed procedure, including salpingostomy, peritoneal platforms, round ligament triplication, and uterosacral ligament plication, is pictured in Figure 21-32.

An alternative suspension is the ventral suspension (Figure 21-33). A synthetic absorbable suture of 0 material is placed as a horizontal mattress suture in the uterus at the top of the fundus. A free tapered needle is threaded on the end of the suture having no needle. Each end of the suture is then passed through its respective peritoneum, rectus muscle, and fascia. At the time of peritoneal closure, the suture is tied, bringing the uterus firmly against the inferior surface of the peritoneum. The suture should incorporate abundant uterine tissue to avoid its being pulled out, and care must be taken to avoid piercing the urinary bladder. This suspension may be used with a vertical or transverse fascial incision. Although it provides a direct and substantial suspension, this procedure may produce significant patient discomfort.

POSTOPERATIVE CARE

At the end of the procedure, one author (RBH) instills 1000 ml of warm lactated Ringer's solution intraperitoneally, providing hydroflotation. In addition, 20 mg dexamethasone and 25 mg promethazine are placed in-

Text cont'd on p. 370.

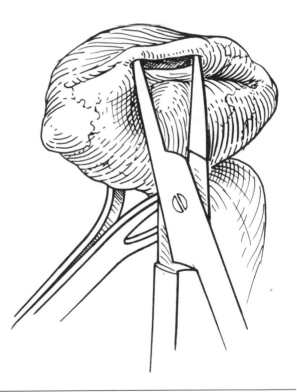

Figure 21-17
The tubal opening is enlarged with a fine hemostat.

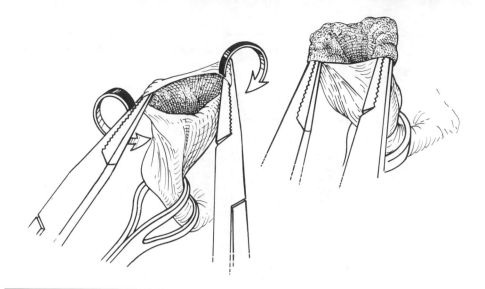

Figure 21-18
A, The mucosal flaps are grasped with fine hemostats and **B,** everted by rotation.

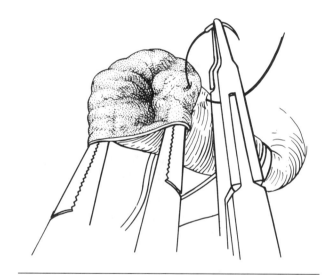

Figure 21-19
The mucosa is fixed to serosa by interrupted 6-0 sutures.

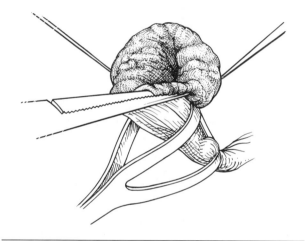

Figure 21-20
The inferior portion of the mucosal flap is grasped with a fine hemostat.

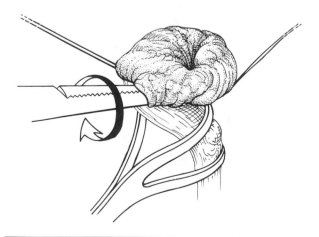

Figure 21-21
The mucosa is everted by rotation of the hemostat.

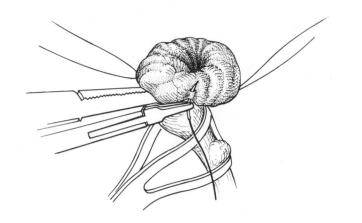

Figure 21-22
The process is continued until all mucosa is everted and fixed with sutures.

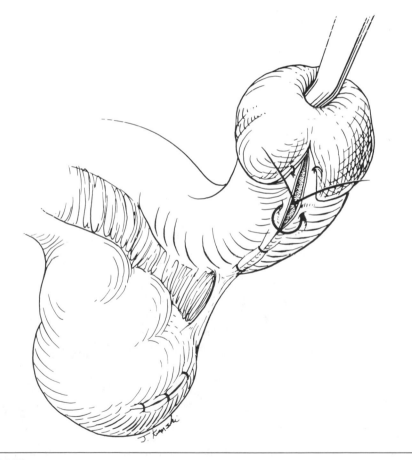

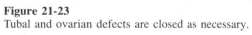

Figure 21-23
Tubal and ovarian defects are closed as necessary.

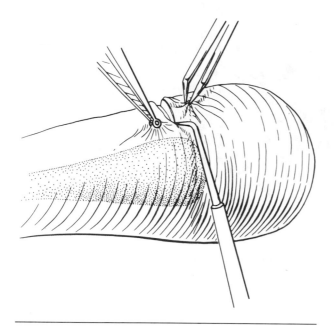

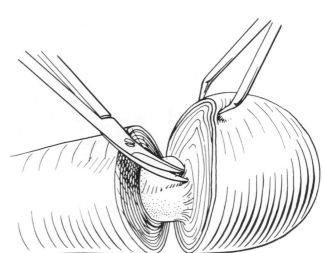

Figure 21-25
Seromuscular layers of the distal tube are excised. Modified from Verhoeven HC et al: Surgical treatment for distal tubal occlusion, *J Reprod Med* 28:293, 1983.

Figure 21-24
Tubal serosa and muscularis are incised in this thick-walled hydrosalpinx. Modified from Verhoeven HC et al: Surgical treatment for distal tubal occlusion, *J Reprod Med* 28:293, 1983.

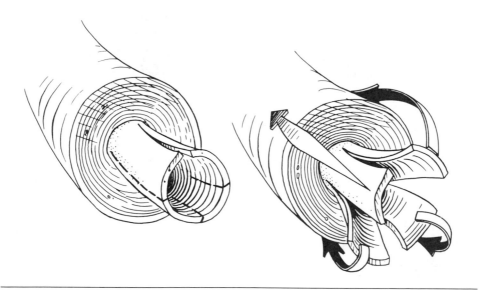

Figure 21-26
Four incisions are made in the mucosa of the tube. Modified from Verhoeven HC et al: Surgical treatment for distal tubal occlusion, *J Reprod Med* 28:293, 1983.

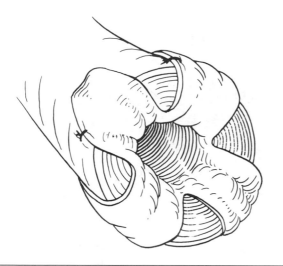

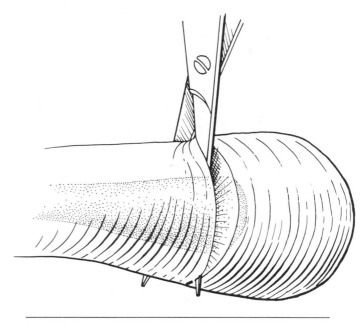

Figure 21-27
Mucosal flaps are sutured to the tubal serosa with fine sutures. Modified from Verhoeven HC et al: Surgical treatment for distal tubal occlusion, *J Reprod Med* 28:293, 1983.

Figure 21-28
The distal tube is excised in this thick-walled hydrosalpinx. Modified from Verhoeven HC et al: Surgical treatment for distal tubal occlusion, *J Reprod Med* 28:293, 1983.

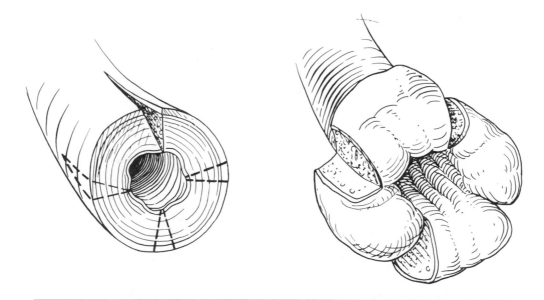

Figure 21-29
Four incisions are made through the full thickness of the tube and the flaps everted and sutured to tubal serosa with fine sutures. Modified from Verhoeven HC et al: Surgical treatment for distal tubal occlusion, *J Reprod Med* 28:293, 1983.

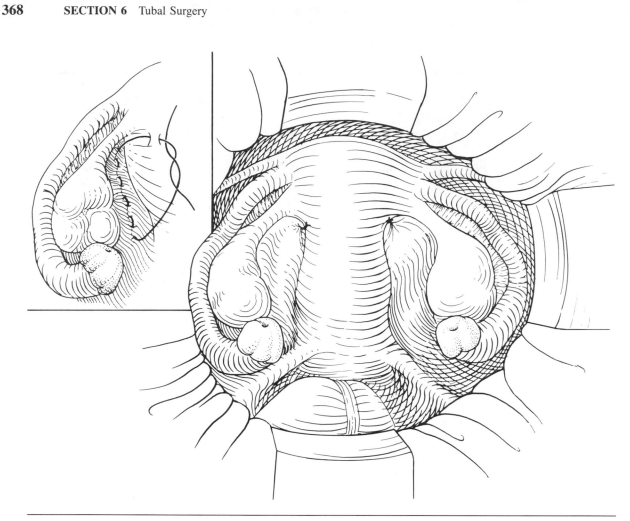

Figure 21-30
Peritoneal platforms are created to prevent the ovaries from adhering to pelvic sidewalls and
posterior broad ligaments.

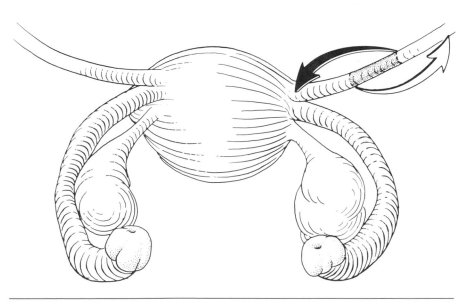

Figure 21-31
The concept of round ligament triplication.

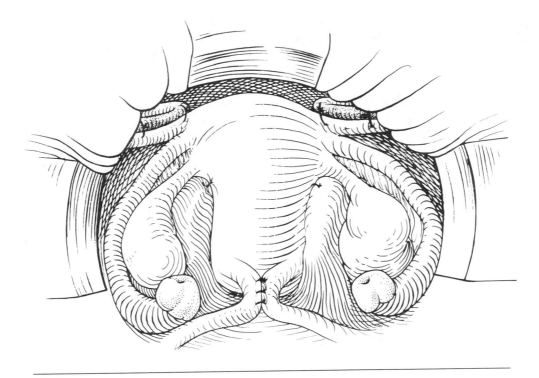

Figure 21-32
A completed procedure, including salpingostomy, peritoneal platforms, triplication of round ligaments, and plication of uterosacral ligaments. If the surgeon elects to perform a plication procedure, great care must be taken to avoid kinking the ureters.

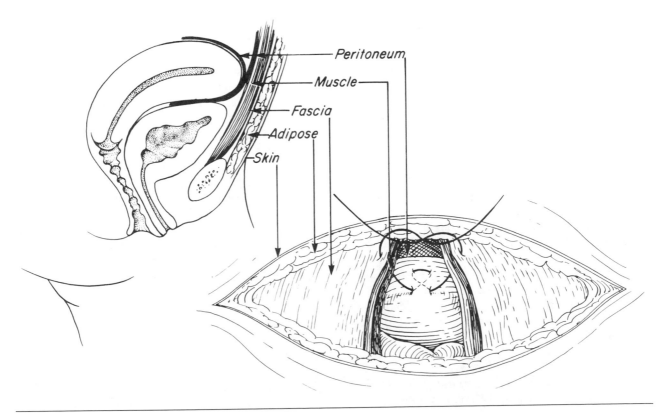

Figure 21-33
The concept of a ventral uterine suspension.

traperitoneally. Ten milligrams of dexamethasone and 12.5 mg promethazine are continued every 4 hours for 7 doses each. The first dose is administered intramuscularly and the remainder by mouth. Each patient receives a prophylactic antibiotic, beginning before surgery. The indwelling Foley catheter is removed on the first postoperative day, intravenous fluids are discontinued, diet is advanced as tolerated, and ambulation is initiated. Hospital discharge is usually on the third or fourth postoperative day. The patient returns for a postoperative visit at 4 weeks and returns to work 4 to 6 weeks after surgery.

PREGNANCY RESULTS

Generally it is difficult to compare results among centers. Reasons include the use of different definitions for salpingostomy and fimbrioplasty, exclusion of patients lost to follow-up, the performance of procedures by surgeons using a variety of techniques, and variations in the use of adjunctive agents. Some surgeons use life-table analysis in calculating outcomes, and others go by actual reproductive performance after surgery, often with inadequate periods of follow-up

It is apparent that we need to standardize definitions of these procedures, agree on guidelines for rating the degree of tubal damage, and establish policies for follow-up. The American Fertility Society has taken a step in this direction with publication of score sheets.

Our results are measured in terms of the number of live births, spontaneous abortions, and ectopic pregnancies. An abortion before or after a term pregnancy is noted. Two or more viable pregnancies in the same patient are reported as only one surgical success, and patients lost to follow-up are considered not pregnant.

That results of female infertility procedures have been poor in the past is highlighted by a survey published in 1937.[18] One hundred and seven surgeons performed 818 infertility procedures and reported a live birth rate of 4.4%. At that time 56% of the respondents were opposed to tubal implantation and salpingostomy procedures.

Prevention of pelvic infection would go far in diminishing the problem of distal tubal disease but seems to be an unlikely development. In the meantime we have learned much about the physiology of conception and the pathogenesis of adhesions; have available excellent antibiotics, superb suture materials, and magnification systems; and are continuing to develop better surgical procedures.

Adhesiolysis results

If tubal patency is unimpaired, and if the infundibulum and fimbriae are conserved, the prognosis after adhesiolysis is favorable. Indeed, if only the mobility of the infundibulum is altered, the procedure offers an excellent prognosis.

Dense adhesions are seldom an isolated finding. Often there is an associated thickness in the tubal wall with damage to tubal mucosa. These morphologic changes undoubtedly influence tubal function and worsen the prognosis.

For adhesiolysis, pregnancy rates vary widely. One author (HCV) found a viable pregnancy rate of 28.4% of 123 patients who had surgery at his clinic.[19] The Mayo Clinic reported a live birth rate of 40% after surgery in patients with prolonged infertility and adhesive disease significantly impairing tubo-ovarian relationships.[20]

Fimbrioplasty results

Partial agglutination and stenosis of the fimbriae probably result from a less severe injury than that producing a hydrosalpinx. It stands to reason that less severely damaged tubes will result in better outcomes.

One author (HCV) achieved a term pregnancy rate of 30% and an ectopic rate of 3.2% in 130 patients undergoing fimbrioplasty by laparotomy.[19] An intrauterine pregnancy rate of 60% and an ectopic pregnancy of 3% were reported in 35 patients.[21] Others reported term pregnancy rates with this procedure are 53% of 29 patients[20] and 60% of 132 patients.[22]

Salpingostomy results

Salpingostomy has a lower success rate than adhesiolysis and fimbrioplasty. The results obtained by microsurgery (including loupes) and surgical laparoscopy for correction of hydrosalpinges show no consistent pattern. Many believe careful surgery performed with any of these modalities will yield equivalent results, since the determinant factor is primarily the quality of the tubal mucosa.[23] Experience has shown the need for prolonged follow-up of these patients to determine accurate term and ectopic pregnancy rates; a minimum of 5 years is necessary.[24]

One author (HCV) noted that the outcome of 143 patients undergoing distal salpingostomy in his clinic were as follows: 19.6% term pregnancies, 4.2% abortions, and 2.1% ectopic pregnancies.[19] A collected series of 692 patients undergoing microsurgical salpingostomy in 7 centers revealed term pregnancy rates between 18% and 31% (median 24%) and ectopic pregnancy rates between 0% and 18% (median 10%).[24]

A collected series taken from 14 centers and including 1275 patients undergoing salpingostomy revealed a term pregnancy rate of 21% and an ectopic pregnancy rate of 8%.[25] Women with a favorable prognosis had a term pregnancy rate of 59%, compared with 4% in those with a poor prognosis. The ectopic pregnancy rate rose predictably in these groups from 4% to 16%, respectively. The authors concluded that patients with poor prognosis should be encouraged to have IVF instead of surgery, whereas surgery seemed most reasonable in those with either a favorable or intermediate prognosis. This recommendation was based on a collected series from 22 IVF centers reporting 7713 cycles in which ova were retrieved, resulting in an overall pregnancy rate of 12%.[25]

A term pregnancy rate of 29% was achieved in 71 patients undergoing salpingostomy.[20] It was 39% in those with moderate adhesions compared with 27% in those with severe adhesions. This is consistent with the finding of a direct correlation of the extent and types of adhesions with successful pregnancy outcome reported elsewhere.[26]

Initial enthusiasm for the use of prostheses has waned, which is in part due to the need for a second laparotomy to remove the device(s). The use of lasers has not shown a significant increase in term pregnancy rates over electrosurgery.[27] Postoperative hydrotubation greatly increased term pregnancy rates in one study.[28] Others found hydrotubation not to be helpful and most surgeons have abandoned it.[29]

Reversal of fimbriectomy for sterilization is thought by some to be inappropriate. However, using macrotechniques and 5-0 suture, one group achieved an intrauterine pregnancy rate of 57% (4 of 7 patients).[23] The same group reported only 15% intrauterine pregnancy rate (3 of 20 patients) in those undergoing salpingostomy to correct postinflammatory hydrosalpinges. Another report included 9 patients having had previous fimbriectomy for sterilization.[30] Three (33%) experienced term pregnancies after salpingostomy. The favorable preoperative findings in these patients were a tubal length of at least 8 cm, an ampullary width of more than 1 cm, mucosal patterns on HSG, and a paucity of peritubal adhesions.

Prognostic factors

The patients most favorable for repair have a small hydrosalpinx, healthy mucosa, thin tubal walls, and filmy adhesions. One group divided 83 patients with complete distal occlusion into three groups, 2, 3, and 4, based on degree of disease as determined by HSG.[22] Ampullary diameters were normal in degree 2, 15 to 25 mm in degree 3, and greater than 25 mm in degree 4 disease. Intrauterine pregnancy rates were 48%, 25% and 22%, respectively, with ectopic pregnancy rates 0%, 6%, and 12%, respectively. The percentages of ciliated cells also decreased progressively, averaging 55.2%, 43.2%, and 28.4%, respectively.

A similar observation was reported by Shirodkar,[31] who divided hydrosalpinges into two groups: those between the small finger and thumb in size (grade 1) and those larger than the thumb (grade 2). Patients with grade 1 hydrosalpinges with near normal mucosa experienced a 50% pregnancy rate, compared with a 10% to 20% in patients with grade 2 hydrosalpinges and poorly preserved mucosa. One author (HCV) had a 29% term pregnancy rate when tubes had a normal diameter, 17% when moderately dilated, and 4% when extremely dilated.[19]

Thick-walled hydrosalpinges seldom result in a successful pregnancy after corrective surgery,[19,22] with figures as low as 1 viable pregnancy in 43 patients.[19] One group developed a rating system that considered five factors in these patients: the nature and extent of adhesions, the appearance of mucosa, the thickness of the tubal wall, and the diameter of the hydrosalpinx. Based on this system, women with a favorable prognosis had an intrauterine pregnancy rate of 77%, intermediate prognosis 21%, and poor prognosis 3%. Those having a combination of many adhesions, thick adhesions, and a thick-walled hydrosalpinx had almost total lack of success after surgery.[32]

In a collected series of 135 patients undergoing repeat salpingostomy reported by 5 centers, term pregnancy rates varied from 8.4% to 33% (median 10%).[24]

Younger patients fare better than older ones. In women between 21 and 25 years of age, primary microsurgical salpingostomy yielded a successful pregnancy of 43.7%, compared with 15.1% to 22.2% in older patients.[19] The groups had similar degrees of tubal damage.

The prognosis was better in patients with distal tubal obstruction and primary infertility than in those with secondary infertility (19.8% vs 11.5%).[19] The rate of conception was essentially the same whether the hydrosalpinx involved one tube (and the other was missing or inoperable) or both. If the patient has proximal and distal tubal obstruction (bipolar block), the prognosis need not be grim (Plates 53 and 54). Surgical correction of this condition in 16 patients resulted in 3 having term pregnancies.[19] Of three patients undergoing correction of bipolar block by one author (RBH), two had successful pregnancies.

The most important prognostic factor is tubal morphology. Patients with healthy mucosa on HSG had a 40% term pregnancy rate; this fell to 10% when the mucosa was destroyed.[19] The results are consistent with research findings on tuboscopy and HSG assessment of ampullary mucosa and pregnancy outcome.[2-4]

Forty-two second-look laparoscopies and HSGs were performed after salpingostomy.[19] Seventy percent of patients had at least one tube open and a paucity of adhesions. The relative low term pregnancy rate implies persistent impairment of tubal function after anatomic corrections.

Follow-up laparoscopy

Some have enthusically supported the concept of lysis of newly formed adhesions soon after laparotomy for distal tubal disease. One group performed laparoscopy 8 days after major surgery.[33] Whereas there was no improvement in intrauterine pregnancy rates, the group undergoing early laparoscopy developed less than half the permanent postoperative adhesions as observed at subsequent laparoscopy. They had an unexplained but significant drop in the rate of subsequent ectopic pregnancies.

No improvement in pregnancy rates was reported among 36 patients undergoing second-look laparoscopy 1 year after salpingo-ovariolysis or salpingostomy by laparotomy, compared with 38 patients having the same procedures but not undergoing second-look laparoscopy.[34] The high frequency of ectopic pregnancies in this study was not decreased in women treated by second-look laparoscopy. The patients in the two groups were randomly assigned in this prospective study.

SUMMARY

Surgery remains an excellent option for management of most patients with distal tubal disease. We must not rest on our laurels, however; continued research and honest reporting of surgical results are essential. Seldom are corrective surgery and assisted reproductive technologies mutually exclusive but should be considered complementary. Appropriate patients should be encouraged to undergo surgery and to take advantage of ART. Surgeons must work closely with ART specialists if infertile couples are to have the best chance of reaching the ultimate success—a healthy baby.

REFERENCES

1. Henry-Suchet J et al: *Chlamydia trachomatis* associated with chronic inflammation in abdominal specimens from women selected for tuboplasty, *Fertil Steril* 36:599, 1981.
2. Young PE et al: Reconstructive surgery for infertility at the Boston Hospital for Women, *Am J Obstet Gynecol* 108:1092, 1970.
3. Ozaras H: The value of plastic operations on the fallopian tubes in the treatment of female infertility, *Acta Obstet Gynecol Scand* 47:489, 1968.
4. Henry-Suchet J et al: Prognostic value of tuboscopy vs hysterosalpingography before tuboplasty, *J Reprod Med* 29:609, 1984.
5. Brosens IA, and Vasquez G: Fimbrial microbiopsy, *J Reprod Med* 16:171, 1976.
6. Fayez JA: An assessment of the role of operative laparoscopy, *Fertil Steril* 39:476, 1983.
7. Mettler L, Giesel H, and Semm K: Treatment of female infertility due to tubal obstruction by operative laparoscopy, *Fertil Steril* 32:384, 1979.
8. Gomel V: Laparoscopic tubal surgery in infertility, *Obstet Gynecol* 26:47, 1975.
9. DeCherney AH: The leader of the band is tired, *Fertil Steril* 44:299, 1985.
10. Levine RL: Economic impact of pelviscopic surgery, *J Reprod Med* 30:655, 1985.
11. Winston RML: Is microsurgery necessary for salpingostomy? The evaluation of results, *Aust NZ Obstet Gynaecol* 21:143, 1981.
12. Fayez JA, and Suliman SO: Infertility surgery of the oviduct: comparison between macrosurgery and microsurgery, *Fertil Steril* 37:73, 1982.
13. Siegler AM, and Kontopoulos V: An analysis of macrosurgical and microsurgical techniques in the management of tuboperitoneal factor in infertility, *Fertil Steril* 32:377, 1979.
14. Pauerstein CJ: From Fallopius to fantasy, *Fertil Steril* 30:133, 1978.
15. Winston RML: Microsurgery of the fallopian tubes: from fantasy to reality, *Fertil Steril* 34:521, 1980.
16. Ellis H: Internal overhealing: the problem of intraperitoneal adhesions, *World J Surg* 4:303, 1980.
17. Kosasa TS, and Hale RW: Treatment of hydrosalpinx using a single incision eversion procedure, *Int J Fertil* 33:319, 1988.
18. Greenhill JP: Evaluation of salpingostomy and tubal implantation for treatment of sterility, *Am J Obstet Gynecol* 33:39, 1937.
19. Verhoeven HC et al: Surgical treatment for distal tube occlusion, *J Reprod Med* 28:293, 1983.
20. Williams TJ: Surgical procedures for infammatory tubal disease, *Obstet Gynecol Clin North Am* 14:1037, 1987.
21. Patton GW Jr: Pregnancy outcome following microsurgical fimbrioplasty, *Fertil Steril* 37:150, 1982.
22. Donnez J, and Casanas-Roux F: Prognostic factors of fimbrial microsurgery, *Fertil Steril* 46:200, 1986.
23. Betz G, Engel T, and Penney L: Tuboplasty—comparison of the methodology, *Fertil Steril* 34:534, 1980.
24. Bateman BG, Nunley WC Jr, and Kitchin JD III: Surgical management of distal tubal obstruction—are we making progress? *Fertil Steril* 48:523, 1987.
25. Marana R, and Quagliarello J: Distal tubal oclusion: microsurgery versus in vitro fertilization; a review, *Int J Fertil* 33:107, 1988.
26. Hulka JF: Adnexal adhesions: a prognostic staging and classification system based on a five-year survey of fertility surgery results at Chapel Hill, North Carolina, *Am J Obstet Gynecol* 144:141, 1982.
27. Mage G, and Bruhat MA: Pregnancy following salpingostomy: comparison between CO_2 laser and electrosurgery procedures, *Fertil Steril* 40:472, 1983.
28. Grant A: Infertility surgery of the oviduct, *Fertil Steril* 22:496, 1971.
29. Rock JA et al: The efficacy of postoperative hydrotubation: a randomized prospective multicenter clinical trial, *Fertil Steril* 42:373, 1984.
30. Novy MJ: Reversal of Kroener fimbriectomy sterilization, *Am J Obstet Gynecol* 137:198, 1980.
31. Shirodkar VN: Factors influencing the results of salpingostomy, *Int J Fertil* 2:361, 1966.
32. Boer-Meisel ME et al: Predicting the pregnancy outcome in patients treated for hydrosalpinx: a prospective study, *Fertil Steril* 45:23, 1986.
33. Trimbos-Kemper TCM, Trimbos JB, and van Hall EV: Adhesion formation after tubal surgery: results of the eight-day laparoscopy in 188 patients, *Fertil Steril* 43:395, 1985.
34. Tulandi T, Falcone T, and Kafka I: Second-look operative laparoscopy 1 year following reproductive surgery, *Fertil Steril* 52:421, 1989.

22

Microsurgical Management of Ectopic Pregnancy

STEPHEN M. COHEN

Ectopic pregnancy (eccyesis) is gestation occurring in an area other than the intrauterine cavity. A pregnancy may implant in the fallopian tube, cervix, and ovary or onto any structure in the abdomen. The majority of ectopic gestations are in the fallopian tube.

During the early part of the century, when blood banks were nonexistent, anesthetics primitive, and surgical techniques crude, it could be shown that salpingectomy decreased morbidity and mortality associated with this condition. Even though the surgical environment long ago progressed from those early years of difficulty, the therapy for ectopic pregnancy remained relatively at a status quo. A transition from extirpative macrosurgical therapy to conservative microsurgical surgery occurred, however, because of significant advances in both diagnostic techniques and surgical therapeutics.

CAUSES OF ECTOPIC PREGNANCY

The worldwide frequency of ectopic pregnancy has been steadily increasing.[1] In the United States the rate has climbed from 1 in 125 to 1 in 80 pregnancies. There are many reasons for this increase, the rising frequency of salpingitis probably being the single most important contributing factor. Gonococcal and nongonococcal infections of the fallopian tube severely damage the delicate mucosa and muscularis. Tubal peristalsis is compromised and ciliated motion disrupted. If complete tubal occlusion does not occur, ectopic gestation is likely to result.

Sterilization is now the most common method of birth control in the United States. The increased demand for permanent sterilization has played a dual role in ectopic pregnancy. It is estimated that 1% of women requesting tubal ligation will subsequently regret their decision and desire reversal. Eccyeses have been reported in up to 10% of patients who have had microsurgical reversal of

sterilization. Tubal ligation failures, occurring at a rate of 6 in 1000 procedures, add a small number of additional ectopic pregnancies to the total.

During the last 2 decades, more women have delayed childbearing into their later reproductive years. This delay results in increased frequency and severity of endometriosis. With its associated adhesion formation and tubal dysfunction, this condition creates an increased risk of ectopic pregnancy.

Even microsurgery itself has increased the prevalence. Pelvic conditions such as pathologic cornual occlusion, previously considered hopelessly uncorrectable, can now be repaired using microsurgical techniques or catheters. Patency of the fallopian tubes can be established in the majority of such cases; however, the tubes do not always function normally. Thus although fertilization can take place, progression of the embryo through the fallopian tube is hindered. Both the frequency and the absolute number of ectopic gestations are increased.

Popularity of the intrauterine device (IUD) in the 1970s has also contributed to the escalating ectopic rate. The IUD increases the risk of salpingitis fivefold to sevenfold; salpingitis, as discussed previously, is a significant risk factor.

Of course, previous ectopic pregnancies predispose to future ones. It has been shown that 25% of patients who conceive after having had one ectopic pregnancy will have another.

DIAGNOSIS

The early diagnosis of extrauterine pregnancy is critical if one is to manage this condition conservatively. If gestation is allowed to progress to the point of advanced tubal rupture, attempts at tubal salvage are most frustrating and unrewarding. The key to early diagnosis is a high index of suspicion on the part of the physician.

Clinicians must constantly be alert to this possibility when treating all females of reproductive age for pain or abnormal bleeding, and be especially aggressive in those with high risk factors, such as a history of salpingitis, endometriosis, IUD use, tubal surgery, infertility, and previous ectopic pregnancy.

The human chorionic gonadotropin (hch) β-subunit radioimmunoassay has made it possible to detect pregnancy within 1 week of conception in almost all circumstances. In the majority of instances, the patient with an early ectopic pregnancy is minimally symptomatic and in stable condition. This assay, which is readily available, becomes an excellent starting point on which to establish the differential diagnosis. In a patient with a condition that requires immediate abdominal surgery, however, this test is not only unnecessary, it is inappropriate.

Ultrasound is of great value in the minimally symptomatic patient with a slightly enlarged uterus and a positive hcg β-subunit test. If an intrauterine gestation is positively identified, the chance of a coexisting ectopic pregnancy is reduced to 1 in 40,000 cases. If the ultrasound examination is equivocal or does not show an intrauterine gestation, the gynecologist must then proceed as the clinical situation dictates. It has been shown that when ultrasound examination does not reveal an intrauterine gestational sac in a patient with a hcg value above 6500 mIU, the gestation is likely to be ectopic.[2,3] Each laboratory must establish values based on its own clinical experience if ultrasound is to be used to its fullest potential. Vaginal ultrasound using endovaginal probes can show intrauterine gestational sacs when values are in the range of 1500 to 2000 mIU.

It has also been shown that hcg values in the normal gestation will double approximately every 2 days. Laparoscopy should be performed in the asymptomatic patient who is at high risk for ectopic pregnancy and whose titers are above 100 mIU but not rising appropriately.

The most significant advance in early diagnosis of ectopic pregnancy is laparoscopy. It carries minimum risk and can even be performed under local anesthesia when necessary. With the addition of this procedure, there is no longer any reason for a patient with a suspected ectopic pregnancy to suffer a delay in diagnosis.

Even though sophisticated diagnostic tools became available in the early 1970s, surgical therapy for ectopic pregnancy remained relatively unchanged until the early 1980s. Advances in therapy, as often occurs, lagged behind improvements in diagnosis; in this case, they awaited new surgical techniques, instruments, and sutures. Although the initial impact of microsurgery in gynecology was an improved method of reversing tubal ligations, it soon became apparent that many other conditions hindering reproduction could be treated using these techniques. Excision of pelvic adhesions, repair of the fallopian tube that had become distally or proximally obstructed by infection, and eradication of endometriosis

are additional applications. It was only a matter of time before these same techniques were applied to the ectopic pregnancy. During this last decade, technologic advances have paralleled those of improved surgical skills. Improvements in instrumentation, sutures, magnification, and lighting have allowed the surgeon significantly to reduce surgical trauma and have made microsurgical procedures the first line of treatment of ectopic pregnancy.

The surgeon must develop a complete data base before performing microsurgery. Without this information, one is faced with the possible intraoperative dilemma of not knowing what course of action the patient would desire. The following information must be obtained from the patient before surgery.

1. Base history (age, gravidity, parity, number of living children)
2. Past medical history
   a. Significant medical problems
   b. Previous surgery
   c. Current medications
   d. Allergies
   e. Blood type and antibody history
   f. Previous transfusion and use of RhoGAM, or Rh(D) immune globulin
3. Contraceptive history
   a. Prior and current contraception use
   b. Plans regarding future pregnancies
   c. Desire for tubal ligation
   d. Wish to maintain an intrauterine pregnancy
   e. History of prior tubal ligation
   f. Wish to repair the ectopic tube (or the opposite tube) during this surgery
4. Gynecologic history
   a. Significant menstrual or pelvic abnormalities
   b. Pelvic surgery
   c. Salpingitis or endometriosis
   d. Infertility
   e. Previous surgery for infertility
   f. History of attempting to conceive
   g. Previous ectopic pregnancy and if so, when, which side, and procedure performed
5. Social history
   a. Objection to blood transfusions or blood products

This information is absolutely necessary if the gynecologist is to make the appropriate intraoperative decisions. If the patient wishes to retain her reproductive potential, the surgeon should attempt conservative surgery if it is not contraindicated by the clinical situation. Tubal ligation should usually be deferred in the patient who has not previously considered permanent sterilization. The emergency created by ectopic pregnancy is not the environment in which to make this most important decision. In the patient who has completed her family and now has become pregnant with an ectopic gestation, it may be most inappropriate to perform conservative surgery. Thus accurate knowledge of each patient's expectations can lead to the appropriate intraoperative judgments.

CHOICE OF PROCEDURE

The most important decision for the gynecologist to make is whether or not the patient with an ectopic pregnancy is physiologically stable enough to undergo the more lengthy conservative microsurgical procedure. If not, it is obvious that the procedure that can be done most expediently should be performed. In the majority of cases, the patient is stable, and the gynecologist can use microsurgical techniques to salvage the fallopian tube and improve her chance of future pregnancy.

There is no argument that when ectopic pregnancy occurs in the sole remaining fallopian tube, one must make all possible attempts to repair this tube. In vitro fertilization excepted, this oviduct may represent the patient's last bridge to fertility. A review of ectopic pregnancy in patients who had only one tube remaining found that conservative surgery resulted in an intrauterine pregnancy rate of 61%.[4] Seventeen percent of patients in this group had repeat ectopic pregnancies. In a similar review, intrauterine and ectopic pregnancy rates were 50% and 21.8%, respectively.[5]

The advantage of conservative microsurgical repair when the opposite tube appears normal is more difficult to demonstrate. Data are accumulating, however, that support the theory that improved pregnancy rates will result. One must remember that the normal-appearing opposite fallopian tube is often not normal, and abnormalities of tubal motility and the tubal muscularis and the presence of mucosal adhesions cannot be determined at the time of surgery. In patients who have had salpingectomy performed, future intrauterine pregnancies are reported at a rate of 30% to 50%.[6-15] Subsequent ectopic pregnancies were seen in 15% to 23% of patients.[7,16,17] The conservative approach has yielded improved intrauterine pregnancy rates of between 50% and 75% and ectopic rates of 9% to 15%.[6,18]

GENERAL SURGICAL GUIDELINES

It is imperative that the gynecologist carefully inspect the pelvis and abdomen for abnormalities at the time of surgery. Descriptions of adhesions and endometriosis and the status of all pelvic structures must be accurate and precisely recorded. All too often, surgical reports lack this information, which is critically important if the patient has difficulty with reproduction in the future. The gynecologist must also describe in great detail the exact surgical procedure performed, including when possible a subjective evaluation of this patient's future reproductive potential.

Microsurgery for ectopic pregnancy can be performed using the standard set of gynecologic instruments. This includes microscope or loupes, low-voltage bipolar or unipolar generators, fine unipolar needles, bipolar forceps, microscissors, microneedle holder, fine forceps, and a fine knife. The carbon dioxide (CO_2) laser, if available, has the added advantage of improving hemostasis during cutting. Nonreactive sutures should be selected, the most popular being nylon, polyglactin, and polyglycolic acid. Plain and chromic catgut sutures should not be used for tubal repair, since these materials are associated with increased inflammatory reaction. The surgeon should work with the smallest-diameter suture that can be handled competently.

An adequate abdominal incision is necessary if one is to manipulate the pelvic structures with minimal trauma. Lint-free sponges, sponges in plastic bags, or silicone pads should be used for positioning the fallopian tube. The tissue should be continually moistened with a heparinized physiologic irrigating solution. Hemostasis should be precise and tissue trauma minimized.

DISTAL AMPULLARY ECTOPIC PREGNANCY
Irrigation

The ampullary ectopic pregnancy may be loosely attached to the fimbriae and mucosa of the tube. On occasion, irrigation with heparinized lactated Ringer's solution will dislodge it. A minimal amount of tissue manipulation is required and an insignificant amount of bleeding is encountered. A special blunt irrigating needle is placed inside of the lumen of the tube and a pressurized stream of fluid is aimed behind the ectopic pregnancy (Figure 22-1). If the pregnancy is dislodged, the rest of the tube should be irrigated to remove blood and debris.

Milking

If implantation has taken place within the distal ampulla, gently squeezing the tube with the fingers may separate the pregnancy from the implantation site and dislodge the pregnancy. This procedure has been called milking the tube (Figure 22-2). It must be done with care, and the surgeon should not persist if it is unsuccessful after a few attempts. The fallopian tube is very vulnerable at this time, and excessive pressure may cause scarring, thus worsening the prognosis for a future intrauterine pregnancy. If milking is successful, the lumen should be irrigated with heparinized lactated Ringer's solution to remove blood and debris.

Linear salpingostomy

In most cases of ampullary ectopic pregnancy, linear salpingostomy with direct removal of the gestation will be necessary. This technique allows careful inspection of the implantation site and accurate hemostasis (Figure 22-3).

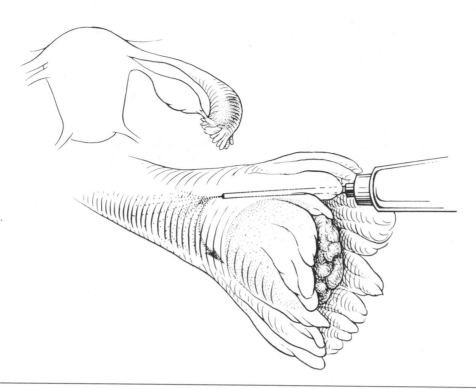

Figure 22-1
Irrigation technique for distal ampullary ectopic pregnancy.

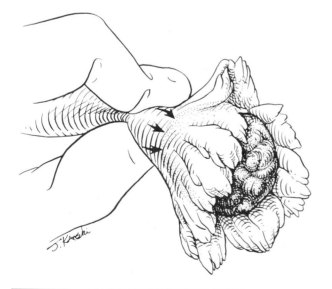

Figure 22-2
Milking technique for distal ampullary ectopic pregnancy.

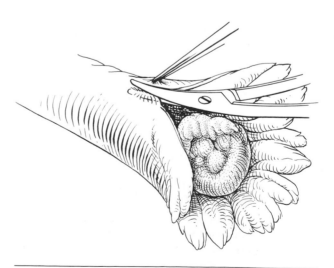

Figure 22-3
Linear salpingostomy for distal ampullary ectopic pregnancy.

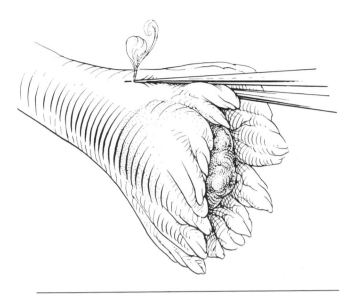

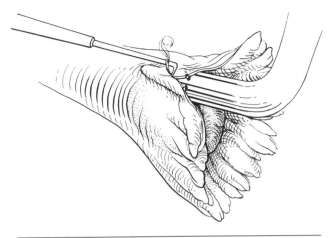

Figure 22-5
Incision is made with low-voltage unipolar coagulator. The tubal wall is attenuated over a dissecting rod to limit thermal damage.

Figure 22-4
Bipolar hemostasis is achieved before placing the incision.

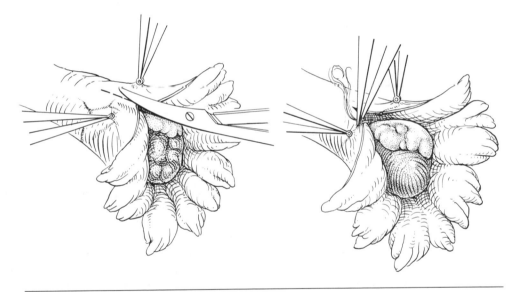

Figure 22-6
Hemostasis is achieved with bipolar coagulation after the incision is made.

The linear salpingostomy is placed along the antimesenteric border. Constant and gentle traction is maintained in a direction perpendicular to the tube to facilitate placement of this incision. Hemostasis must be achieved during the procedure. This can be done before placement of the incision, creating a line of coagulation with the bipolar forcep (Figure 22-4); while the incision is being made, using a fine unipolar needle (Figure 22-5) and blended low-voltage current; or after the incision is placed, using bipolar coagulation along its margin (Figure 22-6). The CO_2 laser is an excellent tool for placing

an incision during surgery for ectopic pregnancy (Figure 22-7). The tube can be opened precisely and hemostasis obtained simultaneously. The products of conception protect the tubal mucosa of the opposite side from laser damage.

After the tube is opened, the pregnancy should be carefully teased from the implantation site using forceps, irrigation, scissors, and unipolar needle when necessary (Figure 22-8). The implant bed itself is usually small, although edema and bleeding may mask this fact. Bipolar forceps are used to secure hemostasis in the implantation

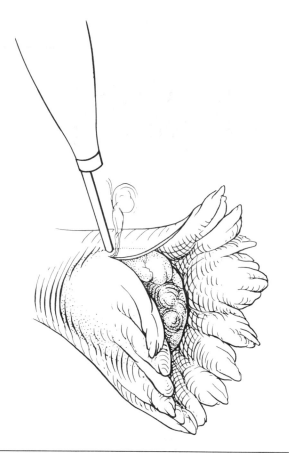

Figure 22-7
The incision is made with the carbon dioxide laser.

site. Magnification allows the surgeon to proceed with precision, accuracy, and minimal tissue destruction. A useful technique while obtaining hemostasis is to compress the vascular supply of the mesosalpinx with the fingers. Using this technique, one can wash the flow of blood away from the field and find the open vessels under direct vision (Figure 22-9). Many gynecologists inject diluted vasoconstrictors into the mesosalpinx under the site of the pregnancy before placing the incision, to help obtain hemostasis.

A linear salpingostomy incision in the distal ampullary section of the fallopian tube need not be closed, as closure may result in stenosis of the lumen and increase the chance of future ectopic pregnancies. The tube will repair itself within a month.

PROXIMAL AMPULLARY ECTOPIC PREGNANCY

Proximal ampullary ectopic pregnancy may be treated either by excising the tube and gestation together or by performing a salpingostomy and removing the gestation. Excision of the portion of the fallopian tube containing

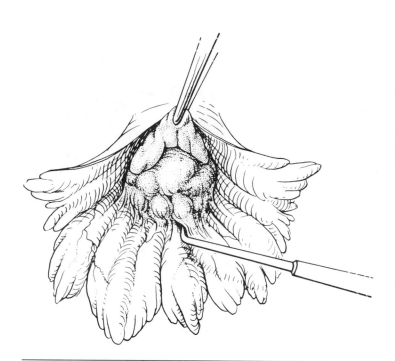

Figure 22-8
The pregnancy is separated from the site of implantation.

the ectopic pregnancy is a procedure that is easily mastered and quickly performed.

Excision

The tube is examined and the location of the ectopic pregnancy is determined. This task is not as easy as it may first appear, as hemorrhage into the tubal lumen and edema of the tubal wall can make it most difficult to locate the implantation site accurately. Often this area is much smaller and more proximal than it first appears.

Permanent nonreactive sutures (nylon, polypropylene) are placed at the proximal and distal ends of the portion of tube containing the gestation. The suture may be placed deep enough in the mesosalpinx to include the vessel arcade just below the tube itself. The surgeon should divide the portion of tube between the permanent sutures proximally and distally. These incisions may be placed using either a knife or CO_2 laser (Figure 22-10). The lumen of the distal and proximal portions should then be carefully examined to confirm that one is clear of the implantation site. Careful inspection after irrigation will usually allow an accurate determination. If the tube or lumen is not clear of the implantation site, more tube should be excised until normal mucosa is observed.

A path through the mesosalpinx is created using bipolar coagulation (Figure 22-11). This small portion of mesosalpinx is then excised using microscissors (Figure 22-12) or CO_2 laser. The tube, together with this portion of mesosalpinx, is then removed.

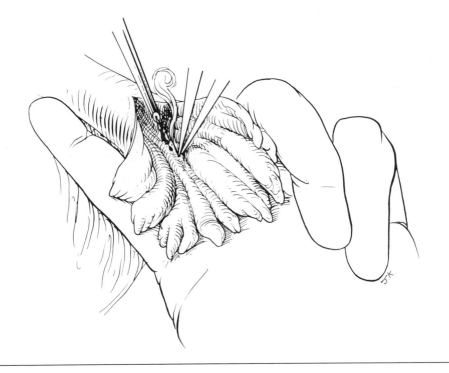

Figure 22-9
Hemostasis is obtained at the site of implantation.

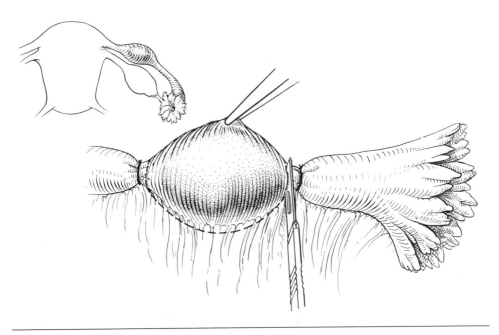

Figure 22-10
Excision technique for proximal ampullary ectopic pregnancy. Care is taken to limit damage to blood vessels in the mesosalpinx.

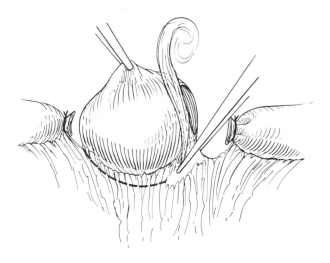

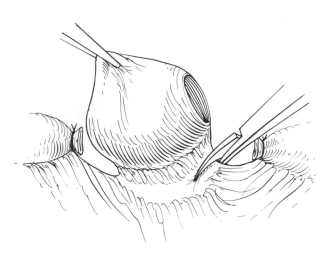

Figure 22-11
Hemostasis of the mesosalpinx is obtained with bipolar coagulation. Nutrient vessels are preserved insofar as practical.

Figure 22-12
The involved tubal segment is excised.

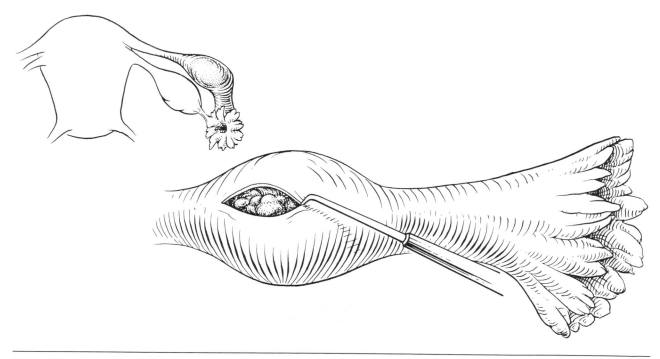

Figure 22-13
Linear salpingostomy is performed with microelectrode.

Under most circumstances, the fallopian tube will be left in this state to be anastomosed at a later time. If the anastomosis is to be performed during the same procedure, the surgeon should excise a portion of tube containing the ectopic pregnancy in exactly the manner described. Permanent sutures, however, would not be placed. Hemostasis is secured with either bipolar coagulator or unipolar needle. The anastomosis then proceeds as described in Chapter 20.

Linear salpingostomy

The fallopian tube is held firmly in place under tension and a linear incision is placed along the antimesenteric border. The incision should be placed directly over the midportion of the ectopic pregnancy and should stop short of the normal-appearing tube. It may be placed with a knife, microelectrode, or CO_2 laser (Figure 22-13). The products of conception should then be removed using forceps, irrigator, scissors, or knife as appropriate

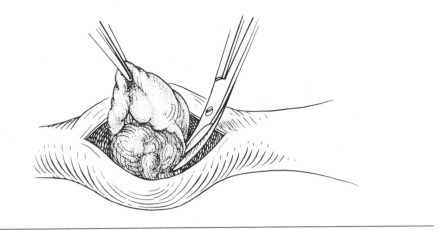

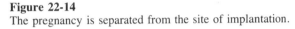

Figure 22-14
The pregnancy is separated from the site of implantation.

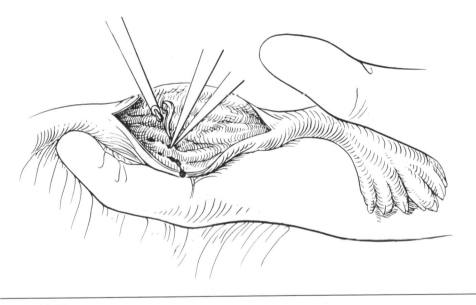

Figure 22-15
Hemostasis is obtained at the site of implantation.

(Figure 22-14). The lumen of the tube is then irrigated with heparinized lactated Ringer's solution. It is not necessary to remove all trophoblastic tissue; if removal will damage the tubal mucosa, the tissue is better left in situ. As with intrauterine trophoblastic tissue, these remnants will be removed by natural processes.

Hemostasis is then obtained along the border of the incision using bipolar electrocoagulation or fine-needle unipolar coagulation as necessary. Hemostasis is secured at the implantation site with bipolar electrocoagulation under constant irrigation (Figure 22-15). Again, manual compression of the vessels in the mesosalpinx with periodic release allows the surgeon better visualization of the bleeding points. It may become necessary to coagulate a portion of the vascular arcade below the fallopian tube. In most cases, collateral circulation to the tube will prevent necrosis and preserve structure and function. Vascular interruption is a preferred alternative to excessive

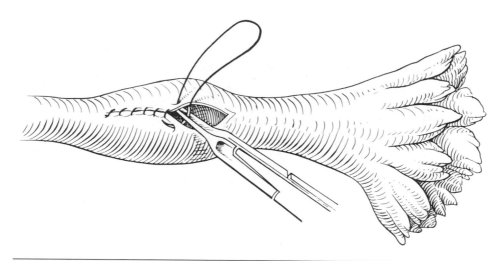

Figure 22-16
Closure of the salpingostomy incision.

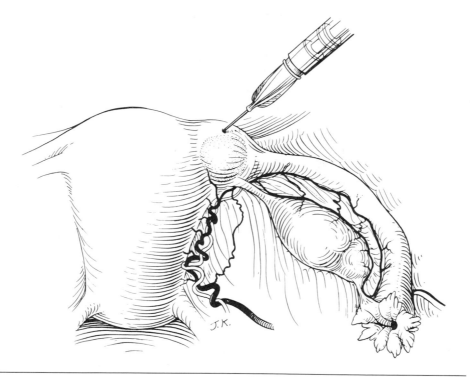

Figure 22-17
Dilute vasopressin is injected in the myometrium overlying an intramural (cornual) ectopic pregnancy.

intraluminal coagulation with damage to the tubal mucosa and muscularis. As with the distal ampullary ectopic pregnancy, vasoconstrictors may be injected before making the incision.

The linear salpingostomy is closed in the same direction that it was opened (Figure 22-16). In this area of tube, a single-layer closure including muscularis and serosa may be performed using fine nonreactive suture.

Present data suggest equally acceptable results with either absorbable or nonabsorbable sutures of polyglactin, polyglycolic acid, nylon, or polydioxanone.

ISTHMIC ECTOPIC PREGNANCY

Ectopic pregnancies occur much less frequently in the isthmus than in the ampulla. Those in the isthmus tend to rupture earlier because of the narrowness of the lumen.

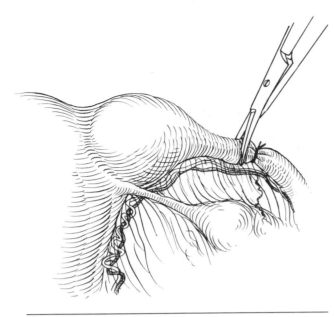

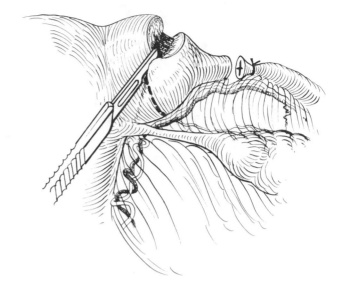

Figure 22-19
An incision is made in the myometrium over the cornual pregnancy.

Figure 22-18
The tube distal to the ectopic pregnancy is ligated and divided. Note the suture is placed to spare the underlying nutrient vessels if feasible.

As in the proximal ampullary ectopic pregnancy, salpingostomy and removal of the pregnancy or partial salpingectomy of the portion containing the pregnancy are both acceptable techniques. The gynecologist will find that in the majority of cases, excision is more practical than salpingostomy for several reasons. First, the lumen is relatively small, which greatly limits the exposure needed to remove the pregnancy successfully and obtain hemostasis. Second, often the isthmic area is in a state of advanced rupture better remediated by excision than repair. Third, although not yet convincingly documented, it appears that isthmic pregnancies are not as easily separated from the tubal mucosa as those that implant in the ampullary area. There are, however, a few occasions in which salpingostomy is appropriate and easily performed. Tubal condition and surgical experience dictate the surgical choice. These procedures have been described and illustrated in the previous section on proximal ampullary ectopic pregnancy.

INTRAMURAL (CORNUAL) ECTOPIC PREGNANCY

Intramural ectopic pregnancies are the most difficult to treat conservatively (Plates 55 and 56). The majority are found in the ruptured state. Major bleeding is usually encountered in this extremely vascularized area.

A vasoconstrictor is injected into the cornu to reduce blood flow (Figure 22-17). The extramural portion of the tube may be separated using a knife or CO_2 laser (Figure 22-18). Hemostasis in the proximal portion of

the distal tube is secured with bipolar coagulation. Manual compression with periodic release allows one to locate the bleeding vessel more easily.

Excision of the cornual section of the uterus is done in a stepwise fashion until normal tubal lumen is visualized (Figures 22-19 through 22-21). Polyglactin or polyglycolic acid sutures of 6-0 are placed transversely across the cornual area to achieve hemostasis (Figure 22-22). The damage created by the ectopic pregnancy and repair will usually require a tubal implantation to be performed later if it becomes necessary to restore the patency of this tube.

CONTROVERSIAL AND UNRESOLVED ISSUES REGARDING MICROSURGICAL REPAIR OF THE ECTOPIC PREGNANCY

In the case of a distal ectopic pregnancy, should the tube be milked or should linear salpingostomy be performed?

The tubal mucosa is fragile and can be easily damaged during any surgical procedure. The fallopian tube then heals with scarring, which will hinder normal function. Both milking the tube and cutting the tubal wall create trauma with subsequent scarring and transmucosal adhesions. Both methods seem appropriate in certain circumstances, but no data exist comparing them.

In a proximal ampullary ectopic pregnancy, should one remove the tubal segment or just the ectopic pregnancy?

A major unresolved issue is whether the gynecologist should remove or preserve the tubal segment that surrounds the ectopic pregnancy when it occurs in the proximal ampullary section. Linear salpingostomy and removal of the products of concep-

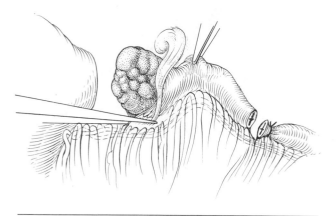

Figure 22-20
The mesosalpinx is coagulated with bipolar coagulation just beneath the involved tubal segment.

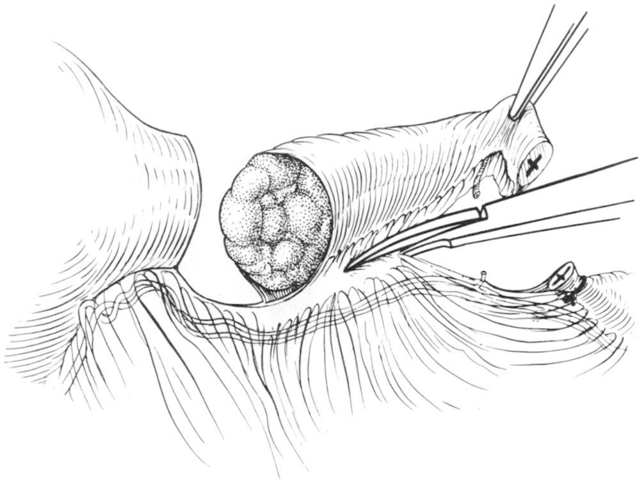

Figure 22-21
The involved tubal segment is excised.

tion create minimal tubal damage, preserve tubal length and function, and eliminate the need for another procedure. The area of damaged tube is left in situ, however, possibly increasing the risk for a subsequent ectopic pregnancy.

The alternative surgical procedure is removal of the portion of tube together with the ectopic gestation. The potential advantage of this procedure is that if the ectopic pregnancy was created by localized tubal pathology, that segment would now be removed, lessening the chance of a future eccyesis. The disadvantage of segmental removal is the necessity to extend surgery time when performing an immediate anastomosis or the necessity to perform a second surgery at a later date. There are no studies to compare these procedures; at the present time we do not know which will result in better patency rates or the greatest number of intrauterine pregnancies.

When performing a linear salpingostomy, should it be left open, be closed transversely, or be closed longitudinally?

All three methods of repair have been reported by various investigators, but no studies are available documenting any advantage of one over the others. A tube left open requires no sutures, and thus the chance of peritubal adhesions probably is decreased (Figure 22-23). The accuracy of healing has not been demonstrated, however, and follow-up patency rates have not been determined. Transverse closure of longitudinal incision produces a larger lumen, thus decreasing the risk of stenosis (Figure 22-24). Disruption of tubal peristalsis is a potential complication in the realignment of the tubal muscularis. Longitudinal closure of a long incision line tends to produce a more accurate approximation, but the potential of tubal stenosis and increased risk of future ectopic pregnancies are of concern (Figure 22-25).

Which suture material should be used for tubal repair of the ectopic pregnancy?

It is not clear which suture material is preferred for tubal surgery. The data extrapolated from general microsurgical research indicate that both permanent and synthetic absorbable sutures create minimal amounts of tissue reaction and inflammation. Catgut sutures and permanent braided sutures should be avoided if possible, as it has been demonstrated that they lead to an increased inflammatory reaction, as well as an increased amount of adhesion formation. Nylon, polypropylene, polyglycolic acid, polyglactin, and polydioxanone seem to be equally acceptable at the present time.

After excision of a tubal segment (isthmic or proximal ampullary), should the anastomosis be performed immediately or delayed for a second procedure?

Both alternatives of surgical repair are acceptable and have been reported in the literature. Obviously, if rupture has occurred and the patient is not in a stable condition, no decision is necessary. In the physically stable patient, the decision is based on whether or not the operating room equipment is available and the crew is prepared to do an unhurried anastomosis. Often, many operating rooms cannot supply optimum conditions when a patient with an ectopic pregnancy arrives at 3 a.m. Under these circumstances, the gynecologist should defer immediate anastomosis. Currently, there are no data comparing immediate anastomosis with a delayed second surgical procedure, and the timing of the repair must be left to the discretion of the surgeon. Further studies are necessary comparing patency and pregnancy rates of immediate versus delayed anastomosis.

LAPAROSCOPIC TREATMENT OF ECTOPIC PREGNANCY

Since the last edition of this book, ectopic pregnancy has been managed conservatively by ambulatory day surgery. The laparoscopic approach is being attempted by gynecologists who have treated other diseases (e.g., endometriosis, obstructed tubes, appendicitis) by endoscopy. One survey reported that 7% of ectopic pregnancies treated by members of the American Association of Gynecologic Laparoscopists were managed by laparoscopy.[19] Early studies reveal similar results to those of open microsurgery. The technique is also similar, except

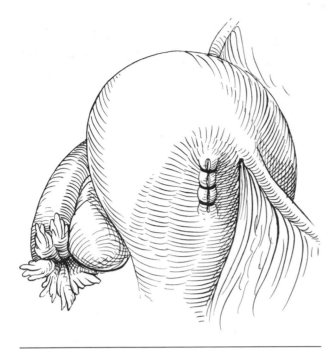

Figure 22-22
The cornu is repaired.

it is performed 30 cm farther away. The laparoscopic approach has yielded intrauterine pregnancy rates of 48% to 64% and ectopic pregnancy rates of 16% to 22%.[20,21]

CONCLUSION

It is time to fine-tune our surgical approaches to ectopic pregnancies. The last decade taught us what procedures to perform; during this decade we need to determine how best to perform them. Controlled scientific studies are necessary to help us decide the surgical procedures, their timing, and the materials to use when performing them.

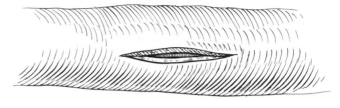

Figure 22-23
Linear salpingostomy: no closure.

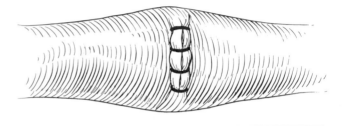

Figure 22-24
Linear salpingostomy: transverse closure.

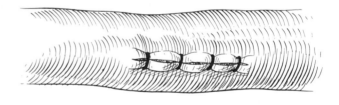

Figure 22-25
Linear salpingostomy: longitudinal closure.

REFERENCES

1. Centers for Disease Control: *Ectopic pregnancy surveillance, 1980-1978,* Atlanta, 1982, U.S. Department of Health and Human Services.
2. Kadar N, DeVore G, and Romero R: Discriminatory hCG zone: its use in the sonographic evaluation for ectopic pregnancy, *Obstet Gynecol* 58:156-161, 1981.
3. Kadar N, Caldwell BV, and Romero R: A method of screening for ectopic pregnancy and its indications, *Obstet Gynecol* 58:162-166, 1981.
4. DeCherney AH, Maheaux R, and Naftolin F: Salpingostomy for ectopic pregnancy in the sole patent oviduct: reproductive outcome, *Fertil Steril* 37:619-622, 1982.
5. Tulandi T: Reproductive performance of women after two tubal ectopic pregnancies, *Fertil Steril* 50:164-166, 1988.
6. Haney AF: Diagnosis and management of ectopic pregnancy. In *Reproductive physiology, endocrinology and infertility,* Braintree, Mass, 1982, Serono Symposia.
7. Bryson SCP: Beta-subunit of human chorionic gonadotropin, ultrasound, and ectopic pregnancy: a prospective study, *Am J Obstet Gynecol* 146:163-165, 1983.
8. Kitchin JD et al: Ectopic pregnancy: current clinical trends, *Am J Obstet Gynecol* 134:870-876, 1979.
9. Kucera E et al: Fertility after operations of extrauterine pregnancy, *Int J Fertil* 14:127-129, 1969.
10. Jarvinen PA and Kinnuen O: The treatment of extrauterine pregnancy and subsequent fertility, *Int J Fertil* 2:131-140, 1957.
11. Schenker JG, Eyal F, and Polishuk WZ: Fertility after tubal pregnancy, *Surg Gynecol Obstet* 135:74-76, 1972.
12. Kallenberger DA, Ronk DA, and Jimerson GK: Ectopic pregnancy: a 15-year review of 160 cases, *South Med J* 71:758-763, 1978.
13. Abrams J and Farell D: Salpingectomy and salpingoplasty for tubal pregnancy: survey of the literature, *Obstet Gynecol* 24:281-285, 1964.
14. Bender S: Fertility after tubal pregnancy, *J Obstet Gynaecol Br Emp* 63:400-403, 1956.
15. Timonen S and Nieminen U: Tubal pregnancy, choice of operative method of treatment, *Acta Obstet Gynecol Scand* 46:327, 1967.
16. Siegler AM: Conservative surgery for tubal pregnancy. In *Microsurgery for the Gynecologist.* Washington, D.C., 1983, American College of Obstetrics and Gynecology.

17. Bronson RA: Tubal pregnancy and infertility, *Fertil Steril* 28:221-228, 1977.

18. DeCherney AH, Romero R, and Naftolin F: Surgical management of unruptured ectopic pregnancy, *Fertil Steril* 35:21-24, 1981.

19. Hulka JF et al: American Association of Gynecologic Laparoscopists' 1985 membership survey, *J Reprod Med* 32:732-735, 1987.

20. DeCherney AH and Diamond MP: Laparoscopic salpingostomy for ectopic pregnancy, *Obstet Gynecol* 70:948-950, 1987.

21. Pouly JL et al: Conservative laparoscopic treatment of 321 ectopic pregnancies, *Fertil Steril* 46:1093-1097, 1986.

OVARIAN SURGERY

23

Surgery of the Ovary, Including Anatomic Derangements of the Fimbrial-Gonadal Ovum-Capture Mechanism

....

BRIAN M. COHEN

SURGICAL ANATOMY

The vascular anatomy of the distal oviduct and ovary is illustrated in Figure 23-1. Note the major artery to the uterine cornu, the subtubal branch of the uterine artery, and the anastomoses of the ovarian artery with branches of the tubal artery at the base of the ovary. One of these branches runs alongside the fimbria ovarica at the distal end of the oviduct.

Two principles of microsurgery must be emphasized:
1. As many of these blood vessels as possible must be preserved to avoid ischemia with subsequent poor tissue healing.
2. Knowledge of the anatomic location of these vessels allows the surgeon to operate in a bloodless manner. This facilitates the first objective and at the same time the reduction in fibrin deposition lowers the frequency of postoperative pelvic adhesions.

Figure 23-2 illustrates the two vascular regions that present problems when performing surgery on the ovary. Multiple fine vessels and capillaries are present in the cortical zone of the ovary just beneath its surface. These are transected with minimal blood loss using a micro-electrode or laser.

Within the cortex, the most significant hemostasis problems are posed by the vessels arising from the hilum that traverse ovarian tissue. These are often difficult to define, since they may be retracted by adjacent stroma. Those that are easily seen may be grasped and coagulated with a bipolar electrode. The others are occluded by using sutures that compress the lateral stroma and thereby secondarily result in pressure occlusion of these blood vessels.

Uterine retroversion may be associated with laxity of round ligaments and ovarian ligaments, and functional elongation of the fimbria ovarica (Figure 23-3). Forward mobilization of the uterus often results in traction of the infundibulopelvic ligament, which causes upward displacement of the distal ampulla and fimbriae. In many cases this is associated with relocation of the tubal ostium alongside the surface of the ovary, even in the face of elongation of the fimbria ovarica. Where such mobilization of the tubal ostium is not achieved by this single measure, it is treated surgically by plication of the fimbria ovarica as described later.

The surgeon must understand that simple plication of the round ligaments with anterior displacement of the uterus may itself result in elevation of the fimbrial ostium onto the gonadal surface, so that the subsequent surgical procedures may not always be necessary.

Figure 23-4, A illustrates the mobility of the fimbrial ostium when in close relationship to a normal-sized ovary. Under these circumstances the patulous fimbrial ostium may have cilial surface contact with half of the ovarian surface. When there is ovarian enlargement, as occurs with chronic cysts or enlarged polycystic ovaries, the fimbrial ostium has close proximity to only a small amount of the ovarian surface (Figure 23-4, B). The net result is a significantly reduced likelihood that there will be ovum pick-up in a single ovulatory cycle. Ovum pick-up may occur from the limited area of ovary close to the fimbrial ostium or occasionally from the pelvic cul-de-sac, but this is less efficacious than direct pick-up from the ovarian surface.

Text cont'd on p. 393.

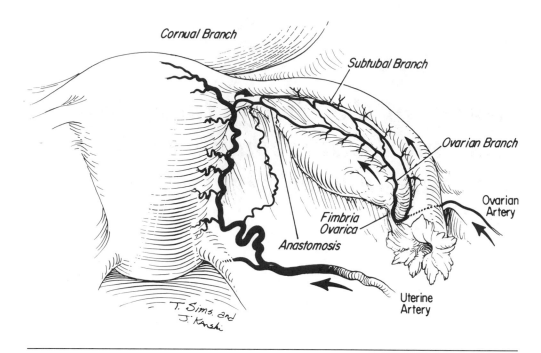

Figure 23-1
Vascular anatomy of the oviduct and ovary. Note cornual branch, subtubal vessels, and artery beside the fimbria ovarica.

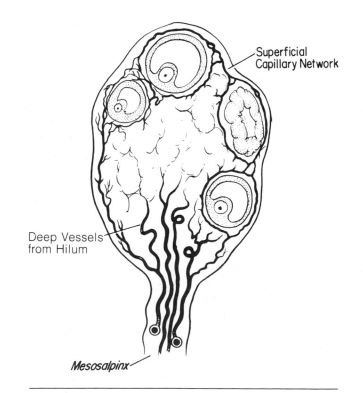

Figure 23-2
Vascular anatomy of the ovary pertinent to ovarian resection and reconstruction.

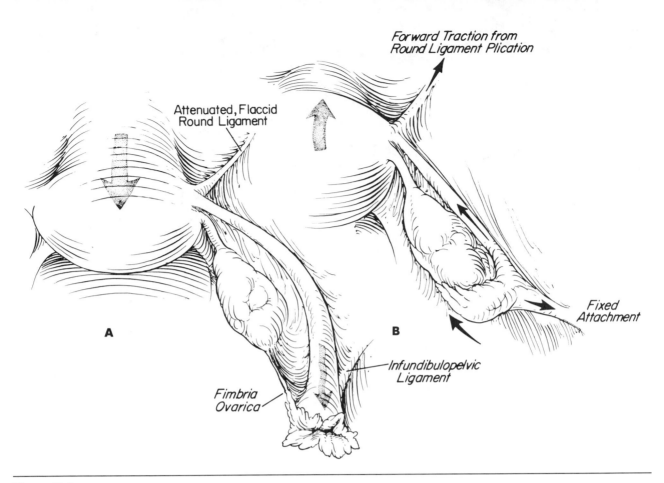

Figure 23-3
The effect of uterine retroversion (related to laxity of pelvic ligaments) on spatial relationship between the ovary and the fimbrial ostium of the oviduct. **A,** Proptosis of the fimbriae away from the ovarian surface. **B,** Anteversion causes traction on infundibulopelvic ligament with elevation of fimbriae over the ovarian surface.

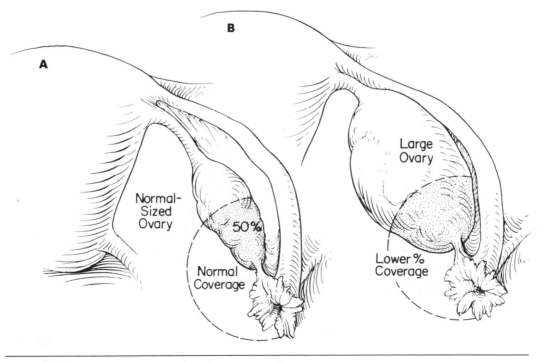

Figure 23-4
Relationship between the tubal ostium and ovarian surface affected by gonadal enlargement.
A, Normal-size ovary and **B,** large ovary.

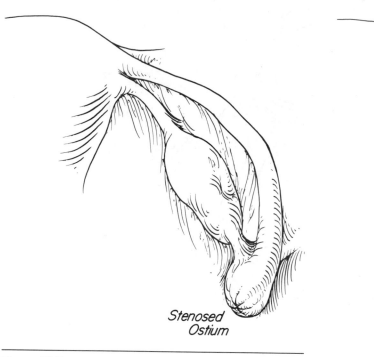

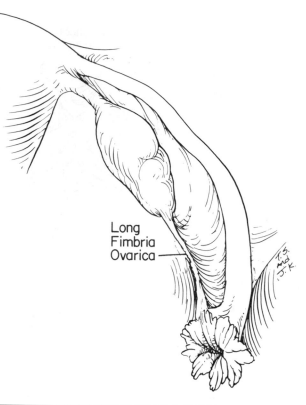

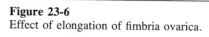

Figure 23-5
Stenosed tubal ostium reduces the likelihood of ovum pick-up.

Figure 23-6
Effect of elongation of fimbria ovarica.

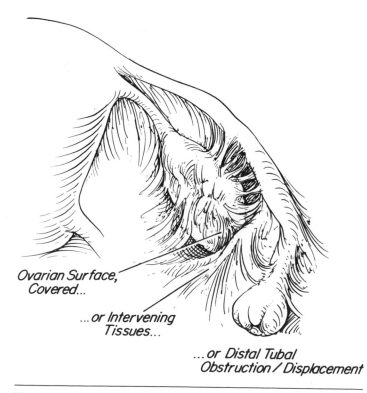

Figure 23-7
Major causes of damage to fimbrial ovum pick-up mechanism.

A truly stenosed tubal ostium is not capable of being widely exposed to a large surface of the ovary (Figure 23-5). Surgical relief of this stenosis with the resultant large widened ostium should provide a more efficient ovum-capture mechanism. Figure 23-6 illustrates the effect of significant elongation of fimbria ovarica (>4 cm). This implies loss of surface contact between the ovary and the tubal ostium. Here, the most likely site of ovum pick-up is from the pelvic cul-de-sac.

The major causes of breakdown in the fimbrial ovum-pick-up mechanism are related to anatomic separation of the ovary and the tubal ostium (Figure 23-7). This may be the result of adhesion formation over the ovarian surface, scar tissue traction, or displacement of the ovary or tubal ostium away from each other, and closure of the oviduct, both complete and incomplete, together with fixity of the tubal ostium away from the ovarian surface.

MICROSURGICAL PROCEDURES

Cysts of the paroophoron may displace the tubal ostium from the ovarian surface (Figure 23-8, *A*; Plates 57 and 58). When less than 1 cm in diameter these are easy to remove, but they may be 2 to 3 cm in diameter, in which case an absolutely meticulous microsurgical approach is mandatory. One must prevent intraoperative bleeding, excessive coagulation, and destruction of the artery to the distal fimbriae with consequent tubo-ovarian distortion resulting from adhesion formation.

There are usually vessels on either side of the mesosalpinx running longitudinally from the undersurface of the tube to the base of the ovary. Branches from these blood vessels often enter the walls of the cysts. The mesosalpinx is opened on its anterior aspect to preserve the broad ligament in direct continuity with the ovarian surface when possible. Using a microelectrode, an incision is made between two blood vessels, transecting only one of the peritoneal surfaces of the broad ligament (Figure 23-8, *B*). Once this is divided, the cyst is defined and delivered from this small opening in the mesosalpinx by gentle traction. As the cyst is elevated, any vessels that supply its sidewall are coagulated with the bipolar electrode, which facilitates removal of the paratubal cyst hemostatically (Figure 23-8, *C*). The opening of the mesosalpinx is now sutured using 8-0 absorbable nonreactive suture material (polyglycolic acid, polyglactin, or polydioxanone on a taper-point needle) (Figure 23-8, *D*).

If the tubal ostium is greater than 4 cm away from the ovary, this displacement is corrected by plicating the fimbria ovarica using a nonabsorbable, nonreactive 7-0 suture (polypropylene) on a taper-point needle.

Infrequently, careful examination of the tubal ostium may reveal that in addition to the primary ostium and its folds, there are accessory redundant fimbrial folds bearing no relationship to those that are directed to the tubal os-

tium (Figure 23-9). Staining these fimbriae (methylene blue or indigo carmine) and observing them under the surgical microscope confirm that their folds end in culde-sacs and that they are redundant and accessory.

Fimbrial folds that are clearly unrelated to the tubal ostium are excised, particularly where they are approximately 1.5 to 2 cm in width and 2 to 3 cm in length, and that displace the tubal ostium well away from the ovarian surface with no primary folds appearing to run from the ovarian surface to the tubal ostium (Figure 23-10; Plates 59 and 60).

At removal, hemostasis is effected by elevating them and repeatedly turning the tissue to be removed from side to side, thereby ensuring that each blood vessel on both inner and outer surfaces is defined and coagulated with the bipolar microelectrode. Once bipolar coagulation of well-defined vessels has been completed, the tissue is excised using a microelectrode or sharply focused laser under the surgical microscope.

When removal of the accessory fimbrial folds has been completed, the primary fimbrial folds are defined. If the tubal ostium is more than 4 cm away from the ovary, it is plicated on its serosal surface, thereby approximating the fimbriae with the ovary. This plication results in a mobile ostium that is within 2 cm of the ovarian surface.

Another distal congenital tubal abnormality is accessory fimbriae on the distal ampulla or close to the tubal ostium. These may be sessile or pedunculated, with pedicles ranging from fine strands to rudimentary tubal stalks. Fimbrial stalks are removed by ligation of their pedicles or by transection with a microelectrode after microbipolar coagulation (Plate 61). Accessory fimbriae may occur on their own or in association with accessory tubal ostia (Figure 23-11, *A*). These ostia may be rudimentary (<0.5 cm in diameter) or truly represent a complete tubal ostium (>1 cm in diameter). They are present primarily in two locations and at varying distance from the end of the oviduct. Surgically, they may be classified as distal (within 1–3 cm of the tubal ostium), or ampullary (>3 cm from the ostium). Minor accessory ostia less than 0.5 cm in diameter are inverted, and seromuscular repair of the infundibulum or ampulla is completed using 8-0 nonreactive suture material on a taper-point needle.

Where major accessory ostia are present and associated with no other cause of infertility in patients who have not conceived despite all other treatment, microsurgical reconstruction of the distal oviduct is completed in the following manner. If the accessory ostium is close to the end of the oviduct, it is used as the main ostium in the reconstruction of a single distal tubal fimbrial ovum-capture mechanism (Figure 23-11, *B*; Plate 62). The incisions are carefully planned, after which distal fimbriae and their folds are excised, thereby ensuring that the new ostium has continuous fimbrial folds that are contiguous with the ovarian surface.

Text cont'd on p. 396.

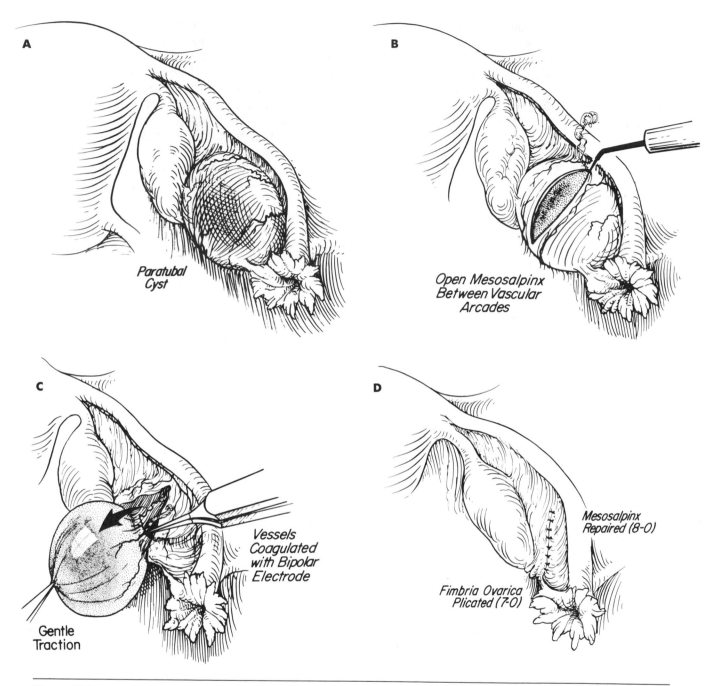

Figure 23-8
Surgical anatomy and microsurgical technique for removal of a large paratubal cyst. **A,** The cyst is bulging medially. **B,** Because of the medial placement of the cyst, the incision is made medially. **C,** The cyst is carefully resected. **D,** The mesosalpinx is repaired and the fimbria ovarica is plicated.

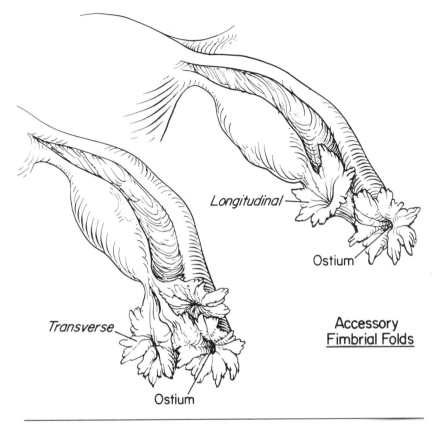

Figure 23-9
Surgical anatomy of accessory fimbriae. Note transverse and
longitudinal accessory folds.

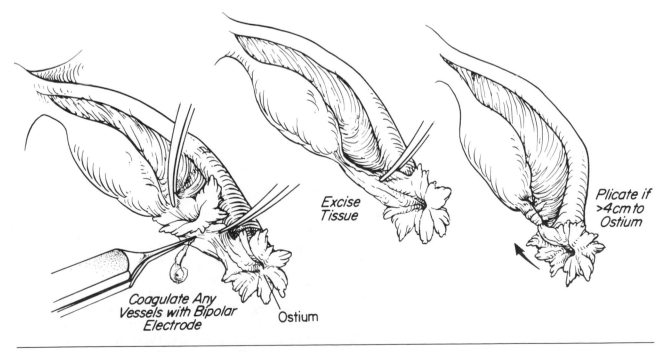

Figure 23-10
Microsurgical technique for resection of accessory redundant fimbriae. Note preservaton of continuous primary fold of fimbria from tubal ostium to ovarian surface.

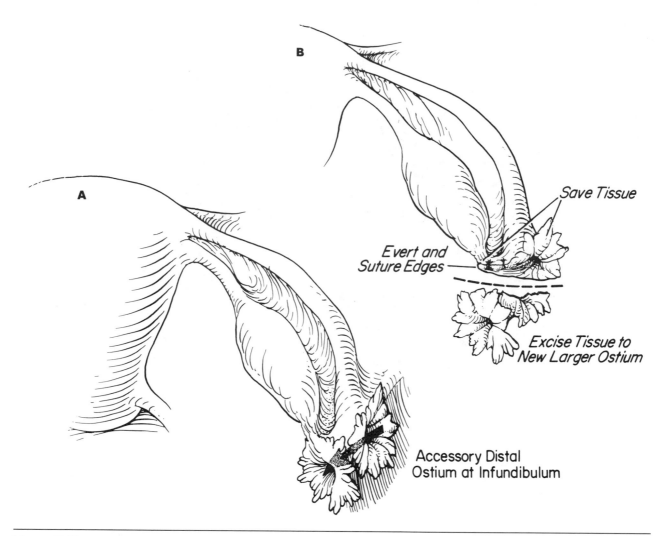

Figure 23-11
Microsurgical repair of major accessory tubal ostium at oviduct infundibulum. **A,** The congenital
anomaly is pictured. **B,** The primary ostium is excised and correct tubo-ovarian relationship established.

Where a large accessory ostium occurs in the midampullary segment of the oviduct (>3 cm from its fimbrial
end), resection of the distal oviduct using the accessory
ostium as the main tubal opening would involve loss of
a major functional segment of the tube (Figure 23-12,
A). Loss of significant proportions of tubal ampulla is
associated with a major decline in achievement of pregnancy after restoration of tubal patency. Thus we are
reluctant to remove this significant distal segment of ampulla with the infundibulum.

If the accessory ostium has minor extruded cilial folds,
these are gently inverted into the ampulla, and seromuscular closure is completed longitudinally. On the other
hand, if major fimbrial folds protrude from the ostium,
these are first excised by gentle traction and microbipolar
coagulation of their vascular pedicles. The accessory ostium is then inverted and seromuscular closure of the

defect is completed using 8-0 nonreactive, absorbable
suture material on a taper-point microsurgical needle
(Figure 23-12, *B*).

SURGERY OF THE OVARY

Resection and reconstruction of the ovary has always
presented difficulty to the gynecologic microsurgeon in
view of the mobility of the ovary, its relatively hard
cortex, and the vascularity of its surface together with
that of the inner ovary.

In previously accepted macrosurgical terms, each of
these factors was of minimal consequence where one
proposed to resect tissue and achieve hemostasis and
relative cortical apposition. The high frequency of multiple intrapelvic adhesions after an ovarian resection is
well documented. To achieve precise resection, reconstruction, and perfect cortical apposition, it is essential

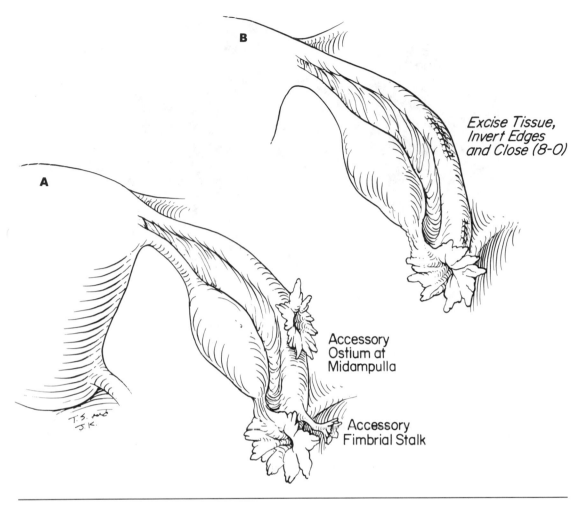

Figure 23-12
Repair of major midampullary accessory ostium and an accessory fimbrial stalk. **A,** The anomalies are pictured. **B,** The accessory ostium is inverted and the fimbrial stalk excised.

that the gonad be immobilized and precise hemostasis effected. These two factors facilitate the subsequent completion of perfect cortical apposition.

In recent years an ovarian clamp has been specifically designed to grasp the ovarian hilum in an atraumatic and gentle fashion. This clamp has very pliable jaws and multiple ratchets that enable the surgeon merely to hold the ovary on a hammock-like surface with partial hemostasis (Figure 23-13).

The ovarian clamp enables an assistant to immobilize the gonad absolutely so that a microelectrode or the focused laser may be used on the ovarian surface to transect the ovarian cortex and its inner stroma in a precise manner.

Basic instrumentation for microsurgery of the ovary is illustrated in Figure 23-14. This includes unipolar electrode, bipolar microelectrode, hand-held laser, and a means of continuous tissue irrigation.

In principle, the inner gonad is explored under irrigation in an effort to define vessels that may be specifically grasped with the bipolar electrode and coagulated. The ovary held in the ovarian clamp is surrounded with lint-free gauze soaked in heparinized solution before beginning the surgery.

Suture materials

Sutures must not tear through the soft inner gonadal tissue. They are placed within the ovary and do not exit the ovarian surface. The inner ovary is repaired using 4-0 an 5-0 sutures placed on a urologic tapered needle. Suture material may include polydioxanone, coated polyglycolic acid, or coated polyglactin; where tissues are extremely friable, chromic catgut is used. All knots are buried deep within the gonad.

Fine approximation of the outer ovarian cortical surface is completed with nonreactive suture materials on

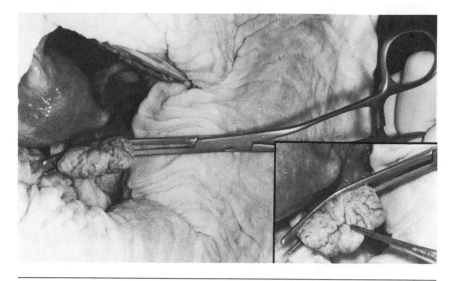

Figure 23-13
Use of the Cohen ovarian clamp for immobilization and partial gonadal hemostasis. Note the smooth atraumatic surface and open condition of instrument. (Clamp manufactured by Codman and Shurtleff.)

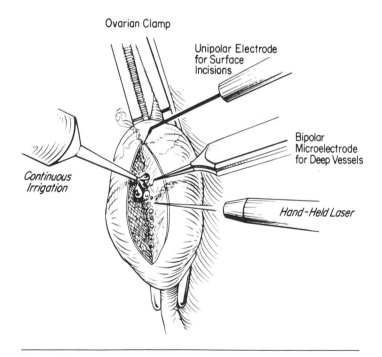

Figure 23-14
Basic instrumentation for microsurgical ovarian resection and reconstruction.

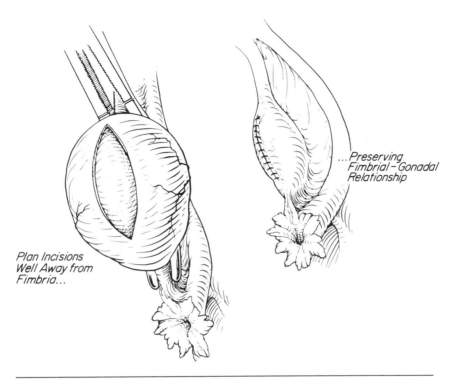

Plan Incisions Well Away from Fimbria...

...Preserving Fimbrial-Gonadal Relationship

Figure 23-15
Overview of planning ovarian incisions and reconstruction to preserve and restore normal fimbrial-gonadal relationship.

taper-point needles. Polydioxanone, polyglactin, and nylon of the 6-0 and 7-0 variety are the sutures of choice.

Surgery on the ovarian surface

Most commonly one is faced with the problem of adhesions on the ovarian surface and/or associated endometriosis. These may be removed using an angled microelectrode in a very fine superficial shaving fashion. If a laser is available, the defocused laser beam can be used in a repeat-pulse modality. This effectively removes the adhesions from the superficial surface of the ovary. It is imperative that adhesions over the ovary are excised and not merely transected, as they may constitute a barrier to ovulation and transfer of the ovum into the oviduct.

Where the ovarian surface must be divided to remove significant cysts or endometriosis and rarely, a wedge of gonadal tissue, it is essential to plan the incisions carefully. The cysts, endometriosis, or wedge should be removed through incisions placed as far away from the fimbrial end of the ovary as possible to reduce the chances of subsequent adhesion formation between the lateral ovarian surface and the oviduct. The volume of material removed is designed to ensure that the ovarian reconstruction restores a normal fimbrial-gonadal relationship with maximal preservation of ovarian cortex (Figure 23-15; Plates 63 and 64).

After resection of the pathologic tissue, it is essential to mobilize the ovarian cortex before attempting the re-

pair. This is achieved by incisions beneath the surface using the microelectrode. Freeing the cortical edges ensures that they may be perfectly opposed when sutured together with minimal tissue tension.

Ovarian reconstruction

The ovarian clamp is used to immobilize the gonad. Lint-free swabs soaked in heparinized physiologic solution are placed around the clamp to prevent contamination of the peritoneum with blood. The abnormal tissue is resected. Angle sutures are placed at either end of the site of ovarian resection (Figures 23-16 through 23-19). An effort is made to achieve coagulation of specific vessels that are defined with irrigation, and these are coagulated with the microbipolar electrode.

The inner ovary is repaired using interrupted sutures placed deep within the ovary. These barely avoid exiting the ovarian cortical surface and their knots are buried deep in the gonad (Figure 23-16).

These sutures facilitate some lateral compression to assist in hemostasis and they ensure support for the subsequent repair of both inner and more superficial ovarian stromal layers.

From the one angle, a continuous suture is run. Maximal amounts of tissue are obtained to facilitate lateral compression of the transected ovarian surface (Figure 23-17).

The running suture is run back in a second superficial layer thereby approximating the superficial cortex of the

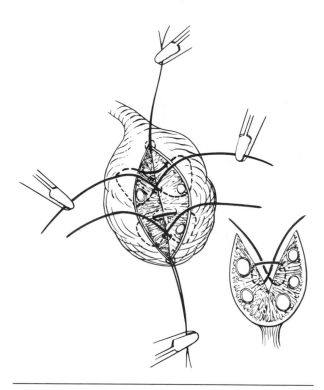

Figure 23-16
Repair of ovary. Note angle sutures and interrupted, deep, inner gonadal layer.

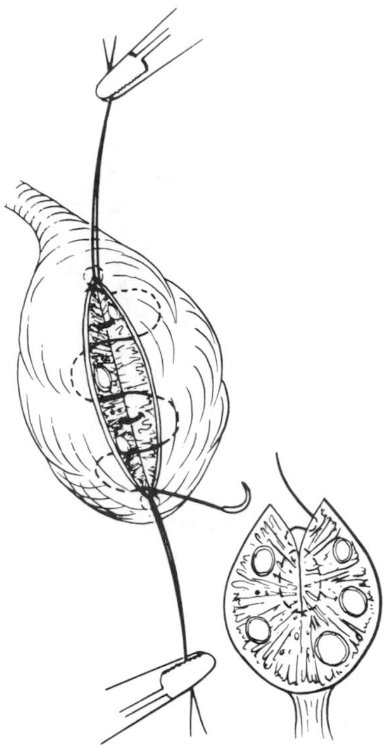

ovary and near perfect apposition of the ovarian surfaces (Figure 23-18).

As shown in Figure 23-19, the ovarian cortex is perfectly approximated using a subcuticular 6-0 polydioxanone suture. Excellent apposition may also be completed using an inversion or baseball suture. Such repair is carried out under the surgical microscope, as magnification facilitates accurate placement of sutures to achieve perfect cortical apposition.

Hemostasis must be absolutely perfect to prevent surface deposition of blood, thereby lowering the risk of formation of tubo-ovarian adhesions.

SURGICAL RECONSTRUCTION OF THE FIMBRIAL-GONADAL RELATIONSHIP AND REPAIR OF THE FIMBRIAL OVUM-CAPTURE MECHANISM

The primary aims of ovarian surgery and the microsurgical approach to anatomic reconstruction of the fimbrial-ovum-capture mechanism are to ensure (1) a healthy free ovarian surface, (2) a widely spread, patulous fimbrial ostium, (3) close proximity between these structures associated with true mobility of the fimbriae over the ovarian surface, and (4) that the primary fimbrial folds run from the ovarian surface to the fimbrial ostium. The surgical anatomy of these principles is summarized in Figure 23-20, which illustrates the steps taken to ensure

Figure 23-17
Repair of ovary. Note running, continuous suture; lateral compression of inner ovarian layers facilitates hemostasis.

proximity of a widely patent fimbrial ostium with a free healthy surface of the ovary.

CURRENT TRENDS
Paratubal cysts

Many paratubal cysts are amenable to laparoscopic dissection or laser or bipolar coagulation of their vasculature and excision or total laser vaporization. Once the vasculature has been coagulated, the cyst is dissected out of the mesosalpinx and removed, usually through a second-puncture cannula (Plates 57 and 58).

In some instances, close proximity to the fimbrial ostium necessitates laser vaporization and marsupialization of the outer surface of the cyst.

Elongated fimbria ovarica

When fimbria ovarica is longer than 4 cm, microsurgery remains the treatment of choice. Alternative options include gamete intrafallopian transfer and in vitro fertilization.

Treatment is directed at the main problem, considered to be failure of ovum pick-up by the distant fimbrial ostium. When less than 4 cm, the fimbria ovarica may be shortened adequately by partial laser coagulation with cicatrization of the peritoneum and fimbrial musculature.

In principle, a defocused, low wattage of laser is rapidly moved from side to side over the peritoneum of the

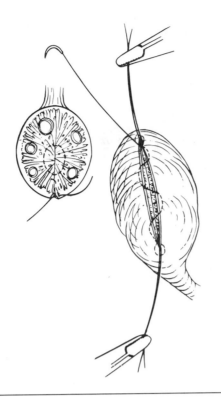

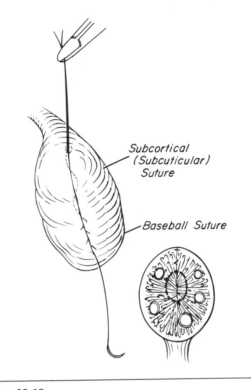

Figure 23-18
Superficial continuous suture completes inner hemostasis and aligns ovarian surface for perfect apposition.

Figure 23-19
Perfect ovarian surface repair with continuous suture line. Note subcuticular, herringbone, and baseball sutures.

fimbria ovarica with resultant shortening of the structure. Alternative methods include use of the bipolar button and the endotherm coagulator in a similar to-and-fro rapid-movement technique.

Polycystic ovary

Failure of medical therapy is an indication for surgery in polycystic ovary disease. Numerous follicles are drained laparoscopically using laser or unipolar coagulator needle methods. Drainage should be done using a totally hemostatic technique avoiding cortical blood vessels. This should minimize the risk of adhesion formation. Particular care must be taken to avoid puncturing the large veins commonly seen at the hilum of these ovaries (Plate 20).

Ovarian cysts

If there is any doubt as to the nature of an ovarian lesion, laparotomy and appropriate pelvic, ovarian, and histologic studies are completed in the routine manner. For benign functional ovarian cysts, on the basis of history of development, physical examination, ultrasound evaluation, and negative blood studies (e.g., CA 125), these cysts are carefully evaluated laparoscopically (Plates 9 through 12).

The cyst wall is rendered hemostatic using the en-

dotherm, bipolar coagulator, or laser technique and subsequently drained using a 16-gauge needle passed through a second-puncture cannula. Atraumatic graspers are used to hold the cyst edges, and the cyst is either peeled out of its bed or a significant piece is excised and submitted for histologic examination. Excision is accomplished with the endotherm, unipolar, or fiberoptic laser, or more simply with laparoscopic scissors. The inner cyst wall is meticulously evaluated, and if any suspicious lesions are noted, laparotomy and routine oncologic evaluation and management are performed.

Once the cyst wall has been resected or the cyst peeled out of its cavity, the ovary is left to heal spontaneously. Meticulous hemostasis is essential, together with mass pelvic irrigation using a solution of heparinized Ringer's lactate consisting of 2000 IU heparin, 100 gm Solucortef, and 100 mg of ampicillin/L.

When cysts or endometriomas are larger than 5 cm or extremely vascular, the surgeon should not hesitate to proceed to laparotomy and use of routine laser and microsurgical reconstructive techniques.

SUMMARY

Surgery of the ovary is facilitated with an atraumatic ovarian clamp, and resection and reconstruction are car-

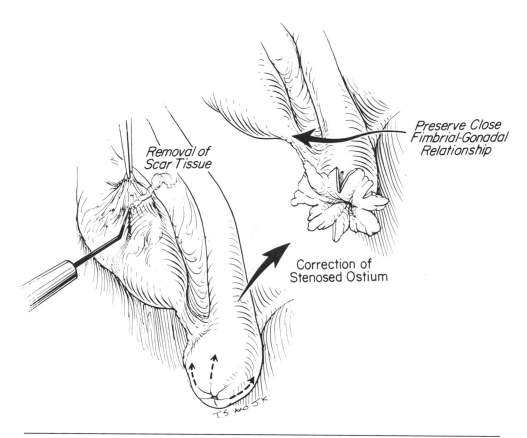

Figure 23-20
Primary aims of microsurgical reconstruction of normal fimbrial-gonadal relationship.

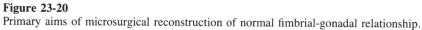

ried out to restore normal fimbrial-gonadal relationships, at the same time preserving a perfect cortical surface of ovary exposed to the fimbrial ostium. Meticulous attention to each of the following details optimizes the chances of subsequent conception in women undergoing surgical restoration of their reproductive organs:

1. Distal tubal surgery is directed to ensure an efficient fimbrial ovum-capture mechanism.
2. When completing each distal oviduct and ovarian surgery, specific attention is directed to reconstruction and repair of the fimbrial-gonadal relationship and ovum-capture mechanism.
3. The fimbrial ostium is always left attached to the upper outer surface of the ovary either by its original, normally located fimbria ovarica, or by re-

construction of this structure using nonabsorbable suture material.
4. This approach to microsurgical reconstruction of fimbrial-gonadal relationships should restore a normal anatomic location of the fimbriae close to the surface of the ovary and maximize the chance of ovum pick-up, as is the case in the normally fertile female.
5. In recent years, operative endoscopy has facilitated surgical correction of distal adnexal disease with the laparoscope. Many patients remain, however, for whom laparotomy, microsurgery, and pelvic reconstruction are simpler, safer, and more effective.

ENDOMETRIOSIS

24

Endometriosis: Surgical Considerations

RONALD E. BATT

JAMES M. WHEELER

Since the mid 1980s substantial changes have occurred in our perception of endometriosis. The stereotype that it affects the thin, white career women has given way to the realization that neither the body habitus nor the racc of women with endometriosis differs from that of other women.[1] Extensive data have accumulated on the immunologic, endocrine, and pathophysiologic changes associated with endometriosis.[2-8] Furthermore, the disease has been underdiagnosed until recently, when subtle forms have been identified.[9-15] A wide spectrum of endometriotic lesions is recognized, of which the classic power-burn peritoneal lesion and the chocolate ovarian endometrioma are the conspicuous forms.

Since the first edition of this atlas, a dramatic shift in surgical treatment from laparotomy to laparoscopic surgery has taken place. Now it is possible to offer surgical removal of endometriosis to patients with all stages of the disease and in most cases, preserve childbearing potential. To realize the full potential of surgery to relieve pain, enhance fertility, and restore health, the surgeon must recognize the varied appearances of endometriosis and the host responses to the disease.

PERITONEAL AND OVARIAN ENDOMETRIOSIS

Peritoneal endometriosis, diagnosed at laparoscopy, presents a wide spectrum of lesions starting with nonpigmented, epithelial, plaque-type implants that replace the normal pelvic peritoneum and are usually not recognized unless searched for with near-contact laparoscopy and peritoneal blood painting.[16-18] Subtle vesicular-type implants look like petechial hemorrhages or single or multiple, clear or pigmented blisters and polyps, less than 5 mm in diameter. The pigmented lesions vary from pink to red, brown, blue, or black.[19,20] They are described as red and purple raspberry, to account for their hemorrhagic

color and polypoid appearance, and as blueberry cysts that are filled with older blood.[21]

With time, the small pigmented peritoneal lesions enlarge into conspicuous lesions that elicit an encircling fibrotic host response, and often coalesce into plaques.[22,23] They appear as the familiar blueberry cysts; puckered black lesions; dark gray, powder-burn lesions; deep, invasive, fibrotic, bluish nodules; thick, white, fibrotic plaques, some with pigmented lesions; moist red adhesions; and dense obliterative adhesions.[22,24,25]

Ovarian endometriosis, visualized at laparoscopy, often appears as superficial, mossy red adhesions or vesicular, polypoid, and cystic implants similar to peritoneal lesions. Endometriomas are smooth or puckered cysts varying from millimeters to several centimeters in size with or without the presence of adhesions. Because of the high concentrations of steroid hormones within the ovaries, the endometriotic implants enlarge to form "chocolate" cysts that invade the surface of the ovary with a predilection for the posterior surface. The inside of an ovarian endometrioma is actually the outside surface of the ovarian cortex.[26] Whereas this may be true for most endometriomas, some at the hilus of the ovary may be caused by lymphatic dissemination.

HISTOLOGIC CRITERIA

Current clinical standards permit the diagnosis of endometriosis based on visualization of the disease at surgery.[27] In our opinion, histologic verification should be attempted in all cases, when it can be done safely.

Strict histologic criteria require the presence of endometrial stroma and epithelium for diagnosis.[28,29] Others accept endometriotic stroma alone as diagnostic.[30] Some of the earliest lesions exhibit only endometriotic epithelium,[31] and at the other end of the spectrum, many lesions that have undergone resorption may have only endometriotic epithelium or stroma or hemosiderin-laden macrophages as the residual; we consider this histologic picture consistent with the diagnosis of endometriosis.[32]

DISEASE PATTERNS

Pelvic endometriosis can be divided into simple and complex patterns. In the simple patterns, the pelvic anatomy is undistorted and simply serves as the stage on which the endometriotic lesions have been imposed. This corresponds to the American Fertility Society revised classification stages I and II.[33] The complex patterns are associated with distorted pelvic anatomy and correspond to stages III and IV.

Endometriosis is a disease with two major pathologic manifestations.[22] The first is invasion of organs by endometrial basal stromal cells that do not respond to cycle hormonal stimulation. When the stromatous elements of the endometrium infiltrate inwardly between the muscle bundles of the uterine wall, they may penetrate into lymphatics and blood vessels to invade other organs by embolization, or they may continue to penetrate more deeply between the muscle bundles to infiltrate the cardinal, uterosacral, and round ligaments by direct extension.

The second manifestation is invasion of organs by glandular and superficial stroma cells that do respond to cyclic hormonal stimulation. When the glandular and stromatous elements of the superficial endometrium, which are responsive to cyclic hormonal stimulation, are shed outwardly into the endometrial cavity, they may spread to sites beyond the uterus by normal menstruation, by retrograde tubal menstruation; and by spill at surgery or obstetric delivery to transplant and invade the surface of the host tissues. Ovarian endometriomas may rupture, spill, and invade host tissues secondarily.

There is much more to endometriosis than implants, cysts, fibrosis, and adhesions (Figure 24-1). Among the many associated pathophysiologic changes that have been recognized are altered prostaglandin secretion, luteinized unruptured follicle syndrome, luteal phase deficiency, anovulation, hyperprolactinemia, autoimmune changes, activation of peritoneal macrophages, and evidence of neuroendocrine dysfunction.[34-38]

Organ involvement

Endometriosis is usually limited to organs of the pelvis and lower abdomen. The susceptible tissues and organs are the peritoneum of the lower anterior abdominal wall, the urinary bladder, round ligaments, uterus, cardinal ligaments, uterosacral ligaments, rectovaginal pouch, posterior cervix at the cervicovaginal angle, rectum, sigmoid colon, fallopian tube, ovary, broad ligament, ureter, vermiform appendix, ileum, cecum, and ascending colon, and occasionally, the diaphragm. In addition, the portio vaginalis of the cervix, posterior vaginal fornix,

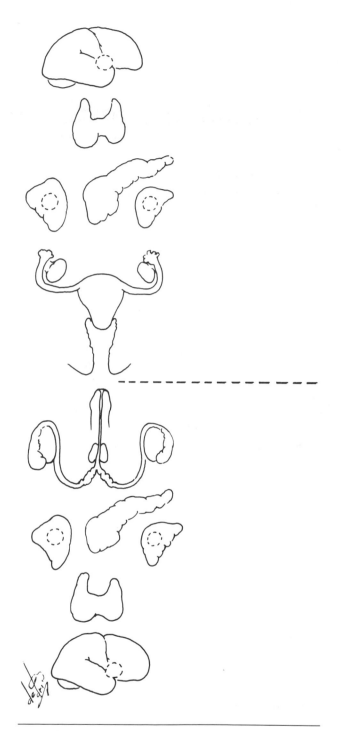

Figure 24-1
Problems of psychoneuroendocrine, medical, and reproductive origin in both partners should be evaluated and treated before surgery for endometriosis is contemplated. This form provides a convenient record of pertinent data.

vagina, and perineum at the site of an episiotomy may be involved.

Nowhere is the host influence of the local pelvic environment better exemplified than in the distribution of endometriosis of the bowel (rectum, sigmoid colon, cecum, appendix, distal ileum) virtually to the exclusion of the remainder of the large and small bowel.[22] These structures all should be examined systematically for endometriotic lesions both at laparoscopy and at laparotomy.

Asymmetry

The disease exhibits lateral as well as anteroposterior asymmetry. Frequently, all or the majority of lesions occupy one side of the pelvis to the left or right of midline with sparing of one adnexa. Since the ovary is so vulnerable to adhesive disease, this adnexal sparing favors the prognosis for fertility. Thus women with severe unilateral adnexal disease and a normal contralateral ovary and tube have a better prognosis for fertility than women with bilateral severe adnexal disease.[39]

Consistent with the hypothesis of retrograde menstruation and implantation,[40] the rectovaginal pouch is the ultimate reservoir for retrograde menstrual detritus. When the uterus is retroverted, the menstrual flow collects predominantly in the posterior rectovaginal pouch of Douglas. However, the anteroposterior distribution depends to some degree on the anatomic position of the uterus.

Endometriosis of the anterior vesicouterine pouch is more common when the uterus is anteverted because some of the menstrual detritus is captured and held in that location.[41] Nevertheless, deep, invasive, nodular, fibrotic endometriotic disease of the posterior pelvis far outweighs deep invasive disease of the anterior vesicouterine pouch. Peritoneal pockets with endometriosis (mullerianosis) are predominantly unilateral and confined to the posterior pelvis.[7]

Invasion

Endometriosis invades but does not digest and destroy tissue as a malignancy does. Instead, it elicits a foreign body reaction that was described as follows: "The radial expansion of fibrosis about a lesion is not a centrifugal invasion by the endometrium itself into the surrounding organs and structures but rather an exhibition of widely recognized foreign body reaction called forth by the irritant nature of the central, active areas."[23] This was confirmed by ultrastructural examination of endometriosis. The authors found "clear definitive junctions between endometrial cells and the scar tissue."[42]

In women with chronic peritoneal and ovarian endometriosis, a well-defined plane of dissection exists between the fibrous and normal tissue that can be identified and dissected easily under magnification at laparoscopic surgery as well as at laparotomy. During the acute and subacute phases of the disease, the host tissues have not walled off the invading endometriosis: the host tissues are soft and vascular, and clinically, the margins of the disease are ill defined, making identification, dissection, and hemostasis difficult.

Acute and chronic endometriosis

Goodall[22] drew the analogy between endometriosis and infection. During the acute phase, raised, red and orange, proliferative lesions and thin-walled blue, chocolate-filled cysts can be seen; the host tissues are soft and hypertrophied, with venous congestion ranging from fine hyperemia to marked dilation of pelvic veins. As the disease progresses through the subacute into the chronic stage, the implants elicit a fibrotic host response to form thick-walled, blue cysts and eventually, firm, fibrous nodules and plaques containing chocolate-colored material. The peritoneum of the rectovaginal pouch and of the bladder often becomes thickened, sclerotic, and white.

During acute exacerbations of chronic disease, two or three generations of peritoneal endometriosis may be observed simultaneously: fresh red and orange implants with surrounding hyperemia among thin-walled, blue endometriotic cysts and older powder-burn lesions, plaques, and nodules embedded in sclerotic, thickened peritoneum.

Acute active endometriosis on the ovarian surface resembles peritoneal lesions or may take the form of tight, red, mossy adhesions that have a predilection for the crevices of the ovary. Active superficial and deep endometriomas of the ovary are thin-walled, friable, and filled with liquid black blood. As the disease progresses through the subacute stage, the blood in the cysts is not renewed as rapidly by repeated ectopic menstruation or by hilar vessel hemorrhages, and the fluid content becomes brown with a thicker consistency. When the disease reaches the late chronic stage, there is minimal to no contribution of menstrual detritus as the last of the ectopic endometrium is destroyed by pressure and fibrosis. The fluid portion of the blood is reabsorbed, leaving behind tarry material inside a thick, fibrous capsule.

Goodall's analogy holds even to treatment. The acute stage of the disease should be treated by medical means, carefully avoiding surgery, whereas the chronic stage, by far the most common variety, is more responsive to surgery. After medical treatment of acute, inflammatory endometriosis, the disease may be excised at laparoscopic surgery or at laparotomy.

Malignancy

The frequency of malignant transformation of extragenital endometriosis (retroperitoneum, rectovaginal space, cesarean section scar, inguinal region, episiotomy) is extremely low.[43] Endometrioid carcinoma has been the most frequent histologic type, and cases of clear cell carcinoma are reported.[43,44]

Numerous case reports implicated the role of estrogens in the malignant transformation of endometriosis. This suggests the danger of giving unopposed estrogen therapy to women with the disease.[43] Malignant transformation involving the obliterated rectovaginal pouch–posterior vaginal fornix was reported not only with use of unopposed estrogen therapy[45-48] but also with Enovid (Searle, Chicago, Ill) and DepoProvera (Upjohn, Kalamazoo, Mich).[49] This may be prevented by surgical excision of the endometriosis followed by cyclic or continuous oral administration of both estrogen and progesterone replacement therapy.

Documented cases of transformation from ovarian endometriosis through the intermediate stages to malignancy are rare, since the cancer rapidly destroys the endometriosis.[50] However, carcinoma arising from the endometriosis of the ovary has been reported,[51-56] occurring in 8 of 950[52] and 3 of 889 women.[57] Endometrioid carcinoma is the most common histologic type of cancer in ovarian endometriosis.

Based on personal experience, Fox[56] reported:

Adenocarcinomatous change appears to take place more commonly in endometriotic cysts than in any other type of cystic lesion in the ovary and the author has personally examined a considerable number of examples of endometrioid and clear cell adenocarcinomas which were clearly arising in endometriotic cysts.

Fox qualified that statement by noting that quite often a suspicion that an endometrioid or clear cell neoplasm has arisen in endometriosis is engendered by the presence of endometriosis either in the contralateral ovary or elsewhere in the pelvis. Using these criteria, Fox estimated that between 15% and 20% of endometrioid adenocarcinomas of the ovary are derived from preexisting endometriosis.

Surgeons should be aware of ovarian malignancy, since more and more women in their forties and fifties are requesting conservative surgery for endometriosis rather than hysterectomy and bilateral salpingo-oophorectomy. Excision of all ovarian endometriosis in this age group followed by histologic examination of the specimens seems preferable to aspiration and medical suppression or laser vaporization or coagulation. We are of the opinion that endometriomas of the ovary should be excised and examined histologically.

HOST RESPONSES TO ENDOMETRIOSIS
Hypertrophy and relaxation

Two of the more commonly recognized host responses to acute and subacute endometriosis are soft hypertrophy of the uterus and relaxation of the round, broad, and uterosacral ligaments, which allow gravity to pull the heavy uterus into the rectovaginal pouch where it becomes susceptible to invasion by endometriosis and to fixation by endometriotic adhesions. As the disease progresses to the chronic state, either naturally or under the influence of medication, the uterus firms, but the supporting ligaments remain relaxed and elongated, resulting in acquired, chronic uterine retroversion.

The ovaries also may respond to hypertrophy, often asymmetrically, attributable to invasion of endometriomas. Whereas endometriomas that invade the hilum of the ovary characteristically adhere to the posterior broad ligament, the deep endometriomas invading the ovary from the antimesenteric or anterior surfaces remain free of attachment to the posterior broad ligament, although they may adhere to the fallopian tube or sigmoid colon.

The ovarian ligaments tend to relax and elongate and permit the enlarged, heavy ovaries to descend deeply into the pelvis where they may adhere to the uterus, uterosacral ligaments, and rectovaginal pouch. When these lesions are bilateral, the enlarged endometriotic sclerotic ovaries may appear to the uninitiated as two large polycystic ovaries sitting in the rectovaginal pouch. In reality this is a centripedal form of the disease in which the uterus, ovaries, uterosacral ligaments, and rectovaginal pouch are mutually involved with endometriosis and endometriotic adhesive disease.

Sclerosis of solid organs

Peritoneal sclerosis involving the rectovaginal pouch and uterosacral, cardinal, and broad ligaments restricts the upward mobility of the uterus and adnexae. At pelvic endoscopic surgery, the white sclerosis of the broad ligaments makes it difficult to identify the ureters. The technique for ureteral identification under such circumstances is described in Chapter 25.

In extreme cases, progressive sclerosis of the tunica albuginea of the ovary results in cartilaginous consistency of the entire ovary. It was postulated that sclerosis of the ovary was one of the causes of ovulatory dysfunction associated with advanced endometriosis.[58] Most women with this problem require ovulation induction.

Sclerosis of hollow organs

Sclerosis and fibrosis are the host responses that finally limit the spread of endometriosis, preserving health at the expense of fertility. The sclerosing response has a particularly unfortunate effect on hollow organs, causing cervical stenosis, cornual angle tubal stenosis, ampullary convolutions, infundibular tubal stenosis, and fimbrial phimosis.

Sclerosis and fibrosis of certain hollow organs can be a threat to health by causing stenosis and in some cases partial obstruction of the ileum, vermiform appendix, and colon. Sclerosis and fibrosis of the ureter lead to ureteral fixation, followed by obstruction with hydronephrosis and atrophy of the kidney.

Stenosis and obstruction of tubular organs by endometriotic sclerosis and fibrosis develop silently. The disease process may escape detection unless the surgeon searches for evidence at history, physical examination, hysterosalpingography, laparoscopy, and selective radiologic examinations of the urinary tract and bowel.

Inflammation

The monthly transient inflammation associated with retrograde menstruation, the episodic inflammation associated with leakage or rupture of an endometrioma, and the inflammation associated with an activated immune system may be due to a systemic autoimmune phenomenon, a defect in the local immune system, or simply to an overwhelming of the local immune system by excessive menstruation.[37]

Considerable attention has been focused on the pelvic peritoneal fluid environment.[59-64] Activated macrophages phagocytose sperm[65] and are associated with a significant decrease in the ability of sperm to penetrate zona-free hamster oocytes.[59,66] The presence of activated macrophages may perpetuate the inflammatory process and also the endometriotic disease. Activated macrophages within the peritoneal fluid are known to secrete prostaglandins that may induce pathologic alteration of mechanisms of follicular rupture, tubal motility, corpus luteum formation, and implantation.[36]

In patients susceptible to endometriosis, direct toxic effects of pelvic peritoneal fluid have been demonstrated on various aspects of the reproductive process such as inhibition of ovum capture,[67] direct inhibiting effect on the sperm-oocyte interaction in the mouse,[68] and decreased sperm survival in peritoneal fluid.[69] Complete aspiration of pelvic peritoneal fluid and thorough lavage of the pelvis with copious amounts of Ringer's lactate solution at the time of pelvic endoscopic surgery or microsurgery, together with thorough flushing of the fallopian tubes by chromotubation or hydrotubation, may have an interval therapeutic benefit.

Inflammatory reaction in the fallopian tubes of patients with advanced endometriosis is probably present more often than surgeons suspect. Review of the histologic specimens from 194 patients with ovarian endometriosis disclosed that in 22% the fallopian tube(s) showed inflammatory and/or ulcerative lesions.[70] The investigators found the oviduct involved with dystrophic salpingitis in association with ovarian endometriosis, and these women may complain of low-grade fever during menses in addition to pelvic pain. Usually the salpingitis was unilateral and associated with deep, locally extensive ovarian endometriosis. This condition is treated by unilateral salpingo-oophorectomy.

Endometriotic adhesions

Endometriosis induces dense, obliterative adhesions between contiguous organs: ovary and posterior broad ligament, ovary and sigmoid colon, ovary and posterior uterus, ovary and uterosacral ligament, ovary and oviduct. The ovary is particularly vulnerable.

From available evidence it seems that endometriosis diminishes plasminogen activator. Ohtsuka[71] studied the pathogenesis of endometriotic adhesions and concluded:

The pathogenic mechanism of adhesions was presumed to be as follows: early lesions of endometriosis were always covered with peritoneum, so adhesions could not be observed. However, enlargement of lesions produced a damage of peritoneum and outpouring of fibrin, causing fibrinous adhesions to other peritoneum. Fibrous adhesions were promoted by a decrease of fibrinolytic activity in the lesions.

The two areas of the pelvis most likely to develop obliterative endometriotic adhesive disease are the rectovaginal pouch and the left adnexa. The rectum is fixed at the pelvic floor and normally lies in contact with the posterior vagina, cervix, and uterus, where undisturbed, except for periodic evacuations of the bowel, the contiguous surfaces are in intimate contact. This permits progression of the obliterative adhesive process.

The sigmoid colon is fixed at the pelvic brim near the left infundibulopelvic ligament and naturally rests against the left adnexa. Thus it is positioned to entrap retrograde menstruation in the left ovarian fossa, which promotes endometriotic adhesions among the left posterior broad ligament, the left ovary and tube, and the sigmoid colon. When this adhesive process is fully developed, a left frozen pelvis results, with the ovary and fallopian tube sandwiched in an obliterative adhesive process between the pelvic wall and the sigmoid colon.

The right ovary occupies a privileged position. Unlike the rectum and sigmoid colon, which have an obligatory pelvic lie, the cecum, vermiform appendix, and ileum usually have an abdominal lie and thus are not in position to adhere to the right adnexa. Consequently, capillary action that sequesters menstrual detritus between the posterior surface of the right ovary and the right posterior broad ligament forms peritoneal-ovarian adhesions only.

The oviduct is less often involved with adhesions or endometriosis; however, adhesions between the ovary and the tube, especially those that involve the fimbria ovarica, are detrimental to fertility. Surgical reconstruction of the damaged, shortened fimbria ovarica is important.[72,73] The normal fimbrial-ovarian relationship must be preserved during resection of ovarian endometriomas.[74]

Based on surrogate embryo transfer experiments in primates and experiments with a single ovary and a single oviduct on opposite sides of the pelvis, it was concluded that eggs are captured most often by the oviduct on the same side as the corpus luteum and that pick-up in the rectovaginal pouch of Douglas is probably insignificant.[75,76] Particular care should be made to preserve and, if necessary, to restore the normal relationship of the fimbria ovarica at surgery.

The omentum seems relatively resistant to invasion by endometriosis. It seldom adheres spontaneously to endometriotic lesions, except in cases complicated by intense tissue anoxia caused by the inflammatory reaction secondary to rupture of a large ovarian endometrioma.

Surgical adhesions

Omental adhesions are more often the hallmark of surgical intervention than a spontaneous host response to endometriosis. Surgical experiments demonstrated that ischemic tissues were a strong stimulant for adhesion formation.[77] A zone of ischemic peritoneum caused by crush injury, tight suturing, strangulation by ligature, or the application of free omental or free peritoneal graft to an area of anoxic tissue produced adhesion formation in 39 of 47 procedures, whereas adhesions formed in only 5 of 58 peritoneal defects left open and raw.

Twenty-one years later, in a review of the prevention and treatment of adhesions, that author stated:

> The thesis that fibrous adhesions develop in relation to areas of ischemia and represent vascular grafts into such tissues explains the great majority of instances in which acquired adhesions are found within the peritoneal cavity. . . . Wherever possible, peritoneal defects should be left open rather than pulled together under tension.[78]

Tension produces ischemia, which provokes adhesion formation.

Adhesions from sexually transmitted diseases

Endometriosis complicated by sexually transmitted disease carries a poor prognosis for conception, as well as increased risk for ectopic pregnancy. An adnexa with greater than 50% enveloping, obliterative, dense adhesions from sexually transmitted disease carries a poor prognosis for conception after reconstructive surgery.[79]

At laparoscopy, the surgeon should consider the possibility of superimposed sexually transmitted disease when (1) generalized pelvic inflammation is found in the absence of a recently ruptured endometrioma; (2) the oviducts are edematous and inflamed; (3) there is a disproportionate amount of peritubal adhesions or distal tubal damage; (4) perihepatic adhesions are found; (5) the extent of adhesions far exceeds the severity of the endometriotic lesions.

Peritoneal pockets and congenital anomalies

Peritoneal pockets associated with endometriosis are, with rare exception, confined to the posterior pelvis, the rectovaginal pouch, and the posterior broad ligaments (Table 24-1). In our experience, 46% of pockets involved only the rectovaginal pouch, 26%, only the broad ligaments, and 28%, both structures.[15]

Peritoneal pockets in the rectovaginal pouch occur in a predictable pattern. They may be unilateral, bilateral, or central in location. The openings are round or elliptical, and laterally they tend to be obscured from casual view by the uterosacral ligaments (Figure 24-2). In many cases, the uterosacral ligaments are markedly attenuated and thinned. The pockets may be simple, baffled, septate, or cryptic. They descend for a variable distance (1.5–5 cm) into the rectovaginal space (Figure 24-3) and are attached to neither the rectum nor the vagina (Figure 24-4). Often a rich vascular network surrounds the orifice of a peritoneal pocket; care must be exercised to avoid excessive bleeding when excising the pocket (Figure 24-5). The pocket floor can be grasped and easily everted like a wind sock for excision and histologic examination for the presence of endometriosis.

Peritoneal pockets in the posterior broad ligament are usually elliptical or oval with an elongated anterior-posterior axis. They may occur lateral or medial to the ureter and are smaller when occupying the medial position. Lateral to the ureter they vary in size from small to large depressions of sufficient capacity to engulf the ovary and tube (Figure 24-7). Within the broad ligaments the pockets may be open, cavernous, or cryptic.

Three subtle, macroscopic, nonpigmented endometriotic lesions may be encountered in association with peritoneal pockets: spider nodules, brim nodules, and organoid lesions. In addition, microscopic lesions have been found. The spider nodule is a highly characteristic lesion usually found in the floor of a peritoneal pocket in the broad ligament and occasionally in the pouch of Douglas (Figure 24-8). The spider lesion is a 1- to 2-mm, raised, firm, tan nodule of cartilaginous consistency from which radiate four to six thick-walled blood vessels. The brim nodule is an endometriotic lesion 2 to 8 mm in diameter on the brim of a pocket in the broad ligament or rectovaginal pouch (Figure 24-9).[32]

Patients with peritoneal pockets should be examined carefully for congenital anomalies of the fallopian tubes and for congenital medial displacement of the ureters. In some patients the ureters are located immediately adjacent to the uterosacral ligaments where they are at increased risk to injury during pelvic surgery.

CLINICAL EPIDEMIOLOGY

Endometriosis may be symptomatic and detectable at laparoscopy from menarche through the menopause. Based on analysis of available data, the incidence was estimated to be 2.5/1000 woman-years and the prevalence at 10% in the general population of the United States.[80]

Incidence is the rate of occurrence of new cases of endometriosis in a population under study or the number of new cases per population over time.[81] Prevalence is

Text cont'd on p. 413.

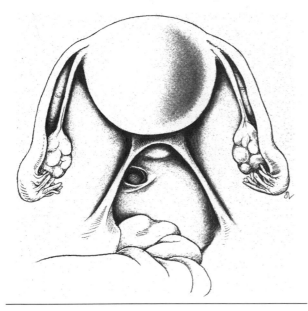

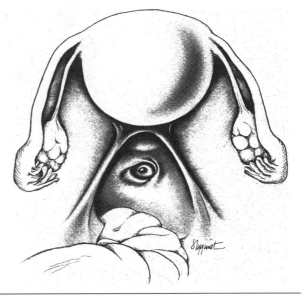

Figure 24-2
Artist's sketch of posterior pelvis showing peritoneal pocket, in left lateral rectovaginal pouch of Douglas, partially obscured by the uterosacral ligament. A peritoneal fold accentuates the posteromedial border and marks the position of the rectum beneath the peritoneal reflection. From Batt RE and Smith RA: Embryologic theory of histogenesis of endometriosis in peritoneal pockets. *Obstet Gynecol Clin North Am* 16:17, 1989.

Figure 24-3
Central pocket in rectovaginal pouch of Douglas shows a baffled passageway extending downward into the rectovaginal space anterior to the rectovaginal septum. Note typical implantation-type endometriosis that sometimes occurs within these recesses. Most often a regressive form of endometriosis is observed as a brim nodule or microscopic disease in the deep portion of the pockets. From Batt RE and Smith RA: Embryologic theory of histogenesis of endometriosis in peritoneal pockets. *Obstet Gynecol Clin North Am* 16:19, 1989.

Table 24-1 Comparison of endometriosis and mullerianosis associated with peritoneal pockets (E/PP) and implantation endometriosis (IE)

Clinical features	E/PP	IE
Clinical course	Regressive	Progressive, invasive
Host response	Atrophy, calcification, inflammation	Hypertrophy, peritoneal fibrosis, inflammation, hemorrhage
Adhesions	Absent	Characteristic and frequent
Distribution	Localized to defined area of posterior pelvic peritoneum	Random distribution; entire pelvis, including peritoneum and ovary
Pouch of Douglas	Open	May be obliterated
Peritoneal pockets	Characteristic	Absent
Chocolate cysts	Absent	Frequent
RAFS classification*	Stage I (minimal)	Stages I–IV

*American Fertility Society: Revised American Fertility Society classification of endometriosis, *Fertil Steril* 1985; 43:351.
From Batt RE and Smith RA: Embryologic theory of histogenesis of endometriosis in peritoneal pockets, *Obstet Gynecol Clin North Am* 16:24, 1989.

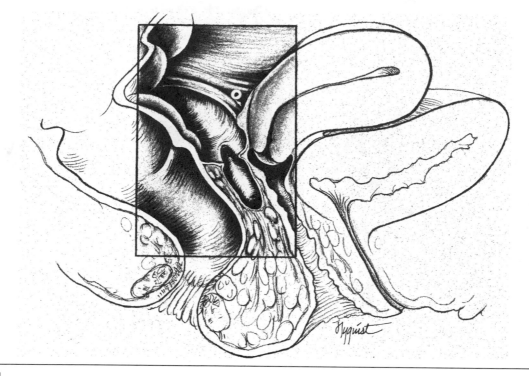

Figure 24-4
Illustration of a sagittal section through the peritoneal pocket in the midpouch of Douglas. The peritoneal pocket descends into the rectovaginal space anterior to the rectovaginal septum, and is not attached to either the vagina or the rectum. From Batt RE, Smith RA, Buck GM, Naples JD, and Severino MF: A case series-peritoneal pockets and endometriosis: Rudimentary duplications of the mullerian system. *Adolesc Pediatr Gynecol* 2:54, 1989.

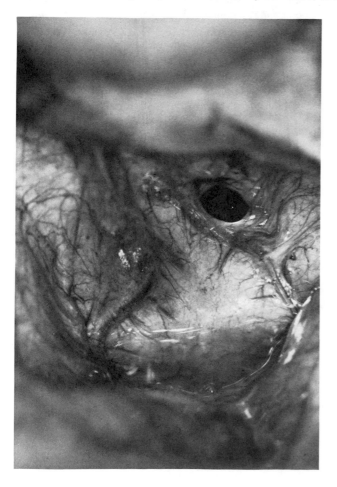

Figure 24-5
Original photograph on which Figure 24-3 was based. Note the rich vascular network on the surface of the peritoneum of the rectovaginal pouch. From Batt RE and Smith RA: Embryologic theory of histogenesis of endometriosis in peritoneal pockets. *Obstet Gynecol Clin North Am* 16:20, 1989.

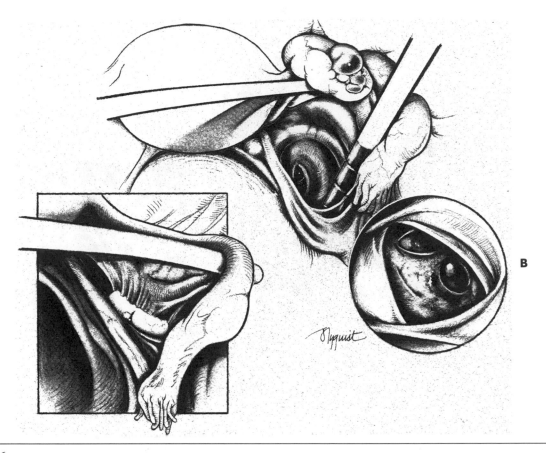

Figure 24-6
(Inset) Illustration of a large broad ligament recess sequestering the right ovary. Note ureter forming medial brim. **A,** Recess with ovary easily removed. Note peritoneal pocket in the floor. **B,** Close-up showing baffles and two deeper recesses. Biopsy revealed endometriosis. From Batt RE, Smith RA, Buck GM, Naples JD, and Severino MF: A case series-peritoneal pockets and endometriosis: Rudimentary duplications of the mullerian system. *Adolesc Pediatr Gynecol* 2:55, 1989.

the percentage of the population that has endometriosis at a given time. For practical day-to-day care of patients, clinicians should be aware of the four groups of women in whom the prevalence is highest: teenagers with intractable dysmenorrhea or pelvic pain; women with the diagnosis of or undergoing treatment for infertility, particularly primary infertility; women with pelvic pain; and women with pelvic masses.

Monthly fecundity and life table analyses that show the quality of the patient follow-up are two desirable methods of presenting the results of endometriosis research.[82] Multivariate statistical analysis techniques for categoric and continuous data are more sophisticated and "robust," meaning able to compensate for less than perfect data in terms of satisfying underlying assumptions. Analyzing available data, Wheeler and Malinak asked, "Does mild endometriosis cause infertility?"[83] More population-based data are needed to confirm this proposed tenuous association.

OFFICE ASSESSMENT OF ENDOMETRIOSIS
Age

Endometriosis may occur from menarche to menopause.[84] It is important to emphasize that it is a common finding at laparoscopy in adolescents who complain of pelvic pain.[9] The youngest with histologic evidence of endometriosis was a 10½-year-old who had menstruated only three times.[85] Most cases are detected during the third and fourth decades of life. The mean ages for patients with mild, moderate, and severe disease and infertility was 27 years.[86] Postmenopausal endometriosis has been recognized for many years.[87-90]

Family history

Less than 10% of patients with endometriosis have a family history of the disease.[91] They do, however, seem to have more severe disease at a younger age. History of endometriosis in a mother, sisters, aunts, or cousins of a patient complaining of pelvic pain or infertility should alert the physician to the possibility of the disease.

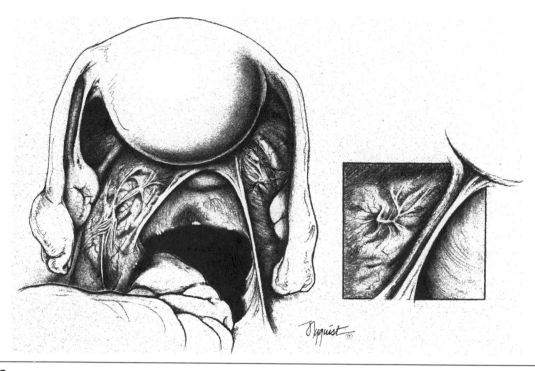

Figure 24-7
Attenuated and sharp-edged uterosacral ligaments. The left broad ligament contains a shallow
elliptical pocket with multiple spider nodules in the floor and posterior edge. Spider nodules are
raised in relief, with endometriosis in the central nodule and thick-walled blood vessels forming
the radiating spider legs. Note the normal coursing ureter lateral to the peritoneal pocket. (Inset
is a close-up from another case showing medially displaced ureter adjacent to the uterosacral
ligament. A spider nodule is in the floor of the broad ligament pocket.) From Batt RE and
Smith RA: Embryologic theory of histogenesis of endometriosis in peritoneal pockets. *Obstet
Gynecol Clin North Am* 16:21, 1989.

Pain

A history of increasing menstrual pain is strongly suggestive of endometriosis.[80] Pain in the adolescent does not
have to be of years duration. Goldstein et al, reporting
on their experience with endometriosis at the Adolescent
Unit of Boston Children's Hospital Medical Center,
stated:

> Certainly, the adolescent female, who has been menstruating
> for six months or more, who reports cyclic pelvic pain occurring
> just prior to or at the onset of menses and who has tenderness
> with or without nodularity on pelvic examination fits the classic
> description.[85]

Deep dyspareunia is usually associated with endometriotic involvement of the uterosacral ligaments or rectovaginal pouch. The surgeon may study the mechanism
of this disorder at laparoscopy by observing the distention
of the posterior vaginal fornix using a sponge stick. The
cervical ends of the uterosacral ligaments are displaced
laterally and superiorly and the uterus is lifted anteriorly
as the pressure of the sponge stick is absorbed by the
vaginal portion of the rectovaginal pouch.[24] Pain with

defecation, crampy abdominal pain, and rectal bleeding
at menses may herald bowel endometriosis.

Bleeding

A controlled epidemiologic study of women with endometriosis associated with primary infertility found that
women with short cycle length (≤ 27 days) and with long
menstrual flow (≥ 7 days) had more than double the risk
of developing endometriosis than those with longer cycles
and shorter duration of flow.[92] Menorrhagia, which is
due to a general hypertrophy of the endometrium or to
endometrial polyps, is common.[93] Premenstrual spotting
is reportedly associated with endometriosis.[94]

Endometriosis-associated infertility

The tentative diagnosis of endometriosis should be en-
tertained in all patients who complain of infertility. Two
studies employing artificial insemination donor in women
with and without endometriosis demonstrated decreased

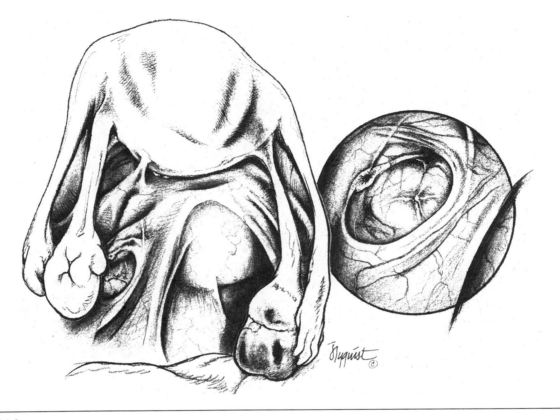

Figure 24-8
Illustration of a longitudinally oriented oval pocket in the left posterior broad ligament with a brim nodule at 9 o'clock and a spider nodule on the floor of the pocket (enlarged view). These are typical gross endometriotic lesions associated with peritoneal pockets. From Batt RE, Smith RA, Buck GM, Naples JD, and Severino MF: A case series-peritoneal pockets and endometriosis: Rudimentary duplications of the mullerian system. *Adolesc Pediatr Gynecol* 2:55, 1989.

fecundity (conception rate per cycle) in those with endometriosis, even minimal disease.[95,96] The risk for infertility is nearly 20 times greater in patients with endometriosis than in women without the condition.[97]

Women with endometriosis and primary infertility, secondary infertility, and pelvic symptomatology were compared with matched friend controls and medical controls.[1] It was found that 41% of patients with endometriosis had primary infertility, 35% had secondary infertility, and 27% had other pelvic symptomatology, including dysmenorrhea, irregular menstrual bleeding, and pelvic pain not associated with menstruation. Twenty-nine percent of the husbands were subfertile by the criteria of the American Fertility Society.

A rapid, structured infertility investigation should be completed before laparoscopic surgery. Time and timing are critical. Evaluation and treatment should be so coordinated that both husband and wife reach their peak fertility potential simultaneously, in this case, at the time of surgery for endometriosis.[98]

The first 15 months after surgery are the optimum times for conception.[99] When donor insemination is required, arrangements should be completed before surgery so that insemination can be performed during the best months for conception.

Health problems

Seven potential major health problems are associated with endometriosis: profuse, unremittant menorrhagia; intractable pelvic pain; bowel pain or obstruction; ureteral obstruction; osteoporosis; pneumothorax or hemothorax; and malignancy. During the course of diagnosis and evaluation of the disease, these disorders should be kept in mind.

Profuse, unremittant bleeding

This may be associated with ovulatory dysfunction, endometrial polyps, submucous fibroids, endometrial hyperplasia, or adenomyosis. Bleeding may be controlled in some women by hysteroscopy and thorough curettage followed by danazol, gonadotropin-releasing hormone

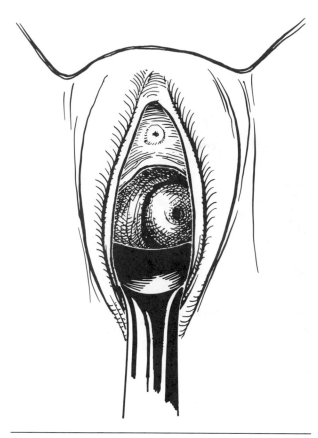

Figure 24-9
Lateral displacement of the cervix to the left or right of midline on inspection of the upper vagina through a speculum is an early and usually reliable sign of pelvic endometriosis.

(GnRH), or cyclic oral medroxyprogesterone or norethindrone. When this treatment is unsuccessful, endometrial ablation or hysterectomy may be required.

Intractable pelvic pain

Deep, infiltrating endometriotic nodules with active stromal and glandular tissue are a particularly important cause of pelvic pain. These lesions especially involve the bladder pillars, uterosacral ligaments, and rectovaginal pouch, penetrating through into the posterior vaginal fornix or deeply into the rectum, or extending laterally in the cardinal ligaments to impinge on the ureters. Although they may respond temporarily to medical suppression, surgical excision of all endometriosis and complete removal of ovarian tissue at hysterectomy are the only means to provide complete relief of pain.

Bowel pain or obstruction

The gastrointestinal tract is the most common site of extrapelvic endometriosis, being present in 8% of patients at laparoscopy and laparotomy.[100,101] Patients usually do not volunteer a history of bowel complaints; this must be sought actively by the physician during a review of systems. Women experiencing pain with bowel movements preceding or during menses should be examined for endometriosis of the rectum and sigmoid colon. Those with a history of endometriosis and crampy abdominal pain should be suspected of having endometriosis of the small or large bowel. Both problems can occur before and after menopause.

Flexible sigmoidoscopy, colonoscopy, barium enema, and small bowel series may be used selectively to study the bowel lumen. In our hands, flexible sigmoidoscopy is the most consistently positive examination, and painful, fixed angulation is the most common finding. Sigmoidoscopy performed premenstrually or during menstruation is ideal to detect endometriosis of the bowel mucosa.

Biopsy at endoscopy differentiates endometriosis from malignancy, but this crucial differential diagnosis really only involves patients with a mucosal lesion. Most lesions of endometriosis of the bowel involve the serosa and muscularis, not the mucosa. The disease starts externally and invades the muscularis and occasionally the mucosa; primary cancer of the bowel starts in the mucosa and invades the muscularis.

Small bowel endometriosis causing intermittent or complete obstruction requires bowel resection.[102] Disease at the appendiceal-cecal junction can cause obstruction requiring appendectomy. Stenosis may be observed, but obstruction of the rectum, sigmoid colon, and cecum is uncommon because of the large caliber of the bowel lumen, and perforation is uncommon.[103] Large or bulky lesions and those threatening partial obstruction should be treated by extraluminal resection when possible, or by wedge resection or segmental bowel resection.[100,104,105] Medical treatment of endometriosis is not without hazard; ischemic colitis was reported with danazol therapy.[106]

With the universal availability of laparoscopy, every gynecologist and general surgeon has an opportunity to diagnose endometriosis of the rectum, sigmoid colon, appendix, ileum, cecum, and ascending colon before the lesions become a health problem. Bowel endometriosis should be staged according to the classification and stages of the extragenital disease.[100]

Ureteral obstruction

Endometriosis may invade the serosa (extrinsic) or muscularis and/or mucosa (intrinsic) of the ureter, causing fixation of the ureter and physiologic obstruction of the peristaltic waves without narrowing or compromising the lumen. Further progression of the disease, however, can cause partial or complete ureteral luminal obstruction.[107-109] The disease may involve the ureteral orifice, the bladder wall, or the pelvic ureter up to the pelvic inlet.

Ureteral obstruction is insidious and should be suspected whenever a patient with endometriosis complains of repeated urinary tract infections, hematuria, or flank pain. Characteristically, the symptoms are related to the menstrual cycle. The disorder should also be sought in patients with locally severe endometriosis that involves the broad ligaments, cardinal ligaments, or uterosacral ligaments, and in those with complete obliteration of the rectovaginal pouch or a left frozen pelvis.

Partial or complete ureteral obstruction may occur from direct invasion by endometriosis or from fibrosis. Complete obstruction is not common but it may occur, leading to silent death of a kidney and hypertension.[110] At every laparoscopy and laparotomy for endometriosis, the ureters should be identified and examined along their entire pelvic course for evidence of endometriotic involvement. Ureteral peristalsis should be observed. The usual treatment is ureterolysis, although segmental resection or reimplantation of the ureter into the bladder may be necessary.

Osteoporosis

Patients with endometriosis seem to be at increased risk for osteoporosis; studies have shown a reduced bone mass and evidence of high-turnover bone loss.[111-113] Other investigators concluded that bone mineral mass of patients with endometriosis was not significantly different from the normal population; however, use of a GnRh agonist for 6 months or more induced significant loss of vertebral bone mineral content.[114]

Preservation of ovarian function is desirable in patients with endometriosis to preserve bone mass. In our opinion, excision of endometriosis at laparoscopy or laparotomy is preferred over repeated courses of medical suppression, which at best are only a temporizing procedure and at worst deplete the bone mineral content.

Women with endometriosis who enter the menopause naturally or surgically should be treated with estrogen and progesterone replacement therapy to prevent osteoporosis. We initially prescribe conjugated estrogen 0.625 to 0.9 mg and medroxyprogesterone 2.5 mg daily, preferably after excision of all endometriosis. This therapy should induce some atrophic changes in microscopic endometriosis, as it does in the endometrium. We have observed exacerbation of the disorder in patients treated with estrogen replacement alone.

Pneumothorax and hemothorax

Endometriosis involving the lung or thoracic cavity occurs in one of four ways: catamenial pneumothorax (22% had concurrent pelvic endometriosis and 95% involved the right chest), catamenial hemothorax (100% involved the right lung and all had concurrent pelvic endometriosis), catamenial hemoptysis (none had concurrent pelvic endometriosis), and asymptomatic pulmonary nodules (20% had concurrent pelvic endometriosis).[100] The evidence suggests that any of these manifestations would support the clinical diagnosis of pulmonary endometriosis until proved otherwise.

Bronchoscopy, thoracentesis, and thoracoscopy may be followed by medical suppression with danazol or GnRH analogs. The most successful therapy of pulmonary nodules and recurrent pulmonary endometriosis includes thoracotomy, excision of endometriosis, and pleurodesis by either chemical or abrasive techniques.[100] This disease is frightening to patients, and in our experience they readily submit to thoracotomy when it is recurrent. Fortunately, it is predominately right sided, so that the risk for bilateral pneumothorax is probably small.

Malignancy

Severe atypia was reported in 3.5% of women with ovarian endometriosis.[115] The lesion is considered potentially malignant. It was proposed that patients with "atypical endometriosis" should be placed under long-term observation.[116] Adenocarcinoma, adenoacanthoma, clear cell carcinoma, and endometrioid carcinoma are the most common ovarian malignancies associated with atypical ovarian endometriosis.

Pathologists should emphasize foci of atypical endometriotic epithelium in their reports, since these lesions might well be the morphologic substrate of epithelium with malignant potential.[55] It might be well for all of us to alert pathologists to highlight reports of moderate and severe atypical changes in endometriotic specimens.

Of 75 endometrioid carcinomas of the ovary, 49 were histologically pure and 26 showed histologic admixtures of other neoplasms of mullerian derivation.[117] Fifty-three percent of ovarian mixed epithelial papillary cystadenomas of borderline malignancy of mullerian type were associated with endometriosis; the patients' average age was 35 years.[54] This report lends further credence to the importance of histologic evaluation of all ovarian cysts and tumors.

Physical appearance

Women with endometriosis cannot be distinguished from other women with gynecologic problems on the basis of their body measurements.

Obstruction of menses

Congenital anomalies of the vagina, cervix, or uterus that partially or completely obstruct the menstrual flow increase the likelihood of endometriosis.[118,119] These conditions should be considered especially in the young adolescent with pelvic pain and slight or absent menstrual flow. Cryosurgery or deep cauterization of the cervix may cause significant cervical stenosis and ultimately endometriosis in women exposed to diethylstilbestrol in utero.[120]

Lateral displacement of the cervix

Normally, the cervix is a midline structure in direct alignment with the urethra and anus. In adolescent and adult women with endometriosis, inspection often reveals the cervix displaced 1 cm or more to the left or right of midline because of shortening of one cardinal ligament that resists efforts to push the cervix back to the midline position. This diagnostic sign is particularly useful in the nulliparous female who has pelvic pain or infertility.

Nodules

Tender nodules in the rectovaginal pouch of Douglas or in the uterosacral ligaments strongly suggest the presence of endometriosis. Clinically, tenderness precedes the development of nodules and may be elicited by vaginal, rectovaginal, or rectal examination, particularly if performed in the premenstrual or menstrual phase of the cycle. In the premenopausal patient, ovarian carcinoma can also cause cul-de-sac and uterosacral ligament nodularity, and should be investigated.

DIAGNOSIS

Until a reliable noninvasive test for endometriosis is clinically available, laparoscopy remains the sine qua non for the diagnosis. When a noninvasive test is available, laparoscopic surgery will still be important for staging, mapping, and treating the disease. A high index of clinical suspicion combined with a concerted effort to make the diagnosis early will render more cases amenable to pelvic laparoscopic surgery with relief of pain, restoration of fertility, and maintenance of health.

Before laparoscopy, the priorities of the patient and her husband may be recorded and compared (Table 24-2).

TREATMENT

Treatment of endometriosis may be discussed rationally with the patient based on Sampson's paradigm of retrograde menstrual dissemination, local inflammation, and implantation.[40,121-123]

Barriers to normal menstruation should be removed: imperforate hymen, transverse vaginal septum, obstructed duplicate vagina, cervical stenosis, and functional blind uterine horn. Endometriosis may be excised from reproductive, urinary, and gastrointestinal organs by laparoscopic or microconservative surgery. Retrograde menstruation and local inflammation may be reduced by prescribing cyclic oral progestogens and regular vigorous exercise. Retrograde menstruation and local inflammation may be eliminated temporarily by pregnancy and lactation or by prescribing continuous progestogens, danazol, or GnRH analogs. Permanent amenorrhea and/or elimination of retrograde menstruation may be obtained by endometrial ablation, hysterectomy, bilateral

Table 24-2 Priorities

	Patient	Husband
Comfort	2	2
Fertility	1	3
Health	3	1

This set of priorities is typical of an infertile couple in whom pain is a significant factor. Seeing them in graphic form is an excellent mechanism for meaningful discussion and understanding, and serves as a bench mark for future discussions.

Table 24-3 Treatment options

Treatment	Patient	Husband	Physician
Expectant	0	0	0
Medical suppression	0	0	0
Laparoscopic surgery	1	1	1
Microconservative surgery	(1)	(1)	(1)
Ovulation stimulation	2	2	2
Intrauterine insemination	2	2	2
Artificial insemination by donor	0	0	(2)
Gamete intrafallopian transfer	3	3	3
In vitro fertilization with embryo transfer	0	0	3
Partial zona drilling	0	0	4
Adoption	(3)	0	(4)

The treatment options shown in Table 24-3 are typical for an infertile couple with severe endometriosis and both ovulatory and semen dysfunction in whom, for financial or religious reasons, IVF/ET is not an option. The graphic form is helpful for working out options and for long-term management. A patient with pelvic pain as the main problem might choose laparoscopic surgery followed by medical suppression.

oophorectomy, 1500 rad of radiation to the ovaries, and partial or complete salpingectomy.

REFERENCES

1. Darrow S: Case-control study of the relationship of reproductive factors to the risk of endometriosis, doctoral dissertation, Department of Social and Preventive Medicine, 1991, State University of New York at Buffalo.
2. Haney AF: Etiology and histogenesis of endometriosis, *Prog Clin Biol Res* 323:1-14, 1990.
3. Halme J and Surrey ES: Endometriosis and infertility: the mechanisms involved, *Prog Clin Biol Res* 323:157-178, 1990.
4. Dmowski WP, Braun D, and Gebel HJ: Endometriosis: genetic and immunologic aspects, *Prog Clin Biol Res* 323:99-122, 1990.
5. Schweppe KW: Endometriotic lesions: location, gross, histologic, and ultrastructural aspects, *Prog Clin Biol Res* 323:33-47, 1990.
6. Brosens IA: Evolution of endometriotic lesions: is endometriosis a progressive disease? *Prog Clin Biol Res* 323:151-156, 1990.

7. Batt RE et al: Mullerianosis, *Prog Clin Biol Res* 323:413-426, 1990.
8. Vernon MW: Experimental endometriosis in laboratory animals as a research model, *Prog Clin Biol Res* 323:49-60, 1990.
9. Goldstein DP, Cholnoky CD, and Emans SJ: Adolescent endometriosis, *J Adolesc Health Care* 1:37, 1980.
10. Chatman DL and Zbella EA: Pelvic peritoneal defects and endometriosis: further observations, *Fertil Steril* 46:711, 1986.
11. Vernon MW et al: Classification of endometriotic implants by morphologic appearance and capacity to synthesize prostaglandin F, *Fertil Steril* 46:801, 1986.
12. Jansen RPS and Russell P: Nonpigmented endometriosis: clinical, laparoscopic, and pathologic definition, *Am J Obstet Gynecol* 155:1154, 1986.
13. Redwine DB: Age-related evolution in color appearance of endometriosis, *Fertil Steril* 48:1062, 1987.
14. Stripling MC et al: Subtle appearance of pelvic endometriosis, *Fertil Steril* 49:427, 1988.
15. Batt RE et al: A case series—peritoneal pockets and endometriosis: rudimentary duplications of the mullerian system, *Adolesc Pediatr Gynecol* 2:47-56, 1989.
16. Murphy A et al: Unsuspected endometriosis documented by scanning electron microscopy in visually normal peritoneum, *Fertil Steril* 46:522-524, 1986.
17. Redwine DB: Is "microscopic" peritoneal endometriosis invisible? *Fertil Steril* 50:665-666, 1988.
18. Redwine DB: Peritoneal blood painting: an aid in the diagnosis of endometriosis, *Am J Obstet Gynecol* 161:865-866, 1989.
19. Vasquez G, Cornillie F, and Brosens IA: Peritoneal endometriosis: scanning electron microscopy and histology on minimal pelvic endometriotic lesions, *Fertil Steril* 42:696, 1984.
20. Cornillie F: The normal peritoneum. Peritoneal endometriosis. Ovarian endometriosis. In Brosens I and Gordon A (eds): *Tubal Infertility*, Philadelphia, 1990, JB Lippincott.
21. Sampson JA: Benign and malignant endometrial implants in peritoneal cavity, and their relation to certain ovarian tumors, *Surg Gynecol Obstet* 38:287, 1924.
22. Goodall JR: *A study of endometriosis, endosalpingiosis, endocervicosis, and peritoneo-ovarian sclerosis: a clinical and pathologic study*, Philadelphia, 1943, JB Lippincott.
23. Sturgis SH and Call BJ: Endometriosis peritonei: relationship of pain to functional activity, *Am J Obstet Gynecol* 68:1421, 1954.
24. Batt RE and Naples JD: Conservative surgery for endometriosis in the infertile couple, *Curr Probl Obstet Gynecol* 6:70, 1982.
25. Martin DC: *Laparoscopic appearance of endometriosis: an atlas*, ed 2, vol 3, Memphis, 1990, Resurge Press.
26. Hughesdon PE: The structure of endometrial cysts of the ovary, *J Obstet Gynaecol Br Emp* 64:481-487, 1957.
27. Barbieri RL: Etiology and epidemiology for endometriosis, *Am J Obstet Gynecol* 162:565-567, 1990.
28. Lauchlan SC: The cytology of endometriosis, *Am J Obstet Gynecol* 94:533, 1966.
29. Clement PB: Endometriosis, lesions of the secondary mullerian system, and pelvic mesothelial proliferations. In Kurman RJ (ed): *Blaustein's pathology of the female genital tract*, ed 3, New York, 1987, Springer-Verlag.
30. Barbieri RL: Endometriosis, *Curr Probl Obstet Gynecol Fertil* 12:9-31, 1989.
31. Stripling MC, Martin DC, and Poston WM: Does endometriosis have a typical appearance? *J Reprod Med* 33:879-84, 1988.
32. Batt RE and Smith RA: Embryologic theory of histogenesis of endometriosis in peritoneal pockets, *Obstet Gynecol Clin North Am* 16:15-28, 1989.
33. American Fertility Society: Revised American Fertility Society classification of endometriosis, *Fertil Steril* 43:351, 1985.
34. Koninckx PR et al: New aspects of the pathophysiology of endometriosis and associated infertility, *J Reprod Med* 24:257-260, 1980.
35. Muse KN and Wilson EA: How does mild endometriosis cause infertility? *Fertil Steril* 38:145-152, 1982.
36. Surrey ES and Halme J: Endometriosis as a cause of infertility, *Obstet Gynecol Clin North Am* 16:79-92, 1989.
37. Dmowski WP, Gebel HM, and Rawlins RG: Immunologic aspects of endometriosis, *Obstet Gynecol Clin North Am* 16:93-104, 1989.
38. Batt RE: Endometriosis: implantation endometriosis and treatment of minimal endometriosis and infertility. In Stangel JJ (ed): *Infertility surgery*, Norwalk, Conn, 1990, Appleton and Lange.
39. Buttram VC Jr: Surgical treatment of endometriosis in the infertile female: a modified approach, *Fertil Steril* 32:635, 1979.
40. Sampson JA: The development of the implantation theory for the origin of peritoneal endometriosis, *Am J Obstet Gynecol* 40:549, 1940.
41. Jenkins S, Olive DL, and Haney AF: Endometriosis: pathogenic implications of the anatomic distribution, *Obstet Gynecol* 67:335, 1986.
42. Lox CD, Word L, and Heine MW: Ultrastructural evaluation of endometriosis. Paper presented at the fortieth annual meeting of the American Fertility Society, New Orleans, April 1984.
43. Ahn GH and Scully RE: Clear cell carcinoma of the inguinal region arising from endometriosis, *Cancer* 67:116-120, 1991.
44. Hitti IF, Glasberg SS, and Lubicz S: Clear cell carcinoma arising in extraovarian endometriosis: report of three cases and review of the literature, *Gynecol Oncol* 39:314-320, 1990.
45. Granai CO et al: Malignant transformation of vaginal endometriosis, *Obstet Gynecol* 64:592, 1984.
46. Reimnitz C et al: Malignancy arising in endometriosis associated with unopposed estrogen replacement, *Obstet Gynecol* 71:444-447, 1988.
47. Berkowitz RS, Ehrman RL, and Knapp RC: Endometrial stromal sarcoma arising from vaginal endometriosis, *Obstet Gynecol* 51:34s-37s, 1978.
48. Orr JW Jr, Holiomon JL, and Sisson PF: Vaginal adenocarcinoma developing in residual pelvic endometriosis: a clinical dilemma, *Gynecol Oncol* 33:96-98, 1989.
49. Addison WA, Hammond CB, and Parker RT: The occurrence of adenocarcinoma in endometriosis of the rectovaginal septum during progestational therapy, *Gynecol Oncol* 8:193, 1979.
50. Sampson JA: Endometrial carcinoma of the ovary arising in endometrial tissue in that organ, *Arch Surg* 10:1-72, 1925.
51. Scully RE, Richardson GS, and Barlow JF: The development of malignancy in endometriosis, *Clin Obstet Gynecol* 9:384, 1966.
52. Mostoufizadeh M and Scully RE: Malignant tumors arising in endometriosis, *Clin Obstet Gynecol* 23:951, 1980.
53. Baiocchi G, Kavanagh JJ, and Wharton JT: Endometrial stromal sarcomas arising from ovarian and extraovarian endometriosis: report of two cases and review of the literature, *Gynecol Oncol* 36:147-151, 1990.
54. Rutgers JL and Scully RE: Ovarian mixed-epithelial papillary cystadenomas of borderline malignancy of mullerian type: a clinicopathologic analysis, *Cancer* 61:546-554, 1988.
55. Moll UM et al: Ovarian carcinoma arising in atypical endometriosis, *Obstet Gynecol* 75:237-239, 1990.
56. Fox H: Malignant potential of benign ovarian cysts: the case against. In Sharp F, Mason WP, and Leake RE (eds): *Ovarian cancer*, New York, 1990, WW Norton.
57. Corner GW Jr, Hu C-Y, and Hertig AT: Ovarian carcinoma arising in endometriosis, *Am J Obstet Gynecol* 59:760, 1950.
58. Grant A: Additional sterility factors in endometriosis, *Fertil Steril* 17:514, 1966.
59. Halme J and Hall JL: Effect of pelvic fluid from endometriosis patients on human sperm penetration of zona-free hamster ova, *Fertil Steril* 37:573, 1982.
60. Halme J and Mathur S: Local autoimmunity in mild endometriosis, *Int J Fertil* 32:309, 1987.

61. Badawy SZ et al: Immune rosettes of T and B lymphocytes in infertile women with endometriosis, *J Reprod Med* 32:194, 1987.

62. Halme J et al: Peritoneal macrophages from patients with endometriosis release growth factor activity in vitro, *J Clin Endocrinol Metab* 66:1044, 1988.

63. Halme J, Becker S, and Wing R: Accentuated cyclic activation of peritoneal macrophages in patients with endometriosis, *Am J Obstet Gynecol* 148:85, 1984.

64. Confino E, Harlow L, and Gleicher N: Peritoneal fluid and serum autoantibody levels in patients with endometriosis, *Fertil Steril* 53:242-245, 1990.

65. Muscato JJ, Haney AF, and Weinberg JB: Sperm phagocytosis by human peritoneal macrophages: a possible cause of infertility in endometriosis, *Am J Obstet Gynecol* 144:503, 1982.

66. Chacho KJ, Anderson PJ, and Scommegna A: The effect of peritoneal macrophage incubates on the spermatozoa assay, *Fertil Steril* 48:694, 1987.

67. Suginami H et al: A factor inhibiting ovum capture by the oviductal fimbriae present in endometriosis peritoneal fluid, *Fertil Steril* 46:1140, 1986.

68. Sueldo CE et al: The effect of peritoneal fluid from patients with endometriosis on murine sperm-oocyte interaction, *Fertil Steril* 48:697, 1987.

69. Oak MK et al: Sperm survival studies in peritoneal fluid from infertile women with endometriosis and unexplained infertility, *Clin Reprod Fertil* 3:297, 1985.

70. Czernobilsky B and Silverstein A: Salpingitis in ovarian endometriosis, *Fertil Steril* 30:45, 1978.

71. Ohtsuka N: Study on pathogenesis of adhesions in endometriosis, *Acta Obstet Gynaecol Jpn* 32:1758, 1980.

72. Winston R: Reconstructive microsurgery at the lateral end of the fallopian tube. In Chamberlain G and Winston R (eds): *Tubal infertility*, New York, 1982, Blackwell.

73. Garcia CR and Mastroianni L Jr: Microsurgery for treatment of adnexal disease, *Fertil Steril* 34:413, 1980.

74. Boeckx W, Gordts S, and Brosens IA: Techniques for microsurgical repair of the ovary. In Phillips JM (ed): *Microsurgery in gynecology,* vol 2, Downey, Calif, 1981, American Association of Gynecologic Laparoscopists.

75. Hodgen GD: Surrogate embryo transfer combined with estrogen-progesterone therapy in monkeys; implantation, gestation and delivery without ovaries, *JAMA* 250:2167-2171, 1983.

76. Hodgen GD: Embryo transfer, implantation, and the uterine endometrium. Paper presented at the fortieth annual meeting of the American Fertility Society, New Orleans, April 1984.

77. Ellis H: The aetiology of post-operative abdominal adhesions—an experimental study, *Br J Surg* 50:10-16, 1962.

78. Ellis H: Prevention and treatment of adhesions, *Infect Surg* 2:803-817, 1983.

79. Hulka JF: Adnexal adhesions: a prognostic staging and classification system based on a five-year survey of fertility surgery results at Chapel Hill, N.C., *Am J Obstet Gynecol* 144:141, 1982.

80. Goldman MB and Cramer DW: The epidemiology of endometriosis, *Prog Clin Biol Res* 323:15-31, 1990.

81. Cramer DW: Epidemiology of endometriosis. In Wilson EA (ed): *Endometriosis*, New York, 1987, Alan R. Liss.

82. Wheeler JM: Statistical methods in evaluating endometriosis, *Prog Clin Biol Res* 323:443-448, 1990.

83. Wheeler JM and Malinak LR: Does mild endometriosis cause infertility? *Semin Reprod Endocrinol* 6:239, 1988.

84. Batt RE and Severino MF: Endometriosis: from menarche to menopause. In Stangle JJ (ed): *Infertility surgery*, Norwalk Conn, 1990, Appleton and Lange.

85. Goldstein DP et al: New insights into the old problem of chronic pelvic pain, *J Pediatr Surg* 14:675, 1979.

86. Houston DE: Evidence for the risk of endometriosis by age, race, and socioeconomic status, *Epidemiol Rev* 6:167, 1984.

87. Kempers RD et al: Significant postmenopausal endometriosis, *Surg Gynecol Obstet* 111:348, 1960.

88. Punnonen R, Klemi P, and Nikkanen R: Postmenopausal endometriosis, *Eur J Obstet Gynecol Reprod Biol* 11:195, 1980.

89. Faulkner RL and Riemenschneider EA: Reactivation of endometriosis by stilbestrol therapy, *Am J Obstet Gynecol* 105:560, 1945.

90. Schram JD: Endometriosis after "pelvic cleanout," *South Med J* 71:1419, 1978.

91. Malinak LR et al: Heritable aspects of endometriosis. II. Clinical characteristics of familial endometriosis, *Am J Obstet Gynecol* 137:332, 1980.

92. Cramer DW et al: The relation of endometriosis to menstrual characteristics, smoking, and exercise, *JAMA* 255:1904-1908, 1985.

93. Beilby JOW, Farrer-Brown G, and Tarbit MH: The microvasculature of common uterine abnormalities other than fibroids, *J Obstet Gynaecol Br Common* 78:361, 1971.

94. Wentz AC: Premenstrual spotting: its association with endometriosis but not luteal phase inadequacy, *Fertil Steril* 33:605, 1980.

95. Rodriguez-Escudero PJ et al: Does minimal endometriosis reduce fecundity, *Fertil Steril* 50:522-524, 1988.

96. Jansen RP: Minimal endometriosis and reduced fecundability: prospective evidence from an artificial insemination by donor program, *Fertil Steril* 46:41-43, 1986.

97. Strathy JH et al: Endometriosis and infertility: a laparoscopic study of endometriosis among fertile and infertile women, *Fertil Steril* 38:667, 1982.

98. Sadigh H, Naples JD, and Batt RE: Conservative surgery for endometriosis in the infertile couple, *Obstet Gynecol* 49:562, 1977.

99. Buttram VC Jr and Betts JW: Endometriosis, *Curr Probl Obstet Gynecol* 2:11, 1979.

100. Markham SM, Carpenter SE, and Rock JA: Extrapelvic endometriosis, *Obstet Gynecol Clin North Am* 16:193-219, 1989.

101. Wheeler JM et al: Gastrointestinal endometriosis. Paper presented at the First International Endometriosis Symposium, Clermont-Ferrand, France, Nov 19-21, 1986.

102. Haines JD Jr: Ileal endometriosis: a difficult preoperative diagnosis, *Postgrad Med* 85:145-146, 1989.

103. Ledley GS, Shenk IM, and Heit HA: Sigmoid colon perforation due to endometriosis not associated with pregnancy, *Am J Gastroenterol* 83:1424-1426, 1988.

104. Weed JC and Ray JE: Endometriosis of the bowel, *Obstet Gynecol* 69:727, 1987.

105. Coronado C et al: Surgical treatment of symptomatic colorectal endometriosis, *Fertil Steril* 53:411-416, 1990.

106. Miyata T, Tamechika Y, and Torisu M: Ischemic colitis in a 33-year-old-woman on danazol treatment for endometriosis, *Am J Gastroenterol* 83:1420-1423, 1988.

107. Moore JG et al: Urinary tract endometriosis: enigmas in diagnosis and management, *Am J Obstet Gynecol* 134:162-172, 1979.

108. Pittaway DE et al: Recurrence of ureteral obstruction caused by endometriosis after danazol therapy, *Am J Obstet Gynecol* 143:720-722, 1982.

109. Appel RA: Bilateral ureteral obstruction secondary to endometriosis, *Urology* 32:151-154, 1988.

110. Davis OK and Schiff I: Endometriosis with unilateral ureteral obstruction and hypertension: a case report, *J Reprod Med* 33:420-422, 1988.

111. Parvizi ST et al: Serum osteocalcin (SBGP) indicates high turnover bone loss in women with endometriosis. Paper presented at the forty-fourth annual meeting of the American Fertility Society, Atlanta, October 1988.

112. Hutchinson-Williams K et al: Disordered calcium homeostasis and decreased bone mass in endometriosis. Paper presented at the forty-fourth annual meeting of the American Fertility Society, Atlanta, October 1988.

113. Comite F et al: Reduced bone mass in reproductive-aged women with endometriosis, *J Clin Endocrinol Metab* 69:837-842, 1989.

114. Dawood MY, Lewis V, and Ramos J: Cortical and trabecular bone mineral content in women with endometriosis: effect of gonadotropin-releasing hormone agonist and danazol, *Fertil Steril* 52:21-26, 1989.

115. Czernobilsky B and Morris WJ: A histologic study of ovarian endometriosis with emphasis on hyperplastic and atypical changes, *Obstet Gynecol* 53:318-322, 1979.

116. LaGrenade A and Silverberg SG: Ovarian tumors associated with atypical endometriosis, *Hum Pathol* 129:1080-1084, 1988.

117. Czernobilsky B, Silverman BB, and Mikut a JJ: Endometrioid carcinoma of the ovary, *Cancer* 26:1141, 1970.

118. Huffman JW: Endometriosis in young teen-age girls, *Pediatr Ann* 10:501, 1981.

119. Hanton EM et al: Endometriosis associated with complete or partial obstruction of menstrual egress, *Obstet Gynecol* 28:626, 1966.

120. Haney AF and Hammond MG: Infertility in women exposed to diethylstilbestrol in utero, *J Reprod Med* 28:851, 1983.

121. Halme J et al: Pelvic macrophages in normal and infertile women: the role of patent tubes, *Am J Obstet Gynecol* 142:890, 1982.

122. Halme J et al: Retrograde menstruation in healthy women and in patients with endometriosis, *Obstet Gynecol* 64:151, 1984.

123. Berger NG and Rock JA: Peritoneal fluid environment in endometriosis, *Semin Reprod Endocrinol* 3:313, 1985.

25

Endometriosis: Advanced Diagnostic Laparoscopy

RONALD E. BATT

JAMES M. WHEELER

Advanced diagnostic laparoscopy requires a three-puncture technique and an intrauterine manipulator, as well as vaginal and rectal probes selectively, for systematic observation and recording of positive and negative findings on a pelvic map.[1] The first laparoscopy is the benchmark by which all subsequent progression, regression, or stability of endometriosis is measured.

At laparoscopy gynecologists have a natural tendency to focus attention on conspicuous ovarian and peritoneal endometriosis and perform little more than a cursory examination of the bowel and ureters. However, the pelvis is a complex conical structure. In addition to the pelvic floor, with its superficial and deep structures, the urinary, reproductive, and gastrointestinal tracts may be involved with significant endometriosis. Only by a rigorous examination of all these structures can one hope to develop a comprehensive view of the disease process in each individual. Successful treatment and follow-up are based on accurate diagnosis.

ALPHA SEQUENCE EXAMINATION

The alpha sequence[2] (Figure 25-1) examination and palpation of the bowel, ureters, and reproductive organs is a precise technique to diagnosis and stage extragenital endometriosis according to the classification of Markham, Carpenter, and Rock,[3] and pelvic endometriosis according to the American Fertility Society revised classification for endometriosis.[4] The organs are examined in a specific sequence:

1. The anterior abdominal wall, bladder, round ligaments, uterus, uterosacral ligaments, rectovaginal pouch, rectum, and sigmoid colon.
2. This naturally leads the surgeon's eye to the left anterior broad ligament, left fallopian tube, left ovary, left posterior broad ligament, and left ureter.
3. The examination is carried to the right anterior broad ligament, right fallopian tube, right ovary, right posterior broad ligament, and right ureter.
4. Finally, the vermiform appendix, distal 50 to 100 cm of ileum, cecum, ascending colon, gallbladder, liver, diaphragms, stomach, and omentum are examined.

ANATOMY
Rectovaginal pouch

We prefer the nomenclature rectovaginal pouch to cul-de-sac because it calls attention to the rectum and pararectal tissues that form the posterior portion and to the vaginal and paravaginal tissues that form the anterior portion of this structure.

The anatomy of the rectovaginal pouch and rectovaginal septum was studied in living humans.[5] The mean depth of the pouch did not differ significantly in nulliparous (5.3 ± 0.5 cm) and multiparous women (5.4 ± 0.4 cm). What is particularly important to understanding endometriosis is that in 93% of women studied, the floor of the rectovaginal pouch normally extended to the middle one third of the vagina; in only 7% was it related to the upper one third (Figure 25-2).

This anatomic configuration allows endometriosis of the rectovaginal pouch to penetrate anteriorly into the vaginal wall or full thickness into the posterior vaginal fornix. Similarly, it may penetrate posteriorly into the rectum or full thickness through the rectal wall.

When disease obliterates the rectovaginal pouch, it is commonly and erroneously referred to as endometriosis of the rectovaginal septum because the lesions are palpated within the tissues between the rectum and the vagina. In reality, the examiner is palpating endometriosis of the obliterated rectovaginal pouch that may include disease of the uterosacral ligaments, rectum, and pos-

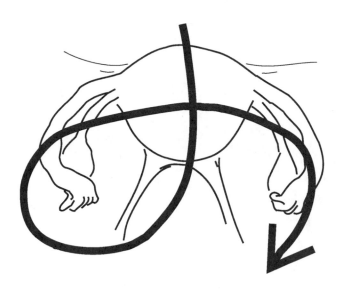

"Alpha" Sequence

Figure 25-1
The alpha sequence examination for endometriosis. From Batt RE, Naples JD, and Severino MF: Endometriosis. In Piver MS (ed): *Manual of gynecology and gynecologic oncology*. Boston, 1989, Little, Brown & Co.

terior vaginal fornix but not of the rectovaginal septum. The rectovaginal septum is a solid fascial structure that begins where the lowermost portion of the rectovaginal pouch ends.

Rectovaginal septum

The rectovaginal septum has been studied in human specimens between 8 fetal weeks and 100 years of age.[6] Formed by the fusion of the walls of the fetal peritoneal pouch, it extends from the caudal margin of the rectovaginal pouch to the proximal edge of the perineal body.[7] Failure of normal fusion during early life may produce a congenitally deep rectovaginal pouch without a rectovaginal septum. This would permit endometriosis to invade the vagina and rectum at a lower level.

During research on endometriosis associated with peritoneal pockets,[8] we found that pockets in the floor of the rectovaginal pouch descended for variable distances into the rectovaginal space, anterior to the rectovaginal septum. They were not attached to the vagina or the rectum. They were easily everted and excised, except in one patient in whom a pocket was fused to the perineal body.

Although menstrual detritus may occasionally settle to the bottom of peritoneal pockets within the rectovaginal space, it is probably an uncommon cause of rectal endometriosis. The pockets are usually potential spaces until they are distended by carbon dioxide and their orifices exposed by upward traction of the rectum at laparoscopy.

Anatomic divisions of the small and large bowel

The small intestine is divided into the duodenum, jejunum, and ileum. The large intestine consists of the cecum and vermiform appendix, ascending colon, transverse colon, descending colon, sigmoid colon, rectum, and anal canal.[9]

The vermiform appendix projects from the cecum. The ileocecal junction marks the division of the cecum below and the ascending colon above. The ascending colon extends upward to the hepatic flexure. The transverse colon runs from the hepatic flexure to the splenic flexure. The descending colon extends from the splenic flexure to the medial border of the psoas muscle, where it becomes the sigmoid colon. The sigmoid colon has a mesentery fixed at the junction with the descending colon above and at the junction with the rectum below, anterior to the third sacral segment. The sigmoid colon lies mainly in the left side of the pelvis and may vary in length from 15 to over 60 cm. Patients with a long sigmoid colon may have a distinct rectosigmoid flexure or angulation. The rectum begins at the third sacral segment and follows the curve of the sacrum and coccyx. As it passes through the levator muscles it becomes the anal canal, which terminates at the anus.

Anatomic divisions of the ureter

The ileopectineal line divides the ureter into abdominal and pelvic portions.[10] The pelvic ureter is divided into three parts: the pars posterior that runs from the level of the sacroiliac joint along the lateral pelvic wall to the entrance of the preformed tunnel in the broad ligament; the pars intermedia, which runs within the broad ligament to the vesicouterine ligament; and the pars anterior, which runs from the entrance into the vesicouterine ligament to the ureteral orifice of the bladder.

The left ureter may be found above the iliopectineal line at the apex of the intersigmoid fossa by displacing the sigmoid colon medially and cephalad with one instrument and the left adnexa anterolaterally with the second lower quadrant instrument. Normal peristalsis should be observed. If the peritoneum is thickened or the ureter is not readily apparent, it may be located lateral to the pulsations of the hypogastric artery. The right ureter crosses the iliac vessels at the bifurcation of the common iliac artery and is easier to locate than the left ureter.

Anatomic landmarks

The following pelvic landmarks keep the surgeon oriented. Deep epigastric vessels determine the location of second and third puncture instruments and are located just lateral to the lateral umbilical folds. The round ligaments bear a constant relationship to the uterus distorted by congenital anomalies, fibroids, or adhesions. The uterosacral ligaments are located medial to the lower pelvic ureters; the hypogastric arteries are located medial

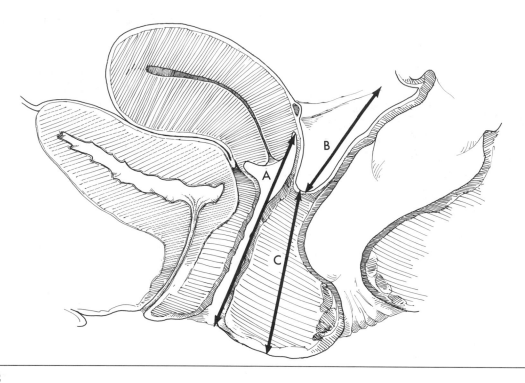

Figure 25-2
Anatomy of the rectovaginal pouch of Douglas and the rectovaginal septum. The dimensions were measured at the time of examination under anesthesia and laparoscopy. A = length of posterior vaginal wall, B = depth of rectovaginal pouch of Douglas, C = length of rectovaginal septum. From Kuhn RJP, and Hollyock VE: Observations on the anatomy of the rectovaginal pouch and septum. *Obstet Gynecol* 59:445, 1982.

to the upper pelvic ureters. The external iliac arteries and the infundibulopelvic ligaments identify the lateral margins of the pelvis. The vermiform appendix marks the distal ileum for examination.

Adolescent pelvic anatomy

Subtle differences in the pelvic anatomy of adolescent females must be appreciated for safe and effective laparoscopic surgery (Figure 25-3). Their bony pelvis and capacity for carbon dioxide (CO_2) are smaller than for adults. Care must be taken to avoid injuring the great vessels both at insertion of the Verres needle and the laparoscopic trocar. We recommend a 10-mm laparoscope for a wider field of vision than that afforded by a smaller laparoscope. A vertical or transverse intraumbilical incision is cosmetically acceptable.

The deep epigastric vessels usually lie more medial in the adolescent. They should be visualized directly through the laparoscope to avoid injury when placing the lateral punctures for the second and third instruments. Transillumination of the abdomen will identify the superficial epigastric vessels so they may also be avoided.

The small volume of CO_2 pneumoperitoneum (1.5 L) may be suctioned out rapidly with loss of control of the

surgical field. Constant-pressure insufflators are helpful; otherwise close attention to maintaining a constant pneumoperitoneum is critical.

Special attention should be paid to detect obstructions to the outflow of normal menstruation, since these may accelerate retrograde menstruation and the progression of the endometriosis. Since the uterus is often small, care must be taken to avoid perforation with the intrauterine instrument used for manipulation.

The rectum is more anterior than in adults. When diagnostic laparoscopy is to be followed immediately by laparoscopic surgery, endometriotic lesions in the foreshortened rectovaginal pouch must be excised with care to avoid injury to the rectum and bleeding from hemorrhoidal vessels. There may be insufficient room to perform a culpotomy to remove large specimens.

The fallopian tubes occupy a more lateral position, exposing the ovaries to direct view. This tends to accentuate the visual impact of adolescent polycystic ovaries that do not require surgical therapy.

Congenital anomalies

A deep congenital fossa in the posterior broad ligament is often associated with medial displacement of the ureter.

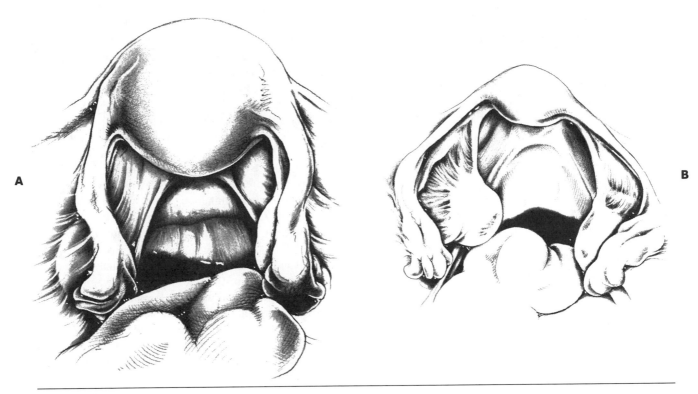

Figure 25-3
Adolescent pelvic anatomy. Compared with the adult pelvis **A,** the adolescent pelvis **B,** is
smaller, the obstetric conjugate shorter, and the carbon dioxide capacity smaller; the cervical
canal is relatively longer and the uterus smaller; the rectum is more anterior, the fallopian tubes
more lateral and the deep epigastric vessels more medial; the ovaries are often polycystic.

Patients with pelvic peritoneal pockets should be examined carefully for endometriosis, congenital anomalies of the fallopian tubes, and congenital medial displacement of the ureter(s). Medially displaced ureters are at increased risk for injury during surgery of the uterosacral ligaments and ovarian fossa.[11]

ENDOMETRIOSIS
Simple disease patterns

The simple disease patterns account for 75% of cases seen in a regional endometriosis and reproductive surgery referral center.[12] The pelvic anatomy is not distorted by the endometriotic process but simply serves as the stage on which the implants have been imposed. This corresponds to stages I and II of the revised classification of the American Fertility Society.[4]

Subtle endometriosis

Patients with pelvic pain and/or infertility may exhibit only nonpigmented and nonclassic pigmented forms of endometriosis. If these lesions are not recognized, the delay in diagnosis may result in continued symptoms and progression of the disease in some women.

Conspicuous endometriosis

The classic powder-burn lesion, blueberry and chocolate cysts, fibrotic nodules, and ovarian endometriomas, are familiar to all gynecologists.

Complex disease patterns

Features of the complex disease patterns include anatomic distortion caused by deep endometriotic invasions, marked host responses, complicated folding, tissue contraction, and obliterative adhesions. This corresponds to moderate, severe, and extensive endometriosis and to stages III and IV of the revised classification of the American Fertility Society. The complex disease patterns account for 25% of cases seen in a regional endometriosis and reproductive surgery referral center.[12] Considerable skill and experience are required to treat the complex problems involved.

Centrifugal pattern

The predominant pattern of endometriosis is the centrifugal pattern with the adnexa adherent to the posterior broad ligaments with or without obliterative disease of the rectovaginal pouch.

Left frozen pelvis

This pattern is characterized by a large ovarian endometrioma fused to the broad ligament over the ureter, with the oviduct adherent between the ovary and the broad ligament or adherent to the tubal pole and antimesenteric border of the ovary, and the whole enveloped by the sigmoid colon in dense obliterative adhesions.[13] It develops spontaneously when the sigmoid colon envelops the left adnexa to contain the chocolate debris from repeated ruptures of left ovarian endometriomas, or it may develop in response to surgical intervention. In both instances the left adnexa is irreparably damaged. An intravenous pyelogram is recommended to detect partial or complete obstruction of the left ureter.

Obliterated rectovaginal pouch of Douglas

Partial obliteration of the rectovaginal pouch usually indicates deep, nodular, invasive disease of one uterosacral ligament and sometimes of the pararectal or rectal tissues adherent to it. Complete obliteration is usually associated with deep, nodular, invasive disease of the uterosacral ligaments, posterior cervix, and rectum.

Centripedal pattern

The centripedal pattern is a less common but more severe form of endometriosis. The uterus is retroflexed, retroverted, and adherent to itself and to the rectum, with complete obliteration of the rectovaginal pouch and adherence of both ovaries to the posterior uterus and sides of the rectum.

Complete frozen pelvis

The frozen pelvis represents the most complex and severe disease pattern. It is the final stage of endometriosis in patients with aggressive disease, impaired immune host defenses, and numerous attempts at medical and surgical treatment. The health of the patient is threatened. This is not the place for heroic surgery,[14] such as radical dissection with preservation of the uterus and one adnexa. Rather, the prudent recommendation is total abdominal hysterectomy, bilateral salpingo-oophorectomy, and excision of pelvic, bowel, and ureteral endometriosis.

Pelvic mapping

The bladder is elevated in the midline by the cervix to form shallow depressions laterally that are the principal sites for bladder endometriosis. These lesions may achieve large proportions and deeply invade the bladder musculature, but full-thickness lesions are uncommon. Invasive disease of the base of the bladder is restricted to women who have undergone a vaginal hysterotomy to terminate pregnancy and, infrequently, after low segment cesarean section.

The round ligaments are the landmarks for identifying congenital and acquired anomalies of the uterus. Deep, invasive endometriosis of the posterior uterus is an enigmatic lesion. The cornual angles of the uterus are drawn posteriorly and medially by retraction of the myometrial disease. The severe form of this lesion is uncommon. The patients complain of significant pelvic pain, and unfortunately, medical suppression is only palliative; this disorder ultimately requires hysterectomy.

The uterosacral ligaments may be thin and attenuated or hypertrophied. They should be examined visually, as well as palpated for deep, nodular, fibrotic lesions, and the information gained correlated with the findings on bimanual pelvic examination. Deep, nodular, fibrotic endometriosis may invade the posterior cervix at the cervical vaginal angle, with penetration into the posterior vaginal fornix. Endometriosis of the posterior vaginal fornix can be differentiated from malignancy by biopsy.

Endometriosis of the floor of the rectovaginal pouch is located anatomically at the level of the midvagina. When the surgeon observes complete obliteration of the rectovaginal pouch, it must be realized that lesions extend downward for at least 5 cm from the level of the uterosacral ligaments and posterior cervix to the floor of the obliterated pouch at midvagina.

On the antimesenteric surface, where the rectal fascia is fused to the muscularis,[15] endometriosis rapidly invades the bowel wall (Figure 25-4). We have observed that lesions as small as 4 to 6 mm in diameter had invaded full thickness through the muscularis. This deep penetration of a small lesion is due to the intimate adherence of the rectal fascia to the muscularis, and the rich vascular supply of the muscularis of the bowel that forms an ideal medium for growth of endometriosis.

Lesions 4 mm and smaller have had little time to elicit a fibrotic host response to wall them off. By the time they have grown to 6 mm in diameter, we have observed that such a response begins to form. With further growth, the surrounding serosa and superficial muscularis contract over the endometriotic lesion to form a stigma, as the lesion penetrates and enlarges within the hypertrophied muscularis of the bowel. In some cases the endometriosis penetrates through the mucosa to become visible at sigmoidoscopy and to bleed at menses. Endometriosis may be differentiated from malignancy by biopsy.

Endometriosis tends to implant on the mesosalpinx between the isthmus of the tube and the utero-ovarian ligament, as well as the ampulla and the fimbria ovarica. Disease of the proximal stump is common after tubal ligation. Ovarian endometriosis can be superficial, mossy red adhesions or vesicular, polypoid, and cystic implants similar to peritoneal lesions. Endometriomas are smooth or puckered cysts varying from millimeters to several centimeters in size, with or without adhesions. Adhesions that fix the ovary to the broad ligament should be considered endometriotic and excised together with all ovarian endometriomas for histologic examination.

The peritoneum may be thickened and opaque, making identification of the ureter difficult. The ureter may be identified lateral to the pulsations of the hypogastric arteries. Ureteral peristalsis should be observed; normal peristalsis is consistent with normal ureteral function. We have observed rapid hyperperistalsis when the lower ureter was fixed and invaded by endometriosis, without narrowing or obstruction of the ureter on intravenous pyelogram; the endometriosis and scar tissue blocked the normal progression of the ureteral peristalsis to the bladder. An intravenous pyelogram is indicated in all patients in whom a ureter is hidden by disease.

Endometriosis causes bulbous swelling of the tip of the appendix and may cause intussusception of the appendix into the cecum. Appendicitis and carcinoid tumor of the appendix are included in the differential diagnosis. Endometriosis is usually confined to the distal 50 cm of the ileum.[16] The surgeon should look for evidence of Crohn's disease (growth of mesenteric fatty tissue onto the ileum, enlarged mesenteric lymph nodes, and hyperemia of the bowel) and for Meckel's diverticulum. Usually the cecum and ascending colon have a pelvic lie when they are involved with endometriosis. The disease is usually confined to implants on the right diaphragm.

PROCEDURE
Informed consent

Informed consent is a process, not an event. The more information the patient has, the better she will be prepared mentally and physically to make an intelligent, informed decision about whether to undergo the proposed surgery.[17] The surgeon's training and credentials should be available for review.

Items to be included in the informed consent process are as follows:

1. Clinical diagnosis of endometriosis based on history and physical examination.
2. Prognosis with expectant treatment.
3. Treatment proposed, such as advanced diagnostic laparoscopy with possible pelvic laparoscopic surgery.
4. Alternative treatment, such as medical suppressive therapy, ovulation stimulation, and microconservative surgery by laparotomy.
5. Risks, benefits, and complications of diagnostic laparoscopy and pelvic laparoscopic surgery.[16]
6. Likelihood of success in terms of relief of symptoms, conception, and recurrence.

Timing of the surgery

The proliferative phase of the cycle is preferable if one is planning to progress to pelvic endoscopic surgery for endometriosis. This will avoid the risk of interrupting a pregnancy and also the inconvenience of bleeding from a corpus luteum and pelvic congestion. These advantages

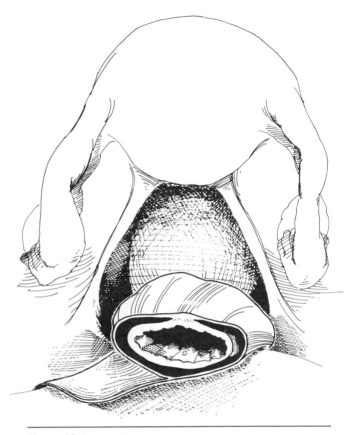

Figure 25-4
Anatomy of the rectum. The rectal fascia is fused to the muscularis on the antimesenteric border of the rectum, but is separated from the muscularis laterally and posteriorly. From v. Peham H, Amreich J: *Operative gynecology*. Philadelphia, 1934, JB Lippincott Co.

more than offset the slightly increased visual prominence of some subtle endometriotic lesions during the luteal phase. Patients who have been receiving suppressive therapy with danazol or gonadotropin-releasing hormone (GnRH) analogs should be withdrawn from medication for a minimum of 4 months before reevaluation laparoscopically so that the suppressed endometriotic lesions can regain visibility.[18]

Preoperative note

The preoperative note should include an assessment of pelvic pain, infertility, and health factors related to endometriosis, as well as positive physical findings such as lateral displacement of the cervix, tenderness or nodularity in the uterosacral ligaments or rectovaginal pouch, fixity of the uterus, and adnexal masses. An abstract of the hysterosalpingogram, office hysteroscopy, pelvic ultrasound,[19] and old operative reports provide indispensable information at surgery.

Equipment

Surgery of the lower genital tract requires the following:
1. Catheter for continuous drainage of bladder.
2. Allis clamp for cervical manipulation.
3. Hank's or Hegar uterine dilator for uterine manipulation.
4. Vaginal probe made from a folded sponge on a sponge stick.
5. Rectal probe.
6. Padded leg holders for low-thigh, dorsal lithotomy position to allow access to the lower genital tract as well as freedom of movement of laparoscopic instruments.

Upper genital tract procedures require the following:
1. Ten-mm, 0-degree, wide-angle laparoscope with bright light source.
2. Ten-mm, 30-degree, wide-angle laparoscope to examine bowel.
3. Video camera and monitor.
4. Constant-pressure insufflator with low and high flow settings.
5. Short, lower quadrant, self-retaining screw trocar sleeves.
6. Laser suction irrigator.
7. Calibrated 5-mm probe.
8. Five-mm atraumatic grasping forceps.
9. Five-mm toothed grasping forceps.
10. Aspirating needle.
11. Five-mm scissors.
12. Bipolar electrocoagulation forceps.
13. Ten-ml syringe with a 20-caliber needle for Palmer test.

Surgical technique

While awake, the patient may be placed in the low-thigh, modified dorsal lithotomy position with padded leg holders and padded elbows. General anesthesia is administered in the supine position and the patient repositioned. Examination under anesthesia is performed. A straight catheter is placed in the bladder and a uterine dilator in the uterus for manipulation.

About 4 L CO_2 are insufflated into the abdomen through a Verres needle. The Palmer test is performed in patients with previous abdominal surgery. The 0-degree, 10-mm diagnostic laparoscope is inserted through an intraumbilical incision, a laser suction-irrigator through a left lower quadrant incision, and a calibrated probe through a right lower quadrant incision. Examination is performed using the alpha sequence. Ideally this examination should be made directly to detect the subtle forms of endometriosis, unless the surgeon has video equipment with color resolution, discrimination, and clarity equal to the human eye.

All gynecologists are capable of performing advanced diagnostic laparoscopy. It is a continuing personal postgraduate course, and surgeons will be rewarded with knowledge of endometriosis and the anomalies and variations in pelvic anatomy that are so essential for refining their surgical skills.

ANALYSIS OF ADVANCED LAPAROSCOPIC TECHNIQUE
Teamwork

Most cases of advanced diagnostic laparoscopy proceed to pelvic laparoscopic surgery immediately. We cannot emphasize too strongly the benefits of a well-trained, dedicated surgical team. Laparoscopic surgery is labor and instrument intense; all planning that eliminates stress, delay, malfunctions, and personality conflicts will reduce surgery time and improve patient care.

A dedicated operating room equipped with all the necessary instruments and facilities coordinated for laparoscopic surgery should be a high priority. Use of the same operating room and the same operating team, month after month, goes a long way to eliminate variables and reduce complications.

Anesthesia

General anesthesia is essential for advanced diagnostic laparoscopy and for laparoscopic surgery. The surgeon must be confident that the patient will not "buck" and push bowel into the surgical field.

Endotracheal intubation

A cuffed endotracheal tube is essential to reduce the risk of aspiration pneumonia, and endobronchial intubation and to maintain good oxygenation in the face of steep Trendelenburg position and intraabdominal CO_2 distention. Gastric secretions can be neutralized preoperatively to reduce further the risks for aspiration pneumonia.

Nasogastric tube

We recommend the nasogastric tube selectively in patients with gastric dilatation and when it is desirable to examine the transverse colon, splenic flexure, and spleen. Visualization of the spleen requires the supine position, right lateral tilt, nasogastric tube, and a left upper quadrant probe.

Position

The patient may be positioned in low-thigh, dorsal lithotomy position while awake to ensure complete comfort and to prevent stress on back, hip, and knee joints, and pressure on nerves and blood vessels of the lower extremities. This position is ideal for access to the lower genital tract, as well as for full range of motion of instruments for examination and surgery of the upper reproductive tract. The operating table is placed in the Trendelenburg position for surgery.

Mechanical cleansing

The bowel, vagina, and abdomen are cleansed the evening before surgery using a Fleet enema until clear, a povidone-iodine vaginal douche, and a pHisoHex shower with mechanical cleansing of the umbilicus. At surgery, the abdomen, umbilicus, and vagina are again cleansed with povidone-iodine scrub.

Antibiotic preparation

A prophylactic antibiotic is administered in anticipation of advanced laparoscopic surgery. One gram of cefazolin or 500 mg of erythromycin is administered intravenously 30 minutes before surgery.

Cervical stenosis

Hydrotubation with a Kahn cannula often dilates the internal os sufficiently, so that it can be located with a silver probe for progressive dilatation. An osmotic cervical dilator may be left in place for 4 hours with benefit. Hysteroscopic instrumentation is required in the more perplexing cases.

Hysteroscopy

Most patients will have had a hysterosalpingogram. We recommend hysteroscopy selectively when the hysterosalpingogram indicates an abnormality, in patients with repeated abortions and in cases with cornual occlusion of the fallopian tubes.

Palmer test

In patients with previous pelvic or abdominal surgery, the Palmer test is performed to determine if the area beneath the umbilicus is free of adhesions. A 20-gauge needle with syringe half loaded with Ringer's lactate solution is inserted vertically and then sequentially toward the pelvic cavity and then laterally with aspiration. If CO_2 bubbles are aspirated from each direction, it is assumed that the area is free of bowel adhesions. Failure to aspirate, or aspiration of blood or bowel contents, signals a solid, vascular, or enteric obstruction that precludes placing the laparoscopic trocar at the level of the umbilicus. An alternative site should be tested.

Open laparoscopy

We use an open laparoscopic technique in patients with a positive Palmer test, in women with a history of abdominal surgery for trauma to the abdomen or pelvis, and in those with several surgical incisions.[20]

Laparoscope: visual control

Optimum visualization is essential for surgery. We recommend a 10-mm, wide-angle 0-degree laparoscope for diagnostic laparoscopy and pelvic laparoscopic surgery with pelviscopy instruments, potassium-titanyl-phosphate (KTP), neodymium:yttrium-aluminum-garnet (Nd:YAG), and second-puncture CO_2 lasers. The 30-degree, 10-mm laparoscope is invaluable to examine the rectum, sigmoid colon, and posterior surface of the ovaries in selected cases.

Placement of lower quadrant instruments

Two lower quadrant instruments placed lateral to the deep epigastric vessels are ideal for diagnostic laparoscopy and for laparoscopic surgery. This separation prevents "dueling" and allows ample space for a lower midline instrument. The use of two instruments is essential to obtain necessary traction and countertraction for examination, biopsy, and surgical treatment.

The deep epigastric vessels can be seen through the laparoscope. By placing one's finger over them and transilluminating the abdominal wall lateral to the vessels, surgeons can identify the superficial epigastric vessels as well. Bleeding can be avoided by inserting the 5-mm trocar in a clear area.

The 5-mm, screw-type, short, second-puncture trocar sleeve designed by Reich[21] is ideal for surgical manuevers and does not pull out when changing instruments (Wolf). The laser suction-irrigator is placed through the left lower quadrant and a 5-mm calibrated probe or atraumatic grasping instrument through the right lower quadrant for a right-handed surgeon.

Videomonitor

This instrument encourages active participation of the surgical team, as well as permits the surgeon to stand erect and avoid back strain. We prefer a videocamera with a beam splitter to have the option to observe directly for subtle, nonpigmented endometriosis and for work in critical areas.

Documentation

A surgical report dictated during surgery is superior to one generated after the procedure. Ideally, the surgeon should wear a lapel microphone to record surgical findings as observed and procedures as performed.

Precise observations are essential to draw an accurate pelvic map of the disease (Figure 25-5). Photodocumentation is desirable using computer-generated videoprints, videotapes, 35mm prints, slides, or Polaroid prints.

Surgical control

The three-puncture technique plus the uterine manipulator and an empty bladder and rectum permit optimum surgical exposure for thorough examination. Vaginal sponge on a stick is used to manipulate the posterior fornix to determine the degree of rectovaginal pouch obliteration. A rectal probe in conjunction with the vaginal probe is helpful to determine whether endometriotic lesions involve the rectal wall.

Text cont'd on p. 431.

Patient's Name _____ Date_____

Stage I (Minimal) - 1-5
Stage II (Mild) - 6-15
Stage III (Moderate) - 16-40
Stage IV (Severe) - >40
Total_____

Laparoscopy_____ Laparotomy_____ Photography_____
Recommended Treatment_____

Prognosis_____

PERITONEUM	ENDOMETRIOSIS	<1cm	1-3cm	>3cm
	Superficial	1	2	4
	Deep	2	4	6
OVARY	R Superficial	1	2	4
	Deep	4	16	20
	L Superficial	1	2	4
	Deep	4	16	20

POSTERIOR CULDESAC OBLITERATION	Partial	Complete
	4	40

	ADHESIONS	<1/3 Enclosure	1/3-2/3 Enclosure	>2/3 Enclosure
OVARY	R Filmy	1	2	4
	Dense	4	8	16
	L Filmy	1	2	4
	Dense	4	8	16
TUBE	R Filmy	1	2	4
	Dense	4*	8*	16
	L Filmy	1	2	4
	Dense	4*	8*	16

*If the fimbriated end of the fallopian tube is completely enclosed, change the point assignment to 16.

Additional Endometriosis: _____

Associated Pathology: _____

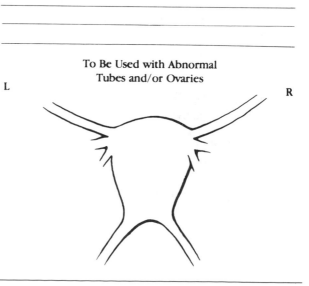

To Be Used with Normal Tubes and Ovaries

To Be Used with Abnormal Tubes and/or Ovaries

Figure 25-5
American Fertility Society revised classification of endometriosis, 1985. From The American Fertility Society: Revised classification of endometriosis: *Fertil Steril* 43:351, 1985.

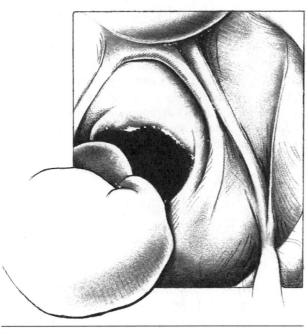

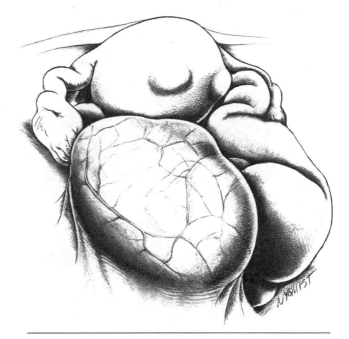

Figure 25-6
Open rectovaginal pouch of Douglas. The peritoneal fluid must be suctioned for cytology and to permit examination. The rectum must be straightened further to facilitate examination for bowel endometriosis. Note the anomalous position of the right ureter, a congenital medial displacement.

Figure 25-7
Left pelvic kidney. Unexpected masses should be examined carefully and gently. Not all large masses are malignant. This was a functioning left pelvic kidney in a patient with a normally placed, functioning right kidney. The examiner should search for congenital anomalies.

Lateral placement of the two lower quadrant instruments facilitates examination of the colon, adnexa, broad ligaments, and ureters, and running the small bowel. This leaves space for a fourth puncture site in the lower midline for a KTP laser or other instrument.

Rectovaginal pouch

The rectovaginal pouch of Douglas is opened by exaggerated anteflexion of the uterus with the intrauterine instrument. The left lower quadrant instrument is used to elevate and straighten the rectum to the level of the sacral promontory; the rectum is held in position with the right lower quadrant probe. A lower quadrant instrument may be required to elevate a prolapsed ovary. All peritoneal fluid should be suctioned.

The vaginal and rectal probes help to distinguish between deep lesions in the anterior and posterior halves of the rectovaginal pouch. Endometriosis may be palpated between the probes and a lower quadrant instrument to estimate the depth or thickness of the disease.

Partial obliteration of the rectovaginal pouch is diagnosed when the rectum adheres to the vaginal portion of the pouch or to either uterosacral ligament. On insertion of the vaginal probe, a bulge will be noted anterior to the rectum, indicating that the obliteration is incomplete.

Complete obliteration of the rectovaginal pouch is diagnosed when the rectum is attached to the posterior cervix and to the arch of the uterosacral ligaments. On insertion of the vaginal probe, there is no bulge anterior to the rectum, and the rectal probe will hit the arch of the uterosacral ligaments, confirming that the obliteration is complete.

Rectum and sigmoid colon

In patients with a large obstetric conjugate, examination of the rectum and sigmoid colon may be adequate with a 0-degree laparoscope, a rectal probe, and an instrument to palpate the rectum. If the obstetric conjugate is small, the view is so tangential that it is useless. In those cases a 30-degree laparoscope is preferable.

Superficial bowel endometriosis has the appearance of peritoneal disease. The deeper lesions have a stigma from retraction and scarring, and on palpation, a much larger lesion than expected may be detected. Appendices epiploicae often adhere to deep bowel lesions and tend to hide them from view. Active inspection and palpation are required to identify bowel endometriosis (Table 25-1).

Fallopian tubes

The oviducts are elevated atraumatically with a blunt probe or by gentle suction with a laser suction-irrigator. All surfaces are examined from the cornual angle laterally, including the fimbriae and fimbria ovarica. The os-

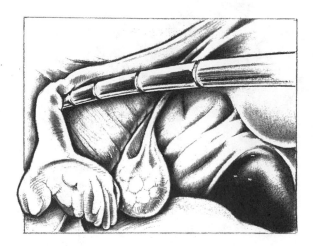

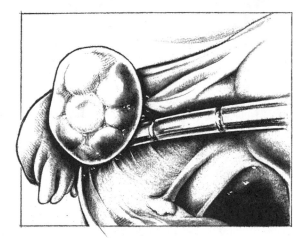

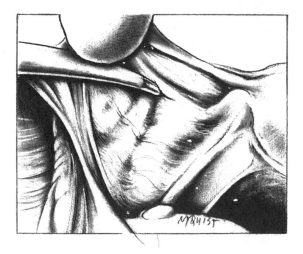

Figure 25-8
Alpha sequence examination. The left oviduct and all surfaces of the left ovary are examined by elevating the left tube and the left ovary with the right lower quadrant instrument. The left ovary is held up and laterally by the left lower quadrant instrument for examination of the left posterior broad ligament.

tium is explored with an atraumatic alligator forceps. Endoscopic examination of the oviduct can be performed selectively.

The fimbriae can be evaluated under a stream of Ringer's lactate solution and by underwater examination. The latter is accomplished by filling the rectovaginal pouch with Ringer's lactate solution and inserting the laparoscope under water to observe the motion and delicacy of the fimbriae. Chromotubation is especially effective under water.

Ovaries

It is essential to examine all surfaces of the ovary. The left adnexa is elevated using the leverage of the right lower quadrant probe and the ovary controlled by sweeping the left lower quadrant laser suction-irrigator under the tubal pole. This allows examination of all surfaces of the ovary. The right adnexa is elevated using the leverage of the left lower quadrant probe, and the ovary is controlled with the right lower quadrant probe. Alternatively, the ovary can be controlled by atraumatic grasping forceps applied to the utero-ovarian ligament or by inserting a spinal needle transabdominally into the ovary.

Endometriosis should be suspected if the ovary is fixed to the posterior broad ligament. The adhesions should be dissected to examine for ovarian endometriomas. The posterior surface near the hilum is the typical location, however, the lesions may occur on any surface. A deep endometrioma may hide within an ovary that is perfectly free of adhesions and surface lesions.

Ruptured endometriomas discovered at laparoscopy should be mobilized and debrided, followed by copious pelvic lavage using several liters of Ringer's lactate solution. After surgery, the patient should be treated with danazol or GnRH analogs for 4 months to suppress the intense inflammatory host response before rescheduling laparoscopic surgery or microconservative surgery. A second-look laparoscopy may be indicated in selected cases.

In contrast, endometriomas ruptured during mobilization of the ovary at laparoscopy can be lavaged to prevent an inflammatory response, and the pelvic endoscopic surgery may be performed immediately.

A preoperative vaginal-abdominal sonogram is recommended in patients with ovarian masses.[22] Selectively, magnetic resonance imaging and tumor markers[23] are suggested for clarification. In a survey of oncologists on the "laparoscopic management of ovarian neoplasms subsequently found to be malignant," 31% of the cases had four "benign" characteristics: less than 8 cm, cystic, unilocular, and unilateral.[24] Fifty percent were stages II to IV at the time of initial laparoscopy or subsequent laparotomy. The invasive epithelial malignancies in the survey occurred at the average age of 44 years, which is 10 years younger than the national average. The ages of the patients with tumors of low malignant potential were even younger. The oncologists recommended that "if there is suspicion of ovarian cancer upon laparoscopic evaluation, the ovarian capsule should not be violated and laparotomy should be initiated."[24] This approach relies on frozen-section diagnosis.

Evidence suggests that aspiration and biopsy do not change the prognosis of patients with ovarian carcinoma.[25,26] In younger women with endometriosis and infertility or pelvic pain in whom malignancy is suspected, we prefer laparoscopic biopsy, permanent histologic sections, and prompt definitive surgery by an oncologist when ovarian cancer is diagnosed. Excision of the intact ovary is recommended in women over 40 years in whom septations are found within an ovarian mass at sonography.[27]

Posterior broad ligaments and ureter

Two probes are necessary for this examination: the left is used to elevate the rectum and sigmoid colon medially and cephalad, and the right to hold them. The left lower quadrant instrument is then swept under the tubal pole of the left ovary to elevate and hold it laterally.

Starting in the intersigmoidal triangle, one should identify the pulsations of the left hypogastric artery. At midpelvis the hypogastric artery disappears laterally under the ureter. The left ureter will be found lying lateral to the hypogastric artery and lateral to the uterosacral ligament. The course of the ureter may be traced from the pelvic brim to the cardinal ligament. Ureteral peristalsis is observed.

The right adnexa is elevated with the lower quadrant laser suction-irrigator and held laterally with the right lower quadrant probe. When the peritoneum is sclerotic and thickened, the peritoneum is depressed medial to the infundibulopelvic ligament to accentuate the pulsations of the hypogastric artery. The peristalsis of the ureter will become evident lateral to the hypogastric artery and lateral to the uterosacral ligament.

Vermiform appendix, ileum, cecum, and ascending colon

A retrocecal appendix may be more easily and quickly found using two lower quadrant probes. Endometriosis is usually confined to the distal 50 cm of the ileum. This length of small intestine can be run easily at laparoscopy using the left and right lower quadrant second puncture instruments.

Liver, gallbladder, diaphragms, stomach, and omentum

These structures should be thoroughly examined and described. The right diaphram must be checked closely in patients who complain of catamenial pneumothorax or hemothorax.

Table 25-1 Classification and stages of extrapelvic endometriosis

Class or stage	Definition
Class	
I	Involves the intestinal tract
U	Involves the urinary tract
L	Involves lungs and thoracic cage
O	Involves other sites outside the abdominal cavity
Stage	
I, no organ defect	Extrinsic—surface of organ (serosa, pleura)
	Lesion <1 cm
	Lesion 1–4 cm
	Lesion >4 cm
	Intrinsic—mucosal, muscle, parenchyma
	Lesion <1 cm
	Lesion 1–4 cm
	Lesion >4 cm
II, organ defect*	Extrinsic—surface of organ (serosa, pleura)
	Lesion <1 cm
	Lesion 1–4 cm
	Lesion >4 cm
	Intrinsic—mucosal, muscle, parenchyma
	Lesion <1 cm
	Lesion 1–4 cm
	Lesion >4 cm

*Organ depends on the organ of involvement and includes but is not limited to obstruction and partial obstruction of the urinary and intestinal tracts and hemothorax, hemoptysis, and pneumothorax resulting from pulmonary involvement.

From Markham SM, Carpenter SE, and Rock JA: Extrapelvic endometriosis, *Obstet Gynecol Clin North Am* 16:214, 1989.

Biopsy technique

The two-instrument technique ensures maximum control. A single-tooth forceps grasps the peritoneum adjacent to the endometriosis and elevates the lesion to the top of a peritoneal fold; the endometriosis is then excised with a biopsy forceps. Maintaining control with the grasping forceps, capillary bleeding may be managed by irrigation and suction until it stops. Significant bleeding should be controlled immediately with bipolar electrocoagulation or laser.

PROCEEDING TO PELVIC LAPAROSCOPIC SURGERY

On completion of the diagnostic laparoscopy, the surgeon must decide whether the patient is a candidate for pelvic laparoscopic surgery or would be treated better by microconservative surgery for endometriosis by laparot-

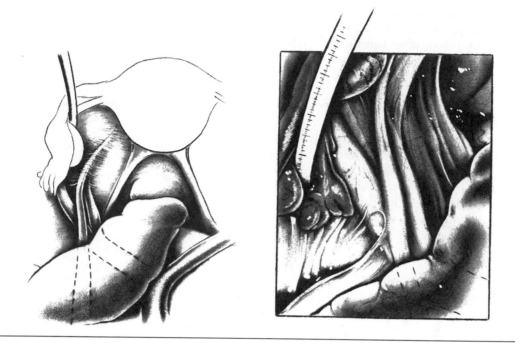

Figure 25-9
The pelvic ureter. The left ureter is shown lateral to the hypogastric artery in the posterior pelvis. Note how the hypogastric artery crosses under the ureter at midposterior pelvis. (See inset). Whenever it is difficult to identify the ureter, look for the pulsations of the hypogastric artery in the posterior pelvis; the ureter will be found lying lateral to the hypogastric artery. Ureteral peristalsis will confirm the location of the ureter.

Table 25-2 Problem-oriented endometriosis treatment algorithm

Disease stage	Pain	Infertility	Health problems*
I, II	1. Laparoscopic surgery ± postop med Rx 2. Med Rx 3. mCSEL ± postop med Rx	1. Expectant Rx 2. Laparoscopic surgery 3. Med Rx 4. mCSEL 5. IVF ± GIFT	1. Laparoscopic surgery + postop med Rx 2. mCSEL + periop med Rx 3. TAH ∓ BSO
III	1. Laparoscopic surgery + postop med Rx 2. mCSEL + periop med Rx 3. Med Rx	1. Laparoscopic surgery 2. mCSEL + periop med Rx 3. Med Rx 4. IVF ± 1 GIFT	1. Laparoscopic surgery + postop med Rx 2. mCSEL + periop med Rx 3. TAH ∓ BSO
IV	1. Laparoscopic surgery + postop med Rx 2. mCSEL + periop med Rx 3. Med Rx	1. Laparoscopic surgery + postop med Rx 2. mCSEL + periop med Rx 3. IVF	1. mCSEL + periop med Rx 2. TAH + BSO

IVF/ET = in vitro fertilization and embryo transfer; GIFT = gamete intrafallopian transfer, if the tubes are perfectly normal; mCSEL = microconservative surgery for endometriosis by laparotomy; TAH = total abdominal hysterectomy; BSO = bilateral salpingo-oophorectomy.
*Health problems include intractable pelvic pain, intractable menorrhagia, bowel endometriosis, ureteral endometriosis, osteoporosis, pulmonary endometriosis, and malignancy.
Modified from Wheeler JM and Malinak LR: *Obstet Gynecol Clin North Am* 16:147, 1989 and Batt RE and Severino MF: *Female Patient* 15:77, 1990.

omy. This decision is based on the patient's priorities, the stage of the disease, confounding variables, and the training and experience of the surgeon (Table 25-2). Ideally, all surgeons performing diagnostic laparoscopy should be capable of performing laparoscopic surgery for endometriosis stages I and II and selectively for stages III and IV. The instruments are in position if it is decided to proceed.

FOLLOW-UP

Successful care of patients with endometriosis requires caring enough to perform thorough diagnosis, individualized management, and prolonged follow-up through menopause.

REFERENCES

1. Wheeler JM: Epidemiology of endometriosis-associated infertility, *J Reprod Med* 34:41-46, 1989.
2. Batt RE, Naples JD, and Severino MF: Endometriosis. In Piver MS (ed): *Manual of gynecologic oncology and gynecology,* Boston, 1989, Little, Brown & Co.
3. Markam SM, Carpenter SE, and Rock JA: Extrapelvic endometriosis, *Obstet Gynecol Clin North Am* 16:193, 1989.
4. American Fertility Society: Revised American Fertility Society classification of endometriosis, *Fertil Steril* 43:351, 1985.
5. Kuhn RJP and Hollyock VE: Observations on the anatomy of the rectovaginal pouch and septum, *Obstet Gynecol* 59:445, 1982.
6. Milley PS and Nichols DH: A correlative investigation of the human rectovaginal septum, *Anat Rec* 163:443, 1969.
7. Nichols DH and Randall CL: *Vaginal surgery,* ed 3, Baltimore, 1989, Williams & Wilkins.
8. Batt RE and Smith RA: Embryologic theory of histogenesis of endometriosis in peritoneal pockets, *Obstet Gynecol Clin North Am* 16:15, 1989.
9. Goligher J and Duthie H: Surgical anatomy and physiology of the anus, rectum and colon. In Goligher J (ed): *Surgery of the anus, rectum and colon,* ed 5, London, 1984, Bailliere Tindall.
10. Zimskind PD, Kelsey DM, and Koppel MM: The anatomy of and surgical approach to the lower urinary tract and genitalia. In Kendall AR et al (eds): *Urology,* vol 1, New York, 1986, Harper & Row.
11. Batt RE et al: A case-series study of peritoneal pockets and endometriosis: rudimentary duplications of the mullerian system, *Adolesc Pediatr Gynecol* 2:47, 1989.
12. Darrow S: Case-control study of the relationship of reproductive factors to the risk of endometriosis, doctoral dissertation, 1991, Department of Social and Preventive Medicine, State University of New York at Buffalo.
13. Batt RE, Severino MF, and Lawton D: Endometriosis: microconservative surgery. In Stangel JJ (ed): *Infertility surgery: a multimethod approach to female reproductive surgery,* Norwalk, Conn, 1990, Appleton & Lange.
14. Batt RE and Naples JD: Conservative surgery for endometriosis in the infertile female, *Curr Probl Obstet Gynecol* 6:58, 1982.
15. Peham HV and Amreich J: *Operative gynecology,* vol 1, Philadelphia, 1934, JB Lippincott.
16. Lansac J, Pierre F, and Letessier E: Digestive endometriosis: results of a multicenter investigation. In Bruhat MA and Canis M (eds): *Endometriosis,* Basle, 1987, Karger.
17. Borten M: Laparoscopic complications: prevention and management, Philadelphia, 1986, BC Decker.
18. Evers JLH: The second-look laparoscopy for evaluation of the result of medical treatment of endometriosis should not be performed during ovarian suppression, *Fertil Steril* 47:502, 1987.
19. Fishman-Javitt MC, Lovecchio JL, and Stein HL: The ovary. In Fishman-Javitt MC, Stein HL, and Lovecchio JL (eds): *Imaging of the pelvis: MRI with correlations to CT and ultrasound,* Boston, 1990, Little, Brown & Co.
20. Hasson HM: Open laparoscopy: a report of 150 cases, *J Reprod Med* 12:234-238, 1974.
21. Reich H and McGlynn F: Short self-retaining trocar sleeves for laparoscopic surgery, *Am J Obstet Gynecol* 162:453-454, 1990.
22. Benacerraf B et al: Sonographic accuracy in the diagnosis of ovarian masses, *J Reprod Med* 35:491-495, 1990.
23. ACOG: Cancer of the ovary, *Technical bulletin* 141, May 1990.
24. Maiman M, Seltzer V, and Boyce J: Laparoscopic excision of ovarian neoplasms subsequently found to be malignant, *Obstet Gynecol* 77:563-565, 1991.
25. Grogan R: Accidental rupture of malignant ovarian cysts during surgical removal, *Obstet Gynecol* 30:718-720, 1987.
26. Dembo AJ et al: Prognostic factors in patients with stage I epithelial ovarian cancer, *Obstet Gynecol* 75:263-267, 1990.
27. Levine RC: Pelviscopic survey in women over 40, *J Reprod Med* 35:597-600, 1990.

26

Endometriosis: Advanced Laparoscopic Surgery

....

RONALD E. BATT

JAMES M. WHEELER

Pelvic laparoscopic surgery consists of a series of operations performed with fine surgical technique. The basic procedures involve the following: coagulation or vaporization of peritoneal and ovarian endometriosis; adhesiolysis; tubal ligation to prevent retrograde menstruation; and debridement in preparation for advanced endoscopic, microconservative, or ablative surgery. These skills can be taught, but advanced operative skills must develop with experience.[1] They are based on complete confidence in diagnostic abilities, intimate knowledge of normal and abnormal topographic anatomy, familiarity with endometriosis and the host responses to the disease, and a firm commitment to perform endoscopic surgery.

In a regional center for reproductive and endometriosis surgery, 75% of patients with endometriosis had minimal to mild disease, and 25% moderate to severe disease.[2] Based on these data, it is reasonable to expect that a large percentage of patients with endometriosis may be treated by advanced laparoscopic surgery.

The advanced laparoscopic surgical techniques presented have evolved from microsurgery with emphasis on excision of endometriosis, minimal trauma, and prevention of ischemia to normal tissues.[3] The techniques are characterized as minimally invasive, invasive, and experimental. Minimally invasive surgery includes excision of peritoneal endometriosis and ovarian endometriomas, ureterolysis, unilateral salpingo-oophorectomy with morcellation, submucous and subserous myomectomy with morcellation, excision of superficial bowel endometriosis, and pelvic lymphadenectomy.[4] Invasive surgery includes minilaparotomy or posterior colpotomy to remove tissue, myomectomy with deep suture reconstruction of the uterus, endoscopically assisted vaginal hysterectomy, and appendectomy. Experimental techniques include enterotomy; extraluminal, wedge, and segmental bowel resections; and staging and treatment of ovarian cancer.[5]

ADVANTAGES AND DISADVANTAGES

Laparoscopic surgery has several advantages over laparotomy; the abdomen remains a closed cavity, with minor portals of entry, no drying, no talc, and no packs. Visual and instrumental access to the rectovaginal pouch are excellent with video display for the surgical team. There may be fewer postoperative adhesions from laparoscopic surgery compared with laparotomy.[6,7] Finally, convalescence is shorter after 1-day ambulatory surgery.

Several problems interfere with the availability and performance of laparoscopic surgery. Sophisticated equipment is extremely expensive. Personnel require a relatively long training time to perform these procedures. A sufficient case load, 80 cases per year, is necessary for the team to maintain expertise. Many insurance companies have not recognized the expertise and time required to perform this surgery and thus do not cover the costs. Access to endometriotic lesions and to pelvic organs is limited by the number and location of secondary portals.

RELATIVE CONTRAINDICATIONS

There are several relative contraindications to laparoscopic surgery. Clomiphene citrate and menopausal gonadotropins cause marked vascular congestion in the pelvic peritoneum and ovaries as well as multiple ovarian cysts; fine surgery is not possible under these adverse conditions. Prolonged administration of progestogens (pseudopregnancy) and ectopic pregnancy cause pelvic congestion that should be allowed to subside for 3 or 4 months before definitive laparoscopic surgery for endometriosis.

The acute pelvic inflammation caused by repeated rupture of ovarian endometriomas should be treated by laparoscopic debridement, thorough lavage, and 2 to 3 months of danazol before definitive laparoscopic surgery. Under ordinary circumstances, surgeons do not like to perform endometriosis surgery under medical suppression. Danazol, gonadotropin-releasing hormone (GnRH) analogs, and progestogens will cause peritoneal endometriosis to regress temporarily, only to reappear after cessation of treatment. Surgery performed during the period of suppression tends to be incomplete; it is preferable to let the effects of suppression subside.[9]

Acute pelvic inflammatory disease (PID) superimposed on endometriosis requires blunt lysis of inflammatory adhesions, drainage of tubo-ovarian abscesses, copious irrigation with Ringer's lactate solution, antibiotic therapy, oral contraceptives or danazol to induce anovulation, and pelvic rest for 6 months before proceeding with laparoscopic surgery.[8]

It is virtually impossible to perform satisfactory laparoscopic surgery for endometriosis that is complicated by extensive pelvic adhesions. These patients are better treated with microconservative surgery by laparotomy. Low posterior cervical leiomyomas and large intramural leiomyomas that require extensive reconstructive surgery are more easily and safely treated by laparotomy.

TRAINING

The basic endoscopic surgical skills are within the capability of most gynecologists; indeed, pressure is growing to insist on these skills from all who perform diagnostic laparoscopy. Prior training in microsurgery is desirable to develop fine motor skills and good surgical habits. Hand-eye coordination may be improved by performing microvascular surgical techniques on the rat, rabbit, and pig, or by practicing on the pelvic trainer and video games.

One can learn the techniques of endometriosis surgery at laparotomy under perfect control and gradually transfer them to laparoscopic surgery with increasing skill. This positive experience can be accelerated by setting aside 1 day each week for laparoscopic surgery, by sharing that experience with another surgeon, and by reviewing videotapes. The learning curve for performing advanced laparoscopic surgery gently and expertly is measured in years.[10]

Advanced endoscopic surgical skills are acquired by experience, repeated postgraduate courses, and observing skilled endoscopic surgeons at work in their own operating theaters. Personality, interest, natural dexterity, and access to patients and proper facilities are the factors that determine the extent to which one will safely and effectively perform these procedures.

OPERATING ROOM AND EQUIPMENT
Flexibility

Duplicate sets of instruments and equipment are not always available. Should the laser fail, the surgeon should be able to work with equal facility using a unipolar elec-tric needle or scissors and biopsy forceps combined with bipolar electrocoagulation.

Constant-pressure insufflator

The Trendelenburg position[11] is unphysiologic and should be maintained for as short a time as possible. A constant-pressure insufflator that removes smoke will prevent overdistention of the abdomen, enhance visualization, and save operating time.

Potassium-titanium-phosphate (KTP) and carbon dioxide lasers

In our hands the laser is used primarily for excision of endometriosis, dissection, and adhesiolysis, and only secondarily for vaporization and coagulation. The advantage of laser is clean, bloodless dissection.

Electrosurgery

Unipolar dissection is also clean and bloodless, but the surgeon must be ever vigilant not to touch two instruments together. Care must be taken when using unipolar electrocoagulation around the bowel and ureter.[12] The unpredictable extent of ischemic necrosis from unipolar electrocoagulation for tubal ligation is familiar to most gynecologists.

Sharp dissection

A third system of energy is scissors and biopsy forceps dissection with bipolar electrocoagulation for hemostasis. Pelviscopy instruments are desirable.

Laparoscope

The 10-mm wide-angle laparoscope with video screen provides maximum control of the surgical field for working through secondary portals. This is the optimal way to deliver potassium-titanyl-phosphate (KTP) fiber laser, mechanical, hydraulic, and electric energy.

Operating laparoscope

The carbon dioxide (CO_2) laser is the optimum mode of energy for delivery through the operating laparoscope. This instrument has a small visual field because of space taken by the operating channel for the laser or scissors. The small visual field is partially compensated by video magnification.

Lower tract and lower quadrant portals

For advanced laparoscopic surgery, a dilator in the uterus for manipulation, a straight catheter in the bladder, and selectively, vaginal and rectal probes are required. In addition, three lower quadrant portals are needed for the laser suction-irrigator, KTP laser, and other pelviscopic instruments. The short self-retaining screw trocar sleeve has two advantages: it remains in place during repeated changes of instruments and it is out of the surgeon's visual field (Wolf).[13]

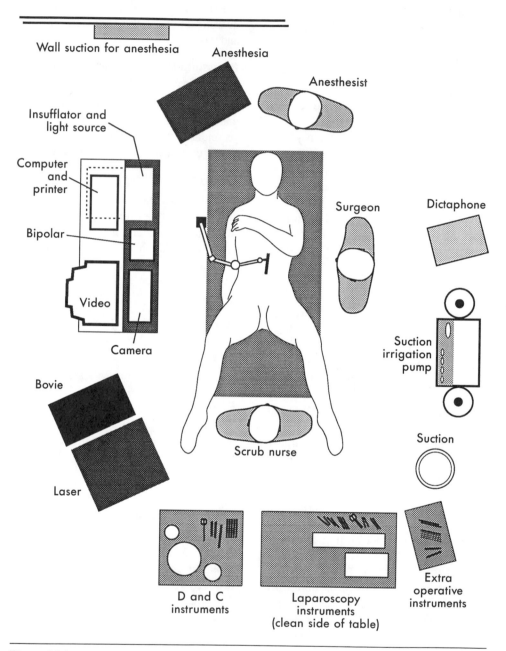

Figure 26-1
Layout of the operating room. The operating theater should be comfortable and efficient with all instrumentation and personnel available.

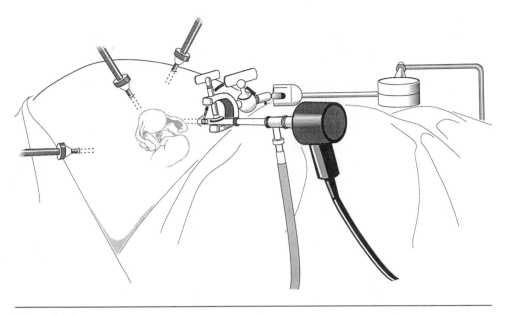

Figure 26-2
Iron Intern. This instrument is used to stabilize the laparoscope on the operative field, enabling the surgeon to operate with both hands. It is especially valuable when no surgical assistant is available.

The "Iron Intern"

The automated surgical robot retractor holder* designed with a ball-and-socket shoulder joint, a hinged elbow joint, and a universal wrist joint is attached to the rail of the operating table above the armboard and to the laparoscopic trocar sheath to fix the laparoscope on the desired field. This is an indispensable instrument when excising deep peritoneal endometriosis and moderate, severe, and extensive disease. The surgeon has both hands free to perform pelviscopic surgery (Figure 26-2).

METHODS OF DISSECTION
Hydrodissection

Ringer's lactate solution is injected by needle and syringe or through a laser suction-irrigator into the retroperitoneal spaces to elevate the peritoneum from the underlying structures. This is a safe way to perform CO_2 laser vaporization of peritoneal endometriosis of the broad ligament.[14] The technique is useful in patients with simple disease patterns where the pelvic anatomy is not distorted by minimal and mild endometriosis.

Aquadissection

This is a combination of mechanical and fluid dissection performed with a suction-irrigation instrument. Its semisharp end and high-pressure fluid-delivery system is used to develop cleavage planes between adherent organs and

tissues. Fibrous bands are identified and incised, and the aquadissection continued. This technique was developed for laparoscopic treatment of extensive pelvic adhesive disease.[15] It is useful in patients with complex disease patterns in whom the pelvic anatomy is distorted by moderate and severe endometriosis.

Scissors

Scissors dissection may be performed through the operating laparoscope or through a second portal of entry. The endometriosis is grasped directly with a single-tooth, dull biopsy forceps and dissected with scissors. The chief advantages are clean, minimally traumatic incisions, and safety around the ureter, bowel, blood vessels, and nerves.

"The significant increase in tissue necrosis and the subsequent foreign body reaction that follows laser incision compared with microscissor incision lead us to conclude that sharp mechanical incision is the modality of choice."[16] However, some of the advantage of sharp dissection of endometriosis is offset by the need for bipolar electrocoagulation. Gomel[17] cautioned, "I think overtreatment of endometriosis with extensive excision leads to very severe pelvic adhesions, and this has been our experience in second-look laparoscopies." He clarified: "We are not referring to excision of endometriomas or endometriotic tissues, but in the presence of mild or moderate disease, to go and remove very large segments of peritoneal surface leads to pelvic adhesions and puts the patient at her worst situation."

*Automated Medical Products, New York, NY.

Biopsy forceps

A single-tooth, dull biopsy (grasping) forceps and a sharp biopsy forceps are introduced through second portals of entry. The endometriosis is maneuvered to the top of a peritoneal fold by grasping the adjacent peritoneum with the grasping forceps; the entire endometriotic lesion is removed by repeated biopsies. Hemostasis is obtained with bipolar electrocoagulation.

CO_2 laser

This is the best cutting laser. It may be used through the operating laparoscope or second portal of entry. Fired directly through the operating laparoscope, it has more coagulation effect because the beam in the primary operating laparoscope is defocused by hitting the wall of the laser channel. Power densities through the CO_2 laser laparoscope diminish above 40 W. In the clinical setting, optimum cutting (vaporization) occurs at low power densities, and cutting plus coagulation occurs at higher power densities.[18]

Fiber laser

The KTP, argon, neodynium:yttrium-aluminum-garnet (Nd:YAG), and homium lasers are introduced through a second portal of entry. This offers the advantage of a full 10-mm wide-angle laparoscopic field of vision augmented by video display. Fiber lasers are popular with many reproductive surgeons because they cut well, produce better hemostasis than the CO_2 laser, are free of alignment problems, and use the familiar eye-hand coordination of open surgery.

Unipolar electrosurgery

Compared with the CO_2 laser, electrosurgical cutting appears to cause a longer-lasting foreign body tissue reaction.[19] Care must be exercised when dissecting around the ureter, bowel, nerves, and blood vessels, since unipolar energy can be conducted by blood vessels and cause delayed ischemic necrosis.

HEMOSTASIS
Preventive

Large blood vessels can be avoided by being thoroughly familiar with the topographic anatomy of the pelvis. Medium vessels may be secured by bipolar electrocoagulation or the GIA stapler before division. Bipolar, unipolar, laser coagulation, or endoclips are effective on small vessels before division. Simultaneous coagulation and division of tiny blood vessels is readily accomplished with the CO_2 and fiber lasers and the unipolar needle. Dilute vasopressin solutions (10 or 20 U in 100 to 200 ml injectable saline) are helpful for preventive hemostasis of the uterus, fallopian tube, and ovary.

Therapeutic

Immediate control of bleeding is essential during laparoscopic surgery to maintain visual and surgical control of the operative field. The flow of blood must be stopped before bipolar, unipolar, laser, or thermal energy can desiccate and seal the vessels, since flowing blood cools the tissues and prevents hemostasis. Grasp and occlude the vessel, irrigate and clear the field with the laser suction-irrigator, and apply one of the modes of hemostasis. The method must withstand the endovascular pressure for 96 hours until complete and permanent sealing of the blood vessel.[20]

Bipolar coagulation should be continued until no current passes through the tissue, indicating complete desiccation. Unipolar electrocoagulation is useful for hemostasis but must be used with caution lest the current travels along undesired alternative pathways. "Once the electrons enter the body they are dispersed through the tissue toward the pathway of least resistance to the return electrode. When the voltage is increased, the electrons have more 'push' to find an alternative pathway."[12] Low-voltage, high-frequency electrogenerators are desirable to prevent electrons following an alternative pathway along blood vessels to cause undesired coagulation and delayed ischemic necrosis in such organs as the bowel and ureter.

Titanium clips do not interfere with magnetic resonance imaging examinations and are useful during laparoscopic surgery. Vascular staples are ideal for the infundibulopelvic ligament and uterine vessels, since they leave vascularized pedicles with less risk for adhesions. In contrast, the Roeder loop causes large, ischemic pedicles that may require neovascularization by omentum, bowel, and adjacent structures, increasing the risk for adhesions. Sutures cause ischemia and adhesions, and should be used only when necessary.[21]

Repeated irrigation with Ringer's lactate solution, suctioning, and observation may be all that is required for spontaneous hemostasis. Laser coagulation with a defocused beam should control persistent minor bleeding. A word of caution: the uterus, uterosacral ligaments, and round ligaments are notorious for delayed bleeding. It is important to recheck the site of excision of endometriosis, since vessels may go into spasm and bleed later.

METHODS OF REPAIR
Leave peritoneal and serosal wounds open

Applying the lessons learned from microsurgery, the excision of endometriotic lesions ensures complete removal of disease and leaves clean wounds with minimal disturbance of tissue vascularity. Most clean, raw peritoneal, and serosal wounds heal without adhesions.[21]

Leave ovarian wounds open

Most reproductive surgeons do not suture the ovary at laparoscopic surgery. Animal studies demonstrated less ovarian adhesions when the ovary was not sutured and more adhesions with suturing of the ovarian cortex.[22-23] This confirmed the earlier work of Ellis that suturing causes ischemia and adhesions. The surgeon may elect to restore the shape of the ovary with internal sutures, leaving the cortical surface free of sutures.

Endoscopic suturing to restore organ integrity and function

When dissection has reached or penetrated the bladder mucosa, a single layer of absorbable sutures will restore muscular integrity. In selected cases, interrupted sutures may be placed in the ureters endoscopically over a ureteral catheter. Both bladder and ureteral suture lines should be covered with Interceed. To restore full muscular integrity of the bowel after deep dissection, the serosa and muscularis are sutured in one layer with interrupted, nonabsorbable suture. We do not recommend applying Interceed to bowel suture lines. After deep myomectomy, reconstruction of the uterine wall with sutures is essential to restore structural and functional integrity for labor. Cover the suture line with Interceed. Mini-laparotomy incisions are sutured to restore integrity of the fascia when large specimens must be removed. Transvaginal suturing of the colpotomy incision is necessary to prevent evisceration.

REDUCING RISKS AND COMPLICATIONS
Bleeding

It is preferable to avoid surgery during the week before menses when the pelvis is congested maximally. Menorrhagia should be controlled by medication and the hemoglobin and hematocrit restored to normal levels before surgery. The bipolar electrocoagulation instrument should be tested every time before surgery. The tired surgeon should reschedule surgery. Precise and fine hemostasis is necessary. If uncontrolled bleeding is encountered, immediate laparotomy is recommended.

Infection

Our practice has been to avoid surgery within 6 weeks of previous surgery. A preoperative physical examination within 1 week of surgery is performed to detect dental, respiratory, urinary, vaginal, and gastrointestinal infections. At surgery, the umbilicus should be thoroughly cleansed with Q-tips and povidone-iodine. Preoperative antibiotics and copious irrigation of the pelvis during and after surgery are recommended to reduce the risk of infection.

Burn

All equipment should be kept in good working order. The laser beam and electrode tips must be kept in full view during surgery. High-voltage electrocoagulation should be avoided. Massive electrocoagulation near bowel or ureter may cause ischemia, delayed perforation, and fistula formation.

Adhesions

Laparoscopic surgery produced less adhesions in animals compared with open laparotomy.[6] A randomized, prospective clinical trial on adhesion formation in humans demonstrated significantly less de novo postoperative adhesions compared with laparotomy.[7]

OPERATIVE SEQUENCE: MINIMALLY INVASIVE SURGERY

The surgeon may proceed to advanced laparoscopic surgery on completing diagnostic endoscopy by placing a fourth portal of entry in the lower midabdomen. The portals of access for instruments are umbilical, left lower quadrant, lower midline, right lower quadrant, uterus, vagina, and rectum. Direct visual control of the ureters is crucial in all operations for pelvic endometriosis.

Pelvic laparoscopic surgery is a series of operations beginning in the rectovaginal pouch. By approaching each adhesiolysis and each endometriotic lesion as a separate operation, some of the more complex disease patterns may be treated effectively. The surgeon should start with the more tedious dissection first, progressing to the easier tasks when fatigue is less a factor in determining outcome. The better adnexa should be operated first.

Anterior abdominal wall

Omental and bowel adhesions should be divided. The surgeon must be able to develop a safe plane of dissection between the bowel and the abdominal wall. If the adhesions are obliterative and the surgeon senses substantial risk, this portion of the procedure should be abandoned. The surgeon may proceed with the pelvic surgery if the abdominal wall adhesions do not prevent good visual control of the operative field.

Peritoneal endometriosis
Excision

We have been committed to excision of peritoneal and ovarian endometriosis because it is not possible to determine the extent of a lesion until it is grasped, elevated, and excised.[24-26] In one study, 42% of lesions were 2 mm or less in depth and could be eradicated by coagulation, vaporization, or excision; 37% were 3 to 5 mm deep and could be treated adequately by thorough laser vaporization or excision; the remaining 21% were 5 to 10 mm deep and required excision.[27]

Undertreatment

Surgeons who treat all peritoneal endometriosis by co-agulation will undertreat 58% of the lesions, and those who treat all peritoneal endometriosis by laser vaporiza-tion will undertreat 21%. Many reproductive surgeons, recognizing the limitations of vaporization and coagu-lation, excise endometriosis.[5,14,28-33]

Adhesion-free healing

Advanced laparoscopic surgery is characterized by ex-cision of all endometriotic lesions. This includes non-pigmented and pigmented peritoneal lesions, as well as the deep, fibrotic, nodular endometriosis in the recto-vaginal pouch and uterosacral ligaments, and ovarian endometriomas. The advantages of excision are the entire lesion is removed regardless of depth; one can ensure histologic verification; a clean, open wound with intact vasculature is achieved; and healing is rapid.

No suturing of superficial or deep peritoneal wounds is required or recommended. The peritoneal defects heal by mesothelialization with minimal adhesion forma-tion.[34] Suturing produces ischemia, which attracts omen-tum, bowel, and adjacent organs to the surgical site to provide neovascularization. All of this can be prevented by simply leaving the peritoneal wounds open to heal.

Energy source

Generally we use the KTP laser at 10 to 14 W on con-tinuous mode, the CO_2 laser at 15 to 35 W superpulse, or the unipolar needle or blade at 20 W cutting current. We prefer the laser as a bloodless scalpel for its speed of application, precision, safety, and simultaneous cut-ting and hemostatic control with minimal tissue damage.

Surgical technique

The two techniques described below leave clean, open wounds with intact vasculature for rapid, adhesion-free healing. The surgeon should not denude large areas of peritoneum in the hope of removing microscopic disease; this promotes adhesion formation.

By using the direct traction technique (grasp, elevate, circumscribe, and dissect), larger endometriotic lesions are grasped with a toothed forceps and traction is applied medially (Figure 26-3). The normal peritoneum/serosa is incised at the periphery of the lesion, and the area underneath is dissected, allowing the normal tissue to fall away. When the endometriotic lesion is grasped ini-tially, it is at the level of the pelvic floor or the serosa of the organ involved. If the surgeon continues to dissect at the same level when the lesion is drawn away, an excessive amount of normal tissue will be removed and deep blood vessels will be at risk of injury. The dissection should "follow the lesion" and allow the normal tissue to retract as the lesion is excised.

With the indirect traction technique (circumscribe, grasp, elevate, and dissect), normal peritoneum/serosa

is incised at the periphery of the lesion; the peritoneal edge of the specimen is grasped, elevated and dissected free (Figure 26-4). This technique has the advantage of delivering an intact specimen undisturbed by the grasping forceps and is preferable when dissecting small lesions. Endometriotic lesions over the ureter may be elevated by hydrodissection and excised by the indirect technique. Using the laser suction-irrigator as a backstop is a mod-ification for excision of endometriosis about the ureter.

Visual control

Visual control is essential. Scissors, and CO_2 and KTP laser dissection are safer than unipolar electrosurgery when operating around the ureter, bowel, blood vessels, and nerves. The laser, with exposures as brief as 0.05 seconds, allows the surgeon literally to cut a few cells at a time.

Uterosacral ligaments

Endometriosis of the uterosacral ligament should be ex-cised after the ureter is identified and under visual con-trol. The ureter is identified through the peritoneum and, if necessary, by surgical dissection. This can be accom-plished by grasping and incising the peritoneum lateral to the ureter, followed by aquadissection until the ureter is in plain view.

A deep endometriotic nodule at the uterine end of the left uterosacral ligament is grasped with a tooth forceps introduced through the right lower quadrant trocar sleeve and pulled toward the midline with constant traction. The KTP laser is inserted through the left lower quadrant trocar sleeve and the laser suction-irrigator through the lower midline trocar. The endometriotic nodule is cir-cumscribed with the laser and excised by following the lesion. Bleeding is controlled immediately with bipolar electrocoagulation as each bleeder is encountered. The wound is left open to heal. The procedure is reversed for the right uterosacral ligament.

Laser uterosacral nerve ablation is effective in treat-ment of central pelvic pain associated with endometri-osis.[35] This procedure may be used in selected cases. A 1-cm by 1-cm-deep crater is vaporized in the uterine end of the uterosacral ligaments. The surgeon must avoid vaporizing laterally to prevent brisk bleeding from the artery within the uterosacral ligament. The ureter must be under direct visual control and safe from harm.

Rectovaginal pouch—open

Excision of endometriosis from the open rectovaginal pouch of Douglas[36] requires control of the uterus and rectum. The rectum is emptied by a mechanical bowel preparation, and if extensive dissection is contemplated, this should be augmented with an antibiotic bowel preparation.

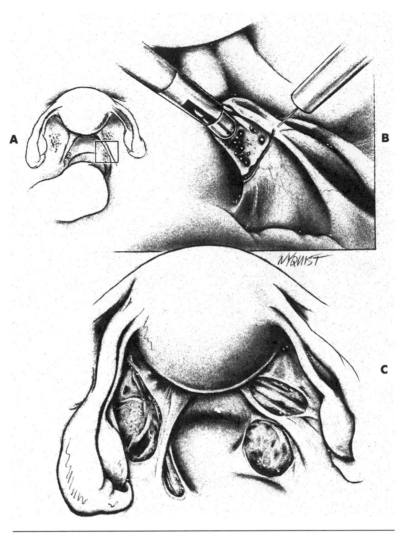

Figure 26-3
Direct traction technique for excision of endometriosis. **A,** Four deep endometriotic lesions. **B,** The direct technique (grasp, elevate, circumscribe and dissect) gives the surgeon control of deep endometriotic lesions and facilitates excision. Dissection should "follow the lesion." **C,** The clean peritoneal wounds are left open to heal.

Vaginal portion

Superficial and deep disease is excised by the direct or indirect traction technique. Subtle forms can be recognized by near contact laparoscopy.[37] Uncommonly, with an open rectovaginal pouch, endometriosis may penetrate into the posterior vaginal fornix. It can be removed by combined laparoscopic and transvaginal dissection.[38]

Peritoneal pockets are everted by grasping the floor with toothed forceps and excised with the KTP or CO_2 laser or unipolar electrode (Figure 26-5). The posterior border of the pockets is formed by the rectum and it is important to follow the lesion to avoid cutting hemorrhoidal blood vessels. The surgeon must be careful of varicosities in the rectovaginal pouch.[26]

Rectal portion

Superficial and deep pararectal endometriotic nodules may be excised if one follows the lesion after it is circumscribed. The hemorrhoidal vessels form a rich supporting vascular network in the pararectal area and should be avoided. Delayed bowel perforation can occur secondary to thermal damage from bipolar coagulation.

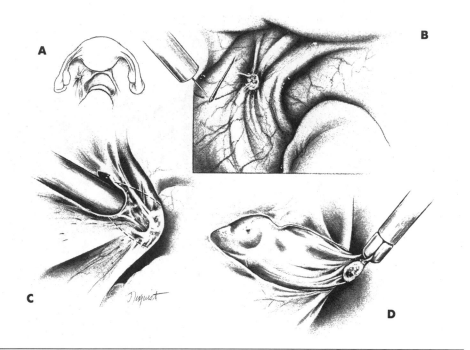

Figure 26-4

Indirect traction technique for excision of endometriosis. The indirect technique (circumscribe, grasp, elevate and dissect) has the advantage of delivering an intact specimen undisturbed by the grasping forceps. **A,** Endometriotic plaque overlying the left ureter. **B,** Incise the peritoneum lateral to the ureter with the CO_2 laser. Separate the endometriotic plaque from the ureter using aquadissection, and perpendicular and parallel spreading with a blunt dissecting forceps. **C,** Using the laser-suction-irrigator to protect the ureter, incise peritoneum on the lateral edges of the lesion with the CO_2 laser. **D,** Grasp the free edge of the peritoneum and excise the specimen.

Rectovaginal pouch—partial obliteration

Endometriosis of the lateral border of the rectum and pararectal tissues adheres to endometriosis of one uterosacral ligament to cause partial obliteration of the rectovaginal pouch. The rectal fascia laterally and posteriorly is separated from the wall of the rectum by a tissue space[39] that tends to protect the rectum from deep invasion by endometriosis. Usually the rectum may be separated from the uterosacral ligament by laser and aquadissection to allow safe excision of deep nodular endometriosis from the rectovaginal pouch and uterosacral ligament.

Before dissection the ureters must be identified at a safe distance or they should be dissected in the following manner. The peritoneum is incised lateral to the ureter. Then the ureter is mobilized by dissecting parallel and perpendicularly with a dissecting forceps and aquadissection. The ureter is displaced laterally before dissecting the uterosacral ligament. This is safer than attempting emergency hemostasis without knowing the location of the ureter.

Rectovaginal pouch—complete obliteration

The antimesenteric border of the rectum adheres to the uterus at the confluence of the uterosacral ligaments with the posterior cervical-vaginal angle. In some cases the rectal adhesions extend upward to the level of the utero-ovarian ligaments. Anteriorly the rectal fascia is weak and intimately connected with the anterior wall of the rectum.[39] Since the rectal fascia and muscularis are fused at the antimesenteric border, endometriotic invasion of the rectum tends to be early and deep. In cases of complete obliteration, endometriosis characteristically invades deeply into the uterus, uterosacral ligaments, and rectum. In some cases, the disease grows through the vaginal wall into the posterior vaginal fornix at the posterior cervical-vaginal angle.

Complete obliteration is differentiated from partial obliteration by the technique of Reich using vaginal and rectal probes.[40] Complete obliteration is diagnosed when only the impression of the rectal and not the vaginal probe can be seen laparoscopically. The ureters are identified by direct visualization, or dissected and displaced laterally. The uterus is put into exaggerated anteflexion using the uterine probe. The rectum is placed in upward traction to identify and incise the line of fusion of the rectum to the uterus, using an electric needle or scissors. The rectum is dissected from the uterus, cervix, uterosacral ligaments, and vaginal portion of the rectovaginal pouch using aquadissection and blunt scissors dissection with a spreading technique. The dissection extends into the areolar tissue of the rectovaginal space, which allows the rectum to be displaced posteriorly. The deep, nodular endometriosis is excised.

Other treatment options for complete obliteration of the rectovaginal pouch

Obliterative rectovaginal pouch disease may be treated expectantly in some patients with infertility, deferring surgical treatment. Medical suppression is acceptable for temporary control of pelvic pain. A third option is to excise endometriosis from the vaginal portion of the rectovaginal pouch, uterosacral ligaments, posterior uterus, and cervix, leaving the bowel lesions untreated. Finally, the patient may be offered laparotomy with extraluminal, wedge, or segmental resection of bowel endometriosis.

Approaching bowel endometriosis and laparoscopic surgery from the viewpoint of reproductive surgeons trained in microsurgery, we recommend resection at laparotomy. In 16 years there have been no pelvic infections and no colostomies. Laparoscopic resection of bowel endometriosis is an investigational procedure. We are reluctant to recommend it until the Society of Reproductive Surgeons of the American Fertility Society considers it a safe and standard procedure equal or superior to laparotomy.

Posterior broad ligaments

In the upper half of the pelvis the ureter lies lateral to the pulsations of the hypogastric artery; in the lower pelvis it lies lateral to the uterosacral ligaments. Posterior broad ligament dissection should be performed with visual control of the ureter and hypogastric artery, and awareness of the large hypogastric vein.

Uterine vessels

Excision of endometriosis from the posterior broad ligament adjacent to the uterus should be undertaken with great care because of the proximity of the uterine vessels, as well as the extensive venous network in the cardinal ligament. At times, it may be prudent to coagulate rather than excise these superficial lesions to avoid the risk of excessive bleeding.

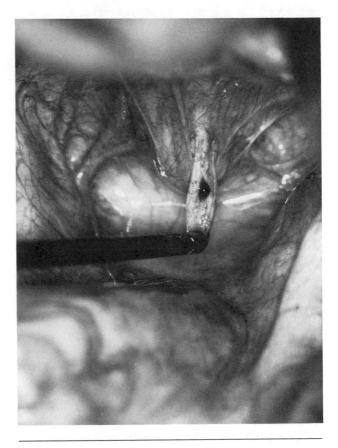

Figure 26-5
Excision of the peritoneal pocket. (See Figure 24-5, which shows this peritoneal pocket before eversion). Peritoneal pockets in the rectovaginal pouch are easily everted from the rectovaginal space for excision, emphasizing the lack of attachment to rectum or vagina. Grasp the floor of the peritoneal pocket, evert and excise. "Follow the lesion" to prevent deep dissection and injury to the hemorrhoidal vessels. From Batt RE and Smith RA: Embryologic theory of histogenesis of endometriosis in peritoneal pockets. *Obstet Gynecol Clin North Am* 16:20, 1989.

Peritoneal pockets

Peritoneal pockets in the posterior broad ligament descend for a variable distance into the pararectal space from a position medial or lateral to the ureter. They do not evert as easily as do those in the rectovaginal pouch. Endometriotic brim nodules or spider nodules in the floor of the pockets are excised by the direct traction technique: grasping, elevation, and excision.[26]

Superficial endometriosis

Superficial endometriosis may be separated from the ureter by hydrodissection and then excised with KTP or CO_2

laser, the scissors, or vaporized with the laser. Hydro-dissection was designed for vaporization of endometriosis with the CO_2 laser because the laser does not penetrate water; care must be taken when the KTP laser is used for coagulation or vaporization because it does penetrate water. We prefer to incise the peritoneum lateral to the endometriotic plaque, use aquadissection to displace the ureter, and excise the endometriosis.

Deep endometriosis

A deep endometriotic plaque overlying the left ureter may be excised using the following technique. The ureter is identified. The endometriotic plaque is grasped and elevated medially with the right lower quadrant instrument. The peritoneum lateral to the ureter is incised, and by aquadissection and parallel and perpendicular spreading forceps dissection, the ureter is separated from the endometriosis. The endometriosis is grasped, pulled medially, and excised with laser or scissors. Hemostasis is achieved by bipolar electrocoagulation.

Deep endometriosis attached to the ureter

When the endometriotic plaque is attached to the ureter, an additional step is required. Scissors or laser dissection and aquadissection are used to cut the endometriosis free of the ureter. Endometriosis that invades deeply into the ureter requires resection and repair at laparotomy.

Ureters

It is mandatory that the laparoscopic surgeon have control of the ureter to prevent injuries.

Congenital ureteral displacement

In the lower pelvis, medial displacement of the lower pars posterior of one or both ureters may occur as an isolated congenital anomaly or in association with peritoneal pockets in the posterior broad ligament or rectovaginal pouch. This is a common congenital anomaly.[26,41] The ureter may form the medial border of a large congenital broad ligament recess.

In the upper pelvis it is important to recognize congenital lateral displacement of the ureter adjacent to the infundibulopelvic ligament when isolating and ligating the infundibulopelvic ligament and when dissecting an adherent ovary. Congenital displacement of the ureter medial to the hypogastric artery is uncommon. Be aware of duplication of the ureter.

Acquired ureteral displacement

In patients with sclerosis and contraction of endometriosis of the cardinal and uterosacral ligaments, the ureter may be pulled medially toward the cervix and uterosacral ligament where it is in danger of injury during surgery.[42]

Deep peritoneal endometriosis with sclerosis in association with ovarian endometriosis may pull the ureter laterally. In this abnormal lateral position the ureter is subject to injury during dissection of the ovary and during division of the infundibulopelvic ligament for salpingo-oophorectomy.

Ureterolysis at the level of the ovary

An endometriotic plaque overlying or invading the ureter is often associated with adherent endometriomas of the ovary. The ureter should be located and controlled before attempting to excise the endometriosis. Elevate the peritoneum lateral to the ureter with a toothed forceps and incise with scissors or laser for a distance of 2 to 3 cm to expose the ureter. Incise dense ovarian adhesions with scissors or laser. Complete the ovariolysis with aquadissection. Displace the ovary laterally and anteriorly. Excise large ovarian endometriomas to improve surgical exposure.

Grasp the lateral edge of the endometriotic plaque with a toothed forceps and reflect medially. Separate the endometriotic plaque from the ureter using aquadissection, and perpendicular and parallel spreading with a blunt dissecting forceps. Cut the dense adhesion bands to the muscularis of the ureter with scissors or laser. Do not tent the ureter. This dissection may be tedious and time consuming. The surgeon should be gentle and persistent, avoiding impulsive moves and rough dissection. Secure blood vessels to the ureter with hemoclips or with fine bipolar forceps. Excise the endometriosis with laser, biopsy forceps, or scissors. Care must be taken not to injure the hypogastric artery or the hypogastric vein. Examine the ureter, and perform additional ureterolysis if necessary. (Deep invasive endometriosis of the ureter requires ureteral resection and repair, for which a laparotomy is recommended.) Leave the raw peritoneal wound open to heal; apply Interceed.

Ureterolysis at the level of the uterosacral ligament

Medial displacement of the ureter to a position adjacent to the uterosacral ligament may occur as a congenital anomaly or from contraction of deep, fibrotic endometriosis in the uterosacral ligament or broad ligament. The ureter should be located and controlled before attempting to excise endometriosis from the uterosacral ligament or broad ligament. Dissection of the ureter must be performed carefully to avoid brisk bleeding from the extensive venous network in the cardinal ligament and from the uterine artery.

With the ureter in full view through the peritoneum or after ureterolysis, the endometriosis may be excised (Figure 26-6). Incise the peritoneum lateral to the ureter 2 cm from the cardinal ligament and extend the incision caudally. Dissect the ureter free with aquadissection and parallel and perpendicular spreading with a blunt dissecting forceps, after the technique of Reich, until it can be displaced with a blunt probe. Cut adhesions to the

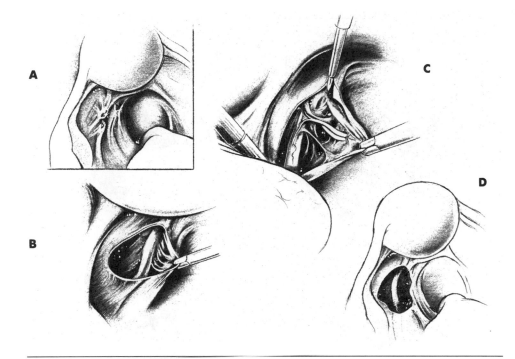

Figure 26-6
Ureterolysis at the level of uterosacral ligament. **A,** Deep endometriosis attached to the left ureter near the cardinal ligament. **B,** Incise the peritoneum lateral to the ureter. Separate the endometriotic plaque from the ureter using aquadissection, and perpendicular and parallel spreading with a blunt dissecting forceps. **C,** With the ureter in view, the large endometriotic lesion is excised with a unipolar 3mm knife. Blood vessels from endometriotic peritoneum to the ureter are ligated wth titanium clips and divided. **D,** Complete the excision by the indirect traction technique. The peritoneal wound is left open to heal.

ureter. Control bleeding with fine bipolar electrocoagulation or hemoclips.

Grasp the endometriosis of the left uterosacral ligament or broad ligament with a toothed forceps from a right lower quadrant portal and maintain constant traction medially. Circumscribe and excise the entire lesion with laser, unipolar needle, or scissors. Secure hemostasis with bipolar electrocoagulation using Kleppinger forceps. The power should be sufficient for hemostasis but low enough to limit lateral spread of thermal energy. Leave the raw peritoneal wound open to heal.

Ureterolysis at the level of the cardinal ligament

Dissection of the ureter within the preformed ureteric tunnel distorted by endometriosis of the cardinal and uterosacral ligaments is beyond the scope of laparoscopic surgery and should be performed at laparotomy.

Ureterolysis of the frozen ureter

When the ureter is firmly embedded in endometriosis, laparotomy is recommended as the mode of access for ureterolysis or resection and implantation into the bladder.

Oviducts

Fallopian tubes may be handled atraumatically with the deactivated Kleppinger bipolar forceps or with suction from a laser suction-irrigator. Peritubal adhesions should be dissected from the cornual angle laterally after the technique of Winston.[43]

Superficial endometriosis of the fallopian tube may be excised by the direct traction technique. Deep lesions may require microsurgical excision. Patients with localized obstruction of the fallopian tube from endometriosis or salpingitis isthmica nodosa should be treated by microsurgical resection and reanastomosis at laparotomy,

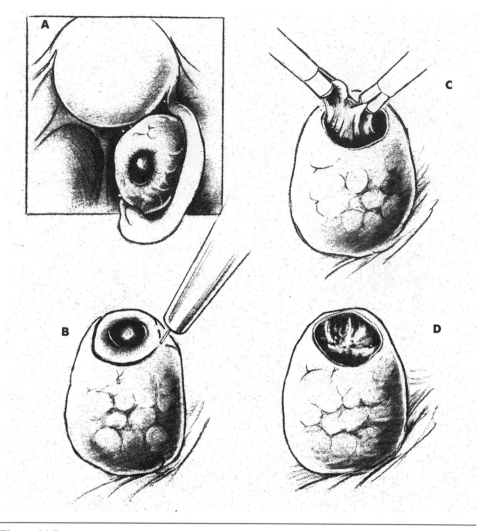

Figure 26-7
Excision of small ovarian endometriomas. **A,** Deep endometrioma less than 2 cm. **B,** Outline the endometrioma by cutting completely through the ovarian cortex with a laser, unipolar needle or scissors. Dissect downward to form an island of endometriosis. **C,** Excise the entire endometrioma with a biopsy forceps. **D,** Secure hemostasis with fine bipolar cautery and leave the ovarian wound open to heal. Interceed may be applied.

or by salpingectomy or salpingo-oophorectomy in selected cases (see Plates 34, 35, 51, and 52).

Ovaries

We recommend permanent histologic sections and second opinion consultations for borderline tumors, especially in the infertile patient. If the biopsies and washings are benign, the patient is rescheduled for endoscopic surgery; if malignant, she is scheduled for an oncology consultation, laparotomy, staging, and selective or complete extirpative surgery.

Some clear cell adenocarcinomas and endometroid carcinomas of the ovary are considered to originate in ovarian endometriomas.[44-46] For that reason we recommend that all endometriomas should be excised and submitted for complete histologic evaluation. We do not believe this is an unreasonable demand on advanced laparoscopists.

Superficial ovarian endometriosis

Excise, vaporize, or coagulate tiny surface lesions and mossy, red endometriotic adhesions. Use short bursts of laser or electrical energy to allow cooling to prevent damaging oocytes.

Endometriomas less than 2 cm diameter

These endometriomas often have a poorly developed fibrous capsule that does not strip from the ovary. They must be excised. Stabilize the ovary by grasping the utero-ovarian ligament, or elevate and stabilize the ovary with the ipsilateral lower quadrant instrument. At laparoscopic surgery, the ovary is stabilized by instruments. This requires dexterity, patience, and skilled assistance. The video monitor reduces fatigue for surgeon and assistant.

Use the intrauterine dilator to maneuver the uterine fundus into the rectovaginal pouch to serve as a platform for the ovary. Circumscribe the endometrioma with laser or unipolar electrode. Dissect down to form an island of endometriosis. Excise the endometrioma completely with biopsy forceps. Secure hemostasis by irrigation, or laser coagulation or bipolar electrocoagulation. Leave the ovarian wound open to heal; do not suture (Figure 26-7).[22,23] Ovarian wounds may be covered with Interceed.

Authors who studied adhesion formation after ovarian surgery in the rabbit model reported:

The results of this study support the contention that a reapproximation of the ovarian cortex is not required after ovarian surgical procedures and, in fact, may be detrimental. If supported by careful observations in women, these findings may help to justify the use of laparoscopic techniques to treat certain ovarian pathologic conditions even though the ovary cannot be reconstructed endoscopically. The ramifications of the reconstruction of the ovarian cortex with sutures after any conservative ovarian surgery warrants further investigation.[22]

Endometriomas 3 to 5 cm diameter

Endometriomas of this size are old enough that a fibrotic host response has developed a fibrous capsule that can be stripped easily from the ovary. The left ovary is elevated and stabilized with the left lower quadrant instrument. Aspirate endometrioma and irrigate with the laser suction-irrigator until clear. Grasp the endometrioma with a right lower quadrant toothed forceps. Outline the endometrioma by cutting completely through the ovarian cortex to identify its capsule. Especially near the hilum of the ovary and also near the utero-ovarian ligament, the capsule must be completely incised to prevent avulsion and hemorrhage when the endometrioma is excised.

Strip the endometrioma from the ovary by applying an upward twisting traction on the lesion and countertraction within the ovary.[47,48] Use aquadissection to separate the capsule from the ovary. Secure hemostasis by irrigation or laser or bipolar coagulation. Reexamine the ovary for deeper "daughter" endometriomas lest significant deep disease go untreated. Leave the ovary open to heal (Figure 26-8).

Endometriomas greater than 5 cm diameter

Large endometriomas are usually adherent to the broad ligament and ureter. Decompress and irrigate the cyst with the laser suction-irrigator until clear to minimize spill before ovariolysis. If spill occurs, copious irrigation

and suction should be done to prevent an inflammatory reaction. Ovariolysis must precede excision. A partial oophorectomy is often required before peeling very large endometriomas from the ovary. Strip the endometrioma from the ovary using aquadissection, traction, and countertraction combined with a teasing, twisting motion.

Endometriomas of this size may adhere tenaciously to the hilar blood vessels, and any attempts to strip or excise them can cause considerable bleeding. Controlling brisk hilar bleeding with electrocoagulation risks devascularization and death of the ovary. To save the ovary, a small portion of cyst wall may have to be left attached to the hilum of the ovary. Coagulate it lightly with the laser or bipolar forceps. The right-handed surgeon is more comfortable working on the hilum of the left ovary from the right side of the patient. (Some of these cases are better treated by microconservative surgery at laparotomy.)

Secure hemostasis within the ovary by defocused laser coagulation or bipolar electrocoagulation. Coagulation shrinks tissue and tends to contract and approximate the edges of the ovary. Leave the ovarian edges open to heal. Internal suture may be desirable to reshape the ovary in selected cases. Use fine sutures and intraovarian, intracorporeal knot tying. Internal sutures should not pierce the ovarian surface.

Unilateral salpingo-oophorectomy

In highly selected cases, unilateral salpingo-oophorectomy may be required for extensive damage to the adnexa.[49] It is important that the other ovary and oviduct be in good condition for fertility. Identify and control the ureter. Proceed with salpingo-ovariolysis. Divide the utero-ovarian ligament and tube. Dissect, isolate, and divide the infundibulopelvic ligament with the GIA stapler device. Complete the salpingo-oophorectomy.

Uterus
Hysteroscopic surgery

Intrauterine adhesions, polyps, submucous fibroids, and septa can be treated by hysteroscopic surgery under laparoscopic control.

Laparoscopic myomectomy

Pedunculated fibroids may be removed easily by coagulating the pedicle and cutting through the stalk. However, laparoscopic removal of intramural fibroids is a controversial procedure. Myomectomy can cause significant uterine bleeding, both immediate and delayed. Adenofibromas and some fibroids are densely adherent to the uterine musculature and may be difficult to dissect. It is more difficult to reconstruct the uterine wall at laparoscopic surgery than at laparotomy.

In excising subserous and intramural leiomyomas, precise surgical closure of the myometrium is required to produce a strong scar to reduce the risk of uterine rupture

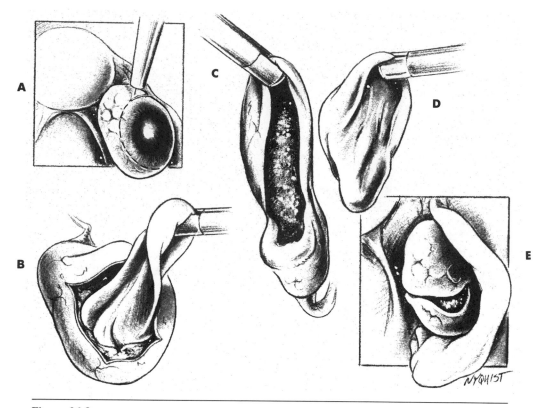

Figure 26-8

Excision of large ovarian endometriomas. **A,** Outline the endometrioma by cutting completely through the surrounding ovarian cortex with a laser, unipolar needle, or scissors. Open, drain and lavage to remove all chocolate material. **B,** Grasp, twist, and gently strip the cyst from the ovary. **C,** Traction must be applied to the cyst from different directions to complete the excision. **D,** The cyst is removed through a 5-mm trocar sleeve. **E,** The ovarian wound falls together without sutures.

during labor. Inject the uterus with a small amount of dilute vasopressin solution, 10 U in 100 ml saline. Make a small incision over the fibroid with a unipolar knife or a CO_2, KTP, or Nd:YAG laser. Exert traction on the fibroid with a corkscrew instrument or a toothed grasping forceps through a secondary port. Isolate the vascular pedicle by combined aquadissection and twisting motion. Desiccate the blood vessels with bipolar electrocoagulation or Nd:YAG laser at 40 to 50 W using defocused, noncontact technique.

Reconstruct the uterus with layers of interrupted deep sutures using an endoscopic curved needle driver.* Curved needles are required to place deep sutures. The endocorporeal knot-tying technique of Topel or the extracorporeal technique of Semm[50] or Reich[15] may be used. Apply Interceed to the suture line to reduce risk of bowel obstruction.

*Cook OB/GYN, Spencer, Ind.

One opinion holds that laparoscopic intramural myomectomy should be avoided as a general rule. Where indicated for health or by size, myomectomy is much easier and safer to perform through a laparotomy incision. Given the substantial risk of transmitting the hepatitis and human immunodeficiency viruses by blood transfusion, patients who are undergoing myomectomy should be prepared for autologous blood transfusions.

External uterine endometriosis

Endometriosis that invades deeply into the serosa and muscularis causing the uterine cornua to retract posteriorly and medially is a formidable lesion that defies conservative surgical treatment. Suppression with GnRH or danazol may be indicated after surgery if the disease is active with an inflammatory host response.

Superficial endometriosis of the posterior uterine wall may be treated, but like fibroids, is associated with uterine adhesion formation. Treatment options are excision, vaporization (electrosurgical, laser), and coagulation (electrosurgical, laser, endocoagulation). Cover wounds with Interceed.

Bladder

Bladder serosa and muscularis

Superficial as well as deep plaques of endometriosis are most commonly found to the left or right of midline. For superficial endometriosis, grasp, elevate, and excise. Leave the wounds open to heal. For deep endometriosis, grasp, elevate, and excise. Use interrupted, absorbable sutures to close deep muscular wounds and full-thickness wounds. Cover the suture line with Interceed.

Bladder base and trigone

Patients who have had vaginal hysterotomy for abortion are susceptible to develop endometriosis of the bladder trigone.[51] Occasionally, deep endometriosis of the base of the bladder develops after cesarean section. Excision of bladder and uterine disease and repair of the organs should be done through a laparotomy incision.

Rectum and sigmoid colon

Laparoscopic resection of bowel endometriosis is an investigational procedure. We are reluctant to recommend it until the Society of Reproductive Surgeons of the American Fertility Society considers it a safe and standard procedure equal or superior to laparotomy.

Superficial bowel endometriosis

Superficial endometriosis may be treated expectantly, excised, vaporized, or coagulated, as one would any superficial peritoneal endometriosis. However, we caution the surgeon that small lesions are not always superficial.

We have observed endometriotic lesions only 4 to 6 mm in diameter that had already penetrated through both muscle layers on the antimesenteric border of the rectum and sigmoid colon. This deep penetration of small lesions is due to two factors: fusion of the weak, anterior rectal fascia to the muscularis in the midline of the large bowel, and the excellent vascular support of the muscularis of the colon that permits rapid and deep invasion. Thus the tendency is for endometriotic lesions on the antimesenteric border of the large bowel, 4 to 6 mm and larger, to be deep. A potential exists for delayed bowel perforation if these lesions are treated with coagulation or vaporization.

Deep bowel endometriosis

The surgeon cannot know until the endometriotic lesion has been dissected whether it can be excised completely by extraluminal resection or will require full-thickness wedge resection or segmental resection and reanastomosis. In our opinion, the risks of pelvic peritonitis and prolonged anesthesia in the steep Trendelenburg position outweigh the benefits of laparoscopic surgery to excise deep bowel endometriosis. Symptomatic disease should be excised at laparotomy after mechanical and antibiotic bowel preparation.

Vermiform appendix

Superficial endometriosis of the appendix in the patient with minimal or mild endometriosis should be treated expectantly to avoid the risk of infecting the other surgical sites.

Deep endometriosis of the tip or middle of the appendix may be confused with a carcinoid tumor. Endometriosis of the base of the appendix may cause obstruction and subacute or acute intraluminal appendicitis. Intussusception of the appendix into the cecum may be associated with endometriosis or a carcinoid tumor. Endometriosis of the tip or mid appendix may be treated by laparoscopic appendectomy using the GIA endoscopic stapling device and antibiotic coverage. Endometriosis of the base of the appendix or endometriosis with intussusception should be resected at laparotomy.

Ileum, cecum, and ascending colon

These organs have thin walls. The potential for delayed bowel perforation and peritonitis exists if endometriotic lesions are treated with coagulation or vaporization. Deep lesions are best handled by extraluminal, wedge, or segmental resection at laparotomy.

Diaphragm

Superficial endometriosis of the right diaphragm may be treated by vaporization or coagulation with a CO_2 laser, taking precautions to avoid blood vessels and the phrenic nerve.

SPECIMENS

Laparoscopic surgery should not be different from other surgery. All tissue specimens should be submitted for histologic examination and verification of diagnosis. Endometriotic lesions that are subjected to formalin rapidly lose their familiar color differentiation. Photographs at laparoscopy will preserve the appearance of the gross pathology for the surgeon, the pathologist, and the patient.

Ideally, each specimen should be sent to the pathologist in a separate, labeled container, identifying it and the location from which it was removed. This will ensure precise clinicopathologic correlation between surgical and histologic diagnosis—benign, atypical, and malignant. This can get expensive, however; alternatively, specimens can be grouped or all submitted together, unless the surgeon is suspicious of cancer.

Morcellation

Large specimens may be removed using one of the morcellators of Semm[50] or by cutting the specimen into smaller pieces with scissors, laser, or electrosurgical knife for removal through the 5- or 10-mm trocar sleeves.

Percutaneous extraction

Medium-size specimens can be removed by enlarging the intraumbilical midline peritoneal and fascial incision after the technique of Reich.[44] The operative laparoscope is withdrawn partially to cut the peritoneum and abdominal fascia with the CO_2 laser. The specimen is grasped with a forceps through the operative laparoscope; instruments and specimen are withdrawn together.

Minilaparotomy

An alternative procedure would be a small lower abdominal incision or a Rocky-Davis lateral transverse incision for removing the specimen.

Posterior colpotomy

Distend the posterior vaginal fornix with a sponge in a ring forceps. Incise transversely through the vaginal portion of the rectovaginal pouch with a unipolar electrode, or with a CO_2 laser at 60 to 100 W, or KTP laser at 20 W for simultaneous cutting and hemostasis. Relatively large specimens (up to 10 cm) may be placed into the cul-de-sac, grasped with a vaginal instrument, and teased through the distensible colpotomy incision.

STAGED PROCEDURES

Laparoscopic debridement and postoperative medical suppression with GnRH or danazol for 3 to 4 months is followed by advanced laparoscopic surgery; by microconservative surgery for endometriosis by laparotomy; or excision of all pelvic endometriosis, total abdominal hysterectomy, bilateral salpingo-oophorectomy, and excision of bowel and ureteral endometriosis.

LAPAROSCOPICALLY ASSISTED VAGINAL HYSTERECTOMY

Advanced laparoscopic surgery for endometriosis may be performed with excision of all pelvic endometriosis preparatory to a standard vaginal hysterectomy with or without vaginal repair.

Laparoscopic surgery

Identify the ureters at all stages of the procedure. Excise the peritoneal endometriosis. Mobilize and excise the adnexa with the GIA stapler. Divide the round ligaments with the GIA stapler. Develop the bladder flap using aquadissection. Divide the uterine vessels bilaterally with the GIA stapler. Use laser for the posterior culpotomy, cutting against the vaginal probe.

Vaginal hysterectomy

Identify the ureters. Open anterior vaginal fornix. Divide and secure the uterosacral ligaments and cardinal ligaments and remove the uterus and adnexae. Support the vagina with the cardinal and uterosacral ligaments. A prophylactic enterocoele repair is performed before closing the vaginal cuff. A sacrospinous fixation and anterior and posterior colporrhaphy are performed if indicated.

REFERENCES

1. Batt RE: Learning basic and advanced laparoscopic surgery. In Martin DC (ed): *Manual of endoscopy,* Downey, Calif, 1990, American Association of Gynecologic Laparoscopists.
2. Darrow S: Case-control study of the relationship of reproductive factors to the risk of endometriosis, doctoral dissertation, Department of Social and Preventive Medicine, State University of New York at Buffalo, 1991, p 96.
3. Batt RE and Naples JD: Microsurgery for endometriosis and infertility. In Hunt RB (ed): *Atlas of female infertility surgery,* Chicago, 1986, Year Book Medical Publishers.
4. Querleu D, Leblanc E, and Castelain B: Laparoscopic pelvic lymphadenectomy in the staging of early carcinoma of the cervix, *Am J Obstet Gynecol* 164:579-581, 1991.
5. Reich H, McGlynn F, and Wilkie W: Laparoscopic management of stage 1 ovarian cancer: a case report, *J Reprod Med* 35:601-604, 1990.
6. Luciano AA et al: A comparative study of post operative adhesions following laser surgery by laparoscopy vs. laparotomy in the rabbit model, *Obstet Gynecol* 74:220-224, 1989.
7. Lundorff P et al: Adhesion formation after laparoscopic surgery in tubal pregnancy: a randomized trial versus laparotomy, *Fertil Steril* 55:911-915, 1991.
8. Reich H and McGlynn F: Laparoscopic treatment of tuboovarian and pelvic abscess, *J Reprod Med* 32:747-752, 1987.
9. Evers JLH: The second-look laparoscopy for evaluation of the result of medical treatment of endometriosis should not be performed during ovarian suppression, *Fertil Steril* 47:502, 1987.
10. Wheeler JM and Reynolds N: When is enough surgery enough? Developing learning curves for new operative techniques. Paper presented at a meeting of CREOG/APGO, New Orleans, Feb 20-23, 1991.
11. Prentice JA and Martin JT: The Trendelenburg position: anesthetic considerations. In Martin JT (ed): *Positioning in anesthesia and surgery,* ed 2, Philadelphia, 1987, WB Saunders.
12. Soderstrom RM: Electrosurgery: advantages and disadvantages, *Prog Clin Biol Res* 323:297-304, 1989.
13. Reich H and McGlynn F: Short self-retaining trocar sleeves for laparoscopic surgery, *Am J Obstet Gynecol* 162:453, 1990.
14. Nezhat C and Nezhat FR: Safe laser endoscopic excision or vaporization of peritoneal endometriosis, *Fertil Steril* 52:149, 1989.
15. Reich H: Laparoscopic treatment of extensive pelvic adhesions, including hydrosalpinx, *J Reprod Med* 32:736, 1987.
16. Filmar S et al: A comparative histologic study on the healing process after tissue transection. II. Carbon dioxide laser and surgical microscissors, *Am J Obstet Gynecol* 160:1068-72, 1989.
17. Gomel V: Advanced operative laparascopy, *ACOG Update* 15:(7):4, 1989.
18. Reich H, MacGregor TS III, and Vancaillie TG: CO_2 laser used through the operating channel of laser laparoscopes: in vitro study of power and power density losses, *Obstet Gynecol* 77:40, 1991.
19. Filmar S et al: A comparative histologic study on the healing process after tissue transection. I. Carbon dioxide laser and electromicrosurgery, *Am J Obstet Gynecol* 160:1062-1067, 1989.
20. Hay DL, von Fraunhofer JA, and Masterson BJ: Hemostasis in blood vessels after ligation, *Am J Obstet Gynecol* 160:737-739, 1989.
21. Ellis H: The aetiology of post-operative abdominal adhesions—an experimental study, *Br J Surg* 50:10, 1962.
22. Brumsted JR et al: Postoperative adhesion formation after ovarian

wedge resection with and without ovarian reconstruction in the rabbit, *Fertil Steril* 53:723-726, 1990.

23. Wiskind AK et al: Adhesion formation after ovarian wound repair in New Zealand white rabbits: a comparison of ovarian microsurgical closure with ovarian nonclosure, *Am J Obstet Gynecol* 163:1674-1678, 1990.

24. Sadigh H, Naples JD, and Batt RE: Conservative surgery for endometriosis in the infertile couple, *Obstet Gynecol* 49:562, 1977.

25. Batt RE and Naples JD: Conservative surgery for endometriosis in the infertile couple, *Curr Probl Obstet Gynecol* 6:1-98, 1982.

26. Batt RE et al: A case-series of peritoneal pockets and endometriosis: rudimentary duplications of the mullerian system, *Adolesc Pediatr Gynecol* 2:47, 1989.

27. Martin DC, Hubert GD, and Levy BS: Depth of infiltration of endometriosis, *J Gynecol Surg* 5:55, 1989.

28. Jansen RPS and Russell P: Nonpigmented endometriosis: clinical, laparoscopic, and pathologic definition, *Am J Obstet Gynecol* 155:1154, 1986.

29. Martin DC and Vander Zwaag R: Excisional techniques with the CO_2 laser laparoscope, *J Reprod Med* 32:753, 1987.

30. Davis GD and Brooks RA: Excision of pelvic endometriosis with the carbon dioxide laser laparoscope, *Obstet Gynecol* 72:816, 1988.

31. Cornillie FJ et al: Deeply infiltrating pelvic endometriosis: histology and clinical significance, *Fertil Steril* 53:978, 1990.

32. Nisolle M et al: Histologic study of peritoneal endometriosis in infertile women, *Fertil Steril* 53:984, 1990.

33. Redwine DB: Laparoscopic excision of endometriosis (LAPEX) by sharp dissection. In Martin DC (ed): *Laparoscopic appearance of endometriosis*, Memphis, 1990, Resurge Press.

34. Ellis H: Prevention and treatment of adhesions, *Infect Surg* 2:803, 1983.

35. Lichten EM and Bombard S: Surgical treatment of primary dysmenorrhea with laparoscopic uterine nerve ablation, *J Reprod Med* 32:37-41, 1987.

36. Kuhn RJP and Hollyock VE: Observations on the anatomy of the rectovaginal pouch and septum, *Obstet Gynecol* 59:445, 1982.

37. Redwine DB: Is "microscopic" peritoneal endometriosis invisible? *Fertil Steril* 50:665, 1988.

38. Martin DC: Laparoscopic and vaginal colpotomy for the excision of infiltrating cul-de-sac endometriosis, *J Reprod Med* 33:806, 1988.

39. Peham H and Amreich J: *Operative gynecology,* vol 1, Philadelphia, 1934, JB Lippincott.

40. Reich H: New techniques in advanced laparoscopic surgery. In Sutton C (ed): *Laparoscopic surgery,* London, 1989, Bailliere.

41. Batt RE and Smith RA: Embryologic theory of histogenesis of endometriosis in peritoneal pockets, *Obstet Gynecol Clin North Am* 16:15, 1989.

42. Grainger DA et al: Ureteral injuries at laparoscopies: insights into diagnosis, management and prevention. *Obstet Gynecol* 75:839-843, 1990.

43. Winston R: Reconstructive microsurgery at the lateral end of the fallopian tube. In Chamberlain G and Winston R (eds): *Tubal infertility,* London, 1982, Blackwell.

44. Scully RE, Richardson GS, and Barlow JF: The development of malignancy in endometriosis, *Clin Obstet Gynecol* 9:384, 1966.

45. Mostoufizadeh M and Scully RE: Malignant tumors arising in endometriosis, *Clin Obstet Gynecol* 23:951, 1980.

46. Moll UM et al: Ovarian carcinoma arising in atypical endometriosis, *Obstet Gynecol* 75:237, 1990.

47. Martin DC and Diamond MP: Operative laparoscopy: comparison of lasers with other techniques, *Curr Probl Obstet Gynecol Fertil* 9:564, 1986.

48. Reich H and McGlynn F: Treatment of ovarian endometriomas using laparoscopic surgical techniques, *Reprod Med* 31:577-584, 1986.

49. Reich H: Laparoscopic oophorectomy and salpingo-oophorectomy in the treatment of benign tubo-ovarian disease, *Int J Fertil* 32:233, 1987.

50. Semm K: *Operative manual for endoscopic abdominal surgery,* Chicago, 1987, Year Book Medical Publishers.

51. Simmons CA: Some peculiarities of endometriosis, *Proc R Soc Med* 61:357, 1968.

27

Endometriosis: Microconservative Surgery

RONALD E. BATT

SALVADOR M. UDAGAWA

JAMES M. WHEELER

Microconservative surgery for endometriosis has evolved from the conservative operation of Wharton.[1] For over 60 years surgeons have refined the procedure through research into the natural history of endometriosis and the host responses to the disease.[2-23]

Since the first edition of this atlas, a major shift to advanced laparoscopic surgery has taken place. Microconservative surgery for endometriosis by laparotomy (mCSEL) is now reserved for patients with severe and extensive disease, bowel and ureteral endometriosis, or large leiomyomas for which precise organ reconstruction is required.

MICROSURGICAL TECHNIQUE

According to Acland: "There are various kinds of seeing that we can practice and only one of them is good enough for microsurgery. Wishing you could see isn't good enough, hoping you can see isn't good enough, only seeing that you can see is good enough to give you the margin of safety and assurance that you need in your microsurgical technique."[24]

Microsurgery places two demands on the surgeon: the use of magnification and exquisitely delicate surgical technique. Those who master microvascular surgical techniques will thereafter perform surgery with profound respect for tissues based on first-hand laboratory experience of the gentleness required to restore vascular integrity and function.

Compared with macrosurgery, microsurgery offers two advantages for the patient: complete resection of endometriosis with less risk of vascular injury[25] and fewer postoperative ovarian adhesions.[26]

PREVENTION OF ADHESIONS

Various ancillary modalities are used by reproductive surgeons to prevent adhesions. We recommend the following techniques.

Microsurgical technique

Magnification with the operating microscope of 1.8- to 2.5-power operating loupes fulfills the requirements for mCSEL. Constant irrigation with warm Ringer's lactate solution is necessary to keep all surfaces moist. We recommend that surgeons own and care for their microsurgical instruments.

Reduce pelvic congestion and inflammation

Less pelvic congestion is encountered and hemostasis is easier when operating chronic endometriosis during the midproliferative phase of the cycle. Preoperative danazol for 8 to 12 weeks or gonadotropin-releasing hormone (GnRH) agonist for 12 to 16 weeks is recommended to treat acute inflammatory host response to endometriosis. We prefer danazol because the course of treatment is shorter and the surgery easier. It is important to treat coexistant sexually transmitted infections before mCSEL. Remote handling of tissues with instruments is recommended. Abrasive surgical sponges should be avoided.

Reduce bacterial colonization

Microconservative surgery for endometriosis by laparotomy should be delayed at least 6 weeks after laparoscopy to reduce risk for infection. A bactericidal soap shower the night before surgery and mechanical cleansing of umbilicus, abdomen, and vagina in surgery are recommended. Prophylactic antibiotics are used in all infertility cases. Mechanical and antibiotic bowel preparation is recommended before bowel surgery.

Extraluminal bowel resection is preferred, especially during infertility operations. We recommend strict indications for segmental bowel resection and appendectomy. Interceed should not be used over the bowel anastomosis suture line. Copious irrigation of the pelvis with Ringer's lactate solution before closing will reduce bacterial colonization below the critical level for infection.

Reduce risk of wound infection and hematoma formation

Electrosurgical entry of all layers except skin produces a clean, hemostatic wound. The 7-inch plastic ring wound protector wraps the wound edges and prevents drying during surgery. A Jackson-Pratt subfascial drain through a separate stab incision is recommended for all Maylard incisions and, selectively, for Pfannenstiel incisions.

Reduce tissue ischemia

Wide surgical exposure permits gentle retraction of wound edges and precise dissection with unipolar microelectrode, scissors, or laser. Bipolar electrocoagulation is recommended for precise hemostasis. Hemostatic staples are preferred to large ligatures. It is best to avoid sutures; peritoneal and ovarian wounds are left open to heal. Where unavoidable, fine synthetic (polydioxanone or polyglactin) internal sutures can be used for organ reconstruction, but no surface sutures should be placed. Fascial edges should be approximated loosely for healing.[27]

Separate wounded surfaces during healing

Uterine suspension is used where indicated. Interceed applied to uterine, ovarian, and broad ligament wounds reduces the risk of adhesions.[28]

Minimize postoperative ileus

The self-retaining wound retractor is adjusted to place minimal tension on the wound. The intestines can be wrapped in omentum and gently displaced cephalad with a warm pack soaked in Ringer's lactate solution. Early oral feeding is recommended to strengthen immunocompetency.[29] Good hydration is maintained with postoperative oral and intravenous fluids. Hydration can be monitored clinically and by a urinary output of 60+ ml/hour. An indwelling Silastic Foley catheter for 24 to 48 hours prevents overdistention of the bladder.

THE MICROCONSERVATIVE PROCEDURE

The immediate objectives of mCSEL are to excise all endometriosis and associated pathologic lesions and to restore reproductive anatomy and function. The twin principles of minimal trauma and prevention of ischemia to normal tissues should be foremost as the surgeon excises endometriosis and prepares tissues for healing. From start to finish, surgery should proceed smoothly with an easy rhythm, using the lowest magnification required to see clearly.

Experienced surgical team

Gynecologic surgeons who assume responsibility for the care of patients with severe and extensive endometriosis are encouraged to develop a surgical team with a colorectal surgeon and a urologist. An integrated surgical team that is experienced in pelvic, bowel, and ureteral endometriosis is desirable to minimize complications and secure consistently good results.

Organ-specific surgery

Microconservative surgery for endometriosis consists of a series of procedures performed in logical sequence. The operative fields should be prepared carefully so that each organ is operated under ideal conditions. We prefer to prepare and operate on the lower pelvis first, then flood this area with Ringer's lactate solution, and prepare and operate the upper pelvis.

PREPARATION OF THE SURGICAL FIELD— LOWER PELVIS

The most difficult dissection occurs in the lower pelvis where the organs are fixed by deep, nodular, invasive disease, by sclerosis and shortening of the cardinal and uterosacral ligaments, and by dense adhesions. We recommend a widely dissected Pfannenstiel, Maylard modification, or midline incision because the surgeon must have wide exposure to perform surgery gently.

Insert the 7-inch plastic ring wound protector and wrap the edges of the wound. Adjust the Kirschner four-blade retractor (Figure 27-1) for the desired exposure. Examine the bowel by inspection and palpation and note all endometriotic lesions for later treatment. Wrap the bowel in the omentum and displace it cephalad with lint-free wet packs.

Place a 2-0 polyglactin countertraction suture through the posterior cervix. Give the suture a half-twist to form a pair of suspenders to displace the uterine fundus up and under the pubic blade of the Kirschner retractor. Anchor the two ends of the suture by artery forceps under the rim of the retractor frame. Put a Silastic pad under the suspenders suture to protect the uterus from abrasion (Figure 27-2). Alternatively, the uterus may be stabilized by a Deavor retractor attached to the "Iron Intern" automated surgical robot retractor holder.*

Use 1.8× or 2.5× wide-angle surgical loupes and 4000-candle-power coaxial headlamp to see peritoneal

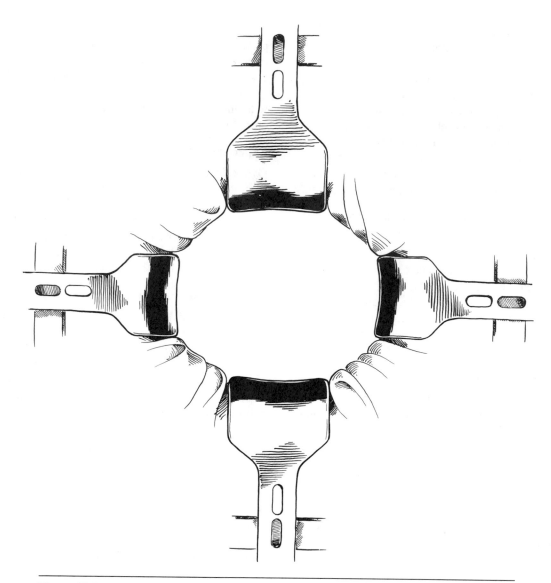

Figure 27-1
Kirschner retractor with a K-4 setting. The 6-cm blades at the pubic and umbilical positions and the 5-cm blades at the left and right positions give an octagonal opening 10 cm long and 12 cm wide, providing 104 cm² of working area with excellent exposure of the lower and upper pelvis for operating extensive endometriosis.

endometriosis clearly. Surgery is more refined and faster when the surgeon and the assistant are comfortable standing or seated using the full range of mobility of the operating table.

Handle tissues remotely with Teflon rods and traction sutures. Use electrosurgical and scissors dissection and keep finger dissection to a minimum. Throughout the procedure, moisten tissues with warm heparinized Ringer's lactate solution.

Rectovaginal pouch of Douglas and uterosacral ligaments
Open rectovaginal pouch

Systematically identify and transfix all endometriotic lesions involving the uterosacral ligaments, posterior cervix, and peritoneum of the vaginal and pararectal portions of the rectovaginal pouch with individual traction sutures (Figure 27-3). Excise each lesion in turn by a separate operation starting in the depths of the pelvis and systematically working outward (Figures 27-4 through 27-8).

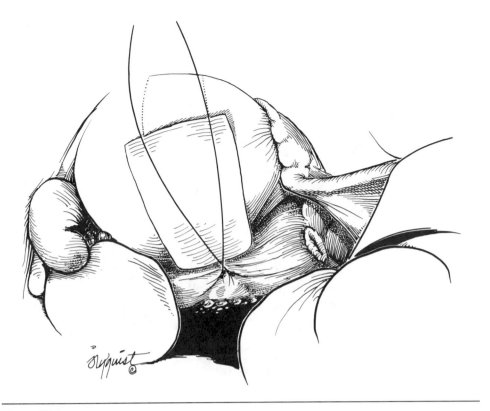

Figure 27-2
The lower pelvis is fully displayed and stabilized for the duration of the operation using a posterior cervical suspenders suture and a protective silicone rubber vest.

Elevate each endometriotic lesion by its traction suture until the peritoneum blanches, and circumscribe with the unipolar electrode. The peritoneum immediately retracts to reveal the breadth of the nodule, plaque, or cyst. The depth of the lesion can be determined only by further dissection. Most electrosurgical excisions are bloodless. Use Ringer's lactate irrigation solution and gentle suctioning to identify bleeding vessels. Preventive and therapeutic hemostasis is obtained with bipolar electrocoagulation to minimize blood loss and tissue necrosis.

Fine electrosurgical or laser dissection produces wounds with intact vasculature. The clean, raw wounds should be left open to heal by mesothelialization. Most will heal without adhesions. Reperitonealization is contraindicated. "Whenever possible, peritoneal defects should be left open rather than pulled together under tension."[30] Careful irrigation of each defect should be performed to remove devitalized tissue.

Dissection of deep pararectal endometriosis inevitably leads to tangential cuts of veins causing bleeding that is difficult and dangerous to control with bipolar electrocoagulation. It may be controlled by grasping the vessel with a fine long forceps and securing with a vascular clip or fine gallbladder clamp and free tie.[18] Unfortunately, this results in devascularized pedicles that invite adhesion formation. Large ischemic pedicles should be avoided;

if unavoidable, they should be trimmed and inverted with minimal tension using 6-0 polypropylene suture material.

Partial obliteration of the rectovaginal pouch

Laterally, the rectal fascia is separated from the muscularis of the rectum by a tissue space.[31] This anatomic arrangement retards endometriotic invasion of the lateral rectal muscularis. Since it is the lateral wall of the rectum that adheres to the uterosacral ligament in most cases of partial obliteration, usually the rectum can be dissected free with minimal risk of entering the bowel lumen. The bulk of the endometriosis is usually located in the uterosacral ligament.

Identify the ureter; dissect it free if necessary. Gently grasp the rectum with a large Babcock clamp and retract it toward the sacral promontory. Transfix and elevate the deep endometriosis. Lightly incise the line of fusion between the rectum and the uterosacral ligament with a unipolar electrode. This opens a plane of cleavage. Use pressurized water dissection and long blunt scissors to separate and displace the rectum to its normal position.

Elevate the endometriosis in the uterosacral ligament until the overlying peritoneum blanches to identify the outer limits of the disease. Circumscribe the disease with a unipolar needle. Dissect deeply with unipolar needle or Metzenbaum scissors, lifting, teasing, and cutting tis-

Text cont'd on p. 462.

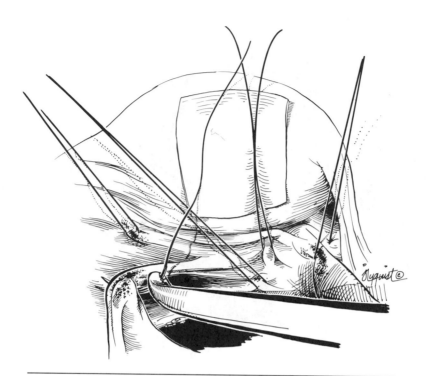

Figure 27-3
Endometriotic lesions of the lower pelvis are identified under magnification and transfixed with individual traction sutures.

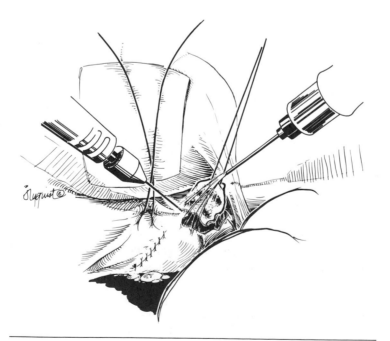

Figure 27-4
Deep nodular endometriosis in the right uterosacral ligament is elevated with traction suture and circumscribed with a microunipolar electrode under magnification.

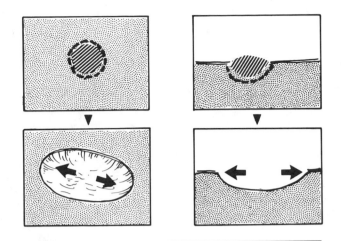

Figure 27-5
When an endometriotic cyst or nodule is circumscribed, the
peritoneum retracts widely. After excision, the clean wound
is left open to heal.

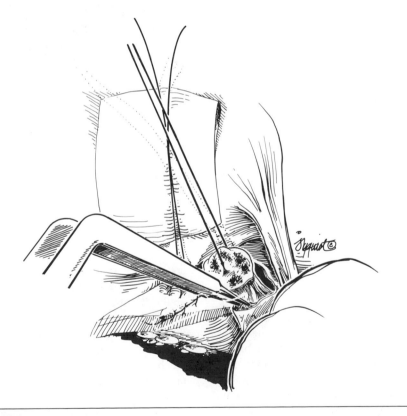

Figure 27-6
Hemostasis is obtained with precise bipolar electrocoagulation as soon as each vessel is encountered. In the lower pelvis, the surgeon maintains traction on the lesion, dissects, and operates
the foot-controlled bipolar forceps; the assistant surgeon irrigates as needed and operates the
suction. The operating field should be free of blood when dissection resumes.

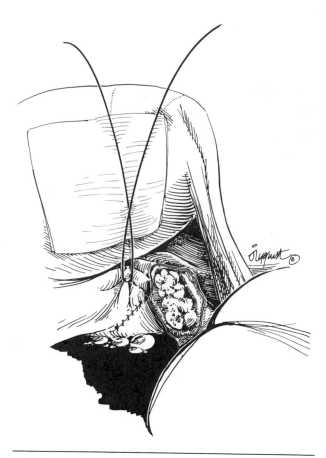

Figure 27-7
Raised edges of the raw wound immediately after meticulous resection of deep endometriotic nodule. Within a few minutes the wound will flatten out. When the dissection is clean, with minimal disruption of the vascularity of surrounding normal tissues, the raw wound is left open to heal. Reperitonealization is unneccessary and undesirable. The raw wound is composed of mesothelial tissue, which rapidly heals by differentiation of new peritoneum from the underlying connective tissue of the entire wound, and without adhesion formation in most instances.

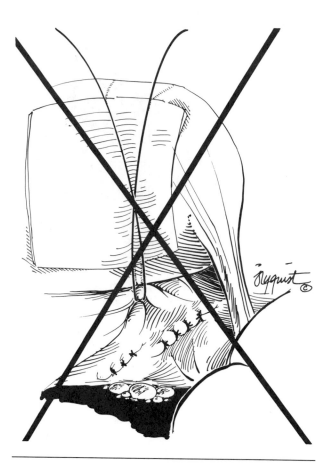

Figure 27-8
Traditionally, surgeons have repaired all peritoneal wounds by interrupted or running sutures, which cause tissue ischemia that leads to adhesion formation. This practice is based on the reparative characteristics of skin, derived from ectoderm, which heals from its edges. If skin edges are not meticulously approximated, an unattractive scar results. In contrast, the peritoneum, derived from mesoderm, heals not from the edges but regenerates from the entire surface of the wound simultaneously to form a smooth, new peritoneal surface when the clean, raw wound is left open to heal.

sue. The scarring is deeper under the central portion of the endometriosis than at the borders. Excise the entire endometriotic focus and surrounding fibrous scar. Leave the wound open to heal after thorough irrigation.

The resulting peritoneal defect in one case measured 4 cm long and 1.5 cm wide. Five years later at laparoscopy it was well mesothelialized without adhesions, and measured 4 cm long and 1.5 cm wide. In the cases where endometriosis does invade the muscularis of the rectum, dissection should be performed with scissors and the muscularis repaired with interrupted sutures.

Complete obliteration of the rectovaginal pouch

Anteriorly, the rectal fascia is fused to the muscularis of the rectum.[31] This anatomic arrangement facilitates direct

and deep endometriotic invasion of the rectal muscularis where the disease extends caudally, cephalad, and laterally. Contraction of the surrounding fibrotic tissue causes shortening of the rectal serosa and muscularis as they are "gathered" into one large lesion.

Complete obliteration of the rectovaginal pouch is a much more serious entity with deep invasion of the rectum. The mother-lode of endometriosis is usually distributed unequally among the uterosacral ligaments, uterus, and rectum. The rectum adheres to the uterus and proximal uterosacral ligaments, and the adhesions may extend all the way up the posterior uterus to the level of the utero-ovarian ligaments. The rectal adhesions are usually dense and their dissection is difficult. It can be accomplished by persistent scissors and blunt dissection.

With the unipolar electrode, incise the line of maximum fibrosis at the junction of the rectum and uterus to establish a plane of dissection; then sweep away the less dense adhesions with aquadissection and finger dissection. Use large, blunt, thoracic scissors dissection against the uterus and blunt countertraction against the rectum to open the obliterated rectovaginal pouch. Once the rectum is free and back in its normal anatomic postion, the excision proceeds as with an open rectovaginal pouch.

We observed a muscular defect 10 cm long after dissecting a large, contracted endometriotic lesion from the rectum. Such large lesions are better treated by wedge resection or segmental bowel resection and reanastomosis than by extraluminal resection. Bowel resection should be performed as the last procedure before closing the abdomen.

Complete obliteration with ovaries adherent to the rectum

In the ordinary case of complete obliteration of the rectovaginal pouch, the ovaries adhere laterally to the pelvic sidewalls—the centrifugal pattern. The more devastating centripedal pattern involves complete obliteration of the rectovaginal pouch, with the uterus retroflexed and retroverted, and the ovaries prolapsed and densely adherent to the posterior uterus and sides of the rectum.

After debridement, surgery is performed on the obliterated rectovaginal pouch. Later the ovarian endometriomas are resected and the elongated utero-ovarian ligaments plicated. The uterus requires a modified Gilliam suspension to hold it anterior and the ovaries laterally during healing.

Complete obliteration: endometriosis of posterior vaginal fornix

Complete obliteration of the rectovaginal pouch may be complicated by endometriosis that penetrates into the posterior vaginal fornix with invasion of the portio vaginalis of the cervix. Surgery on patients with this complex condition should be performed with the patients in the low-thigh, frog-leg, lithotomy position, which permits simultaneous transabdominal and transvaginal surgical access to the lesion.

Open the obliterated rectovaginal pouch and displace the rectum posteriorly. Transfix and excise the lesions of the posterior uterus and uterosacral ligaments. Transfix, elevate, and dissect the endometriosis of the cervical-vaginal angle from the cervix entering the posterior vaginal fornix. Repair the cervix. Resect the vaginal portion of the rectovaginal pouch full thickness posterolaterally and detach the specimen from the rectal wall. Dissect the endometriosis within the rectal muscularis. Repair the rectum. Close the defect in the vagina transvaginally with interrupted sutures.

Posterior broad ligaments and ureters

The ureters are in jeopardy at three levels during surgery for endometriosis: above the pelvic inlet during presacral neurectomy, at the ovarian fossa, and at the uterosacral ligaments during excision of endometriosis or laser uterosacral nerve ablation.

Normally the ureters traverse the pelvis lateral to the hypogastric arteries and 1.5 to 2 cm lateral to the uterosacral ligaments. However, the surgeon should be aware of congenital anomalies in the lower pelvis, where one or both ureters encroach on the lateral border of the uterosacral ligaments.[32]

Both ureters should be identified before resecting endometriosis of the uterosacral and the broad ligaments (Figure 27-9). If a ureter is obscured by sclerosis, endometriosis, or adhesive disease, the peritoneum lateral to the ureter should be opened and the ureter identified. Preoperative ureteral catheters are helpful in extensive disease.

When the ovary is fused to the peritoneum overlying the ureter, open the peritoneum, and identify and displace the ureter from harm (Figure 27-10). Mobilize the ovary and oviduct by unipolar needle dissection against Teflon rods. Displace the ovary upward and laterally by a traction suture through the endometrioma. Keep all tissues moist. Excise the peritoneal endometriosis. Use pinpoint bipolar hemostasis. Leave the wounds open to heal.

Left-frozen pelvis

In severe cases of endometriosis, reproductive surgeons encounter the left-frozen pelvis: a large ovarian endometrioma fused to the broad ligament and ureter, with the oviduct sandwiched between the ovary and the broad ligament, or adherent to the tubal or antimesenteric border of the ovary, and the whole completely enveloped by the sigmoid colon in obliterative adhesive disease (Figure 27-11).

The right adnexa should be evaluated carefully, and if it is normal, the surgeon may proceed directly to remove the left adnexa. If, however, there is the least question about the status of the right adnexa, the surgeon should leave the left adnexa undisturbed, returning to remove it only when the right ovary and oviduct are functional.

The left-frozen pelvis is approached by retroperitoneal dissection. Free the sigmoid colon from the infundibulopelvic ligament and anterior broad ligament. Incise the peritoneum lateral to the infundibulopelvic ligament and open to the left round ligament (Figure 27-12). Dissect retroperitoneally with blunt instrument dissection or scissors. Identify the ureter. Divide the infundibulopelvic ligament (Figure 27-13). Expose the full length of the pelvic ureter by retroperitoneal dissection. Dissect the sigmoid colon from the oviduct, ovary, and the peritoneum, with the ureter in full view and safe from injury.

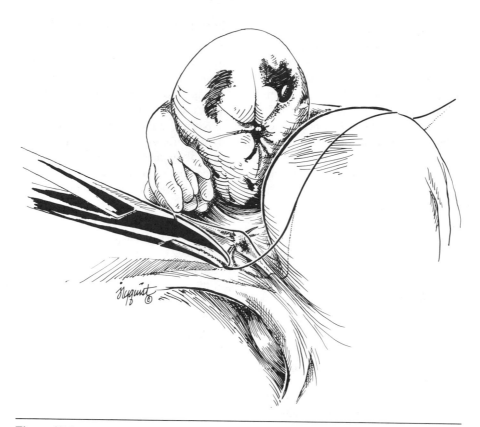

Figure 27-9
Transfixion of a flat endometriotic plaque overlying the left uterine vessels and ureter. With traction, the peritoneum blanched to reveal a retroperitoneal "iceberg" endometriotic nodule much wider than the surface plaque. Dissection was necessary to identify the vessels and ureter and to disclose the depth of retroperitoneal invasion to ensure complete removal. These lesions should be excised, not coagulated. The chocolate endometriotic cyst involved the posterior surface of the left ovary.

Next, dissect the ovary and tube from the peritoneum (Figure 27-14).

Starting at the infundibulopelvic ligament, incise the lateral wall peritoneum medially toward the ureter and then caudally along the ureter to the base of the cardinal ligament. Cut the left tube and left utero-ovarian ligament from the uterus. Then incise the peritoneum downward to the ureter at the base of the cardinal ligament to complete the dissection. The specimen is removed en bloc (Figure 27-15). The dissection is rapid and nearly bloodless. Any compression of the ureter can be relieved by direct retroperitoneal dissection. The large triangular peritoneal defect is left open to heal; alternatively, a redundant rectosigmoid can be used to cover the defect.

Ovarian remnant syndrome

The ovarian remnant syndrome usually causes pelvic pain with or without a mass.[33,34] Incomplete surgery of the left-frozen pelvis is a common cause of the syndrome, especially with the transperitoneal rather than retroperitoneal approach to the ovary. Laparoscopic salpingo-oophorectomy or oophorectomy with ligatures is another cause of this syndrome.

PREPARATION OF THE SURGICAL FIELD— UPPER PELVIS

Adjust the uterine suspenders suture or the Iron Intern. Loosely fill the lower pelvis with lint-free wet packs to form a level platform for the adnexae. Insert a silicone rubber pad to provide a smooth working surface.

Prepare the surgical field carefully. We recommend sitting on the side of the patient opposite the ovary and oviduct to be treated since the most difficult dissection is always the posterior surface of the ovary. The better ovary and tube are examined and treated first, using the operating microscope or operating loupes (Figure 27-16).

Oviduct

Salpingolysis should precede ovariolysis. Start the dissection at the cornual angle and proceed laterally, freeing the oviduct from the ovary and restoring the fimbria ovarica (Figure 27-17). We prefer the unipolar microelectrode or carbon dioxide (CO_2) laser for dissection. Hemostasis is secured with unipolar electrocoagulation or bipolar jeweler's forceps. Serosal and peritoneal wounds are left open to heal. Fimbrial phimosis should be dilated slowly. Occasionally, an incision is required.

Text cont'd on p. 466.

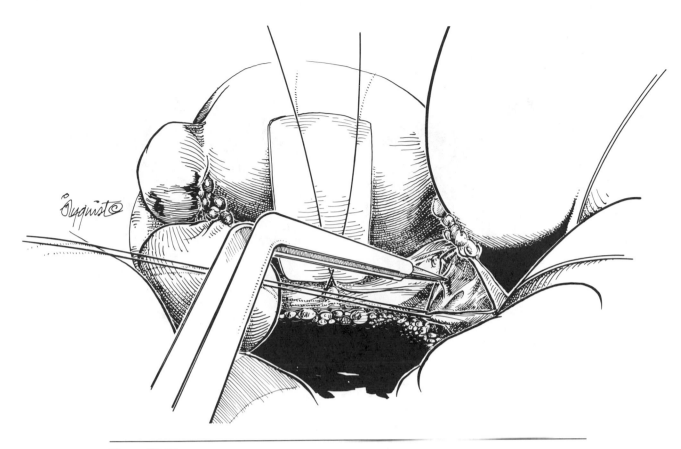

Figure 27-10
A large defect in the right broad ligament resulted from mobilizing the ureter, freeing the adherent ovary, and resecting the peritoneal endometriosis. The raw wound is clean; hemostasis is precise with bipolar electrocoagulation; no devascularized ligated pedicles are present. This wound is left open to heal.

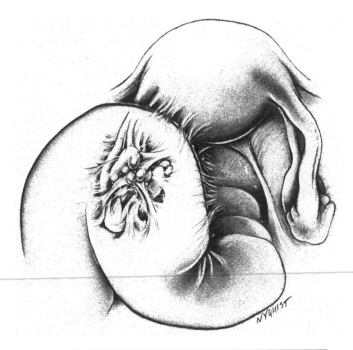

Figure 27-11
Left-frozen pelvis. The left adnexa is irreparably damaged by extensive endometriosis and adhesive disease.

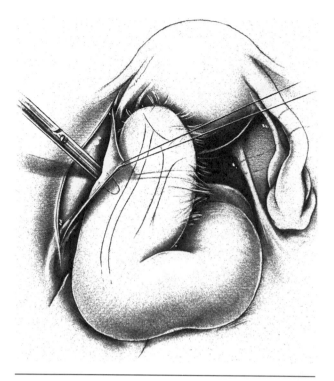

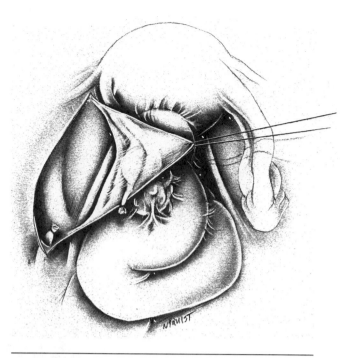

Figure 27-12
Left-frozen pelvis. Dissect the sigmoid colon from the left anterior broad ligament and infundibulopelvic ligament. Then incise the left anterior broad ligament laterally from the infundibulopelvic ligament to the round ligament. Identify the ureter by blunt and sharp retroperitoneal dissection using long, blunt-tipped scissors.

Figure 27-13
Left-frozen pelvis. Ligate the infundibulopelvic ligament and expose the full length of the pelvic ureter by further retroperitoneal dissection.

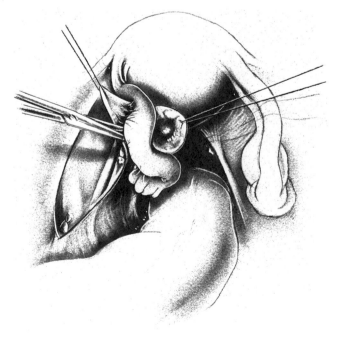

Figure 27-14
Left-frozen pelvis. With the ureter under direct vision, dissect the sigmoid colon from the left oviduct, ovary and pelvic peritoneum; then dissect the oviduct and ovary from the posterior peritoneum.

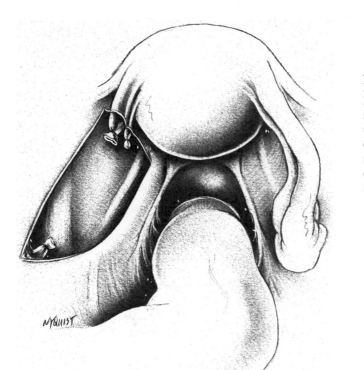

Figure 27-15
Left-frozen pelvis. Starting at the left infundibulopelvic ligament, incise the lateral wall peritoneum medially toward the ureter and then caudally along the ureter to the base of the cardinal ligament. Cut the left tube and utero-ovarian ligament and incise the peritoneum downward to the ureter to complete the dissection. Remove the specimen en bloc, leaving a large triangular peritoneal defect.

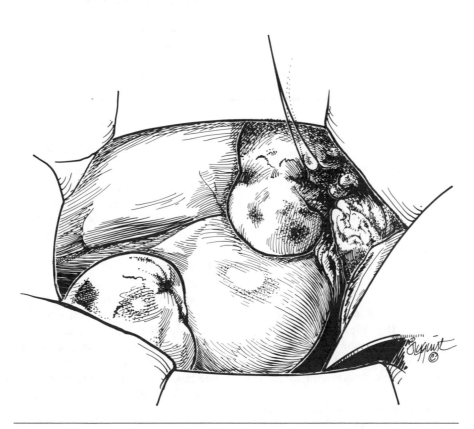

Figure 27-16
Ovarian endometriosis. Unequal adnexal damage from endometriosis. There is an endometrioma in the left ovary, and the right ovary and oviduct are severely damaged. The severely damaged right adnexa is displaced upward and laterally by a traction suture through one of the endometriomas, to be kept moistened while the lesser involved adnexa is repaired. The better ovary should be repaired first before the severely damaged ovary is removed. This way the surgeon does not inadvertently render the woman castrate should unexpected problems be encountered in the attempt to repair the better ovary.

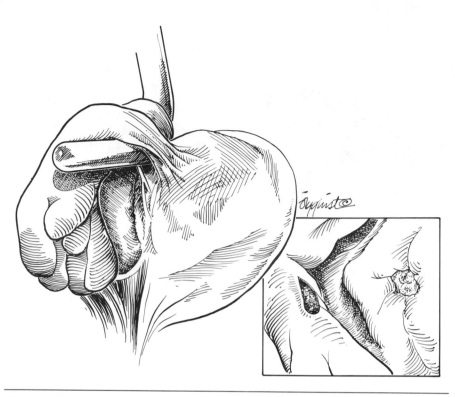

Figure 27-17
Oviduct adhesions. Vascularized immobilizing adhesions between the ampulla of the oviduct and the ovary interfere with the ovum capture. The adhesions are excised and the clean, raw surfaces are covered with Interceed to reduce reformation of adhesions between the two contiguous surfaces.

Endometriotic nodules or cysts may involve any portion of the tubal serosa and muscularis. Each lesion should be transfixed, elevated, and circumscribed with a unipolar microelectrode. Dissection is performed under high magnification with either a microelectrode or microscissors. Secure hemostasis with bipolar jeweler's forceps. Obstructing lesions require segmental resection and microsurgical tubal reanastomosis.

Ovary

Perform ovariolysis under magnification before excising endometriomas (Figure 27-18). Float the enveloping adhesions with Ringer's lactate solution. Grasp the adhesions with jeweler's forceps and excise with the unipolar microneedle. Use pinpoint hemostasis with the same instrument.

Begin surgery on the healthier ovary first. A deeply invasive hilar endometrioma requires meticulous dissection to ensure complete removal of the disease with preservation of the ovarian blood supply. Microsurgical technique can make the difference between a functional ovary and ischemia-induced premature ovarian failure.

Ideally, all ovarian endometriomas should be excised through an elliptical incision in the long axis of the ovary. Those that invade posteriorly may require an oblique elliptical incision extending from the mesovarium toward the antimesenteric border of the ovary.

Endometriomas 2 cm or smaller

Endometriomas 2 cm or smaller in diameter have a poorly defined fibrous capsule and must be dissected from the ovary (Figures 27-19 through 27-24). Transfix the endometrioma with a traction suture and outline with a shallow elliptical incision using the unipolar microelectrode. The tunica albuginea of the ovary does not retract like the peritoneum. Therefore a second and even a third wider elliptical incision may be required to expose the endometrioma without having to undercut normal ovarian tissue. Place a countertraction suture of 5-0 polypropylene inside the ovary. Under magnification, dissect the endometrioma and any deep daughter cyst from the ovary with scissors. Secure hemostasis with a foot-controlled fine bipolar forceps as the bleeding vessels are encountered. Leave the ovarian wound open to heal.[35]

Endometriomas 2 cm and larger

A larger endometrioma will have a well-defined fibrous capsule and can usually be peeled from the ovary. Transfix the endometrioma with a traction suture and outline with a shallow elliptical incision using the unipolar microelectrode and strip it from the ovary. Use fine scissors dissection near the hilum of the ovary. Obtain hemostasis with irrigation, suction, and pinpoint bipolar electrocoagulation (Figures 27-25 through 27-28). Control ex-

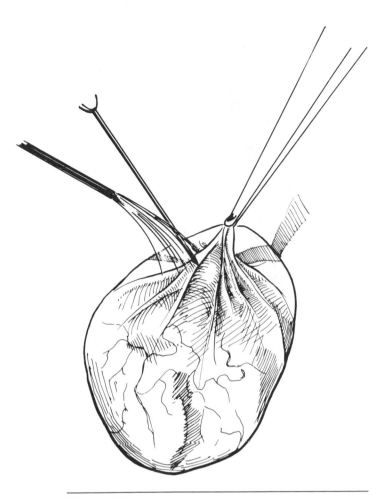

Figure 27-18
Ovarian adhesions. Tentlike enveloping adhesions of the ovary are elevated with a fine forceps and floated with irrigating solution. Under magnification, the adhesions are dissected from the ovary with a unipolar microelectrode. As with all microsurgery, the surgeon's wrists must be stabilized and dissection performed with fingertip control to keep from lacerating the ovarian surface.

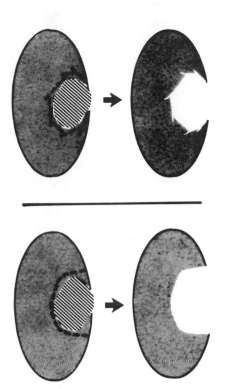

Figure 27-19
An ovarian endometrioma in the posterior surface of the ovary often extends into the hilum and mesovarium. The surgeon should sit on the opposite side of the table to see this lesion well. A wide elliptical incision to unroof the endometrioma permits easy dissection of the side walls and floor of the lesion. A small elliptical incision gives poor exposure, leading to numerous undercuts during dissection. Not only does the surgeon risk incomplete removal, but bleeding in the crevices caused by undercutting is difficult to control.

cessive bleeding temporarily with a rubber-shod cardiovascular clamp applied to the mesovarium, and place 5-0 nylon sutures at 5- to 10-mm intervals within the ovary for permanent hemostasis and deep closure of the ovarian wound. Reconstruct the ovary to present the largest surface area to the fimbriae for ovum pick-up. Bring the edges of the ovarian cortex into approximation with a second layer of deep sutures. Use no sutures in the tunica albuginea.[36]

Special attention is required when the only functional ovary contains a large endometrioma (Figures 27-29 and 27-30). When both ovaries are equally damaged, repair both. If one ovary and oviduct are normal or easily repaired and the contralateral ovary is severely damaged, remove the latter rather than repair it. The decision to perform a unilateral salpingo-oophorectomy can be made with more confidence if the surgeon has examined both adnexa and repaired the better one first (Plates 51 and 52).

Malignancy

Surgeons should be vigilant for ovarian neoplasms. Infertile women with a unilateral tumor of borderline malignant potential may be treated by unilateral salpingo-oophorectomy, lymph node dissection, and contralateral microconservative surgery for endometriosis.

Uterus

Fibroids should be excised through a midline uterine incision, using secondary intramural incisions to remove lateral growths. The midline incision is less vascular and farthest from the ovaries. A modified Gilliam suspension elevates the ovaries laterally and further reduces the risk of ovarian adhesions to the uterus.

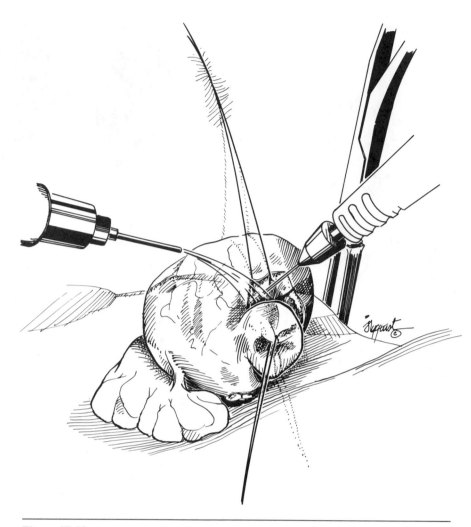

Figure 27-20
Endometrioma less than 2 cm in diameter. The left ovary is elevated and displayed on
a silicone rubber operating pad. A traction suture through the endometrioma and a
countertraction suture inside the ovary facilitate initial dissection with the unipolar
electrode under magnification with operating microscope or loupes.

Inject the uterus with a dilute pitressin solution, 10 U
in 200 ml saline. Incise the serosa and myoma with
scalpel, laser, or unipolar needle. Transfix the myoma
with a traction suture or Lahey thyroid clamp. Twist the
myoma and complete the dissection. Clamp and suture
ligate the vascular pedicle. Sophisticated ultrasound techniques are available to visualize the nutrient blood vessels
to the myoma.[37] Close the wound with interrupted 3-0
polyglactin sutures deep and 5-0 superficially. Apply
Interceed to the suture line just before closing the abdomen to reduce bowel adhesions but only if hemostasis
is complete.

Large fibroids are bisected and each half is dissected
with scissors from inside outward. The nutrient vessels
are clamped and the specimen excised. The endometrial
cavity is seldom entered using this technique.

In our opinion, posterior uterine fibroids should not
be removed through an anterior uterine incision that tra-
verses the uterine cavity. Not only is there potential for
intrauterine adhesions, but the surgical exposure is poor
and the resulting uterus probably is at greater risk of
rupture during pregnancy.

Round ligaments and bladder

The cystic, nodular, and flat lesions of endometriosis
involving the round ligaments and bladder are transfixed,
elevated, and excised.

Rectum and sigmoid colon

Serosal lesions may be excised without suture repair.
Deep bowel endometriosis should be resected only when
the patient has had full mechanical and antibiotic bowel

Text cont'd on p. 474.

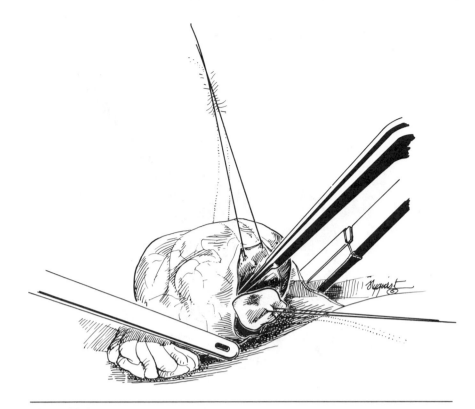

Figure 27-21
Endometrioma less than 2 cm in diameter. Traction and countertraction sutures give the required exposure for precise hemostasis with bipolar electrocoagulation under magnification as the bleeding vessels are encountered. The surgeon controls the fine suction and foot-operated bipolar forceps; the assistant surgeon provides exposure and intermittent irrigation.

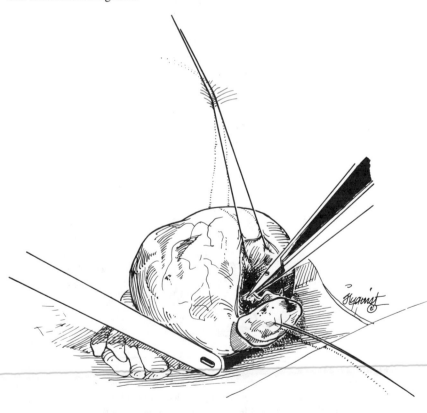

Figure 27-22
Endometrioma less than 2 cm in diameter. Magnification by operating loupes or microscope permits precise scissors or unipolar dissection of the endometrioma and daughter cysts without undercutting the ovary.

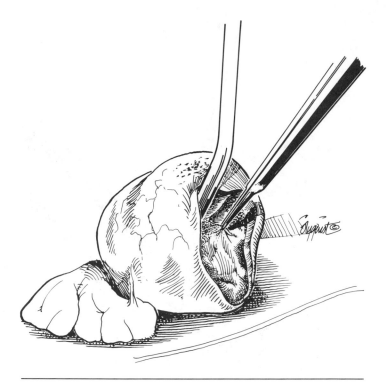

Figure 27-23
Endometrioma less than 2 cm in diameter. Bleeding vessels are identified and coagulated with fine bipolar forceps.

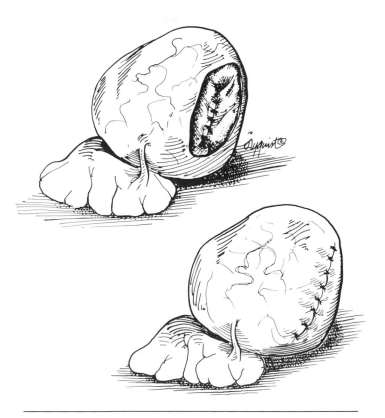

Figure 27-24
Endometrioma less than 2 cm in diameter. Sometimes bleeding vessels retract and defy hemostasis by electrocoagulation. In such cases, hemostasis can be achieved and ischemic necrosis prevented by placing one or two rows of closely spaced 5-0 polypropylene sutures, which are covered with Interceed. We no longer recommend suturing the ovarian cortex.

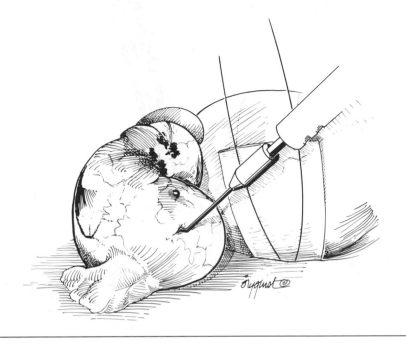

Figure 27-25
Endometrioma greater than 2 cm in diameter. The ovary is elevated and displayed on a silicone rubber operating pad. A wide initial elliptical incision is made with the unipolar microelectrode to unroof a well-encapsulated ovarian endometrioma.

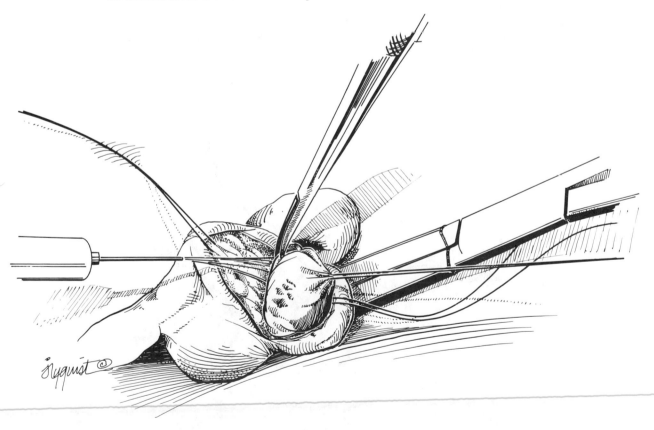

Figure 27-26
Endometrioma greater than 2 cm diameter. Endometriomas this size usually strip easily from the ovary. However, precise microscissors dissection may be required to separate an adherent endometrioma from the ovarian hilar blood vessels.

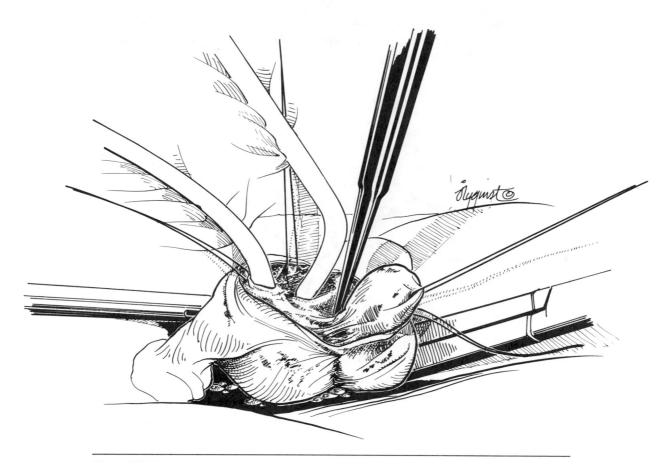

Figure 27-27
Endometrioma greater than 2 cm diameter. Tips of Teflon retractors rest in cavities that remain after dissecting out appendages of the endometrioma. Microbipolar electrocoagulation controls a bleeding vessel at the base of the endometrioma.

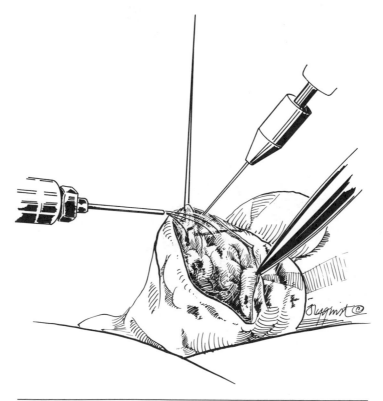

Figure 27-28
Light touch unipolar microelectrocoagulation of tiny bleeding vessels within the ovary. The ovarian wound is left open to heal, or the ovary may be reconstructed with deep, fine sutures covered with Interceed. Surface sutures are not used.

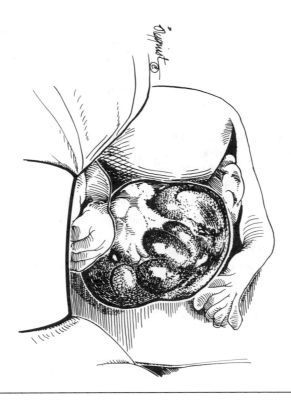

Figure 27-29
A 7-cm endometrioma of the left ovary with only a remnant
of right ovary after resection of a dermoid cyst during ado-
lescence. The endometrioma is resected and the ovarian remnant excised.

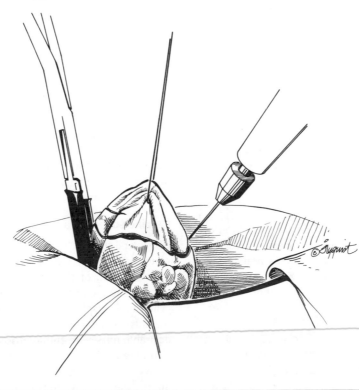

Figure 27-30
Unlike the peritoneum, the ovarian cortex does not retract when incised. A second, wider, cortical incision may be required to unroof the endometrioma and gain direct access to its side walls.
This wider exposure permits precise deep dissection with microscissors near the hilum of the
ovary.

preparation. The surgeon should be prepared for wedge resection or segmental resection and reanastomosis if the lesion cannot be excised by extraluminal resection.

Extraluminal bowel resection

Most bowel endometriosis does not penetrate the submucosa and mucosa and consequently can be excised by extraluminal resection (Figure 27-31). It is the procedure of choice for all cases of colonic endometriosis with normal mucosa at sigmoidoscopy or colonoscopy. It is an acceptable procedure during infertility surgery, since it essentially eliminates the risk of infection. Mechanical and antibiotic bowel preparation is essential, however, to protect against inadvertent entry into the bowel lumen.

Place two to four stay sutures in the rectal wall at the 12, 3, 6, and 9 o'clock positions and traction sutures in the endometrioma. Incise the normal bowel serosa around the endometrioma with a unipolar electrosurgical needle at low voltage. Excise the endometrioma by scissors dissection, making every effort to avoid cutting the mucosa. Numerous large bleeding vessels in the mesentery of the rectum are individually clamped and ligated with 3-0 polyglactin. A long, diamond-shaped muscular defect remains, with the submucosa and mucosa intact (Figure 27-32).

The repair is carried out in the horizontal diameter to avoid stricture. The first suture divides the wound into equal left and right halves. Use a single-layer closure with interrupted 3-0 nylon sutures, avoiding the mucosa to preserve sterility of the surgical field.

Wedge resection of bowel

A transmural endometrioma may be removed by full-thickness wedge resection of the bowel wall, with a single-layer, interrupted suture closure excluding the mucosa. A hand-sewn anastomosis carries minimal risk of leakage and infection (Figure 27-33). Nevertheless, the surgeon who recognizes the benefits of extraluminal resection will find few indications for elective wedge resection of bowel endometriosis.

Segmental bowel resection

Rectal endometriosis rarely develops below the level of the rectovaginal pouch; consequently, anterior resection is not as low as in rectal malignancy. This reduces the risk of leakage from the anastomosis. Segmental resection would be indicated where the entire sigmoid colon showed many sharp angulations and fixations to its mesentery, with deep infiltration of the bowel musculature that caused partial bowel obstruction in several areas. A segmental bowel resection is preferred to several wedge resections (Figures 27-34 through 27-36).

Open the posterior peritoneum to the peritoneal reflection and mobilize the entire sigmoid colon and upper rectum. Visualize and protect the left ureter. Display the

anatomy so that all structures are easily identified. Outline, clamp, divide, and doubly ligate the mesenteric vessels with no. 1 polyglactin sutures. Similarly outline, clamp, divide, and doubly ligate the superior hemorrhoidal vessels distally.

Protect the pelvic area with moist gauze. The bowel is divided between intestinal clamps placed one and one-half finger-breadths below the lowest endometriotic lesion and proximally at the junction of the descending and sigmoid colon. Both ends of the bowel must have satisfactory blood supply and approximate without tension. Bowel continuity is reestablished by an open end-to-end coloproctostomy using a single layer of interrupted 3-0 nylon sutures excluding the mucosa. Alternatively, an EEA stapler can be used. Irrigate with copious amounts of Ringer's lactate solution and verify hemostasis. Position a nasogastric tube in the stomach.

Cecum and ileum

Advanced diagnostic laparoscopy was designed to identify endometriosis of the cecum and ileum. If all the pelvic endometriosis can be excised by laparoscopic surgery, the cecal and ileal lesions can be removed at a subsequent laparotomy.[38] This allows time for the ovarian and peritoneal wounds to heal. Intact organs can withstand bacterial contamination better than wounded organs. Bowel surgery is often best delayed if ovarian surgery was required because of the risk of ovarian abscess.

Superficial lesions may be excised extraluminally. Deeper lesions require wedge or segmental resection and reanastomosis. If bowel endometriosis must be removed during microconservative surgery, a mechanical and antibiotic bowel preparation is mandatory.

Vermiform appendix

Intussusception of the appendix requires wedge resection of the cecum and appendectomy. Bulbous and fusiform endometriotic lesions require appendectomy. Prophylactic appendectomy is contraindicated during infertility reconstructive surgery.

Uterine suspension

Consider uterine suspension selectively to separate wounded surfaces until healing is complete.

Triplication of the round ligaments will antevert the uterus. The modified Gilliam uterine suspension will elevate and displace the ovaries laterally away from wounds in the rectovaginal pouch and uterus. This is desirable for severe endometriosis with a centripedal pattern (Figure 27-37).

A ventral uterine suspension will pull the ovaries medially away from wounds in the posterior broad ligament. This is useful in extensive disease with the centrifugal pattern. Pass one 2-0 nylon suture superficially through

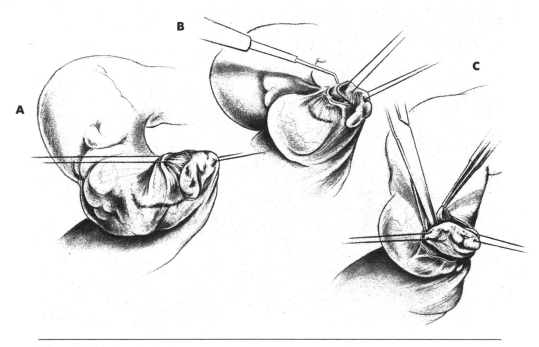

Figure 27-31
Extraluminal bowel resection. (This procedure is the same for the ileum and the colon.) **A,** A solitary deep endometriotic nodule of the ileum is transfixed and elevated with two traction sutures. **B,** Using a unipolar needle, the seromuscular layer is incised to circumscribe the nodule. **C,** The nodule is then dissected from the bowel wall using blunt-tipped Metzenbaum scissors.

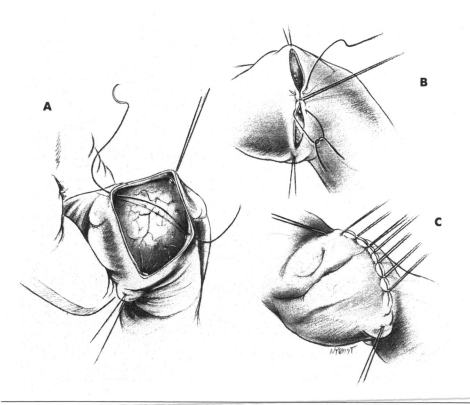

Figure 27-32
Extraluminal bowel resection. **A,** Two lateral traction sutures are placed to facilitate transverse closure of the seromuscular defect. Note the bulging, intact intestinal mucosa. The first seromuscular suture is placed in the midline. **B,** Additional interrupted 3-0 nylon sutures are placed to close the bowel wall. **C,** The single layer seromuscular closure preserves the normal diameter of the bowel wall lumen.

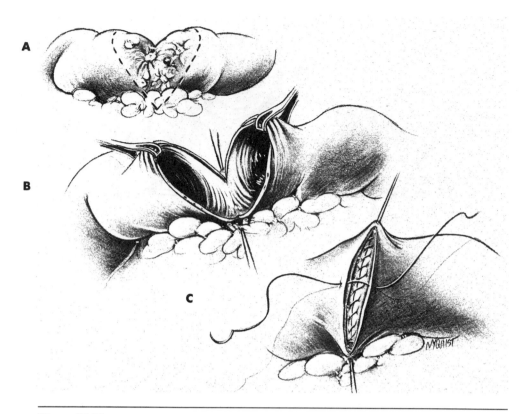

Figure 27-33

Wedge resection of the bowel. (This procedure is the same for the ileum and the colon.)
A, A localized endometrioma of the sigmoid colon is transfixed and elevated with two traction sutures. A stay suture is placed on either side to outline the extent of the endometrioma.
B, After incision of the seromuscular layer with a unipolar needle, gross infiltration of the mucosal layer is recognized and a full-thickness wedge resection is completed using Metzenbaum scissors. Active mesenteric bleeders are individually ligated with 3-0 polyglactin.
C, The bowel wall is closed in two layers: a mucosal layer repair of continuous interlocking 3-0 gastrointestinal chromic catgut is followed by a seromuscular repair using interrupted 3-0 nylon sutures. The closure is performed in the horizontal diameter to preserve the integrity of the bowel lumen.

the midsagittal plane of the uterine fundus and secure it to the anterior fascia on closing the abdomen. The suspension will stretch and, after 1 year, the uterus will be attached to the abdominal wall by an attenuated muscular band 7 to 8 cm long. This procedure is seldom indicated.

Presacral neurectomy

Presacral neurectomy has been advocated for treatment of central pelvic pain associated with endometriosis.[39] No differences in conception rates were noted in patients who underwent conservative surgery for endometriosis, with or without it.[5,10,40] Some of the worst surgical adhesions we have observed attended presacral neurectomy. Stainless steel thumbtacks and fibrin glue can be used to control life-threatening hemorrhage that may be encountered.[41,42]

Presacral neurectomy destroys the early warning system for recurrent peritoneal endometriosis. In our opinion, surgery should be directed toward complete excision of endometriosis rather than relying on presacral neurectomy for pain relief.

Closure

The surgeon makes a final inspection of each operative site. The rinse solution should be clear. Several hundred milliliters of Ringer's lactate solution are left in the pelvis. The abdomen is closed in layers with loose approximation of the fascia. A subfascial Jackson-Pratt drain is placed through a small stab incision for 48 hours.

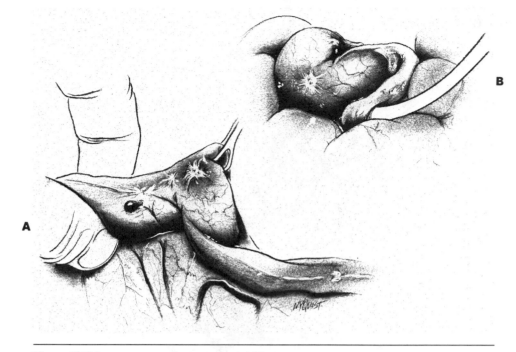

Figure 27-34
Segmental bowel resection. (This procedure is the same for the ileum and the colon.) **A,** A partial obstruction of the ileum caused by deep endometrosis. The dilated bowel segment is held by examining fingers. **B,** Viewed from another perspective, the same obstructing lesion has a "U" or "omega" configuration with the collapsed bowel segment indicated by the Teflon elevator.

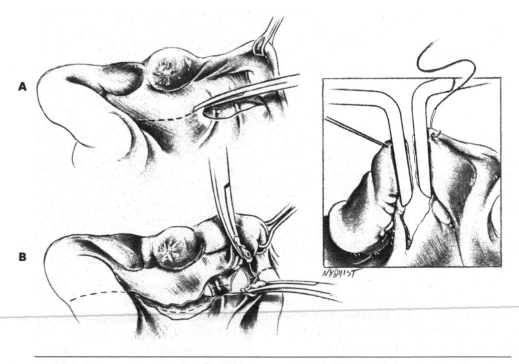

Figure 27-35
Segmental bowel resection. **A,** The mesentery of the ileum is incised with scissors to identify the mesenteric vessels. **B,** The mesenteric vessels are clamped, divided and ligated with 2-0 polyglactin. *(Inset)* The diseased bowel is resected between intestinal clamps. Stay sutures are placed at the antimesenteric border of the bowel.

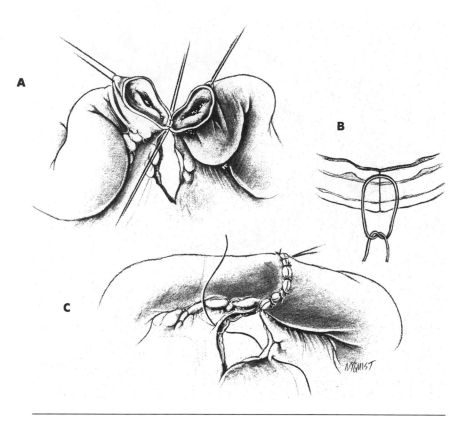

Figure 27-36
Segmental bowel resection. **A,** Continuity of the bowel is re-established by a single layer end-to-end anastomosis using interrupted 3-0 nylon sutures. **B,** The seromuscular suture excludes the mucosa. **C,** The anastomosis is completed without tension. A hand-sewn, single layer anastomosis preserves the internal diameter of the bowel. The mesentery of the bowel is closed with interrupted sutures of 3-0 nylon sutures.

RECURRENT ENDOMETRIOSIS AND INFERTILITY: CONSERVATIVE PROCEDURES

Advanced laparoscopic surgery is particularly applicable in patients with less severe endometriosis but also is valuable treatment for some women with recurrent endometriosis after microconservative surgery.

The experienced reproductive surgeon will recognize patients who may benefit from repeat mCSEL. It is frequently successful in selected patients.[43]

RECURRENT ENDOMETRIOSIS AND INFERTILITY: LESS CONSERVATIVE PROCEDURES

Where conservation of one ovary and the uterus only is possible, in vitro fertilization with embryo transfer (IVF/ET) is required for fertility. Where conservation of one ovary only is possible, IVF/ET and surrogate uterus are required for fertility. When only the uterus can be conserved, husband insemination of the surrogate is required, with recovery of embryo and transfer to wife's uterus. A second option is IVF using the husband's semen and donor eggs with embryo transfer into the wife's uterus. Because of the high pregnancy rate under these conditions, the uterus should be preserved if possible.[44]

We are firmly opposed to scheduling an infertile patient for laparotomy, possible conservative surgery, or possible hysterectomy. In our opinion, hysterectomy should not be performed until both husband and wife have had sufficient time to resolve their infertility and accept the idea, as well as the indication for hysterectomy.

RECURRENT ENDOMETRIOSIS AND HEALTH PROBLEMS: INCOMPLETE PROCEDURES

Experienced surgeons recognize the hazards of heroic attempts to perform complete procedures under adverse circumstances. Profound inflammatory host response at laparotomy, with or without partial bowel obstruction, dictates an incomplete procedure. Postoperative medical suppression will prepare the pelvis for complete excision of endometriosis and associated pathology under controlled conditions.

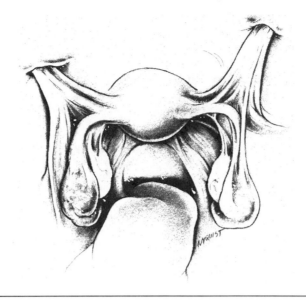

Figure 27-37
Gilliam uterine suspension. At surgery the round ligaments had
been pulled through incisions in the anterior fascia and sutured
in place. Observed through a laparoscope one year later, the
round ligaments have stretched but the uterus remains anteverted
and the ovaries and oviducts are free of adhesions.

Under adverse surgical conditions, bilateral salpingo-
oophorectomy with or without bowel resection may be
the treatment of choice. Subtotal hysterectomy with bilateral salpingo-oophorectomy is much preferred to sew-
ing uterosacral ligaments with endometriosis into the vaginal cuff.

RECURRENT ENDOMETRIOSIS AND HEALTH PROBLEMS: COMPLETE PROCEDURES

Complete extirpation of endometriosis and the reproductive organs may be necessary to preserve health and
quality of life at the cost of fertility.[45] The operations are
often difficult and require a surgical team to minimize
complications. All endometriosis should be excised before proceeding with hysterectomy.

Complete procedures include total abdominal hysterectomy with bilateral salpingo-oophorectomy; excision
of all endometriosis by laparoscopic surgery, laparo-
scopic-assisted vaginal hysterectomy, and bilateral salpingo-oophorectomy; and modified radical hysterectomy
and bilateral salpingo-oophorectomy.

The technique for modified radical hysterectomy requires four steps, which follow:

1. Transfix the infundibulopelvic, uterosacral, and
   round ligaments peripheral to the endometriosis and
   carry the dissection toward the uterus.

2. Dissect the preformed ureteric canals in the cardinal
   ligaments to mobilize endometriosis within the cardinal ligaments.
3. Excise all endometriosis.
4. Complete the hysterectomy, bilateral salpingo-
   oophorectomy, and reconstruction of the pelvic
   floor.

POSTHYSTERECTOMY CUFF VAGINECTOMY

Endometriosis of the vaginal cuff is a complication of
intrafascial hysterectomy for endometriosis without excision of the disease from the uterosacral ligaments, rectum, and rectovaginal pouch. The persistent disease
causes pelvic pain and deep dyspareunia. Cuff vaginec-
tomy under these circumstances can be a difficult procedure. The procedure requires a bowel preparation. Bilateral ureteral catheters are desirable.

Mobilize the ureters to the ureteric canals. Divide the
round ligaments and mobilize the bladder anteriorly. Unroof the ureters in the ureteric canals and secure the
uterine vessels bilaterally.

Dissect the rectum from the posterior vaginal cuff using the unipolar electrode initially. Continue dissecting
into the rectovaginal space with large blunt scissors. Divide the uterosacral ligaments, leaving the endometriosis

attached to the vagina. Open the vagina in the midline and excise the entire vaginal cuff, removing involved cardinal and uterosacral ligaments and the vaginal portion of the rectovaginal pouch. Close the vagina with interrupted sutures, incorporating the cardinal ligaments into the angles for support. Excise the rectal endometriosis.

IMMEDIATE AND LONG-TERM FOLLOW-UP
Comfort

After excision of endometriosis, women may be treated with cyclic combination oral contraceptive pills to reduce retrograde menstruation until pregnancy is desired. Women who do not wish to become pregnant and those over 35 years of age may be offered laparoscopic tubal ligation to eliminate retrograde menstruation and to protect them from further exposure to implantation endometriosis.

Fertility

All other infertility factors should have been corrected before endometriosis surgery so that both husband and wife are at their peak fertility potential during the postoperative months. If conception has not occurred within 12 to 15 months, the couple should be reevaluated and laparoscopic surgery performed. In cases of extensive endometriosis, second-look surgical laparoscopy in 6 months is encouraged.

Women should be encouraged to breast-feed their baby, and if a second child is desired, to attempt pregnancy when nursing is discontinued. Women treated for endometriosis do not have unlimited fertility; we recommend they have two children before using contraception.

Health

At menopause 0.625 mg of conjugated estrogen and 2.5 mg of medroxyprogesterone may be prescribed to prevent osteoporosis. In patients with endometriosis we prefer the balanced combination so that microscopic endometriotic deposits are not stimulated by unopposed estrogen.

After hysterectomy for extensive disease, a period of estrogen deprivation may be desired before starting hormonal replacement therapy. During that interval, 100 mg of danazol given daily will prevent hot flushes and also ameliorate bone loss by its androgenic activity.[46]

REFERENCES

1. Wharton LH: Conservative surgical treatment of pelvic endometriosis, *South Med J* 22:267, 1929.
2. Green TH: Conservative surgical treatment of endometriosis, *Clin Obstet Gynecol* 9:293, 1966.
3. Rogers SF and Jacobs WM: Infertility and endometriosis: conservative surgical approach, *Fertil Steril* 19:529, 1968.
4. Ranney B: Endometriosis. II. Emergency operations due to hemoperitoneum, *Obstet Gynecol* 36:437, 1970.
5. Spangler DB, Jones GS, and Jones HW Jr: Infertility due to endometriosis, conservative surgical therapy, *Am J Obstet Gynecol* 109:850, 1971.
6. Acosta AA et al: A proposed classification of pelvic endometriosis, *Obstet Gynecol* 42:19, 1973.
7. Kistner RW: Management of endometriosis in the infertile patient, *Fertil Steril* 26:1151, 1975.
8. Hammond CB, Rock JA, and Parker RT: Conservative treatment of endometriosis: the effects of limited surgery and hormonal pseudopregnancy, *Fertil Steril* 17:756, 1976.
9. Weed JC and Holland JB: Endometriosis and infertility: an aggressive surgical approach. In da Paz AV (ed): *Recent advances in human reproduction*, Amsterdam, 1976, Excerpta Medica.
10. Garcia CR and David SS: Pelvic endometriosis: infertility and pelvic pain, *Am J Obstet Gynecol* 129:740, 1977.
11. Sadigh H, Naples JD, and Batt RE: Conservative surgery for endometriosis in the infertile couple, *Obstet Gynecol* 49:562, 1977.
12. Brosens IA, Boeckx W, and Gordts S: Conservative surgery of ovarian endometriosis in infertility, *Eur J Obstet Gynecol Reprod Biol* 8:277, 1978.
13. Schenken RS and Malinak LR: Reoperation after initial treatment of endometriosis with conservative surgery, *Am J Obstet Gynecol* 131:416, 1978.
14. Buttram VC Jr: Surgical treatment of endometriosis in the infertile female: a modified approach, *Fertil Steril* 32:635, 1979.
15. Malinak LR: Infertility and endometriosis: operative technique, clinical staging, and prognosis, *Clin Obstet Gynecol* 23:925, 1980.
16. Rock JA et al: The conservative surgical treatment of endometriosis: evaluation of pregnancy success with respect to the extent of disease as categorized using contemporary classification systems, *Fertil Steril* 35:131, 1981.
17. Kistner RW and Patton GL: *Atlas of infertility surgery*, Boston, 1975, Little, Brown & Co.
18. Batt RE and Naples JD: Conservative surgery for endometriosis in the infertile couple, *Curr Probl Obstet Gynecol* 6:1, 1982.
19. Gordts S, Boeckx W, and Brosens I: Microsurgery of endometriosis in infertile patients, *Fertil Steril* 42:520, 1984.
20. Batt RE and Naples JD: Microsurgery for endometriosis and infertility. In Hunt RB (ed): *Atlas of female infertility surgery*, Chicago, 1986, Year Book Medical Publishers.
21. Wheeler JM and Malinak LR: The surgical management of endometriosis, *Obstet Gynecol Clin North Am* 16:147, 1989.
22. Buttram VC Jr: Principles of conventional conservative surgery, *Prog Clin Biol Res* 323:269, 1990.
23. Batt RE, Severino MF, and Lawton D: Endometriosis: microconservative surgery. In Stangel JJ (ed): *Infertility surgery: a multimethod approach to female reproductive surgery*, Norwalk, Conn, 1990, Appleton & Lange.
24. Acland RD: Basic techniques for microvascular surgery (instructional videotapes), Louisville, Ky, 1983, Microsurgical Laboratory, University of Louisville.
25. Boeckx W, Gordts S, and Brosens IA: Techniques for microsurgical repair of the ovary. In Phillips JM (ed): *Microsurgery in gynecology*, vol 2, Downey, Calif, 1981, American Association of Gynecologic Laparoscopists.
26. Eddy CA, Asch RH, and Balmaceda JP: Pelvic adhesions following microsurgical and macrosurgical wedge resection of the ovaries, *Fertil Steril* 33:557, 1980.
27. Stone IK, von Fraunhofer JA, and Masterson BJ: The biomechanical effects of tight suture closure on fascia, *Surg Gynecol Obstet* 448-452, 1986.
28. Adhesion Barrier Study Group: Prevention of postsurgical adhesions by Interceed (TC 7), an absorbable adhesion barrier: a prospective, randomized multicenter clinical study, *Fertil Steril* 51:933, 1989.
29. Andrassy RJ: Preserving the gut mucosal barrier and enhancing immune response, *Contemp Surg* 32:21-27, 1988.
30. Ellis H: The aetiology of post-operative abdominal adhesions— an experimental study, *Br J Surg* 50:10-16, 1962.
31. Peham H and Amreich J: *Operative gynecology*, vol 1, Philadelphia, 1934, JB Lippincott.

32. Batt RE et al: A case-series study of peritoneal pockets and endometriosis: rudimentary duplications of the mullerian system, *Adolesc Pediatr Gynecol* 2:47, 1989.

33. Pettit PD and Lee RA: Ovarian remnant syndrome: diagnostic dilemma and surgical challenge, *Obstet Gynecol* 71:580-583, 1988.

34. Price FV, Edwards R, and Buchsbaum HJ: Ovarian remnant syndrome: difficulties in diagnosis and management, *Obstet Gynecol Surv* 45:151-156, 1990.

35. Brumsted JR et al: Postoperative adhesion formation after ovarian wedge resection with and without ovarian reconstruction in the rabbit, *Fertil Steril* 53:723-726, 1990.

36. Wiskind AK et al: Adhesion formation after ovarian wound repair in New Zealand white rabbits: a comparison of ovarian microsurgical closure with ovarian nonclosure, *Am J Obstet Gynecol* 163:1674-1678, 1990.

37. Kurjak A: *Transvaginal color Doppler,* Park Ridge, NJ, 1991, Parthenon.

38. Stahl C and Grimes EM: Endometriosis of the small bowel: case reports and review of the literature, *Obstet Gynecol Surv* 42:131-136, 1987.

39. Tjaden B et al: The efficacy of presacral neurectomy for the relief of midline dysmenorrhea, *Obstet Gynecol* 76:89-91, 1990.

40. Polan ML and DeCherney A: Presacral neurectomy for pelvic pain and infertility, *Fertil Steril* 34:557, 1980.

41. Patsner B and Orr JW Jr: Intractable venous sacral hemorrhage: use of stainless steel thumbtacks to obtain hemostasis, *Am J Obstet Gynecol* 162:452, 1990.

42. Malviya VK and Deppe G: Control of intraoperative hemorrhage in gynecology with the use of fibrin glue, *Obstet Gynecol* 73:284-286, 1989.

43. Wheeler JM and Malinak LR: Recurrent endometriosis. In Nichols DH (ed): *Reoperative gynecologic surgery,* Chicago, 1991, Mosby-Year Book.

44. Zamloni L, Meldrum DA, and Buster J: Extracorporeal fertilization and embryo transfer in the treatment of infertility, *West J Med* 144:195-204, 1986.

45. Pratt JH and Williams TJ: Indications for complete pelvic operations and more radical procedures in the treatment of severe and extensive endometriosis, *Clin Obstet Gynecol* 23:937, 1980.

46. Foster GV, Zacur HA, and Rock JA: Hot flashes in postmenopausal women ameliorated by danazol, *Fertil Steril* 43:401, 1985.

ADDITIONAL CONSIDERATIONS

28

Complications of Infertility Surgery

ROBERT B. HUNT

Pelvic surgery is associated with some specific problems. Whereas this presentation by no means includes all complications, those discussed can assist the surgical team in reviewing its own procedures from the standpoint of safety. Additional complications related to laparoscopy are discussed in Chapters 16 and 17.

INTRAOPERATIVE TECHNIQUE
Neurologic Complications

Hyperextension of the upper extremity may result in permanent injury to the brachial plexus. Improper padding of the lower extremity also may produce neurologic deficit, particularly when the patient is in stirrups during prolonged procedures. Great care must be exercised in positioning the patient on the operating table to lessen this risk.

When a Pfannenstiel incision is chosen, the surgeon must be cognizant of the location of the ilioinguinal nerve to avoid damaging it (Figure 28-1). If the nerve is severed, the innervated area becomes permanently numb. If ligated, the patient will experience a burning sensation in the area of nerve distribution that may persist for months.

The iliohypogastric nerves accompany the perforating vessels through the anterior fascia into the subcutaneous tissue (Figure 28-2). If the surgeon dissects widely between the rectus muscles and fascia or the fascia and subcutaneous tissue, a large area of skin numbness will be noted after surgery. An effort should be made to preserve these perforating vessels and accompanying sensory nerves.

Serious damage to the femoral nerve may occur if it is subjected to undue pressure for a prolonged period. One culprit is the deep blades present on some retractors. The surgeon should select a retractor with curved blades, thus avoiding such pressure (Figure 28-3). The same complication has been reported with positioning at laparoscopy. Every effort should be made to prevent damage to the femoral nerve. The injury, manifested by foot drop, may persist for many months or be permanent.

Peroneal nerve injury secondary to pneumatic compression stockings used during surgery has been reported.[1] The patient mostly recovered from the resulting foot drop after 2 months of physical therapy.

Intestinal complications

The abdomen is opened meticulously to avoid intestinal damage. Care must be taken to prevent a crush injury to the bowel as the abdominal retractor is being positioned. In addition, bowel may be entered or devascularization may occur when loops of bowel are being dissected away from pelvic structures. To prevent this the surgeon must identify and dissect along the "white lines" that demarcate the planes of dissection.

A particularly difficult task is dissecting the bowel away from the posterior surface of the uterus and cervix when the cul-de-sac is obliterated with dense adhesions. Superb lighting, excellent assistance, and loupe magnification are helpful. When bowel injuries occur, appropriate consultation is sought and the bowel repaired.

Urinary tract complications

The proximity of ureters and bladder may result in damage to these structures when the pelvic anatomy has been distorted from adhesions or endometriosis. The surgeon must be aware of their locations before initiating the dissection. If the patient has had extensive pelvic surgery in the past, it may be prudent to perform a preoperative intravenous pyelogram or ultrasound examination of the urinary tract.

When dissecting the ovary and fallopian tube from their adhesed bed, the ureter is frequently attached to these structures. Often the adnexa can be gently dissected away from the pelvic sidewall without entering the extraperitoneal space (Figure 28-4). Occasionally the surgeon will have to identify the ureter at the pelvic brim and mobilize it away from the adnexa to accomplish a safe dissection.

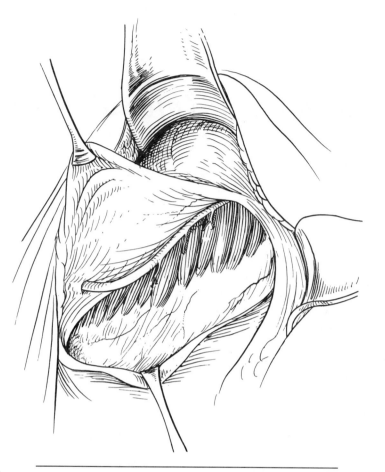

Figure 28-1
The ilioinguinal nerve as it exits through the external oblique
aponeurosis.

Advanced laparoscopic procedures designed to remove adhesions and endometriosis have resulted in ureteral injuries. These injuries have serious consequences, often associated with electrosurgery and frequently resulting in loss of a kidney.[2]

When peritoneal platforms are developed, care is taken to prevent the ureter from being distorted by the suture (Figure 28-5).

To reduce the chance of a bladder injury, the bladder is kept deflated by continuous or intermittent catheter drainage. Urinary bladder injuries may occur during laparoscopy or when the secondary trocar is inserted. The surgeon must identify the location of the bladder before inserting these secondary trocars. If the location is unclear, the surgeon may fill the bladder transurethrally, then deflate it before inserting the trocar. An additional safeguard is to avoid placing the secondary trocar inferior to a previously existing transverse lower abdominal incision, since the bladder is sometimes retracted to the scar.

Similarly, the bladder may be injured at the time the abdomen is opened. To achieve an ample peritoneal in- cision, the surgeon will sometimes have to open the peritoneum lateral to the bladder (Figure 28-6). The proximity of the bladder must be kept in mind at wound closure to prevent its being incorporated in the peritoneal suture (Figure 28-7).

Bladder injuries may also occur at the time of dissection, particularly when dense adhesions are involved, as in the case of endometriosis or previous surgery. Also uterine suspension procedures involve surgery adjacent to the bladder, placing the organ in jeopardy.

If the surgeon is unsure whether a ureteral injury has occurred, indigo carmine dye may be injected intravenously and the site in question observed for its egress. Similarly, indigo carmine may be injected into the urinary bladder to identify an occult opening in the bladder. When the injury is recognized, appropriate consultation is sought and repair of the urologic defect effected.

Thermal injury

Many thermal injuries can be avoided by properly grounding the patient, ensuring adequate insulation of microelectrodes, avoiding contact of an activated elec-

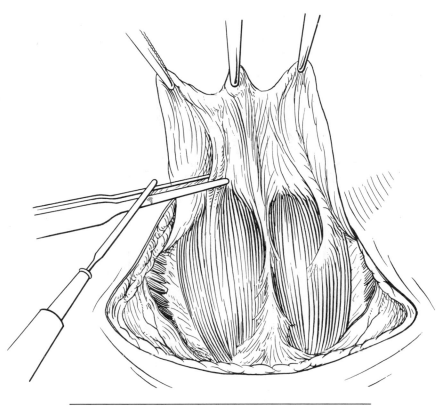

Figure 28-2
Perforating vessels and sensory nerves as they penetrate the
external oblique aponeurosis.

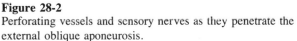

trode with a metal instrument, keeping bowel and other structures remote of the activated electrode, and choosing an alert first assistant. A thorough understanding of the physics of unipolar, bipolar, and thermocoagulation units, as well as resulting tissue effects, is mandatory (see Chapter 6).

Foreign bodies

The problem of instrument counts and retained foreign bodies is compounded by the large number of instruments required and the small sutures used in restorative procedures. To lessen this problem, several comments are in order.

When placing an intrauterine catheter, the surgeon must be aware that some models have parts that detach. All parts must be accounted for when the device is removed from the vagina.

When displacing the bowel out of the pelvis, sponges are never used, only large abdominal packs. When placing a Kerlix gauze in the posterior cul-de-sac, only one gauze is used (see Figure 28-3). If additional packing is required, a large abdominal pack may be added on top of the gauze.

One microsuture is used at a time, and it is passed to the nurse when it is no longer needed. The nurse then places the needle in bone wax or the sponge in which the needle was packaged. If the needle does disengage from the needle carrier or drop into the wound, its migration into the abdomen is unlikely if one uses the exposure techniques shown in Figure 28-3.

Occasionally a needle will be lost. To prepare for such an event the surgeon should consult with the radiology department and obtain a written opinion for the operating room staff as to whether a film of the abdomen should be taken to determine its location. The three hospitals in which I operate do not recommend obtaining an abdominal film for sutures of 8-0 or 9-0 material. If such a needle is lost, we do nothing further than to conduct a careful search.

Of concern is the loss of sutures or breakage of instruments in surgical laparoscopy.[3] Careful inspection of these often fragile instruments before surgery is essential. Also when cutting a suture that has been tied intraabdominally, the surgeon should leave at least 4 cm on the needle and extract the needle through the secondary tro-

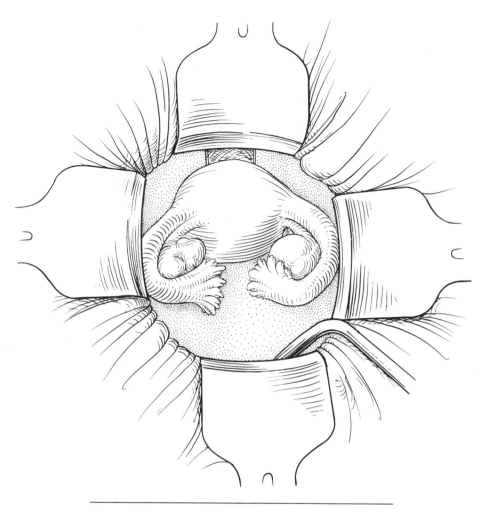

Figure 28-3
Pelvic exposure is complete. Note the cul-de-sac packing over a sump drain, the wound protector, and the curved blades of the Kirschner retractor.

car slowly and under direct vision. This lessens the chance of the needle being dropped and provides a better chance of retrieving it laparoscopically if it is.

Deposition of solid particles intraabdominally from CO_2 tanks at the time of insufflation for laparoscopy is a possibility.[4] A suggested remedy is use of a filter.

An interested and informed operating room staff supported by a schedule that minimizes staff changes during surgery may reduce mishaps.

SHORT-TERM POSTOPERATIVE COMPLICATIONS
Wound

Blood vessels in the abdominal wound may be tamponaded by the retractor. When the retractor is removed, care must be taken to identify these open vessels and ligate or coagulate them appropriately. Failure to do so may result in a wound hematoma.

Dissection in the subcutaneous space may result in the accumulation of fluid, resulting in a seroma. A wound drain is used to lessen the chance of this happening (Figure 28-8).

If high-molecular-weight dextran is used intraabdominally, care should be taken to irrigate the subcutaneous space copiously to prevent any residual dextran, since it can lead to a seroma by virtue of its high osmotic pressure.

Extreme abdominal and vulvar edema may develop after surgical laparoscopy or laparotomy when significant quantities of fluid are placed in the abdomen at the time of wound closure. The fluid leaks through fascial openings into the subcutaneous tissue and may travel to the vulva. The soft mass that results is often unilateral. Once

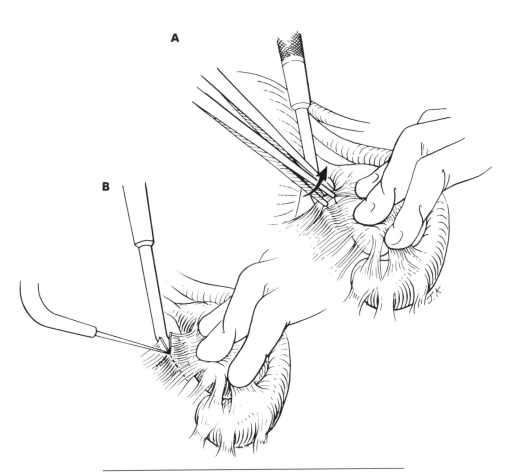

Figure 28-4
The adnexa are being dissected away from the pelvic sidewall by **A**, bipolar forceps and **B**, dividing adhesions with a
needle electrode over a dissecting rod.

hematoma is ruled out and the diagnosis made, the patient
is reassured and asked to rest. The swelling usually abates
after approximately 2 days.

Wound infections do occur, but fortunately, are unusual. The use of a wound protector should keep the
abdominal wall tissue moist and lessen damage. When
the skin is closed, Steri-strips or a similar adhesive should
be placed across the incision to support the wound edges.
They can be removed by the patient approximately 1
week after surgery.

Wound dehiscence may also occur. Careful hemostasis, use of substantial synthetic sutures, incorporating
ample amounts of fascia into the sutures, not placing an
overabundance of sutures, and ensuring complete fascial
closure should make this a rare complication.

Intraabdominal hemorrhage

Surgical procedures are dependent on the patient having
an intact clotting mechanism. If there is a history of
unusual bleeding or bruising associated with previous
surgery or mild trauma, appropriate hematologic workup

is in order. We advise each of our preoperative patients
to avoid aspirin-containing medications for 2 weeks before surgery.

Major hemorrhage can occur after procedures described in this atlas. An example is partial omentectomy
(Figure 28-9). The surgeon must be cognizant always of
unsecured blood vessels. They should be dealt with effectively by coagulation or ligation, since they can bleed
significantly after surgery.

Infection

Fortunately, peritonitis after surgery to restore or maintain fertility is unusual. Care must be taken to avoid gross
contamination from use of cameras, microscopes, and
other ancillary equipment.

Surgeons should consider not removing the appendix
except in situations where it is diseased, since appendectomy presents an opportunity for potentially harmful
bacteria to enter the abdomen.

Urinary tract infections occasionally occur. A urine
culture should be obtained when an indwelling Foley

Text cont'd on p. 492.

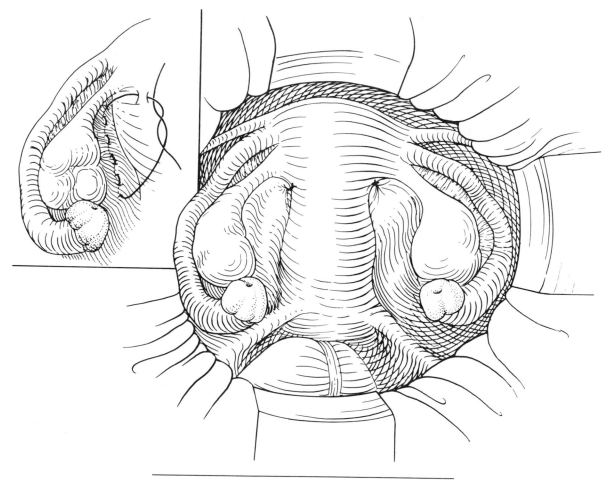

Figure 28-5
Peritoneal platforms are developed *(inset)* to prevent adnexa
from adhering to the pelvic sidewalls.

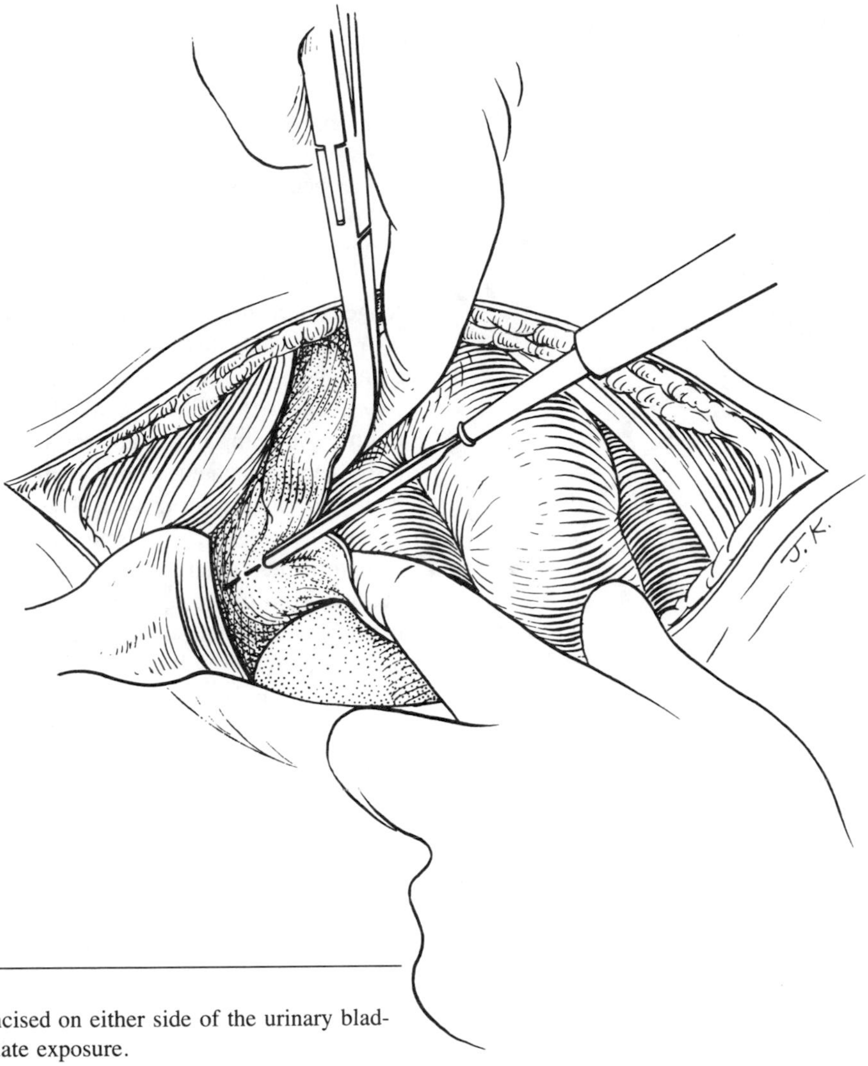

Figure 28-6
The peritoneum is incised on either side of the urinary bladder to provide adequate exposure.

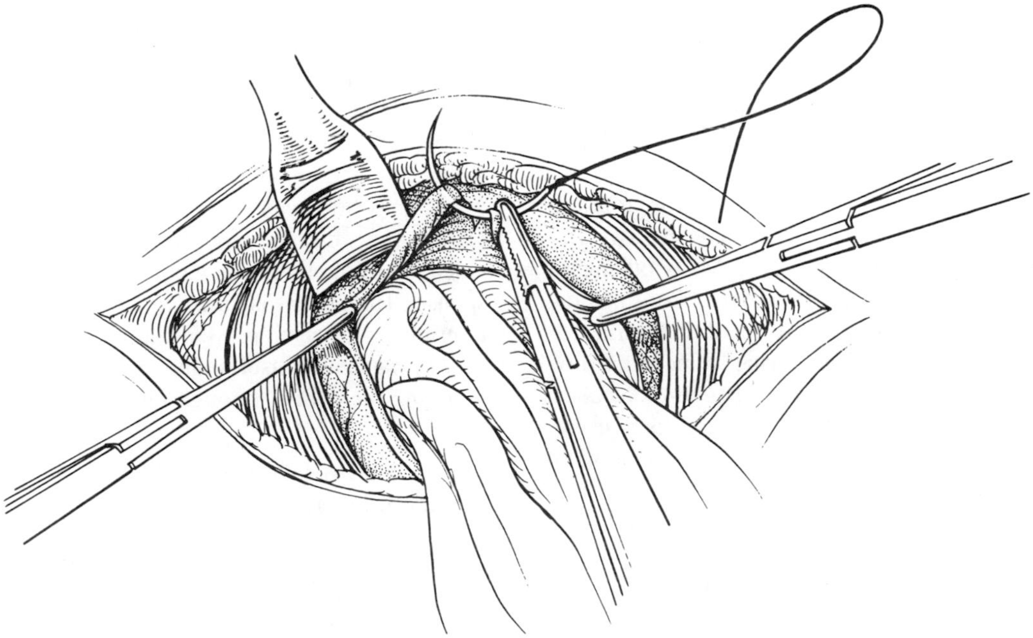

Figure 28-7
Peritoneal closure is begun inferiorly alongside the urinary bladder.

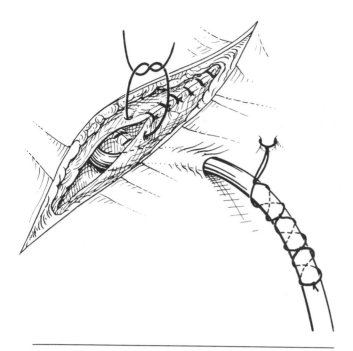

Figure 28-8
A Hemovac drain is positioned in the subcutaneous space to evacuate accumulating postoperative fluids.

catheter is removed after surgery and the offending bacteria treated specifically.

I treat each patient with a prophylactic antibiotic unless she requests otherwise. The value of such practice in these procedures is not known.

Cardiovascular complications

To detect underlying cardiovascular disorders, a careful history and physical examination are basic. If the patient has been taking diuretics, electrolytes are checked. If she has a history of mitral valve prolapse or a physical examination that suggests such, she is given the appropriate prophylactic antibiotic regimen. These are just two examples of relatively common problems. Many other cardiovascular conditions can be important. Consultation with a cardiologist is obtained as deemed appropriate.

Significant fluid shifts occur during some infertility procedures. One example is the use of high-molecular-weight dextran intraabdominally. Because of its high osmotic pressure, this agent attracts additional tissue fluid into the abdominal cavity.[5] If too much dextran 70 is placed intraperitoneally, the patient may suffer hypovolemic shock. Conversely, if the same agent is used to distend the uterine cavity for surgical hysteroscopy, and significant intravasation occurs into the pelvic veins, the patient may develop fluid overload (Figure 28-10). Similarly, use of excessive volumes of other fluids for uterine distention, such as dextrose and water, can place the patient into profound electrolyte imbalance (hyponatre-

mia) and fluid overload. To prevent serious complications, the surgeon must be aware of the volumes of these agents being absorbed and fluid shifts that are occurring.

Postoperative pulmonary emboli are rare in infertility patients, which is perhaps due in part to early ambulation. It is advisable to use compression stockings during the longer microsurgical procedures.

A potentially disastrous complication is the development of acute compartment syndrome in the leg. This poorly understood phenomenon has been associated with trauma and being in stirrups for a prolonged time. It has also been associated with a malfunctioning pneumatic boot and, in the arm, with a pneumatic cuff used in orthopedic surgery.[6,7] Muscle tissue contained in fascial compartments undergoes swelling that obstructs venous outflow from the compartment, resulting in more swelling and eventual muscle necrosis. The patient will complain of pain and will have swelling of one or both legs with arterial pulses intact. Myoglobin levels are extraordinarily elevated. Immediate fasciotomy should be considered, or else the involved extremity(ies) may be lost.

Adverse reactions

With the number of agents used during the course of these procedures, it is a wonder that we do not see more adverse reactions. Examples are allergies to dextran or antibiotics, hematologic problems associated with methylene blue or indigo carmine, and activation of a duodenal ulcer with steroids.

If a steroid-antihistamine regimen is used, the patient may appear quite flushed in the postoperative period. She may also appear inappropriately happy and pain free. This reaction is generally short lived and harmless, disappearing within 3 days.

Pain

When intraabdominal high-molecular-weight dextran is used, the patient may experience severe chest or shoulder pain for the first 2 days after surgery. Intraabdominal balanced salt solutions sometimes produce a similar response. The patient is assessed appropriately to rule out a serious complication. Medication, a heating pad, massage of trapezius muscles, and reassurance go a long way in aiding the patient through this period of discomfort.

LONG-TERM COMPLICATIONS
Ectopic pregnancy

When a patient conceives after reparative pelvic surgery, that pregnancy should be considered to be ectopic until proved otherwise. Prevention of the potentially disastrous effects of a neglected ectopic pregnancy begins with the informed consent process (see Appendix A). Each patient must be aware of this possibility and is instructed to call the office as soon as she thinks she

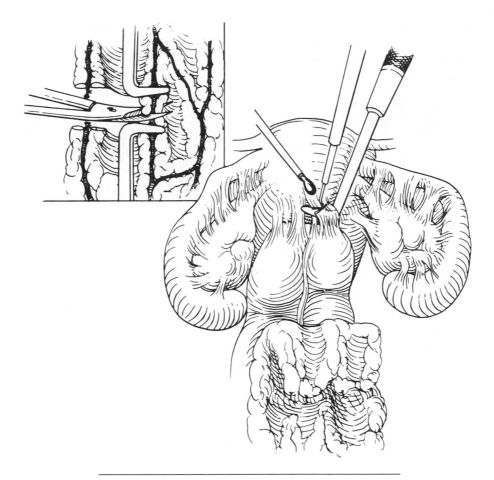

Figure 28-9
(Inset) Diseased omentum is being resected. An omentopexy is shown for comparison.

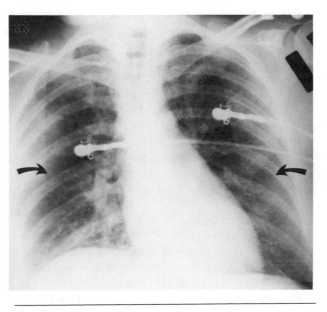

Figure 28-10
Hyskon-induced pulmonary edema *(curved arrows)* as a sequela to hysteroscopic lysis of severe intrauterine adhesions.

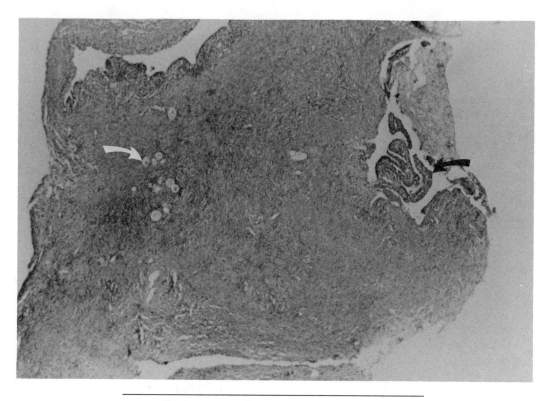

Figure 28-11
Histologic view (20 ×) of an ovarian endometrial cyst that
has been resected from the ovary. Note the endometrial
glands *(black arrow)* and the ovarian follicles *(white arrow)*
make up the cyst wall. There is no cleavage plane between
the endometriosis and ovarian tissue.

is pregnant. Once the pregnancy is confirmed, she is
monitored carefully by quantitative measurement of human chorionic gonadotropin levels and serial ultra-
sounds until the fetal heart beat is detected in the uterus
(see Chapter 22).

Genetic abnormalities

If the patient has a history of several miscarriages, or if
either she or her partner has a strong family history of
genetic abnormalities, appropriate genetic testing should
be encouraged. The increasing frequency of genetic abnormalities in offspring, particularly trisomy 21 (Down
syndrome), in the female patient 35 years old or older
is well established. The patient should consider genetic
testing of the pregnancy once she has conceived.

Premature ovarian failure

This complication may occur naturally or as a result of
ovarian surgery. The surgeon should consider obtaining
baseline levels of follicle-stimulating and luteinizing hormones in the infertile patient with oligomenorrhea or one
who is 40 years of age or older.

If an ovary is removed, it is possible the remaining
ovary will not function. Another cause of postoperative
ovarian failure is in the removal of endometriomata with
ovarian preservation, especially when the cysts are
greater than 5 cm and bilateral. When the endometrial
cyst wall is studied microscopically, one will observe
that there is no cleavage plane between the resected endometrial cyst and the normal ovarian tissue. Follicles
will be incorporated in the cyst wall (Figure 28-11). If
enough follicles have been removed, ovarian failure will
occur. I have observed a similar histologic finding after
resection of a dermoid.

Tubal occlusion and adhesion formation

Postoperative adhesions and tubal closure are serious
complications. Although it appears that individual variation in the tendency to form postoperative adhesions
is wide, the surgeon should make every effort to use
the surgical principles discussed in this atlas. I strongly
believe that ischemia is the most significant cause of
postoperative adhesions, as reported by Ellis,[8] and
every effort must be made to prevent it. The steps taken

to discourage adhesion formation are thoroughly discussed in Chapter 29.

Uterine rupture

Fortunately, rupture of the uterus is an unusual complication. When the uterus has been opened or dissection carried out deep into the wall of the uterus, as in metroplasty, myomectomy, resection of an adenomyoma, cornual anastomosis, or tubal implantation, subsequent uterine rupture during the prenatal and intrapartum phases of pregnancy is possible. The surgeon should determine at the time of infertility surgery whether a cesarean delivery should be performed and the couple and obstetrician so informed.

Psychologic complications

Infertility can be devastating. It is tempting to treat the affected couples in a somewhat cookbook fashion and remain insensitive to their psychologic needs. I encourage each reader to review the emotional stages these couples go through, as outlined in Chapter 3. This information will help us understand some of the irrational statements and actions we observe frequently. We will be in a much better position to interact with these patients and recognize when counseling is in order. It is our duty to provide these couples with reasonable emotional support as we evaluate and treat their infertility.

SUMMARY

The surgeon and the entire hospital and office staff involved in the care of the infertile couple should constantly review complications, both potential and real, and discuss ways to prevent them. This surveillance should reduce their frequency and allow surgeons and staffs to enjoy many tension-reduced years in the care of these patients.

REFERENCES

1. Cohn GM et al: A complication associated with pneumatic compression stockings used for gynecologic surgery, *J Gynecol Surg* 5:389, 1989.
2. Grainger DA et al: Ureteral injuries at laparoscopy: insights into diagnosis, management, and prevention, *Obstet Gynecol* 75:839, 1990.
3. Whitman GF and DiLauro S: Morbidity from in vitro fertilization secondary to instrument failure: a case report, *Fertil Steril* 53:375, 1990.
4. Biomedical Safety & Standards Bulletin: Contaminated CO_2 gas could injure laparoscopy patients, 20:49, 1990.
5. Pfeffer WH: A surgeon's guide to preventing adhesions, *Contemp Obstet Gynecol* 19:1, 1982.
6. Werbel GB and Shybut GT: Acute compartment syndrome caused by a malfunctioning pneumatic compression boot, *J Bone Joint Surg* 68:1445, 1986.
7. Green TL and Louis DS: Compartment syndrome of the arm: a complication of the pneumatic tourniquet, *J Bone Joint Surg* 65:270, 1983.
8. Ellis H: The cause and prevention of postoperative intraperitoneal adhesions, *Surg Gynecol Obstet* 133:497, 1971.

29

Adjunctive Agents in Infertility Surgery

GARY HOLTZ

Peritoneal adhesions cause infertility by encasing the ovary, covering the fimbriae, distorting the tubal-ovarian relationship, or by kinking and thereby occluding the fallopian tube. Their development or postoperative reformation after lysis is a major cause of failure of reconstructive surgery. To meet this challenging problem, the surgeon must understand how peritoneal injuries normally heal adhesion-free, be cognizant of factors that impede this process, and be familiar with modalities that may reduce adhesion development.

NORMAL PERITONEAL HEALING

A serosal injury causes the release of vasopermeability factors and chemotactic mediators that initiate the inflammatory reaction.[1] An immediate transient increase in vascular permeability is produced by histamine and rapidly resolves. A second, delayed alteration occurs over 3 to 6 hours and is not dependent on the previous one. This may be mediated by anaphylatoxins, bradykinin, and prostanoids. Chemotactic factors induce the movement of leukocytes to the site of injury, cause production of peroxide and superoxide radicals, and initiate enzyme release, causing further tissue damage. Thromboplastin is released and activates the clotting cascade. As a result, serosanguineous exudate is produced that coagulates within a period as short as 3 hours, causing fibrinous agglutination of peritoneal surfaces.

Normally, fibrinous attachments are lysed within 72 to 96 hours of formation.[2] Plasminogen activators located in the mesothelium and submesothelial blood vessels covert plasminogen, present in blood and fibrinous exudates, to plasmin, a fibrin-splitting enzyme. Other proteases are likely to be involved as well. Only fibrinous attachments that persist for 3 days or longer are susceptible to fibroblast migration and proliferation, producing permanent adhesions. Factors that impair fibrinolysis or produce excessively heavy fibrin deposits are therefore causative of adhesion formation.

Repair of the peritoneal defect also begins promptly. Although controversy exists regarding the source of the new mesothelial cells, they are present at the base of the defect within 2 to 3 days of injury. Complete healing by a single cell layer occurs as rapidly as 5 days after injury.[3] Large defects heal as rapidly as smaller ones, since repair occurs from the base, rather than from the sides of the defect.

PATHOGENESIS OF ADHESIONS

Formation of peritoneal adhesions is largely dependent on factors that cause inadequate fibrinolysis. Foremost among these is the production of ischemic tissue by coagulation, ligation, crushing, or devascularization.[2,4,5] Ischemia impairs the intrinsic ability of the peritoneum to lyse fibrin by reducing plasminogen activator activity.[5] The rapidity with which this occurs, the extent of reduction, and its duration vary with the injury.[6] Inhibition can extend to adjacent undamaged tissue as well. Abrasion of the serosal surface also impairs fibrinolysis.[5]

Drying of the serosa is another common intraoperative insult that causes the production of fibrinous attachments; however, these are usually lysed within 2 to 3 days of formation. Similarly, in the absence of any other insult, fresh unclotted blood does not consistently induce adhesion formation. When both drying and subsequent contact with blood occur, adhesion development usually follows.[7] Plasma induces slightly fewer adhesions in the presence of an injured serosa; defibrinated blood and heparinized blood products do not cause adhesion development. Blood provides an additional source of fibrin and contains cellular elements that make lysis more difficult. Platelets stimulate the serosal inflammatory reaction and fibroblastic proliferation.[8] Large preformed clots may cause adhesion development in the absence of any other serosal injury, presumably because of high concentrations of diffusable permeability factors and fibrin.

Keeping the peritoneum moist seems a logical solution to this problem. However, wetting the serosa with a physiologic solution before exposure to blood does not prevent adhesion formation. Rather, a wetting injury is simply substituted for the drying.

The majority of postoperative adhesions contain foreign bodies.[9] The most frequently noted are powder from surgical gloves; lint from packs, drapes, or gowns; and suture material. Their role in the pathogenesis of adhesions is probably substantially less than their frequent presence implies.

When fluff from packs is allowed to fall into the abdominal cavity of rats, minimal adhesions form; however, when packs are placed within the abdominal cavity, presumably abrading the serosa, adhesions develop.[10,11] Similar observations have been made regarding suture materials. Sutures do not consistently cause adhesions regardless of their chronic reactivity when placed loosely in the peritoneum.[12] When employed to reapproximate peritoneal defects, producing tension and ischemia along the line of closure, adhesions usually are caused. However, there are other reasons to employ the least reactive suture material available.

Infectious peritonitis is responsible for many pelvic adhesions. Bacteria release enzymes that induce inflammatory exudates and impair fibrinolytic activity. The duration of an infectious process is a significant variable in determining whether these attachments are lysed before fibroblasts migration into them. Infections that persist for more than 3 days permit this to occur.[13]

The pathogenesis of adhesion reformation after lysis has not been evaluated and may vary among patients. Clearly, the propensity for this to occur is greater.[14] Perhaps fibrinolytic activity is reduced in these areas. The sites of injury may also simply be more likely to be apposed.

SURGICAL CONCEPTS

To keep adhesions from forming, the surgical technique should lessen factors associated with their induction. Specifically, every effort should be made to minimize the amount of tissue rendered ischemic and to avoid abrasion of serosal surfaces. Whenever possible, only tissue to be resected should be handled. Reapproximation of the peritoneum is not appropriate unless it can be performed without undue tension along the suture line. Closure is indicated only when it is necessary to obtain hemostasis or to reestablish crucial anatomic relationships. Meticulous closure of the ovarian cortex is also not required and is probably detrimental.[15] Hemostasis must be achieved as precisely as possible to limit the production of ischemic tissue.

Packing the bowel out of the pelvis is often required to obtain adequate exposure. Moist packs may be somewhat less traumatic than dry ones; however, gentle insertion is really the key element. Irrigation rather than sponging to remove blood is optimal, since it reduces the opportunity to abrade the serosa. Controversy exists as to what solution is best for this purpose. Many surgeons use heparinized lactated Ringer's solution.[16] This irrigant greatly reduces the amount of clot formation, but may not significantly decrease fibrin deposition or adhesion formation.[17] Some reconstructive surgeons also add corticosteroids, believing that their topical use may inhibit the inflammatory response; the efficacy of this practice has not been evaluated. Regardless of the irrigant employed, the solution should be at body temperature to reduce possible thermal injury and its impact on body core temperature.

Although the role of foreign bodies in the pathogenesis of postoperative adhesions has been overemphasized, every effort should be made to avoid this additional serosal insult. Glove powder is a major contaminant. Simply washing gloves with a moist pack is not sufficient; rather, they should be washed repeatedly and rinsed.[18] Highly reactive suture materials should not be used. Also important is the use of small, atraumatic needles to reduce the trocar-induced acute inflammatory response to suture placement.

Microsurgery has been established to reduce adhesion formation; however, the benefit derived may not extend to the management of preexisting lesions. No clinical study comparing this technique to a macrosurgical one and subjecting the patients to second-look procedures has been reported. In a primate model, microsurgical technique was marginally superior in reducing adhesion reformation.[19] There is similarly no documentation that the use of any type of laser has a significant impact on adhesion development after lysis.

Evaluations have established that endoscopy reduces de novo adhesion formation but not whether it actually decreases reformation.[20-22] This is probably because of reduced peritoneal injury secondary to abrasion and the reduced opportunity to create large areas of ischemic tissue. Another interesting concept is that delayed ambulation associated with laparotomy is responsible for some of the difference.[23]

Ancillary surgical techniques

Numerous ancillary procedures have been performed in attempts to reduce the occurrence and significance of adhesion formation. Uterine and adnexal suspension are most commonly employed, although the efficacy of neither is established. The latter has been advocated when an early second-look laparoscopy may also allow the suspending sutures to be cut. Uterine suspension has been most widely performed when severe posterior cul-de-sac adhesions are encountered. It may induce chronic pelvic pain, bowel incarceration, and adhesion formation if performed improperly. Simply plicating the round ligaments reduces these risks.

Early (2-12 wks) postoperative laparoscopy for lysis of adhesions has gained considerable popularity, but its benefit is not clearly confirmed. Adhesions are less dense and vascular in the immediate postoperative period[24] and therefore more readily lysed, but the extent to which they reform is less clear. In two studies, third procedures were performed to assess reformation after the early postoperative laparoscopy. Both suggested improvement.[25,26]

Partial omentectomy or omental plication may be performed when extensive omental adhesions are encountered. Once more, benefit is likely but not established. The use of free peritoneal or omental grafts to cover areas of gross abrasion or peritoneal defects unfortunately continues. These devascularized grafts are more likely to induce adhesions than unrepaired areas.

Hydrotubation

Before the application of microsurgery to reconstructive pelvic surgery, hydrotubation was a near universal practice after surgery for distal tubal obstruction. It is intended to flush fibrinous exudate from the tubal lumen and to separate agglutinated surfaces (mucosal or serosal) until fibrinolysis had occurred. Numerous solutions have been employed for this purpose, most containing corticosteroids, antibiotics, and/or proteolytic enzymes.

Grant's[27] study is frequently cited by advocates, since he reported that repetitive postoperative hydrotubation was associated with a substantially greater pregnancy rate than occurred in his preceding series of patients in whom it was not used. This was not a randomized study, and there are several reasons to question its validity. Rock et al[28] also reported a nonrandomized series of patients who had salpingostomies performed and in whom hydrotubation did not increase the frequency of pregnancy when the severity of tubal disease was considered. This procedure is therefore not endorsed, since it clearly is associated with a risk of causing infectious sequelae and is often most uncomfortable for the patient.

Prosthetic devices

Numerous prosthetic devices have been employed to prevent adhesion formation or reformation or to maintain tubal patency. The use of intraoperative stents to facilitate tubal reanastomosis remains widespread. They have been used to optimize tubal patency rates by ensuring luminal alignment and by preventing mucosal adherence. Long-term splinting results in fibrosis and loss of cilia in rabbit lumina.[29,30] Short-term splinting is probably not associated with these adverse sequelae. Moreover, excellent pregnancy rates were described after reversal of sterilization in patients who had splints in situ for 4 weeks after surgery.[31]

Prophylactic agents

The use of ancillary agents to inhibit adhesion development has become nearly universal in reconstructive surgery.[16] Their clinical application has often preceded documentation of efficacy. The adjunct most frequently used is a prophylactic antibiotic.[16] In 1985, 73% of reproductive surgeons surveyed administered a prophylactic antibiotic when performing female reconstructive surgery of any type. An additional 17% did so only during surgery on patients with distal tubal disease. Fifty-nine percent of the surgeons administered a therapeutic regimen (3 doses or 24 hours of therapy). A cephalosporin was the most frequently used drug; however, doxycycline and penicillins were also commonly employed.

Chlamydia may be found in the fallopian tubes of a significant percentage of patients undergoing surgery for distal tubal abnormalities.[32,33] This has been the basis for recommending the use of doxycycline, a drug active against this infectious organism. A 3-day course of therapy is often advocated; however, the benefit of this or any prophylactic regimen has not been evaluated.

Corticosteroids were the most commonly administered drugs for adhesion prophylaxis during the 1970s. Their use continues to be quite widespread. They decrease alterations in vascular permeability, stabilize lysosome membranes, and inhibit the synthesis and release of histamine and other mediators of the inflammatory response.[34] In animal models they inhibit fibroblast migration and proliferation, but they have been reported to stimulate human fibroblast growth. In addition, they reduce the intrinsic fibrinolytic activity of the peritoneum.

Promethazine, an antihistamine, is frequently given concurrently. This drug, a histamine receptor antagonist, limits the release of histamine, inhibits the permeability alterations induced by this and other factors, stabilizes lysosome membranes, and may inhibit fibroplasia.[34] No study has evaluated the effectiveness of promethazine as the sole agent.

Studies in small animals suggested that corticosteroids can reduce adhesion formation and reformation if very large doses are administered in the immediate perioperative period; however, only a small number of primate studies have been conducted, with variable results.[35] Only two human studies have been reported in which second-look procedures were consistently performed. Hydrocortisone (200 mg) was administered as a single intraperitoneal dose in patients undergoing surgery for ectopic pregnancy.[36] Laparoscopy was performed 3 months later to assess adhesion formation. The women who received hydrocortisone had significantly less adhesion formation than did the controls; however, treatment was not randomized among the surgeons involved, raising the possibility that variation in surgical technique was a factor. In a recent study, steroids failed to have an impact on adhesion formation or reformation.[37]

Although the effectiveness of steroids is questionable, their use is not associated with significant morbidity. Wound healing is potentially impaired, and the use of either permanent or synthetic absorbable sutures in the fascial closure is appropriate. Because of their immunosuppressive capabilities, concurrent antibiotic therapy is recommended. The mood elevation associated with steroids has often been considered favorably by surgeons; however, depression manifested after the therapeutic regimen is the most common adverse effect. Malaise, and bone or joint pain after therapy are the next most frequent adverse reaction attributed to their use.[16]

During the 1980s the most frequently used agent for adhesion prevention was 32% dextran 70 in dextrose (Hyskon, Pharmacia).[16] This high-molecular-weight solution was initially developed for uterine distention during hysteroscopy and remains approved only for this application.

The primary action of dextran is thought to be separation of fibrin covered surfaces. Unlike many fluids previously employed, it is absorbed slowly from the peritoneal cavity and does not induce a foreign body reaction.[38] Moreover, it causes an influx of fluid into the abdominal cavity because of the osmotic gradient produced. Dextran also alters the structure of fibrin formed in its presence, facilitating lysis,[39] and it may have a "siliconizing" action on damaged surfaces. Limited evidence suggests that it may impair shedding of plasminogen activator activity from the peritoneum and that it is an immunosuppressant.

Small-animal laboratory studies consistently suggested that Hyskon reduced adhesion development after a peritoneal injury, but it was less effective in impeding reformation after lysis.[35] In the only primate study, it reduced adhesion formation.[40] Four clinical studies with second-look procedures evaluated efficacy in the human.[37,41-43] Two reported positive results and the others failed to confirm effectiveness. There is no obvious reason for the discrepancy; perhaps substantially more severe adhesions were encountered in the negative studies.

The use of dextran intraperitoneally is not without risk. Adverse reactions include labial edema, fever of unknown origin, ileus, and wound complications. Reports of severe allergic reactions have appeared; cul-de-sac aspiration and standard medical measures have been effectively used for treatment.[44] Conflicting data exist as to whether Hyskon is a good bacterial culture medium.[45,46] Consequently, routine prophylactic antibiotic administration is appropriate. Clinically significant impairment of hemostatic mechanisms has not been noted, but Hyskon is contraindicated in the presence of active bleeding. Extravasation into the vulva has been the most frequently reported adverse effect.[16] Although disconcerting for the patient, it is generally not uncomfortable. Shoulder pain and abdominal bloating are also common complaints. Drainage into the wound and collection there can create chronic leakage.

Two barriers have obtained approval from the Food and Drug Administration (FDA) for adhesion prevention. Gore-Tex Surgical Membrane* is a permanent, nonporous sheet of expanded polytetrafluoroethylene. It was developed as an antithrombogenic pericardial membrane substitute. The implant is essentially nonreactive. It received approval for clinical use in 1983, but there had been little interest in or application within the abdominal cavity until recently. This may be attributed to the lack of active marketing to reconstructive surgeons and to the fact that the material is not absorbable. The latter limits sites of application unless a second procedure is performed to remove it. The material also must be sutured in place, and frequently, significant numbers of sutures are necessary to make it conform to a compound curve. These present a risk for adhesion induction if they produce significant areas of ischemia adjacent to the implant. The use of small-caliber sutures, limited in number and tied loosely, is therefore required. It has the distinct advantage that it may be employed safely and probably effectively at sites with less than perfect hemostasis. An optimal use might be over a myomectomy incision. Although relatively costly, unused portions may be resterilized. No clinical series of pelvic applications with second-look procedures has been reported as of 1990; unpublished data confirming efficacy have impressed the author.

Interceed (TC 7)† has been more widely employed since its approval in 1990. This soft, knitted, absorbable material was derived from Surgicel and consists of oxidized, regenerated cellulose. However, there are substantial differences in its porosity, density, and rate of absorption. The material forms a gel after becoming wet and is completely absorbed within 2 weeks of application. It is not intended to be a topical hemostat; in fact, its effectiveness is lost if it becomes saturated with blood. The need for meticulous hemostasis and the fact it should not be employed in the presence of infection are the major limitations encountered. It may be laid over areas of concern and slightly moistened to aid in adherence. It can be displaced by further contact and can float off if excessive volumes of fluid remain in the abdominal cavity. The material can safely be overlapped, but optimum application is with a single layer. Endoscopic usage is also not particularly difficult if the material is backloaded into the surgical channel of the laparoscope for insertion into the abdomen. In contrast to its use at laparotomy, placement of several small pieces, as opposed to a single large one, facilitates application.

*W.L. Gore and Associates, Flagstaff, AZ.

†Ethicon, Inc, Somerville, NJ.

Table 29-1 Comparison of Gore-Tex surgical membrane, Interceed, and Hyskon

Feature	Gore-Tex	Interceed	Hyskon
Ease of use	Requires sutures	Reasonable	Pour or inject
Efficacy for reformation	Probable	Probable	Possible
Area of efficacy	Limited to application	Limited to application	Diffuse
Safety	Inert	Inert	Some rare complications

A well-designed, prospective, multicenter study with second-look laparoscopies confirmed this agent's effectiveness in reducing reformation of pelvic sidewall adhesions. It also reduced the severity of those that did recur.[47]

I currently use Hyskon, Gore-Tex Surgical Membrane, and Interceed, making the decision as to which of the three, if any, during surgery. This is based on how widespread the areas at risk are, their locations, if endoscopic or major abdominal surgery has been performed, and whether minimal oozing is thought to contraindicate use of dextran or Interceed. Knowledge of the advantages and limitations of each agent is crucial when making these decisions (Table 29-1).

FUTURE DEVELOPMENTS

Numerous areas are being investigated. Some interest remains in newer nonsteroidal antiinflammatory agents, although results of evaluations of ibuprofen in the early 1980s were mixed. Calcium channel blockers have been impressive in early animal evaluations, as has tissue plasminogen activator. One of the most clever concepts is the use of a polymer that is instilled into the abdomen as a liquid at room temperature and becomes a gel at the higher body temperature. Other liquids and physical barriers are also being studied.

REFERENCES

1. Ward PA and Yurt RW: The acute inflammatory response and the role of complement, *Infect Surg* 2:759-767, 1983.
2. Buckman RF et al: A physiologic basis for the adhesion-free healing of deperitonealized surfaces, *J Surg Res* 21:67-76, 1976.
3. Raftery AT: Regeneration of parietal and visceral peritoneum: an electron microscopical study, *J Anat* 115:375-392, 1973.
4. Ellis H: The aetiology of post-operative abdominal adhesions: an experimental study, *Br J Surg* 50:10-16, 1962.
5. Buckman RF et al: A unifying pathogenetic mechanism in the etiology of intraperitoneal adhesions, *J Surg Res* 20:1-5, 1976.
6. Raftery AT: Effect of peritoneal trauma on peritoneal fibrinolytic activity and intraperitoneal adhesion formation, *Eur Surg Res* 13:397-401, 1981.
7. Ryan GB, Groberty J, and Majno G: Postoperative peritoneal adhesions, *Am J Pathol* 65:117-148, 1971.
8. Lawler MM et al: Antiplatelet therapy in the prevention of adhesion formation, *Surg Forum* 32:464-465, 1981.
9. Weibel MA and Majno G: Peritoneal adhesions and their relation to abdominal surgery, *Am J Surg* 126:345-353, 1973.
10. Down RHL, Whitehead R, and Watts JMcK: Do surgical packs cause peritoneal adhesions? *Aust NZ J Surg* 49:379-382, 1979.
11. Down RHL, Whitehead R, and Watts JMcK: Why do surgical packs cause peritoneal adhesions? *Aust NZ J Surg* 50:83-85, 1980.
12. Holtz G: Adhesion induction by suture of varying tissue reactivity and caliber, *Int J Fertil* 27:134-135, 1982.
13. Jackson BB: Observations on intraperitoneal adhesions, *Surgery* 44:507-514, 1958.
14. Holtz G, Baker E, and Tsai C: Effect of thirty-two percent dextran 70 on peritoneal adhesion formation and re-formation after lysis, *Fertil Steril* 33:660-662, 1980.
15. Brumsted JR et al: Postoperative adhesion formation after ovarian wedge resection with and without ovarian reconstruction in the rabbit, *Fertil Steril* 53:723-726, 1990.
16. Holtz G: Current use of ancillary modalities for adhesion prevention, *Fertil Steril* 44:174-176, 1985.
17. Jansen RPS: Failure of peritoneal irrigation with heparin during pelvic operations upon young women to reduce adhesions, *Surg Gynecol Obstet* 166:154-158, 1988.
18. Yaffe H et al: Potentially deleterious effects of corn-starch glove powder in tubal reconstructive surgery, *Fertil Steril* 29:699-701, 1978.
19. Holtz G and Kling OR: Effect of surgical technique on peritoneal adhesion reformation after lysis, *Fertil Steril* 37:494-496, 1982.
20. Luciano AA et al: A comparative study of postoperative adhesions following laser surgery by laparoscopy versus laparotomy in the rabbit model, *Obstet Gynecol* 74:220-224, 1989.
21. Nezhat CR et al: Adhesion reformation after reproductive surgery by videolaseroscopy, *Fertil Steril* 53:1008-1011, 1990.
22. Operative Laparoscopy Study Group: Postoperative adhesion development following operative laparoscopy: evaluation at early second-look procedures, *Fertil Steril* 55:700-704, 1991.
23. Das K, Penney LL, and Critser JK: Effects of passive motion and early vs. delayed ambulation on adhesion formation in rat uterine surgery, *Int J Fertil* 35:245-248, 1990.
24. DeCherney AH and Mezer HC: The nature of post-tuboplasty pelvic adhesions as determined by early and late laparoscopy, *Fertil Steril* 41:643-646, 1984.
25. Trimbos-Kemper TCM, Trimbos JB, and van Hall EV: Adhesion formation after tubal surgery: results of the eight day laparoscopy in 188 patients, *Fertil Steril* 43:395-400, 1985.
26. Jansen RPS: Early laparoscopy after pelvic operations to prevent adhesions: safety and efficacy, *Fertil Steril* 49:26-31, 1988.
27. Grant A: Infertility surgery of the oviduct, *Fertil Steril* 22:496-503, 1971.
28. Rock JA et al: Factors influencing the success of salpingostomy techniques for distal fimbrial obstruction, *Obstet Gynecol* 52:591-596, 1978.
29. Khoo SK and MacKay EV: Reactions in rabbit fallopian tubes after plastic reconstruction. I. Gross pathology, tubal patency and pregnancy, *Fertil Steril* 23:201-206, 1972.
30. Winston RML: Microsurgical reanastomosis of the rabbit oviduct and its functional and pathological sequelae, *Br J Obstet Gynaecol* 82:513-522, 1975.

31. Jones HW Jr and Rock J: On the reanastomosis of fallopian rubes after surgical sterilization, *Fertil Steril* 29:702-704, 1978.

32. Shepard MK and Jones RB: Recovery of *Chlamydia trachomatis* from endometrial and fallopian tube biopsies in women with infertility of tubal origin, *Fertil Steril* 52:232-238, 1989.

33. Marana R et al: High prevalence of silent chlamydia colonization of the tubal mucosa in infertile women, *Fertil Steril* 53:354-356, 1990.

34. Replogle RL, Johnson R, and Gross R: Prevention of postoperative intestinal adhesions with combined promethazine and dexamethasone therapy, *Ann Surg* 163:580-588, 1966.

35. Holtz G: Prevention and management of peritoneal adhesions, *Fertil Steril* 41:497-507, 1984.

36. Swolin K: Die einwirkung von grossen, intraperionealen dosen glukokortikoid auf die bildung von postoperativen adhasionen, *Acta Obstet Gynecol Scand* 46:204-218, 1967.

37. Jansen RPS: Failure of intraperitoneal adjuncts to improve the outcome of pelvic operations in young women, *Am J Obstet Gynecol* 153:363-372, 1985.

38. Krinsky AH, Haseltine FP, and DeCherney AH: Peritoneal fluid accumulation with dextran 70 instilled at time of laparoscopy, *Fertil Steril* 41:647-649, 1984.

39. Tangen O, Wik KO, and Almquist IAM: Effects of dextran on the structure and plasmin-induced lysis of human fibrin, *Thromb Res* 1:487-492, 1972.

40. diZerega GS and Hodgen GD: Prevention of postoperative tubal adhesions: comparative study of commonly used agents, *Am J Obstet Gynecol* 136:173-178, 1980.

41. Adhesion Study Group: Reduction of postoperative pelvic adhesions with intraperitoneal 32% dextran 70: a prospective, randomized clinical trial, *Fertil Steril* 40:612-619, 1983.

42. Rosenberg SM and Board JA: High-molecular weight dextran in human infertility surgery, *Am J Obstet Gynecol* 148:380-385, 1984.

43. Larsson B et al: Effect of intraperitoneal instillation of 32% dextran 70 on post-operative adhesion formation after tubal surgery, *Acta Obstet Gynecol Scand* 64:437-441, 1985.

44. Borten M, Seibert CP, and Taymor ML: Recurrent anaphylactic reaction to intraperitoneal dextran 70 used for prevention of post-surgical adhesions, *Obstet Gynecol* 61:755-757, 1983.

45. Bernstein J et al: The potential for bacterial growth with dextran, *J Reprod Med* 27:77-79, 1982.

46. Elkins TE et al: Potential for in vitro growth of common bacteria in solutions of 32% dextran 70 and 1.0% carboxymethylcellulose, *Fertil Steril* 43:477-478, 1985.

47. Interceed Adhesion Barrier Study Group: Prevention of postsurgical adhesions by INTERCEED (TC7), an absorbable adhesion barrier: a prospective, randomized multicenter clinical study, *Fertil Steril* 51:933-938, 1989.

DOCUMENTATION

30

Operating Room Photography and Videography

JAMES F. GREEN

Surgical photodocumentation has become an extremely important part of the surgical process. It has numerous applications.

DIAGNOSIS

Photodocumentation allows video tapes and still photographs to be reviewed without real-time physical presence during the surgical procedure. Thus geographically separate and clinically diverse specialists can be consulted.

DOCUMENTATION

Photographs are often attached to the patient's permanent medical record. This facilitates periodic evaluation of continuing infertility problems. It also aids in verifying quality assurance.

PATIENT TEACHING

Photodocumentation allows infertility conditions to be explained clearly to patient and families. When photographs or video tapes of the patient's condition are used, teaching is improved, options are clearly illustrated, and informed consent is facilitated.

MEDICAL EDUCATION

Live video monitors permit simultaneous observation of laparoscopy and microsurgery by all members of the surgical team. Photodocumentation demonstrates pathologic conditions as well as the appropriate surgical protocol. In addition, photographs and video tapes can be used with referring physicians as a teaching tool. Reportable cases can be documented for journal or seminar presentation.

INVOLVEMENT

An added bonus, particularly during laparoscopy and microsurgery, is that live video involves all of the operating room team. This often results in increased efficiency, reduced response time, and improved operating room team morale.

PHOTOGRAPHIC PRINCIPLES

Quality photodocumentation requires an understanding of several basic principles. Because these principles apply to still photography and videography, they are discussed together.

Light quantity

All photographic process requires different light energy to produce an image. In still photography (slides and prints), the amount of light striking the film is controlled by the shutter speed and the $f/$stop working in combination. The shutter speed is the amount of time the camera's shutter remains open. As long as the shutter is open, light is allowed to strike the film. The shutter speed is most often expressed in whole numbers that represent fraction of a second: $60 = 1/60$ of a second; $500 = 1/500$ of a second. The $f/$stop represents the size of the lens diaphragm opening. The higher the number, the smaller the opening. For example, $f/22$ lets in less light than $f/16$. These numbers vary by a mathematical constant: $f/32$ lets in half as much light as the next $f/$stop, $f/22$; conversely, $f/5.6$ lets in twice as much light as $f/8$. The shutter speed and $f/$stop work in unison to control light access to the film stock.

In videography the concept of $f/$stop works the same as in still photography, but the concept of shutter speed is lost. Video signals are processed at a continuous rate. While film is the image-forming surface in still photography, the pick-up tube or chip (CCD) is the image-forming surface for videography.

The purpose of light control is to regulate the amount of light striking the film or video imaging surface. Too much light results in washed-out video or slides (overexposed); too little results in dark images (underexposed). Different films have various sensitivities; it takes different quantities of light to produce quality images on different film stocks. The relative sensitivity of film can be determined by checking the film's American Standards Association (ASA) or Internal Standards Organization (ISO) rating. All popular film stocks have these ratings clearly displayed on their package. The higher this rating number, the more sensitive the film. For example, ASA/ISO 400 film requires less light than does ASA/ISO 64 film. These ratings also vary by a constant: ASA/ISO 200 film requires half the light ASA/ISO 100 does. It should be noted that as sensitivity increases, so does grain size. Images produced on ASA/ISO 400 film will be more grainy than those produced on ASA/ISO 64 film stock. Small grain size enhances photographic clarity.

In videography the more lines equipment is able to resolve, the sharper the picture. For most fertility applications, equipment that produces a minimum of 300 lines is considered acceptable. It should be noted that line reproduction is only as good as the lowest-grade component. For example, a camera that produces 600 lines is unable to demonstrate this superior resolving power if recorded or played back on a system capable of resolving only 325 lines.

To produce the optimum image, a balance must be struck between the amount of light available and the amount allowed to strike the imaging surface. Once this balance of quantity has been reached, the quality of that light must be considered.

Light quality

The quality of light refers to the type of light by which the subject is to be photographed.

The human brain partially corrects for color shifts under different light sources. Humans are able to recognize red as red whether under sunlight or fluorescent light. Photographic film and videotape do not possess this ability. A video camera must be adjusted to the light source and balanced so that it produces images with correct color (hue and saturation). It is imperative that the camera, not the monitor, be adjusted. If color balance is corrected only on the monitor, there is no correction to the image recorded on the video tape.

A simple procedure for camera-monitor adjustment is as follows: the monitor should be adjusted to a standard signal generally referred to as bars; bars consist of a series of colors; many industrial-grade cameras have a switch that produces them (Figure 30-1). If the camera in use does not have this ability, prerecorded bars can be used

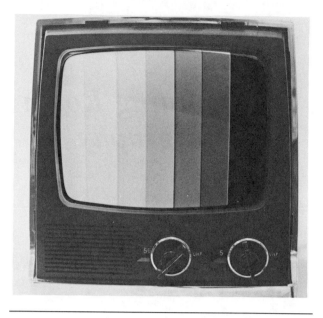

Figure 30-1
Standard color bar signal produced by an industrial-grade television camera.

(they can be played back). Once the signal is obtained (from the camera or by tape playback), the monitor can be adjusted. If bars are not available, the monitor-receiver should be set for good skin tone. This can be done from regular television broadcast signals.

After the monitor-receiver is properly adjusted, all further color modifications should be made to the camera. The camera must be balanced to the light source. If it has a filter wheel, the proper filter should be dialed in. Many industrial- and medical-grade cameras have a white-balance feature that allows the camera to be pointed at a white object; then the white-balance button is pushed and the camera adjusts itself. It is critical to do the white-balancing under the same light source that will be used for the photography. Cameras lacking the white-balance feature should be adjusted according to the manufacturer's recommendations. Often this means adjusting a color-temperature dial until acceptable color results.

Color still photography requires the proper combination of light source and film stock. When using existing operating room lighting, tungsten-balanced film is usually required. This film, balanced to render color properly under incandescent illumination, can be corrected further using color-correcting (CC) filters. Fast films (ASA 160 or above) should be used as they permit the use of shutter speeds of 1/60 or above, which reduces the effect of camera shake. Although passable results can be obtained using tungsten film and existing operating room lighting, daylight film and an electronic flash (strobe) are recommended for optimum results. The strobe light is in perfect balance with daylight color film.

Medium-powered strobes improve picture quality in a number of ways. Because of their relative power and proximity to the subject, they permit the use of slow, fine-grained films. With use of small $f/$stops the film is exposed primarily by the strobe. This exposure eliminates concerns about mixed light sources existing in the operating room. Strobes also can increase the depth of focus. For the purposes of this chapter, depth of focus is designated as the area between the point closest to the camera and the point farthest from the camera where the subject is in focus.

The strobe's power permits the use of small $f/$stops, which increases depth of focus. This concept is important during microsurgery, where under magnification, depth of focus is very shallow.

Use of small $f/$stops is also encouraged during videography; therefore the desirability of a camera capable of low light is clear. It should be noted that in addition to $f/$stop use, depth of focus can be augmented by placing the subject parallel to the camera.[1]

EQUIPMENT SELECTION AND IMPLEMENTATION

The subject to be photographed, as well as the quality and quantity of light, will determine the selection of appropriate equipment. Given their widespread use, relative economy, and ease of use, 35mm still photography and industrial- and medical-grade video equipment are featured in this chapter. Equipment selection and use for surgical photography depend on the surgeon's requirement, which is generally close-up, intraoperative microscope, or laparoscope photography.

Close-up photography

Close-up photography is defined as subjects that are approximately 1 to 90 cm from the camera. This range includes photography of the entire surgical field, instrumentation, and radiographs. For still photography of this type, a macro lens is recommended, since it permits the camera to be focused very close to the subject. This often allows the image on the film (negative or transparency) to be the same size as it is in life (e.g., a 1-cm specimen measures 1 cm on the photographic negative or transparencies). These images are frequently enlarged further during printing or projection. Macro lenses are available in focal lengths ranging from 50 to 200 mm. The longer the focal length, the farther the camera's position from the subject. For operating room photography, a lens in the 90- to 150-mm range is often preferable, since it allows the photographer to remain outside the sterile field but still obtain quality close-up views.

Again, a strobe light is recommended for close-up photography. The type used depends on the subject being

recorded. If the subject is a narrow cavity (e.g., vagina), a ringlight is recommended (Plates 23 through 35, 40 and 41, 53 through 56, 63 and 64 were photographed with a ringlight) to produce an even, flat light that will illuminate the cavity (Figure 30-2). Subjects that allow a less obstructed view, such as gross specimens, are best photographed with one to two small portable strobes. If a single strobe is used, it should be mounted to the side of the camera lens; this type of lighting emphasizes contour and texture. If interest, budget, time, and subject permit, a second strobe light can be added to fill in (add light) to the harsh shadow created by the single light source. The second strobe should be weaker than the main strobe to prevent double shadows (Figure 30-3).

Exposure values for these strobe systems should be calculated before clinical photography is begun. Automatic-exposure strobes offer great promise; however, their adaptability to close-up use should be tested. Often strobe-mounted light sensors are inaccurate in close-up photography. The photographer who wishes to use an automatic system should expose several test rolls using the full range of magnification. These test rolls should be evaluated for accuracy and consistency of proper exposure. Camera-strobe combinations are available that permit sensors to be located inside the camera, thus simplifying close-up exposure. These simplifying systems are referred to as through-the-lens metering (TTL). Many primary and secondary manufacturers have released these systems; if new equipment is to be purchased, this technology should be considered.

If a manual system is to be used, both ringlights and side-mounted strobes can be easily calibrated. The procedure for manual calibration is as follows:

1. Set the strobe(s) to the manual mode.
2. Perform the initial tests at full power. This allows maximum depth of focus and use of fine-grain films. If full power produces overexposed results, gradually cut power until proper exposure-power setting is obtained.
3. Make a series of exposures at $\frac{1}{2}$-$f/$stop increments. Repeat at different magnifications. Magnifications should be noted from the lens barrel (Figure 30-4). Keep accurate records of each exposure-magnification.
4. Process film normally.
5. Project (or print) processed film. Note accurate exposure-magnification combinations.
6. These accurate exposure combinations will remain consistent for all exposures taken at that magnification with the film and that camera-strobe combination.
7. Draw up an exposure table. Attach it to the camera and/or strobe (Figure 30-5).

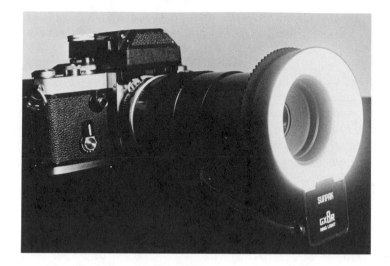

Figure 30-2
105mm macro lens fitted with electronic flash ringlight. A
ringlight is preferable to illuminate cavities.

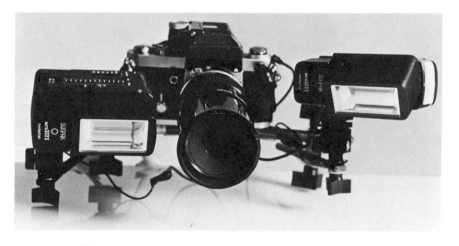

Figure 30-3
Electronic flash double light source. Second strobe light acts
as "fill" light to illuminate shadows created by the main
light.

When videotaping gross surgical procedures, a zoom
lens of approximately 10 to 1 is recommended. With this
lens the videographer can remain outside the sterile field
and still achieve excellent results. When a video program
is to be produced, the videographer should be positioned
as close as possible to the principal surgeon's location.
A wide shot should be recorded before close-ups. Proper
camera position and wide shots help orient the viewer to
the patient's position and anatomy. Macro lenses are used
if extreme close-ups are required. Inexpensive close-up
supplementary lenses are also available that screw onto
the video camera lens. They come in +1, +2, and +3
diopters.

The most common problem with radiographic photography is color shift, typically, a green or blue cast. Slides
and video tapes should reproduce the full tonal range.
Color shifts can be easily eliminated by using the proper
film and filter (still photography) or filter/white-balance
technique (videography). In video, a simple way to
achieve proper rendition is to point the camera at an
empty illuminated view box and then press the automatic
white-balance switch. Lacking this, the camera's color-
temperature dial should be adjusted until proper tonality
is obtained.

Black-and-white transparencies with full tonal range
can be obtained without filtration using a 50mm macro

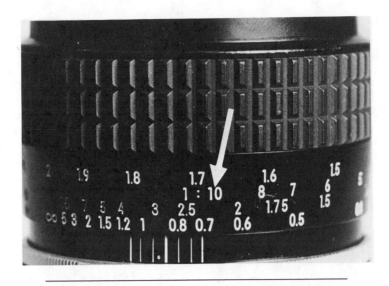

Figure 30-4
Reproduction ratio scale(s). Predetermined reproduction ratios can be determined using these scales. Arrow indicates the setting for a film stock reproduction of one-tenth the subject size.

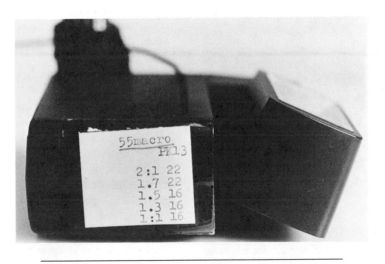

Figure 30-5
Exposure table. Once calibrated, exposure tables facilitate consistent, quality photographs.

lens and Kodak RPC651 film. This film can be processed in X-Omat processing machines available in many radiology departments. The only drawback to this film is its relatively long exposure time of 60 to 90 seconds, which necessitates the use of a copystand or tripod. If the photographer wishes to use daylight color film, filtration is required. Often an inexpensive fluorescent daylight (FLD) filter will produce acceptable results. Black-and-white print film requires no filtration. Good results can be obtained with a relatively fine-grained film (e.g., ASA 32).

Intraoperative microscope photography

Photography through the surgical microscope is both challenging and rewarding. The use of a beam splitter and photoadapter provides the photographer with a surgeon's-eye-view of the procedure.

Photoadaptors are available that permit either a still or video camera to be used (Designs for Vision); also available are adaptors that permit both still photography and videography to be used simultaneously (Zeiss/Urban). It should be noted that the surgeon's binocular view is in stereo while the resulting photographs are monocular.

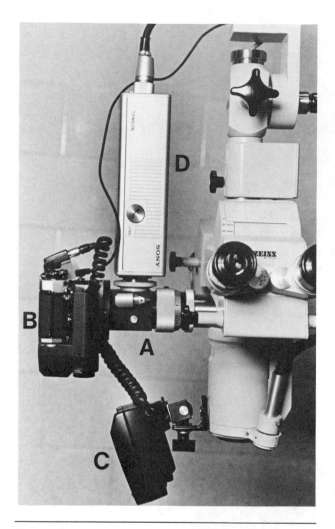

Figure 30-6
Video and still cameras attached to an undraped microscope.
A, Photoadapter. **B**, 35mm camera with auto-winder and remote shutter release. **C**, TTL electronic flash. **D**, Video camera.

For this reason, the photoadaptor should be mounted on the principal surgeon's side of the scope.[2] In addition, the surgeon should compose the photographs and video with one eye; that is, the eye on the same side as the photoadaptor.[3] For best results, the surgeon should place the subject in a plane parallel to the camera, whenever possible. This placement increases the depth of focus.

Still photography

The still camera attached to the intraoperative microscope must be equipped with the proper camera fitting, a motordrive/auto-winder, and a remote shutter release. The photoadaptor fitting must match that of the still camera to be coupled. These camera adaptors can be removed if necessary.

A draped sterile microscope requires a motor drive or auto-winder. This device advances the film and cocks the shutter. Sterile draping also calls for a method of remote

shutter release. An infrared trigger/sensor is often used, as are long shutter-release cables that attach directly to the camera motor drive. Both of these devices require nonscrubbed personnel to trigger the camera. A third alternative is a foot-pedal device that can be operated by the surgeon.

When existing light from the microscope is used for primary illumination, tungsten film should be loaded. To increase the depth of focus (smaller f/stop) or enhance motion-stopping ability (faster shutter speed), the film may be "pushed." Pushing refers to special development procedures that result in increased ASA/ISO ratings, resulting in acceptable images with less light. It is usually done in f/stop increments; each stop is the equivalent of doubling the ASA/ISO rating. Thus ASA/ISO 160 film can be pushed to ASA/ISO 320 (one stop) or 620 (two stops). Two stops is the practical limit for most films. Grain size increases with pushing, and thus sharpness decreases. It is imperative that the processing laboratory be notified that the film has been pushed so that the film will be given special handling.

A reticule should be used to ensure proper focus and to check for relative motion during photographic exposures.[4] The less relative motion between subject and microscope, the sharper the photographic results. The reticule should also be used to center the subjects in the photographic frame.

Although the available light-tungsten film combination will produce acceptable results, superior still photographs can be obtained using daylight film and a portable strobe light. The strobe light allows the use of a smaller f/stop, resulting in increased depth of focus. It also freezes action, thus avoiding blurs caused by patient-microscope relative motion. The strobe light can be attached to the microscope barrel (Figure 30-6). A manual system of exposure can be calibrated using the procedure outlined for small-object photography; however, the previously mentioned TTL system offers great promise. To be used effectively, it requires that the strobe be mounted off camera on the microscope barrel. Because the exposure sensor is not located on the strobe but in the camera body, light quantity is measured after it passes through the microscope's optics. This camera-mounted sensor permits consistent, optimum exposure at all magnifications.

A third alternative for intraoperative still photography is TTL flash delivered through a fiberoptic cable. The TTL-controlled flash is supplied through the same fiberoptics as the continuous surgical light. This system has potential for photographic subjects requiring coaxial illumination.[5]

Videography

Intraoperative microscope videotaping can provide dramatic images. Patency of tubes can be demonstrated

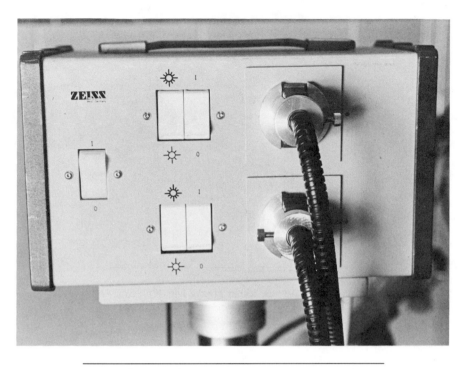

Figure 30-7
Double incandescent microscope light source increases illumination and improves the video signal.

clearly with indigo carmine dye, and surgical and suturing protocols can be demonstrated accurately. The video camera is attached directly to the microscope by means of the photoadapter. Proper lighting is essential, and a double light source is commonly used (Figure 30-7). This additional light improves depth of focus and ultimately reproduction quality. The same photographic and camera set-up techniques outlined for the still photographer should be used by the videographer. Camera and subject placement, as well as critical focus, are essential.

A light-weight camera with at least 300 lines of reproduction is recommended. The camera should be color balanced according to the manufacturer's recommendations. Balancing should be done using the same illumination source employed during the surgical procedure. It is important to note that adjusting the color on the video monitor does not affect the quality of the recorded video tape.

The use of video monitoring during microsurgery enhances surgical team involvement and may improve productivity. Many surgeons monitor the entire procedure, taping only portions that are of particular interest. Selective taping saves tape expense and editing time.

Laparoscope video and still imaging

Because of the relatively low light conditions during laparoscopic photography, sensitive video cameras are recommended. It is imperative that these cameras be color balanced using the laparoscopic light source. Some surgeons forego the laparoscopic eyepiece and use the video monitor to perform these procedures. Systems are available that allow the eyepiece and the camera to be used simultaneously.

Still photography during laparoscopy requires high-speed tungsten film or use of a strobe light source and daylight film. The latter combination is recommended. Several manufacturers produce viewing-strobe light sources with TTL metering capability (Figure 30-8). These use tungsten light for viewing and composing. When the photographic exposure is made, the tungsten light source is extinguished and a strobe light is activated. When used in combination with TTL cameras, these light sources provide consistently good results. The most difficult aspect of laparoscopic photography is equipment interface: light source must match eyepieces, cameras must adapt to eyepieces, and TTL cables must properly activate camera-light source. Once the properly interfaced system is in place, quality photographs can be produced consistently.

ADDITIONAL CONSIDERATIONS
Safety

Patient safety is of primary importance during surgical photography. Whenever possible, battery-operated equipment should be used. When this is not available, all

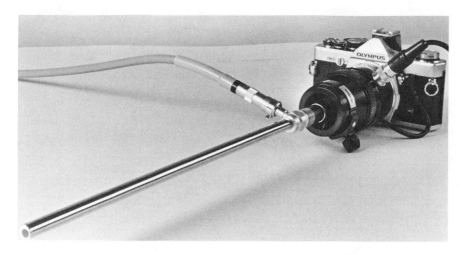

Figure 30-8
Laparoscope attached to a 35mm camera with TTL capability.

electrical photographic equipment should be checked and approved by the hospital's biomedical division. To maintain the sterile field, lenses should be selected to allow the photographer to keep at a reasonable distance. All attachments (lens, filters, scrims, and strobes) should be secured to avoid contaminating the sterile field. The photographer must come prepared so as not to delay the surgical procedure.

Patient privacy

All patients to be photographed must sign a photographic consent form. Once photographs or video tapes have been produced, every effort should be made to protect their right to privacy, including masking identification of names and numbers. All out-takes, extra prints, negatives, and work prints should be considered confidential medical records and treated accordingly.

Image protection

When film has been exposed it is unloaded and sent promptly for processing. Video tape should be protected from accidental erasure. All film and video tapes must be clearly marked and properly filed to avoid loss. Special images and videoproductions can be protected by copyright. A fellow surgeon-photographer's copyrights should be respected.

REFERENCES

1. Lefkowitz L: *The manual of close-up photography,* Garden City, NY, 1979, Amphoto.
2. Rheton AL Jr and Leaky CJ: Preparing movies of microsurgical operations, *Clin Neurosurg* 28:259, 1980.
3. Katzenberg B: Photographing microsurgery-still and dynamic techniques, *J Microsurg* 2:244, 1980.
4. Kilbourne S: Photography through the operating microscope, *J Biol Photog Assoc* 50:9, 1982.
5. Rover J and Muller-Hermann E: Intraocular photography with TTL (through-the-lens) computer-controlled flash, *Graefes Arch Clin Exp Ophthalmol* 219:253, 1982.

Appendix A

· ·

INFORMED CONSENT FORMS

At the time a patient is scheduled to undergo a procedure, she receives the appropriate consent form(s). She reads the form(s), initials each page, signs the final page and writes in restrictions, has it witnessed, and returns it to us. These are forms the editor has developed and used for several years. They have been informative for the patient and serve as superb documentation for legal purposes. The reader may wish to use them as a guide to develop his or her own documentation.

INFORMED CONSENT FOR HYSTEROSALPINGOGRAPHY

Purpose

Hysterosalpingography is a valuable study from a diagnostic as well as a therapeutic standpoint. It provides information about the uterus and fallopian tubes, allowing the diagnosis of conditions such as scar tissue or growths in the uterine cavity and tubal blockage. It is considered therapeutic, since some patients conceive soon after the procedure. The examination should be performed before ovulation but after the menstrual period has ended.

Technique

The procedure is performed in the radiology department. After donning a gown provided by the radiology staff, the patient is positioned on the examining table and a gentle pelvic examination performed. The cervix is visualized by means of a vaginal speculum and stabilized with an instrument known as a tenaculum. A hollow tube (cannula) is placed in the cervical opening, and radiopaque dye (water contrast medium) is slowly injected into the uterus. Appropriate radiographic films are taken to document the findings.

If the fallopian tubes are open, a small amount of a different type of radiopaque dye (oil contrast medium) is injected. Research has shown this particular dye to be effective in enhancing fertility for several months. The water contrast medium is excreted through the patient's kidneys within a couple of hours, but the oil contrast medium may persist.

The procedure does produce cramping and is followed by light bleeding for a few hours. The patient should have a responsible adult accompany her to and from the radiology center. However, the following day intercourse is permitted and she may return to work.

Complications

1. Infections: infections may occur after the hysterosalpingogram. To lessen this possibility, antibiotics may be prescribed, beginning the night before the procedure. Should the patient experience persistent or increasing pain or bleeding over the succeeding hours or days, she must report to our office.

2. Allergic reactions: the patient may be allergic to the radiopaque dye. These reactions are infrequent and usually of little consequence; however, they may be severe, accompanied by a drop in blood pressure and shortness of breath. If the patient has experienced a previous allergic reaction to dye materials used in radiologic procedures, she must alert our office before this test is scheduled.

3. Death: catastrophic complications resulting in death of the patient have been reported but are exceedingly rare.

Summary

The hysterosalpingogram provides the physician with valuable information on the status of the uterus and fallopian tubes. On balance it is an excellent procedure for the properly selected patient.

INFORMED CONSENT FOR HYSTEROSCOPY

Purpose

Hysteroscopy may be performed for diagnostic as well as therapeutic purposes. An example of diagnostic use would be to assess the extent of scar tissue within the uterus. An example of therapeutic use would be to remove these adhesions. Ordinarily the procedure is done in the first portion of the menstrual cycle but after menses have ceased. Pregnancy must be avoided during the cycle in which the hysteroscopy is to be performed.

Technique

Depending on the goal to be achieved, the patient may be asleep (general anesthesia) or may have a spinal, epidural, local, or no anesthesia. The cervix is exposed and dilated if necessary. A small telescope (hysteroscope) is inserted in the uterine cavity. The cavity is distended either with a gas (carbon dioxide) or an appropriate fluid. A light attached to the telescope allows the surgeon to view the interior of the uterus. If the hysteroscopy is therapeutic, the surgeon will correct any problems that can be rectified. For some conditions, a simultaneous laparoscopy is advisable to monitor the hysteroscopic procedure. In addition, it is sometimes necessary to scrape the interior of the uterus (D&C). When hysteroscopy is performed as an outpatient procedure and an anesthetic is used, the patient must arrange for a responsible adult to transport her home after discharge.

Complications

1. Anesthesia: anesthesiologists have made significant advances in improving patient safety; however, anesthetic accidents still occur. If the patient has had prior anesthesia, she should acquire those records for the anesthesiologist.

2. Allergic reaction: the patient may be allergic to distending fluid and medications used. Fortunately, this is an unusual event with hysteroscopy. The reaction is treated with medication and sometimes requires removal of the responsible fluid.

3. Carbon dioxide embolus: this gas could pass into the uterine veins and travel to the lungs, inducing shortness of breath and disturbance in blood pressure. For this reason, the hysteroscopic equipment delivers the carbon dioxide to the uterine cavity at a low rate and pressure, making such a potentially disastrous complication rare.

4. Uterine perforation: the uterine wall can be very thin with certain disease processes, making perforation with the hysteroscope more likely. If this complication occurs, a laparoscopy may be done to repair any damage that might have resulted. This complication usually is not a serious one but may occasionally require major surgery.

5. Infections: although infrequent, infections have been observed after hysteroscopy. Treatment involves administration of the appropriate antibiotic.

6. Death: catastrophic complications resulting in death of the patient are rare.

Summary

We have an advanced surgical team. Our equipment is modern. We are constantly reviewing our techniques and instrumentation to maximize patient safety. The patient is encouraged to ask as many questions as necessary to clear up doubts.

INFORMED CONSENT FOR DIAGNOSTIC AND OPERATIVE LAPAROSCOPY

Purpose

Laparoscopy is an extremely valuable procedure in gynecology and infertility. It may be performed to establish a diagnosis such as determining the cause of infertility or pelvic pain. It is often used as therapy such as removing adhesions (scar tissue) or destroying endometriosis. Pregnancy must be avoided during the menstrual cycle when the procedure is to be performed.

Procedure

The procedure is usually performed with the patient asleep (general anesthesia). In certain instances it may be performed under local anesthesia. With the patient appropriately anesthestized, an instrument (cannula) is placed in the cervix and secured with a tenaculum. These instruments enable the surgeon to position the uterus and aid in the pelvic assessment. A catheter is placed in the urinary bladder to drain it.

The abdomen is inflated with a gas (usually carbon dioxide or nitrous oxide) to allow adequate intraabdominal visualization. An incision is then made at the navel, through which a telescope (laparoscope) is inserted. One to four incisions are then placed in the lower abdomen. These incisions leave scars that are one-fourth to one-half inch in length. Through these incisions the surgeon inspects the pelvic structures and performs indicated procedures, including removing some pain nerves behind the uterus to alleviate menstrual cramps and suspending the uterus forward to enhance fertility and reduce pelvic discomfort. A photograph of the pelvic structures is often taken to document the findings. This also helps the patient to understand what was found and done.

After the procedure has been completed, the gas is allowed to escape from the abdomen, all instruments are removed, and the abdominal incisions are closed with sutures. Often fluid and medications are placed in the abdomen to prevent adhesion (scar tissue) formation. Sometimes a dilatation and curettage (D&C) is required.

Follow-up

The patient will frequently experience pain in her shoulder, chest, and upper abdominal areas caused by the gas. She will also experience tenderness at the incision sites. These discomforts usually diminish markedly after 2 days. Because fluids are often left in the abdomen to prevent adhesion formation, the patient will frequently leak fluid from the incisions and observe swelling in these areas. This fluid leakage and swelling should disappear within 2 days. There is usually some bruising at the incision sites. This disappears in approximately 2 weeks. Many patients go home the day of surgery but must be transported by a responsible adult.

3. Gastrointestinal injuries: injuries to the intestinal tract occur approximately 1 per 500 procedures. This may happen when establishing the portals of entry for the instruments, as well as during pelvic dissection. This is a serious complication and must be rectified. The repair usually requires major surgery. Although a colostomy is a possibility, it is a remote one.

4. Urologic injury: because much dissection is done around the drainage tubes from the kidney (ureters) or the urinary bladder, there is always the possibility of injury to one of these structures. These may be minor or serious, resulting in major surgery and even, rarely, loss of a kidney.

5. Gas embolli: a serious complication is passage of gas used to inflate the abdomen into a major blood vessel, from which it may travel to the patient's heart and lungs. The surgeon uses several checks to lessen this possibility.

6. Phlebitis: the patient may experience tenderness along the vein used for intravenous administration of fluids and medications. Warm compresses are applied, and such tenderness is usually temporary. Occasionally, a small lump at the intravenous site will persist.

7. Incisions: infrequently an incision will become infected, requiring warm compresses, antibiotics, and drainage.

8. Pelvic infections: the patient will sometimes develop a pelvic infection after surgery. She usually receives an antibiotic during surgery to lessen this prospect. When infection develops, she must notify the physician immediately.

9. Allergic reactions: several medications are used during surgery, and there is always a possibility of a reaction to one or more of them. Appropriate steps are taken to counteract it.

10. Ovarian failure: the ovary(ies) may go into permanent failure after surgery. This is usually associated with extensive ovarian surgery such as removal of cysts.

11. Neurologic injuries: pelvic nerve injuries may occur when extensive pelvic dissection is required. These are most often characterized by temporary numbness or tingling in the abdomen or lower extremities, but permanent muscle weakness rarely occurs. Similarly, weakness of the upper extremity has been reported, although infrequently.

12. Failed procedure: occasionally the surgeon will have to end the procedure because of a technical problem or because the procedure is inappropriate for the disease, as in the discovery of a pelvic malignancy. Major surgery would be performed at that time only for an urgent problem and if appropriate, after consultation with the family.

13. Death: catastrophic complications resulting in death of the patient are rare.

Continued.

INFORMED CONSENT FOR DIAGNOSTIC AND OPERATIVE LAPAROSCOPY—cont'd

Complications

1. Anesthesia: anesthesiologists have made significant advances in improving patient safety; however, anesthetic accidents still happen. If anesthesia is required, the anesthesiologist should discuss these complications with the patient before surgery. If the patient has had prior anesthesia, she should acquire those records for the anesthesiologist at the time of the preoperative consultation.

2. Hemorrhage: excessive bleeding can occur when developing the portals of entry in the abdominal wall, as well as during pelvic dissection. Both events are infrequent and can usually be dealt with laparoscopically, but laparotomy is sometimes required. Although the necessity for blood transfusions in laparoscopy is uncommon, the patient should inquire as to the advisability of donating her own blood before the procedure to avoid receiving blood from donors, thus lessening the chance of such sequelae as hepatitis and AIDS.

Follow-up

The patient should call the office the first day after surgery to advise us of any problems and to make her return appointment for 3 weeks later. She should remain out of work for 1 week and should report any unusual signs or symptoms such as unusual vaginal discharge, fever, or increasing pain.

Summary

We have an advanced surgical team. Our equipment is modern. We are constantly reviewing our techniques and instrumentation to maximize patient safety. The patient is encouraged to ask as many questions as necessary to clear up doubts.

INFORMED CONSENT FOR PELVIC RECONSTRUCTIVE SURGERY BY LAPAROTOMY

Purpose

Pelvic reconstructive procedures are often performed to enhance fertility, alleviate pain, or remove tumors such as fibroids and cysts.

Procedure

The patient is usually asleep for the procedure (general anesthesia), but sometimes a spinal or epidural (regional anesthesia) is used. A catheter is often placed in the uterine cavity to check tubal patency, and a drainage tube is inserted in the urinary bladder to prevent bladder distention. An abdominal incision is then made. This is usually approximately 5½ inches in length. Where reasonable, the incision is just beneath the bikini line; however, sometimes it is advisable to make it vertically.

To perform the necessary procedures, combinations of equipment and techniques are available, such as the surgical microscope and laser. Sometimes it is advisable to remove a fallopian tube and/or an ovary if they are severely damaged by disease. If menstrual cramps are a problem, nerves behind the uterus can be divided or vaporized with laser to lessen pain. If the uterus is tipped, it is sometimes suspended forward.

Occasionally, unexpected disease processes are found, such as endometriosis of the appendix or intestinal adhesions. The initial plans for the procedure may have to be changed to manage these unexpected findings and additional procedures performed to correct them.

Several steps are taken to discourage adhesions (scar tissue) formation after surgery. One is to have each patient take an antibiotic before surgery. Another is to administer a combination of steroid and antihistamine (dexamethasone and promethazine) before, during, and after surgery. All irrigating fluids used in surgery contain a blood thinner (heparin) to prevent blood clotting about the pelvic structures. Incisions in pelvic organs are sometimes covered with a fabric (Interceed) that disappears in 30 days. A final step is to place a solution (lactated Ringer's) in the abdomen at the end of the procedure to encourage the pelvic structures to float apart (hydroflotation) and prevent their adherence.

After the procedure is completed, the abdomen is closed with sutures and a drain is usually placed in the incision for 1 to 2 days to prevent fluid accumulation. The catheter in the uterus is withdrawn at the end of the procedure, and the drainage tube in the urinary bladder is removed on the first day after surgery.

Photographs of the pelvic structures are often taken to assist the patient and her referring doctor to understand the surgery.

Complications

1. Genetic abnormalities: when a woman conceives at an older age, she is subject to an increased chance of having a genetically abnormal child. The advisability of undergoing amniocentesis should be discussed with the doctor.

2. Age: fertility lessens as the patient becomes older, particularly after age 40. The patient should be given a realistic estimation of her chance of having a successful pregnancy, as well as the chances of an ectopic pregnancy or miscarriage, before deciding to undergo surgery. The patient should inquire about alternative routes such as adoption and in vitro fertilization.

3. Pain: if the purpose of the procedure is to alleviate pain, the patient must have a realistic expectation of achieving this end before opting for surgery. In my experience, pain relief after surgery is very unpredictable. Also certain conditions can recur, such as endometriosis.

4. Anesthesia: anesthesiologists have made significant advances in improving patient safety; however, anesthetic accidents still occur. If anesthesia is required, the anesthesiologist should discuss these complications with the patient before surgery. If the patient has had prior anesthesia, she should acquire those records for the anesthesiologist.

5. Urinary tract problems: urinary tract infections may occur. They are infrequent, due in part to early removal of the urinary catheter. Injuries to the urinary bladder or drainage tubes from the kidneys (ureters) may occur during dissection. This occurs most often when the patient has severe pelvic endometriosis or extensive pelvic adhesions. When the problem is diagnosed, consultation is obtained and appropriate treatment carried out. Loss of a kidney is a remote possibility.

6. Intestinal injury: the intestinal tract may be injured during dissection. This occurs most often when dissection for severe adhesions or advanced endometriosis is required. The intestinal tract is usually involved in these disease processes. This is a major complication and must be corrected at the time it is recognized. Rarely, a colostomy is required to manage this complication. Bowel obstruction requiring major surgery to correct it is infrequent.

7. Neurologic damage: nerve injuries may occur and are most often characterized by temporary numbness or tingling in the abdomen or lower extremities. Muscle weakness may sometimes occur, but is rarely permanent. Similarly, weakness of the upper extremity has been reported, but, fortunately, is very infrequent. If certain nerves to the uterus are divided purposely to alleviate pelvic pain (presacral neurectomy), the patient may experience some decrease in bowel function and slowing in urinary bladder emptying. This is infrequent and usually temporary. The patient may experience pain or numbness at injection sites. This, too, is usually temporary.

Continued.

INFORMED CONSENT FOR PELVIC RECONSTRUCTIVE SURGERY BY LAPAROTOMY—cont'd

8. Hemorrhage: the surgeon may encounter significant intraoperative or postoperative bleeding requiring blood transfusions and occasionally additional surgery. The patient should inquire as to the advisability of donating her own blood before the procedure to avoid receiving blood from donors, thus lessening the chance of such sequelae as hepatitis and AIDS. In addition, the blood a patient loses may be collected and given back to her through an apparatus called a *cell saver*. To avoid interfering with her own clotting mechanism, the patient should not take aspirin or aspirin-containing medication during the 2 weeks preceding surgery.

9. Heart and blood vessel problems: blood clots may develop in the veins of the pelvis and lower extremities. These are potentially serious because they can travel to the lungs. This complication is unusual and is due in part to our policy of early ambulation after surgery. Phlebitis can occur at the site of the intravenous needle, leaving a small, tender lump that may persist.

10. Allergic and other adverse reactions: the patient receives a variety of substances while hospitalized and sometimes after discharge. Allergic reactions may occur sometimes with one or more of these medications. The patient should alert the hospital staff of any prior allergic reactions.

11. Wound: occasionally a patient develops a collection of fluid or an infection in the wound. An appropriate antibiotic and/or drainage is usually required. The patient will experience numbness near the incision, which usually lasts approximately 6 weeks but can be permanent. Also, a hernia or persistent pain may develop in the wound.

12. Postoperative pain: the patient may experience pain after surgery. Although usually temporary, it may persist.

13. Ovarian failure: the ovary(ies) may go into permanent failure after surgery. This is usually associated with extensive ovarian surgery, such as removal of cysts.

14. Pregnancy: the patient should inquire as to when she can attempt conception after surgery. Also she must report to her doctor immediately as soon as pregnancy is suspected. This is the only reasonable way to lessen the possibility of an advanced ectopic pregnancy, which could be fatal.

15. Death: catastrophic complications resulting in death of the patient are rare.

Follow-up

The patient is usually hospitalized for 4 to 5 days. She may resume driving, as well as intercourse, at 3 weeks, exercise at 4 weeks, and work at 4 to 6 weeks after surgery. She should report any unusual signs or symptoms such as unusual vaginal discharge, fever, or increasing pain. In addition, she should schedule a postoperative visit for 4 weeks after surgery.

Summary

We have an advanced surgical team. Our equipment is modern. We are constantly reviewing our techniques and instrumentation to maximize patient safety. The patient is encouraged to ask as many questions as necessary to clear up doubts.

INFORMED CONSENT FOR LAPAROSCOPIC SURGERY*

The laparoscope, a surgical instrument similar to a telescope, is inserted through a small incision in the bellybutton. The abdomen is distended with a gas called carbon dioxide. The scope allows the doctor to visualize the pelvic organs and allows other instruments to be used under direct vision. Small second, third, and fourth incisions are occasionally made at the pubic hairline for scissors, coagulator, or laser to perform major closed surgery at laparoscopy.

Hysteroscopy is the use of a small optical tube that is inserted through the vagina into the uterus without incision to visualize the uterine cavity. It is usually performed with laparoscopy to determine (1) the size and depth of the uterine cavity; (2) the presence of congenital abnormalities within the uterus; (3) the presence of polyps or fibroid tumors in the uterine cavity; and (4) whether specific abnormalities of the endometrium (lining of the uterus) are present, such as hyperplasia (build-up the lining of the uterus), tuberculosis, or cell changes that indicate early cancer. Dilatation and curettage (D&C) may also be performed if indicated.

Video or pictures may be taken during surgery and used to show you what was seen and done. They are also used for teaching other patients, and demonstrating these techniques to other surgeons.

The doctor performs advanced laparoscopic surgery that includes procedures considered investigational and may include modified instrumentation. These are relatively new techniques not commonly undertaken elsewhere, and can include laparoscopic oophorectomy, hysterectomy, and tubal reversal. Laparoscopic treatment of ovarian neoplasms, benign or malignant, is considered investigational.

Antibiotics, anticoagulants, and other medications may be used with surgery to aid in healing. These medications are not labeled (neither approved nor disapproved) by the Food and Drug Administration for adhesion prevention.

Although laparoscopy is generally an outpatient procedure, you may be asleep from 1-4 hours, occasionally longer.

Plan to avoid any activities that require concentration for at least 2 days. You can usually return to work and moderate activities by the third day. You may require 1-3 weeks to return to heavy activities and for full recovery.

Shoulder pain from the carbon dioxide gas and abdominal distention are common. Your throat may be sore from the endotracheal tube. About 1 in 40 patients is admitted for overnight stay due to nausea, drowsiness, or pain.

Complications from laparoscopic surgery are very uncommon, but they do sometimes occur. It is also possible that because of complications, or because of the discovery of life-threatening abnormalities, immediate major abdominal surgery might be necessary. The chance of severe complications such as hysterectomy, colostomy, paralysis, or death is rare. With respect to your life, this operation is 6 times safer than driving a car and 2-3 times safer than being pregnant.

INFORMED CONSENT FOR LAPAROSCOPIC SURGERY
PAGE 2

Some of the possible complications are the same as those of regular surgery. They include bleeding; infection, particularly of the navel; generalized disease; inflammation of the lining of the abdomen; injury to the stomach or intestines; gas embolism to the lung from the carbon dioxide; abnormal gas collections underneath the skin and in the chest; ruptures or hernias in the surgical wound and through the breathing muscles (diaphragm); burns on the skin of the abdomen and inside the abdomen; damage to the kidney and urinary systems; blood clots in the pelvis and lungs; and allergic and other bad reactions to one or more substances used in the procedure.

Some of these complications may require major surgery; some can cause poor healing wounds, scarring and permanent disability, and very rarely, some can even cause death.

The alternative procedure to laparoscopic surgery is major surgery. However, this alternative method also carries the same risks, requires a much longer period to recover, and causes more pain and discomfort. Therefore, in patients in whom laparoscopic surgery is possible, the procedures provide diagnosis and treatment at low risk and less discomfort. Your doctor cannot and does not guarantee the success of this procedure, that is, that pain will be totally resolved or that pregnancy will occur after surgery, but believes that the procedure is in your best interest.

I understand that during the course of the operation or treatment, unforeseen conditions may be revealed requiring an extension of the original procedure(s) or different procedure(s) than specifically discussed. I hereby authorize the above-named surgeon, his associates, and assistants to perform such other laparoscopic surgical procedures and if necessary laparotomy (abdominal surgery) and to remove any tissue or organs that may be necessary or medically desirable as determined by the surgeon's professional judgment. This authority shall extend to treatment of conditions not previously known by my physicians.

My signature below constitutes my acknowledgement (1) that I have read or had read to me the contents of this form; (2) that I understand and agree to the foregoing; (3) that the proposed operation(s) or procedure(s) have been satisfactorily explained to me, including possible risks and alternatives; (4) that I have all the information that I desire and have had ample opportunity to ask questions on specific points; and (5) that I hereby give my authorization and consent.

I am aware that visiting surgeons may observe and/or participate in my operative care, always under the direct supervision of my doctor.

DO NOT SIGN THIS FORM UNLESS YOU HAVE READ IT, UNDERSTAND IT, AND AGREE WITH WHAT IT SAYS.

---

*This form was developed by Harry Reich, M.D.

Appendix B

. . . .

DIRECTORY OF SURGICAL SUPPLY COMPANIES

Apple Medical
93 Nashaway Road
Bolton, MA 01740
(508) 779-2926
(800) 255-2926
Fax (508) 897-0695

Applied Fiberoptics, Inc.
East Main Street
Southbridge, MA 01556
(508) 765-9121
(800) 225-7486
Fax (508) 764-3639

ASSI—Accurate Surgical and Scientific Instruments Corporation
(United States distributor and representative for Springer and Tritt)
300 Shames Drive
Westbury, NY 11590
(516) 333-2570
(800) 645-3569
Fax (516) 997-4948

Baxter Healthcare (Baxter Hospital Supply Division)
26 Wiggins Avenue
Bedford, MA 01730
(617) 275-1100
(800) 456-5690
Fax (617) 275-6126

Baxter V. Mueller
1500 Waukegan Road
McGaw Park, IL 60085
(800) 323-9088
Fax (708) 473-3165

Cameron-Miller, Inc.
3949 South Racine Avenue
Chicago, IL 60609
(312) 523-6360
(800) 523-6360
Cable: CAMSURGO

Codman and Shurtleff, Inc. (Division of Johnson & Johnson)
41 Pacella Park Drive
Randolph Industrial Park
Randolph, MA 02368
(617) 961-2300
(800) 343-5966
Fax (617) 986-5285

Conkin Surgical Instruments Ltd.
P.O. Box 6707, Station "A"
Toronto, Ontario, Canada M5W 1X5
(416) 922-9496
Fax (416) 922-3501

Cook Ob/Gyn
P.O. Box 271
Spencer, IN 47460

Cuda Products Corp.
6000 Powers Avenue
Jacksonville, FL 32217
(904) 737-7611
Fax (904) 733-4832

Daly Hospital Supply Company
66 Broadway
Route 1
Lynnefield, MA 01940
(617) 595-6300
(800) 388-9000
Fax (508) 532-6916

Davis and Geck
One Casper Street
Wayne, NJ 07470
(201) 831-4236
(800) 243-7421
Telex: 219136

Davol, Inc.
P.O. Box 8500
Cranston, RI 02920
(401) 463-7000
(800) 626-8266
Telex: 927521

Deseret (Becton Dickinson Acute Care)
One Becton Drive
Franklin Lakes, NJ 07417
(201) 848-6762
(800) 333-4813
Fax (201) 848-7066

Designs for Vision, Inc.
760 Koehler Avenue
Ronkon Koma, NY 11779
(516) 585-3300
(800) 345-4009
Fax (516) 585-3404
Telex: 238413 DVI

Downs Surgical PLC
Church Path, Mitcham, Surrey, CR4 3UE
England
Telephone: 01-648 6291
Telex: 927045

Elmed, Inc.
60 West Fay Avenue
Addison, IL 60101
(708) 543-2792
Fax (708) 543-2102

Ethicon, Inc. (Johnson & Johnson)
P.O. Box 151
Somerville, NJ 08876-0151
(201) 218-0707

Ethox
251 Seneca Street
Buffalo, NY 14204-2088
(716) 842-4000
(800) 521-1022
Fax (716) 842-4040

Haemonetics Surgical Products Division
400 Wood Road
Braintree, MA 02184
(617) 848-7100
(800)-225-5242
Fax 848-7950

Johnson & Johnson Medical Inc.
New Brunswick, NJ 08903
(800) 526-5572

Keeler Instruments, Inc.
456 Park
Lawrence Park Industrial District
Broomall, PA 19008
(215) 353-4350
(800) 523-5620

Kendall Co. (Hospital Products Division)
1 Federal Street

Boston, MA 02101
(617) 574-7000
(800) 225-2600
Telex: 940503

Luxtec Corp.
P.O. Box 225
Technology Park, Rte 20
Sturbridge, MA 01566-0225
(508) 347-9521
(800) 325-8966
Fax (508) 347-5704

3 M Health Care (Medical-Surgical Division)
3 M Center Building 225-55-01
St. Paul, MN 55144
(612) 736-9477
(800) 228-3957

Marlow Surgical Technologies & Gynescope Corp.
36212 Euclid Avenue
Willoughby, OH 44094
(216) 946-2453
(800) 992-5581
Fax (216) 946-1997

Martin USA (Division of Gebruder Martin)
2050 Mabeline Road
North Charleston, SC 29418
(803) 569-6100
(800) 243-5135
Fax (803) 569-6133

Gebruder Martin
Ludwigstalerstrasse 132
Postfach 60
D-7200 Tuttlingen
Germany
Telephone: (17461) 706-0
Telex: 762 696 gema d

Medical Workshop
P.O. Box 461
9700 AL Groningen
Holland

Neward Enterprises
Cucamonga, CA 91730

Precept
Division of Work Wear Health Care Group
6624 Jimmy Carter Boulevard
Norcross, GA 30071

Sharpoint
2850 Windmill Road
Reading, PA 19608
(215) 670-2060
(800) 523-3332
Telex: 836425

J. Sklar Manufacturing Co.
3804 Woodside Avenue
Long Island, NY 11101
(212) 599-8489

Surgikos, Inc.
P.O. Box 122
Arlington, TX 76010
(800) 433-5009

Storz Instrument Co.
3365 Tree Court Industrial Boulevard
St. Louis, MO 63122
(314) 225-5051
(800) 325-9500
Fax (314) 225-7365

Karl Storz Endoscopy Inc. (United States
  distributor for Karl Storz GMBH)
10111 West Jefferson Boulevard
Culver City, CA 90230
(800) 421-0837
Telex: 763 656 storz d

Target Therapeutics
Santa Monica, CA 90406

Unimar (United International Marketing Resources,
  Inc.)
475 Danbury Road
Wilton, CT 06897
(203) 762-9550

Valleylab, Inc. (division of Pfizer)
5920 Longbow Drive
P.O. Box 9015
Boulder, CO 80301
(303) 530-2300
(800) 255-8522
Fax (303) 530-6313

Edward Weck and Company, Inc.
Weck Drive
P.O. Box 12600
Research Triangle Park, NC 27709
(919) 544-8000
(800) 334-8511

Richard Wolf Instruments Corp.
7046 Lyndon Avenue
Rosemont, IL 60018
(708) 298-3150
(800) 323-9653
Telex: 726408

Xomed-Treace Inc.
6743 Southpoint Drive North
Jacksonville, FL 32216
(904) 737-7900
(800) 874-5797

Carl Zeiss, Inc. (United States representative for
  Zeiss, West Germany)
One Zeiss Road
Thornwood, NY 10594
(914) 747-1800
Telex: 221834

ZSI (Zinnanti Surgical Instruments)
21540-B Prairie Street
Chatsworth, CA 91311
(818) 700-0090
(800) 223-4740

Wild/E Leitz, Inc.
24 Link Drive
Rockleigh, NJ 07647
(201) 767-1100
Fax (201) 767-4196
Telex: 6853354/Leitz UW

Index

. . . .